D1479563

THE PULMONARY CIRCULATION
AND
ACUTE LUNG INJURY

Edited by

SAMI I. SAID, M.D.

Professor of Medicine
Chief, Pulmonary Disease
and Critical Care Section
University of Oklahoma Health Sciences Center
and Veterans Administration Medical Center
Oklahoma City, Oklahoma

With a Foreword by

Sir John Vane, F.R.S.

Nobel Laureate, Medicine/Physiology, 1982
Group Research and Development Director
The Wellcome Research Laboratories
Beckenham, Kent, England

 Futura Publishing Company, Inc.
Mount Kisco, New York
1985

Library of Congress Cataloging in Publication Data
Main entry under title:

The Pulmonary circulation and acute lung injury.

Includes bibliographies and index.
1. Lungs--Wounds and injuries--Complications and
sequelae. 2. Pulmonary circulation. I. Said, Sami.
[DNLM: 1. Lung--injuries. 2. Pulmonary Circulation.
WF 600 P9824]
RD539.P85 1985   617'.542044   84-73110
ISBN 0-87993-249-X

Published by
Futura Publishing Company, Inc.
295 Main Street
Mount Kisco, New York 10549

L.C.#: 84−73110
ISBN#: 0−87993−249−X

*Dedicated to my teachers, associates,
and students over the years,
to Wadie, Mufeed, and Nadia,
and to my mother and the memory of my father.*

Contributors

Richard K. Albert, M.D.
 Associate Professor of Medicine, Assistant Chief, Pulmonary/Critical Care Medicine, VA Medical Center, University of Washington, Seattle, Washington

Jacques Benveniste, M.D.
 INSERM U 200, Université Paris-Sud, Clamart, France

Richard D. Bland, M.D.
 Associate Professor of Pediatrics, Cardiovascular Research Institute, University of California, San Francisco, California

Kenneth L. Brigham, M.D.
 Joe and Morris Werthan Professor of Investigative Medicine, Director, Pulmonary Circulation Center and Division of Pulmonary Medicine, Vanderbilt University School of Medicine, Nashville, Tennessee

Charles P. Cox, Ph.D.
 Assistant Professor of Research, Department of Medicine, University of Oklahoma Health Science Center, Oklahoma City, Oklahoma

Robert H. Demling, M.D.
 Associate Professor of Surgery, Harvard Medical School, Director, Longwood Area Trauma Center, Boston, Massachusetts

Richard D. Dey, Ph.D.
 Assistant Professor, Department of Cell Biology, University of Texas Health Science Center at Dallas, Dallas, Texas

Lee Frank, M.D., Ph.D.
 Associate Professor, Department of Medicine, University of Miami School of Medicine, Pulmonary Division, Miami, Florida

Jørgen Frøkjaer-Jensen, Ph.D.
 Niels Bohr Established Investigator, Institute of Medical Physiology, The Panum Institute, Copenhagen, Denmark

Thomas N. Hansen, M.D.
 Cardiovascular Research Institute, University of California, San Francisco, California

Takahito Hirose, M.D.
 Chief of Internal Medicine, The National Minami Fukuoka Chest Hospital, Fukuoka, Japan

James C. Hogg, M.D., Ph.D
Professor of Pathology, University of British Columbia, Director, Pulmonary Research Lab, St. Paul's Hospital, Vancouver, British Columbia, Canada

Albert L. Hyman, M.D.
Professor of Clinical Medicine, Professor of Research Surgery, Adjunct Professor of Pharmacology, Director, Surgical Cardiopulmonary Research Laboratory, Tulane University School of Medicine, New Orleans, Louisiana

Louis J. Ignarro, Ph.D.
Professor of Surgery, Pharmacology, and Medicine, Tulane University of Medicine, New Orleans, Louisiana

Rosemary Jones, Ph.D.
Assistant Professor of Pathology, Department of Pathology, Harvard Medical School and Children's Hospital, Boston, Massachusetts

Philip J. Kadowitz, Ph.D.
Professor of Pharmacology, Tulane University School of Medicine, New Orleans, Louisiana

David Langleben, M.D.
Research Fellow, Canadian Heart Foundation, Department of Pathology, Harvard Medical School and Children's Hospital, Boston, Massachusetts

Howard L. Lippton, M.D.
Instructor in Pharmacology, Tulane University School of Medicine, New Orleans, Louisiana

Asrar B. Malik, Ph.D.
Professor of Physiology, Albany Medical College, Albany, New York

Denis J. Martin, Ph.D.
Assistant Professor, Laboratoire de Physiologie, Faculté de Médecine de Grenoble, La Tronche, France

Dennis B. McNamara, Ph.D.
Associate Professor of Pharmacology, Tulane University School of Medicine, New Orleans, Louisiana

Jean Michel Mencia-Huerta, Ph.D.
INSERM U 200, Université Paris-Sud, Clamart, France

Mohammad Mojarad, M.D.
Assistant Professor of Medicine, Department of Medicine, University of Oklahoma Health Science Center, Oklahoma City, Oklahoma

Bernard Poitevin, M.D.
INSERM U 200, Université Paris-Sud, Clamart, France

John T. Reeves, M.D.
Professor of Medicine, Cardiovascular Pulmonary Research Laboratory, University of Colorado Health Science Center, Denver, Colorado

Lynne M. Reid, M.D.
S. Burt Wolbach Professor of Pathology, Harvard Medical School, Pathologist-in-Chief, The Children's Hospital, Boston, Massachusetts

John E. Repine, M.D.
Professor of Medicine and Pediatrics, University of Colorado Medical Center, Denver, Colorado

Regine Roubin, Ph.D.
INSERM U 200, Université Paris-Sud, Clamart, France

Una S. Ryan, Ph.D.
Professor of Medicine, University of Miami School of Medicine, Miami, Florida

Sami I. Said, M.D.
Professor of Medicine, Chief, Pulmonary Disease and Critical Care Section, University of Oklahoma Health Sciences Center and Veterans Administration Medical Center, Oklahoma City, Oklahoma

Maya Simionescu, Ph.D
Professor, Institute of Cellular Biology and Pathology, Bucharest, Romania

James R. Snapper, M.D.
Associate Professor of Medicine, Pulmonary Circulation Center, Vanderbilt University School of Medicine, Nashville, Tennessee

Kurt R. Stenmark, M.D.
Assistant Professor of Pediatrics, University of Colorado Health Sciences Center, Cardiovascular Pulmonary Research Laboratory, Denver, Colorado

Aubrey E. Taylor, Ph.D.
Professor and Chairman, Department of Physiology, University of South Alabama, College of Medicine, Mobile, Alabama

Gerd O. Till, M.D.
Associate Professor, Department of Pathology, The University of
Michigan Medical School, Ann Arbor, Michigan

Mary I. Townsley, Ph.D.
Instructor, Department of Physiology, College of Medicine, University
of South Alabama, Mobile, Alabama

Norbert F. Voelkel, M.D.
Assistant Professor of Medicine, Cardiovascular Pulmonary Research
Lab and Pulmonary Division, University of Colorado Health Sciences
Center, Denver, Colorado

Peter A. Ward, M.D
Professor and Chairman, Department of Pathology, The University of
Michigan Medical School, Ann Arbor, Michigan

Keith S. Wood, B.S.
Research Associate, Department of Pharmacology, Tulane University
School of Medicine, New Orleans, Louisiana

Foreword

It is now well established that the pulmonary circulation has another function apart from that associated with the exchange of gases. This is a pharmacokinetic one, in which the cells and enzyme systems of the pulmonary vascular bed change the biological activity of a variety of substances presented to them via the pulmonary circulation.

Our own contribution to this field started in the 1960s with a study of the metabolic fate of several vasoactive amines, peptides, and prostaglandins. For this, we used a dynamic bioassay system, the blood-bathed organ technique, which allows a continuous and immediate estimation of the inactivation (or activation) of any musculotropic substance in the few seconds that it takes to cross a particular vascular bed. At that time, there were already a few scattered reports in the literature showing that some substances, such as 5-hydroxy-tryptamine, were inactivated on passage through the lungs. It was, however, the concentrated effort by my colleagues in the Department of Pharmacology at The Royal College of Surgeons of England that allowed some general principles to be proposed and also provided the stimulus for much of the future work.

We developed the concept that inactivation or removal of vasoactive substances from the venous blood was an important cleansing function of the lungs, protecting the arterial circulation from the potent and sometimes deleterious effects of these substances. Thus, we showed that not only 5-hydroxytryptamine but also bradykinin, noradrenaline, prostaglandins E_1, E_2, and $F_{2\alpha}$ were all inactivated or removed, whereas some substances, often very closely related, were allowed free passage through the pulmonary circulation. These included adrenaline, angiotensin II, oxytocin, and vasopressin.

The removal of some substances but not of others enhanced the idea that vasoactive hormones could be classified either as local or as circulating, depending on whether they were removed by the lungs. A local hormone would be released at or near the target cells, have its effect, and be inactivated before reaching the arterial circulation. Any of the local hormones that escaped immediate inactivation and spilled over the venous blood would be inactivated within a few seconds either in the blood itself or, if it reached the lungs, by the pulmonary circulation. A circulating hormone would be released into the venous blood and then distributed through the arterial circulation, without loss of activity on passage through the lungs.

The other side of the story began with our work in 1967, which showed that rapid conversion of angiotensin I to the much more active angiotensin II was not in the bloodstream, as previously supposed, but in the pulmonary circulation. This activation of angiotensin I by conversion to angiotensin II in the pulmonary circulation forced us to look at the lungs as a potential "endocrine" organ, which could contribute vasoactive hormones to the circulation as well as remove them. In this context, I stressed the analogy between the respiratory and metabolic functions of the lung. Just as by the physical processes of diffusion and filtration the lung removes carbon dioxide, emboli, and cellular debris from the

blood, so by biochemical processes it removes 5-hydroxytryptamine, bradykinin, and prostaglandins. Just as the respiratory function of the lung adds
oxygen, so the metabolic functions can add angiotensin II and, after specific
types of stimulation, histamine, prostaglandins, rabbit aorta contracting substance (RCS, now known as thromboxane A_2), and perhaps other spasmogens.

It is always pleasing to see a new field develop and grow, particularly if one
is fortunate enough to contribute at an early stage to its development and
growth. The discovery that aspirin inhibited prostaglandin biosynthesis in 1971
and the discovery of prostacyclin in 1976 distracted our attention from the
lungs, but the growth of the arachidonic acid cascade and the identification of
the leukotrienes by Samuelsson has once more brought them into sharp focus.
The isolation and identification of active lung peptides has further emphasized
the role of the lung in producing and modifying biologically potent compounds.

The editor and authors of this book have been among those physicians and
scientists who were quick to recognize the importance of metabolic activities of
the lung in physiological regulation as well as in lung disease. The chapters
presented here give up-to-date and authoritative accounts of the rapid progress
in research in this area and of its applications to the understanding and management of acute lung injury. I commend the reader to this work.

Sir John Vane, F.R.S.
Nobel Laureate, Medicine/Physiology, 1982
Group Research and Development Director
The Wellcome Research Laboratories
Beckenham, Kent, England

Contents

IV. MECHANISMS OF LUNG INJURY: ROLE OF GRANULOCYTES, FREE OXYGEN RADICALS, LIPIDS, AND PEPTIDES (COMPLEMENT)

Introduction and Overview

CHAPTER 1

The Pulmonary Circulation and Acute Lung Injury: Introduction and Overview

Sami I. Said

In addition to its vital role in oxygenating blood and removing carbon dioxide, the pulmonary circulation serves important metabolic functions, including the generation, activation or inactivation of biologically potent compounds that affect vascular and airway smooth muscle, and microvascular permeability.[2,3,28,43,44,56]

Many disorders of the lung, heart, and respiration are associated with reversible or irreversible alterations of the pulmonary circulation. Of these disorders, perhaps none is as closely related in its pathogenesis to the pulmonary circulation as acute, diffuse lung injury. Pulmonary vascular endothelium is a key and early target of acute lung injury, and endothelial damage is the basis of one of the principal lesions in lung injury—high permeability pulmonary edema. Further, because of stimulated release of certain vasoactive and bronchoactive compounds (including lipids, peptides, and oxygen metabolites), or their impaired metabolism, acute lung injury is commonly associated with pulmonary vasoconstriction, bronchoconstriction, and systemic hypotension.[47] Much of the study of the mechanisms of lung injury, therefore, focuses on pulmonary vascular endothelium and smooth muscle, and on the production, metabolism, and biological effects of agents that can modify the structure and function of pulmonary vessels and microvessels, especially with respect to pulmonary vascular injury.

The recently accelerated pace of investigation into experimental pulmonary injury and the related clinical syndrome of "adult respiratory distress" (ARDS) has been catalyzed by rapid and major advances in the isolation, characterization, and identification of biologically active substances, the availability of more selective pharmacologic inhibitors and antagonists, and the development of improved morphologic and immunocytochemical techniques. This monograph reports recent and ongoing advances along the frontiers of research into the morphologic, functional, biochemical, pharmacologic, and pathologic aspects of acute lung injury. Much of the material is concerned with

From Said, S.I. (ed.): *The Pulmonary Circulation and Acute Lung Injury.* Mount Kisco, N.Y., Futura Publishing Co., Inc., 1985.

mechanisms by which the initial lung injury may be produced and by which it may progress to pulmonary edema and other grave abnormalities. The following comments highlight some of the developments discussed in greater detail in subsequent chapters. The comments touch on those areas that my associates and I have participated in or followed most closely over the past two decades.

Metabolic Function and Dysfunction of the Pulmonary Circulation

Among the major metabolic activities of the normal lung are (1) the activation of angiotensin I to angiotensin II; (2) the inactivation of bradykinin, serotonin, norepinephrine, and certain prostaglandins (PGE and PGF compounds);[14,44,56] and (3) the synthesis and release of a variety of biologically active compounds, including amines (e.g., histamine), peptides (e.g., bombesin, vasoactive intestinal peptide "VIP," substance P), and complement,[45] prostaglandins (PGD_2, PGE_2, $PGF_{2\alpha}$, and other arachidonate metabolites (prostacyclin, thromboxanes, and leukotrienes),[1,29,48] as well as other lipids (e.g., platelet activating factor).[4] The lung normally also elaborates dipalmityl phosphatidyl choline (dipalmityl lecithin), the principal surface active ingredient of alveolar surfactant, which protects alveoli against instability (atelectasis) and, to some extent, against pulmonary edema.[8]

These metabolic events in the lung are abnormally altered in disorders of the lung, particularly in the setting of acute lung injury. As a result, there may be excessive formation and reduced degradation of such compounds as prostaglandins,[6] thromboxanes,[6,55,59] leukotrienes,[1,48] platelet-activating factor, and activated complement,[25,32,52] as well as proteolytic enzymes, including thrombin[33] and oxygen free radicals.[11] Considerable evidence links these substances to the pulmonary and systemic responses of acute lung injury,[47] although much remains unknown about the initial lesion that triggers the chain of reactions, the sequence of activation or release of mediators, the interactions among them, and their relative importance in eliciting various reactions in different types of injury. Impaired synthesis and release of alveolar surfactant, known to play a primary pathogenetic role in neonatal respiratory distress ("hyaline membrane disease"),[8] probably contributes to the pathophysiology of other forms of acute lung injury, though its precise contribution is at present uncertain.

Neurohumoral Control of Pulmonary Vessels

It has been known for some time that pulmonary vascular tone is strongly affected by alveolar O_2 and CO_2 tensions and arterial blood pH.[9] In more recent years, the regulatory influence of endogenous humoral substances and of autonomic innervation has been actively investigated. Naturally occurring compounds that tend to contract pulmonary vascular smooth muscle include histamine, serotonin, $PGF_{2\alpha}$, thromboxane A_2, leukotrienes, and platelet activating factor. Pulmonary vasodilators make up a shorter list that includes prostacyclin and VIP.[46] The histochemical distribution, physiology, and pharmacology of adrenergic and cholinergic innervation of pulmonary vessels are now better understood: α-adrenergic agonists contract and β-adrenergic (and usually also cholinergic) agonists relax pulmonary vascular smooth muscle, especially if the vascular tone has been previously raised, as by hypoxia. In addition to the adrenergic and cholinergic components, a nonadrenergic, noncholinergic component of neurogenic relaxation (induced by electrical field stimulation in vitro) has been demonstrated in the pulmonary vessels;[19] the same relaxant system is known to exist in the airways, gastrointestinal tract, and other systems in several mammals, including humans.[39a] Finally, a number of biologically active peptides present in the lung have been localized within neuronal cell bodies, nerve fibers, and nerve terminals innervating airways and pulmonary vessels.[45] Growing evidence suggests that neuropeptides make up a "peptidergic" nervous system that interacts closely with the "classical" neurotransmitters of the central and peripheral nervous systems, and that the peptidergic system forms a third component of autonomic innervation in the lung and in many other organs and tissues.[23a]

The Central Importance of Pulmonary Endothelium in Pulmonary Vascular Responses

Long viewed as a passive "membrane" for the transfer of O_2 and CO_2 between alveolar gas and blood, pulmonary endothelium is now recognized as the site of many important metabolic activities.[41] In many conditions leading to acute lung injury, notably O_2 toxicity, pulmonary endothelium is the first part of the lung to show injury.[7,30] Furthermore, damage to endothelium is an essential prerequisite to the development of "leaky" microvessels—the *sine qua non* of acute lung injury and high permeability pulmonary edema.

Within the past few years, convincing evidence has become available that intact endothelium is required for the vasodilator responses of systemic vessels to numerous agents, including acetylocholine, histamine, ADP, thrombin, bradykinin, and Ca^{++} ionophore A23187.[13] A similar role for endothelium, i.e., endothelium-dependent relaxation, also exists in pulmonary vessels (E. Kubota, T. Saga, and S. I. Said, unpublished observations).

Pulmonary Responses to Acute Injury

The main responses to lung injury are vascular, namely endothelial damage and pulmonary hypertension.[60] Other commonly associated responses include airway constriction and alveolar duct closure, intravascular coagulation, complement activation, and aggregation of granulocytes and platelets.[47,51] In severe instances of acute lung injury, abnormal systemic responses occur, including systemic hypotension, coronary vascoconstriction, and impaired myocardial function.[47]

After the initial acute phase of the injury has passed, other responses set in that promote repair and regeneration. These reparative responses include proliferation of alveolar type II cells (the only alveolar epithelial cells with regenerative potential) to replace damaged alveolar type I cells, followed by inflammatory cell infiltration and fibrosis.[40] Pulmonary vessels undergo structural "remodeling," with obliteration of precapillary units and increased muscularization of the arterial bed.[27,39]

Detection and Assessment of Lung Injury

Improved methods for the detection and the assessment of lung injury are the objective of much investigation. This objective is relatively more easily achieved in experimental animal models where pathologic evidence can be obtained by weighing the lungs after, or even during, the induction of lung injury; the wet weight of the lungs is then compared to their dry weight, or to the predicted normal weight. Similarly, functional evidence of damaged pulmonary microvessels can be inferred from measurements of pulmonary lymph flow and its protein content relative to that of plasma.[50] The evaluation of the extent and severity of lung injury by noninvasive methods is far less easy, specific, or precise.[23] The detection of early lung injury is an even more difficult goal to accomplish. Among the means of detecting early lung injury that have been proposed in recent years are increased serum levels of activated complement (C5a),[20] diminished ability of the lung to metabolize serotonin,[5,14] and the release of certain endothelial enzymes, such as angiotensin-converting enzyme[15,24,37] and neutral metallo-endopeptidase (A.R. Johnson and E.G. Erdos, personal communication).

Mediators of Lung Injury

The intensive efforts to identify the mediator mechanisms of acute lung injury have begun to pay off. Thus, thromboxane A_2, the leukotrienes, platelet activating factor, and active oxygen metabolites are now recognized as likely mediators of the pulmonary vasoconstriction, bronchoconstriction, and other altered lung mechanics associated with several experimental models of acute lung injury.[6,12,16,17,21,26,42,47,55,59] As potential mediators of endothelial injury and high permeability pulmonary edema, only the leukotrienes, platelet activating factor, activated complement, and free oxygen radicals qualify as likely candidates.[17,32,35,36,42,47,52,57] In most forms of experimental lung injury (except those resulting from direct and immediate physical or chemical burns), the presence of activated granulocytes is required for the production of the injury; granulocytes are the primary source of many of the humoral and free radical mediators.[10,34,51] Platelet aggregation and activation may be an important factor in the pathogenesis of acute lung injury, though platelet depletion did not attenuate the pulmonary response of sheep to endotoxemia.[49]

Despite progress in identifying the mechanisms and mediators of lung injury, it is a safe guess that additional compounds, including some that are still to be discovered, participate in the sequence of reactions culminating in full-blown lung injury.

Prevention and Modulation of Lung Injury

Certain endogenously produced compounds may be able to modulate or attenuate lung injury. One compound with such potential is prostacyclin; its protective effect was suggested in experimental *E. coli* endotoxemia and in pulmonary microembolism.[22,31] VIP, an endogenous bronchodilator[45,58] and pulmonary vasodilator that counteracts the effects of leukotrienes,[18] may have similar activity. Naturally occurring antioxidants and free-radical scavengers counteract the toxic effects of oxygen free radicals. Red blood cells, rich in such scavengers, have been found to reduce lung injury due to H_2O_2.[53] The infusion of superoxide dismutase with α-naphthyl thiourea (ANTU) reduced the pulmonary edema induced by ANTU in dogs,[38] and the intravenous administration of liposome-entrapped catalase and superoxide dismutase increased survival of rats exposed to 100% oxygen.[54] Clearly, the identification of compounds that can prevent, reduce, or limit lung injury is an objective with considerable therapeutic potential.

Acknowledgments

My thanks to Marlene McVey, Dixie Seegmiller, and Janice Lambert for help with the manuscript. Supported by VA medical research funds, NIH grant HL30450, and NIH grant HL31039.

REFERENCES

1. Bach, M.K.: The leukotrienes: Their structure, actions, and role in diseases. *Current Concepts*. Kalamazoo, Upjohn, 1983.
2. Bakhle, Y.S. and Vane, J.R.: Pharmacokinetic function of the pulmonary circulation. *Physiol. Rev.* 54:1007–1045, 1974.
3. Bakhle, Y.S. , Vane, J.R. (eds.): *Metabolic Functions of the Lung*. Lenfant, C., ed. Vol. 4 in series on Lung Biology in Health and Disease. New York, Marcel Dekker, 1977.
4. Benveniste, J. and Vargaftig, B.B.: An ether-lipid with biological activities: platelet-activating factor (PAF acether). In *Ether-Lipids: Biochemical and Biomedical Aspects*. Mangold, H.K., Paltauf, H., eds. New York, Academic Press, 1983, pp. 355–376.
5. Block, E.R. and Fisher, A.: Depression of serotonin clearance by rat lungs during oxygen exposure. *J. Appl. Physiol.* 42:33–38, 1977.
6. Demling, R.H.: Role of prostaglandins in acute pulmonary microvascular injury. *Ann. N.Y. Acad. Sci.* 384:517–534, 1982.
7. Deneke, S.M. and Fanburg, B.L.: Normobaric oxygen toxicity of the lung. *N. Engl. J. Med.* 303:76–86, 1980.
8. Farrell, J.P.M.: *Lung Development: Biological and Clinical Perspectives*, Vols. I & II. New York, Academic Press, 1982.
9. Fishman, A.P.: Hypoxia and its effects on the pulmonary circulation. *Circ. Res.* 38:221–231, 1976.
10. Flick, M.R., Perel, A., and Staub, N.C.: Leukocytes are required for increased lung microvascular permeability after microembolization in sheep. *Circ. Res.* 48: 344–351, 1981.
11. Fridovich, I.: The biology of oxygen radicals. *Science* 201:875–880, 1978.
12. Frolich, J., Ogletree, M., and Brigham, K.: Gram-negative endotoxemia in sheep: Pulmonary hypertension correlated to pulmonary thromboxane synthesis. *Adv. Prostaglandin Thromboxane Res.* 7:745, 1980.
13. Furchgott, R.F.: Role of endothelium in responses of vascular smooth muscle. *Circ. Res.* 53:557–573, 1983.
14. Gillis, C.N. and Pitt, B.R.: The fate of circulating amines within the pulmonary circulation. *Ann. Rev. Physiol.* 44:269–281, 1982.
15. Gorin, A.B., Hasagawa, G., Hollinger, M., et al.: Release of angiotensin converting

enzyme by the lung after *Pseudomonas* bacteremia in sheep. *J. Clin. Invest.* 68: 163–170, 1981.

16. Gurtner, G.H., Knoblauch, A., Smith, P.L., et al.: Oxidant- and lipid-induced pulmonary vasoconstriction mediated by arachidonic acid metabolites. *Appl. Physiol.: Respir. Environ. Exercise Physiol.* 55:949–954, 1983.

17. Hamasaki, H., Mojarad, M., Saga, S., et al.: Platelet activating factor raises airway and vascular pressures and induces edema in lungs perfused with platelet-free solution. *Am. Rev. Respir. Dis.* 129:742–746, 1984.

18. Hamasaki, Y., Saga, T., Mojarad, M., and Said, S.I.: VIP counteracts leukotriene D4-induced contractions of guinea pig trachea, lung and pulmonary artery. *Trans. Assoc. Am. Physicians* 96:406–411, 1983.

19. Hamasaki, Y., Saga, T., and Said, S.I.: Autonomic innervation of pulmonary artery: Evidence for nonadrenergic, noncholinergic relaxation. *Am. Rev. Respir. Dis.* 127(4):300, 1983.

20. Hammerschmidt, D.E., Weaver, L.J., Hudson, L.D., et al.: Association of complement activation and elevated plasma C5a with adult respiratory distress syndrome: Pathophysiological relevance and possible prognostic value. *Lancet* I: 947–949, 1980.

21. Harlan, R.W.J., Nadir, B., Harker, L., et al.: Thromboxane A_2 mediates lung vasoconstriction but not permeability after endotoxin. *J. Clin. Invest.* 72:911–918, 1983.

22. Hirose, T., Aoki, E., Ishibashi, M., et al.: The effect of prostacyclin on increased hydraulic conductivity of pulmonary exchange vessels following microembolization in dogs. *Microvasc. Res.* 26:193–204, 1983.

23. Hogg, J.C.: The assessment of pulmonary microvascular permeability and edema. In *The Pulmonary Circulation and Acute Lung Injury.* Said, S.I., ed. Mount Kisco, N.Y., Futura Publishing Co., 1985.

23a. Hökfelt, T., Johansson, O., Ljungdahl, A., et al.: Peptidergic neurones. *Nature* 284:515–521, 1980.

24. Hollinger, M.A., Giri, S.N., Patwell, S., et al.: Effect of acute lung injury on angiotensin converting enzyme in serum, lung lavage, and effusate. *Am. Rev. Respir. Dis.* 121:373–376, 1980.

25. Hosea, S., Brown, E., Hammer, C., et al.: Role of complement activation in a model of adult respiratory distress syndrome. *J. Clin. Invest.* 66:375–382, 1982.

26. Hüttemeier, P.C., Watkins, W.D., Peterson, M.B., et al.: Acute pulmonary hypertension and lung thromboxane release after endotoxin infusion in normal and leukopenic sheep. *Circ. Res.* 50:688–694, 1982.

27. Jones, R., Zapol, W.M., and Reid, L.: Progressive and regressive structural changes in rat pulmonary arteries during recovery from prolonged hyperoxia. *Am. Rev. Respir. Dis.* 125:227, 1982.

28. Junod, A.F.: Metabolism, production, and release of hormones and mediators in the lung. *Am. Rev. Respir. Dis.* 112:93–108, 1975.

29. Kadowitz, P.J., Gruetter, C.A., Spannhake, E.W., et al.: Pulmonary vascular responses to prostaglandins. *Fed. Proc.* 40:1991–1996, 1981.

30. Kistler, G.S., Caldwell, P.B., and Weibel, E.R.: Development of the fine structural damage to alveolar and capillary lining cells in oxygen poisoned rat lungs. *J. Cell Biol.* 33:605–628, 1967.

31. Krausz, M.M., Utsunomiya, T., Feuerstein, G., et al.: Prostacyclin reversal of lethal endotoxemia in dogs. *J. Clin. Invest.* 67:1118–1125, 1981.

32. Larsen, G.L., McCarthy, K., Webster, R.O., et al.: A differential effect of C5a and C5a des arg in the induction of pulmonary inflammation. *Am. J. Pathol.* 100: 179–192, 1980.

33. Malik, A.B.: Pulmonary microembolism. *Physiol. Rev.* 63:1114–1207, 1983.

34. Martin, W.J., II.: Neutrophils kill pulmonary endothelial cells by a hydrogen-peroxide-dependent pathway. *Am. Rev. Respir. Dis.* 130:209–213, 1984.

35. Mojarad, M., Blalock, J.M., Cox, C.P., et al.: Leukotriene C4 increases pulmonary

lymph flow in awake sheep, probably by increasing vascular permeability. *Am. Rev. Respir. Dis.* 129:A103, 1984.

36. Mojarad, M., Said, S.I., and Hamasaki, Y.: Platelet-activating factor increases pulmonary microvascular permeability and induces pulmonary edema. *Bull. Eur. Physiopathol. Respir. (Clin. Respir. Physiol.)* 19:253–256, 1983.

37. Nukiwa, T., Matsuoka, R., Takagi, H., et al.: Responses of serum and lung angiotensin-converting enzyme activities in the early phase of pulmonary damage induced by oleic acid in dogs. *Am. Rev. Respir. Dis.* 126:1080–1086, 1982.

38. Parker, J. C., Martin, D. J., Rutili, G., et al.: Prevention of free radical-mediated vascular permeability increases in lung using superoxide dismutase. *Chest* 83: 52S–53S, 1983.

39. Reid, L.: The 1978 J. Burns Amberson Lecture. The pulmonary circulation: Remodelling in growth and disease. *Am. Rev. Respir. Dis.* 119:531–546, 1979.

39a. Richardson, J. and Beland, J.: Nonadrenergic inhibitory nervous system in human airways. *J. Appl. Physiol.* 41:764–771, 1976.

40. Rinaldo, J.E. and Rogers, R.M.: Adult respiratory distress syndrome: Changing concepts of lung injury and repair. *N. Engl. J. Med.* 306:900–909, 1982.

41. Ryan, U.S. and Ryan, J.W.: Correlations between the fine structure of the alveolar-capillary unit and its metabolic activities. In *Metabolic Functions of the Lung*. Bakhle, Y.S., Vane, J.R., eds. Vol. 4 in series on Lung Biology in Health and Disease. Lenfant, C., ed. New York, Marcel Dekker, 1977, pp. 197–232.

42. Saga, T., Yoshii, K., and Said, S.I.: Protection by FPL 55712 or indomethacin of leukotriene D4-induced pulmonary edema and airway constriction in guinea pig. *Am. Rev. Respir. Dis.* 129:A333, 1984.

43. Said, S.I.: The lung as a metabolic organ. *N. Engl. J. Med.* 279:1330–1334, 1968.

44. Said, S.I.: Metabolic functions of the pulmonary circulation. *Circ. Res.* 50:325–333, 1982.

45. Said, S.I.: Peptide hormones and neurotransmitters of the lung. *The Endocrine Lung in Health and Disease*. Becker, K.L., Gazdar, A., eds. Philadelphia, W.B. Saunders, 1984, pp. 267–275.

46. Said, S.I.: Peptides, endothelium and pulmonary vascular reactivity. *Chest* (In press).

47. Said, S.I.: Peptides and lipids as mediators of acute lung injury. In *Acute Respiratory Failure*. Zapol, W.R., ed. In Lung Biology in Health and Disease series. Lenfant, C., ed. New York, Marcel Dekker (In press).

48. Samuelsson, B.: Leukotrienes: Mediators of immediate hypersensitivity reactions and inflammation. *Science* 220:568–576, 1983.

49. Snapper, J.R., Hinson, J.M., Jr., Hutchison, A.A., et al.: Effects of platelet depletion on the unanesthetized sheep's pulmonary response to endotoxemia. *J. Clin. Invest.* 74:1782–1791, 1984.

50. Staub, N.C.: Pathophysiology of pulmonary edema. In *Edema*. Staub, N.C., Taylor, A.E., eds. New York, Raven Press, 1984, pp. 719–746.

51. Tate, R.M. and Repine, J.E.: Neutrophils and the adult respiratory distress syndrome: State of the art. *Am. Rev. Respir. Dis.* 128:552–559, 1983.

52. Till, G.O., Johnson, K.J., Kunkel, R., et al.: Intravascular activation of complement and acute lung injury. *J. Clin. Invest.* 69:1126–1135, 1982.

53. Toth, K.M., Clifford, D.P., Berger, E.M., et al.: Intact human erythrocytes prevent hydrogen peroxide-mediated damage to isolated perfused rat lungs and cultured bovine pulmonary artery endothelial cells. *J. Clin. Invest.* 74:292–295, 1984.

54. Turrens, J.F., Crapo, J.D., and Freeman, B.A.: Protection against oxygen toxicity by intravenous injection of liposome-entrapped catalase and superoxide dismutase. *J. Clin. Invest.* 73:87–95, 1984.

55. Utsunomiya, T., Krausz, M.M., Levine, L., et al.: Thromboxane mediation of cardiopulmonary effects of embolism. *J. Clin. Invest.* 70:361–368, 1982.

56. Vane, J.R.: The release and fate of vasoactive hormones in the circulation. *Br. J. Pharmacol.* 35:209–242, 1969.

57. Ward, P.A., Till, G.O., Kunkel, R., et al.: Evidence for role of hydroxyl radical in complement and neutrophil-dependent tissue injury. *J. Clin. Invest.* 72:789–801, 1983.
58. Wasserman, M.A., Griffin, R.L., and Malo, P.E.: Comparative in vitro tracheal relaxant effects of porcine and hen VIP. In *Vasoactive Intestinal Peptide*, Advances in Peptide Hormone Research Series. Said, S.I., vol. ed. New York, Raven Press, 1982.
59. Watkins, W.D., Huttemeir, P.C., Kong, D., et al.: Thromboxane and pulmonary hypertension following *E. coli* endotoxin infusion in sheep: Effects of an imidazole derivative. *Prostaglandins* 23:273–285, 1982.
60. Zapol, W.M. and Snider, M.T.: Pulmonary hypertension in severe acute respiratory failure. *N. Engl. J. Med.* 296:476–480, 1977.

II

Structural, Functional, and Pharmacological Background

Cellular Organization of the Alveolar-Capillary Unit: Structural-Functional Correlations

Maya Simionescu

Introduction

Due to a large number of data accumulated in the last two decades, the lung, once viewed as performing solely gas exchange, is now recognized as a complex organ of defined multiple vital functions (exchange of gases, metabolic and endocrine activities) that interrelate and most probably influence each other. The lung fulfills its functions because of (1) its special position in the organism, (2) its location in the circulatory system, and (3) its structural organization.

(1) Considering the whole body, the lung is one of the few organs that has direct contact with the external milieu via a system of tubes—the airways. They secure a continuously renewed and rapid inflow of O_2 and discharge of CO_2; at the same time, exposure of the lung cells to atmospheric air and potential antigens is a continuous challenge that requires an efficient protective mechanism.

(2) In the circulatory system, the lung is strategically situated so as to convert the venous blood, which is received from the right ventricle, into arterial blood, which is returned to the left atrium. Virtually the entire cardiac output passes each time through the lungs before returning to the body. The venous blood pumped into the lungs is characteristically rich in CO_2 and also contains the lymphatic drainage, which empties into the superior vena cava its chylomicrons, lipoproteins, and proteins collected from the interstitial spaces of the body. After passing and being processed through the lungs (pulmonary circulation), the blood returned to the left atrium is further pumped by the left ventricle via the aorta into the arterial system (systemic circulation).

(3) The organization of the lung was differentiated to accommodate the cardiac output within an extensive capillary network in a rather small volume. The air and the blood are confined to two different compartments, each one lined by specialized epithelia. For an efficient exchange of O_2 and CO_2 between air and blood, the structure of the lung has been adapted so as to fulfill two main conditions: (1) a large surface area of contact, and (2) an attenuated barrier

From Said, S.I. (ed.): *The Pulmonary Circulation and Acute Lung Injury.* Mount Kisco, N.Y., Futura Publishing Co., Inc., 1985.

between the two media. The surface area available for exchange is ~120 m², and the barrier between the air and blood is reduced to ~0.5 μm thickness. The lung parenchyma is made up of a large number of cell types (about 40); however, at the level of the repeating functioning units of the lung, "the alveolar-capillary units" that occupy the majority of lung parenchyma, this large number of cell types is markedly decreased.

General Structure of the Lung

The air diffuses through the nose and a system of sequential tubes, the larynx, trachea, and bronchi; the latter enter the lung and divide in several orders of bronchioles. Small bronchioles (~0.5 mm diameter) become endowed along their wall with outpouchings, the alveoli, where the gas exchange between air and blood takes place, and are accordingly termed respiratory bronchioles. The latter continue to divide in smaller tubes invested almost continuously with alveoli; these are the alveolar ducts, which continue with blind-end alveolar sacs, constituted by clusters of alveoli (Figs. 1, 2). The mean diameter of an alveoli is about 250 μm.[12]

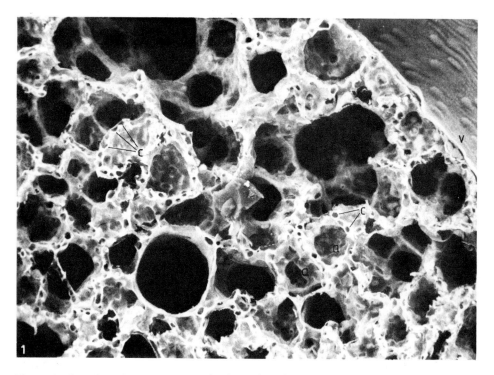

Figure 1: *Scanning electron micrograph of a rat lung fragment, the vasculature of which was washed free of blood. Alveoli (a) are separated by septa that contain a network of blood capillaries (c) appearing in cross-section as small empty cavities. In the upper right corner, part of a large blood vessel (v) exposes on its luminal aspect the nuclei of endothelial cells aligned parallel to the direction of the blood flow. Original magnification, ×350.*

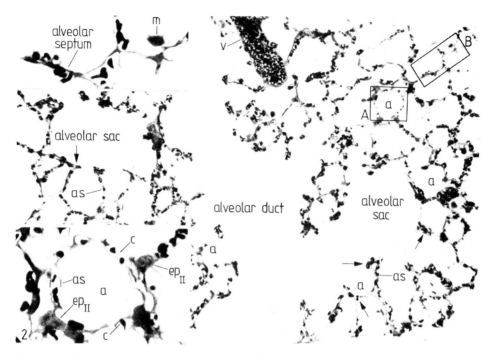

Figure 2: *Mouse lung: low power micrograph illustrating an alveolar duct continuing with alveolar sacs on which several alveoli (a) open. The latter are separated from each other by alveolar septa (as) endowed with blood capillaries recognized by the presence of red blood cells (arrows). v = blood vessel. Original magnification, ×150. Lower inset: An alveolus (a) surrounded by capillaries (c) contained within the alveolar septa (as). ep_{II} = type II epithelial cell (enlarged area of rectangle A). Original magnification, ×400. Upper inset: An alveolar macrophage (m) is apparently free in the airspace (enlarged area of the rectangle B). Original magnification, ×400.*

The venous blood is transported to the lung by the pulmonary artery at low hydrostatic pressure (40 mmHg). The artery branches enter the respective lung and continue to divide up into arterioles, which eventually give rise to an extensive network of capillaries located within the septa separating adjoining alveoli. Oxygenated blood returns to the heart via venules and pulmonary veins.

Blood vessels and air pathways branch in parallel and all alveoli are surrounded by a closely packed capillary network (Figs. 2, 3), resulting in an enormous area of contact and a very close apposition of the cells involved in diffusion of gases. In the adult human lung, there are about 300×10^6 alveoli securing an aggregate exchange surface estimated at about 120 m^2.[44]

The alveolus and the surrounding meshes of capillaries constitute the "alveolar-capillary unit"; the aggregate volume of these units occupies ~80% of the lung parenchyma.[12]

As in all vascular beds, the lung vessels are lined up by *endothelium*, a continuous layer of squamous epithelial cells which in arteries, arterioles, large venules, and veins is backed by smooth muscle cells and, depending on dimension and location, also by elastic elements and an outermost connective tissue

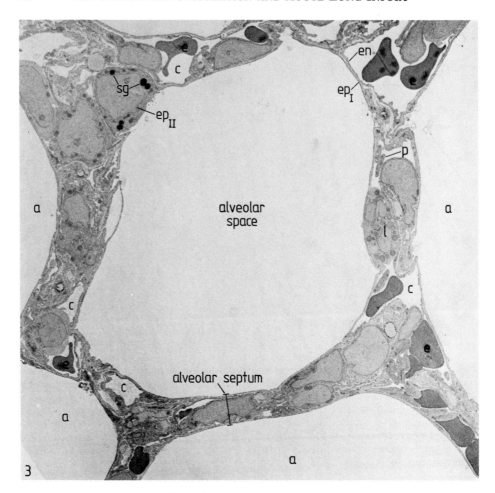

Figure 3: *Cross-section through an alveolus (rat lung) separated from the adjoining alveoli (a) by alveolar septa displaying numerous capillaries (c) marked by erythrocytes (e), platelets (p), and rare leukocytes (l). Although the organization of the alveolar epithelium can be hardly distinguished at this magnification, portions of the thin type I epithelial cell (ep_I) can be noticed facing a comparable region of capillary endothelium (en) to form the air-blood barrier. A cuboidal secretory type II epithelial cell (ep_{II}) can be recognized because of its osmophilic secretory granules (sg). Original magnification, ×2900.*

layer. In capillaries, the endothelium represents the only cellular layer interposed between the blood and the interstitial fluid.

The air passageway is lined by an *epithelium*, which is pseudostratified or cuboidal in the upper segments (trachea, primary bronchi, bronchioles), and becomes progressively simple and squamous at the level of alveoli. In the latter, about 95% of the surface is occupied by the large, squamous *type I epithelial cells*, the rest being constituted by the cuboidal *type II epithelial cells*. Although the type II cells are relatively numerous (~50%), due to their small size, they occupy only a small fractional area of the alveolar surface (Fig. 4). Apparently free in the alveolar space are the *alveolar macrophages*, occurring in a position par-

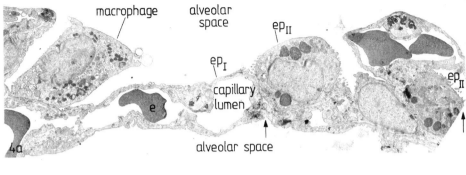

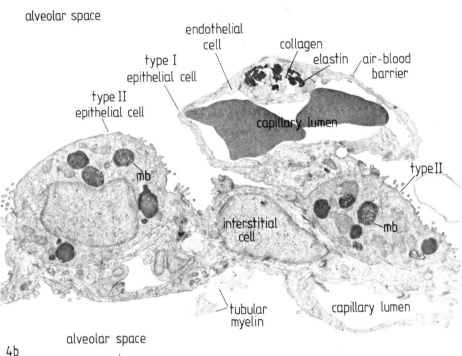

Figure 4.a, b: *Cellular components of the alveolar-capillary unit (rat lung).* **a:** *An alveolar septum separating adjacent alveolar spaces;* **b:** *represents an enlarged area of a consecutive section through the region between the arrows in Figure 4a. epI = type I epithelial cell; epII = type II epithelial cell.* **a,** *original magnification,* ×3600; **b,** *original magnification,* ×7500.

ticularly important for maximum efficiency for defense of the cells of the alveolar-capillary unit (Fig. 2, inset). The *interstitium*, rather reduced in size, is represented at the level of the alveolar-capillary unit by connective tissue elements (fibroblasts, collagen, elastic elements, ground substance), and by numerous contractile interstitial cells and smooth muscle cells (occurring at the tip of the alveolus) (Fig. 4). Collagen and elastic elements form a fibrillar network that extends from the visceral pleura to the major vessels and airways as a "fibrous continuum" interweaving among capillaries.[50] This three-dimensional meshwork is important in maintaining the fragile and relatively lax structure of lung parenchyma.

A detailed analysis of the structural components of the alveolar-capillary unit and their ascribed functions can bring a better insight into the general physiology of the lung.

The Alveolar-Capillary Unit: The Air-Blood Barrier

Endothelium

Of mesodermal origin, these cells account for about 40% of the total pulmonary cells.[51] They are a continuous type of endothelium (no fenestrae) and lie on a basal lamina (basement membrane) that they produce. These large and thin cells are provided with a nucleus and the organelles (although less conspicuous) commonly encountered in all epithelial cells. Close to the nucleus are the Golgi complex, mitochondria, rare endoplasmic reticulum elements, ribosomes and, scattered throughout the cytoplasm, numerous plasmalemmal vesicles opened to the lumen, to the interstitia, or apparently enclosed in the cytoplasm, (Figs. 5, 6). Such vesicles, common to all epithelial cells, appear in endothelial cells as the predominant organelle. In rabbit lung capillaries, morphometric studies have reported 131 vesicles/μm^3.[16]

A peculiarity of the alveolar capillary endothelium is the existence in its peripheral region of two clearly defined zones. One thin area (35 to 65 nm thick) that has few or no plasmalemmal vesicles (*the avesicular zone*) is in close apposition with type I epithelial cell (Fig. 6a). Opposite to it, the endothelium has a mean thickness of about 200 nm and is provided with vesicles (*the vesicular zone*) (Fig. 6b). The thin avesicular zone together with the corresponding part of the epithelial type I cell and their fused basal laminae constitute the *air-blood barrier* (Figs. 4, 6a), at which level the major exchange of O_2/CO_2 takes place.

From the lung capillaries, as in other organs, water and water-soluble macromolecules are continuously transported to the interstitia and surrounding tissues.[37] Studies using exogenous macromolecular tracers have shown that plasmalemmal vesicles are involved in the bulk transport of water-soluble molecules from the plasma across the endothelium to the interstitial spaces.[33] This process, which is common to all endothelial cells, is different from pinocytosis. In the latter process, vesicles take up soluble molecules and transport them to the lysosomes at the level of which the incorporated molecules are digested and ultimately made available for cell use. In the endothelial cells, vesicular transport takes place across the cell, most probably in both directions, bypassing other cellular compartments, a process known as transcytosis.[40] True pinocytosis is a rare event in capillary endothelium, whereas transcytosis probably occurs continuously in order to maintain homeostasia of the interstitial fluid.

Endothelial cells are joined by tight junctions which, in thin sections, appear as points of close contact (Fig. 6c) or fusion of the outer membrane leaflets of the adjoining cells (Fig. 6d). These junctions form belts (presumed to be continuous) around the cells and are of major importance in restricting the passage of water-soluble macromolecules along the intercellular space. Some intercellular junctions appear open to a space of ~5 nm wide.[32] The exact

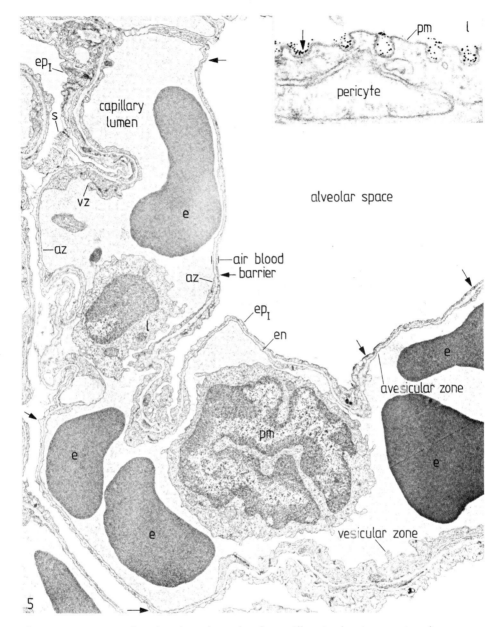

Figure 5: *Longitudinal section through an alveolar capillary (rat lung) occupying almost completely the alveolar septum lined by type I epithelial cells (ep$_I$). The capillary establishes on both sides several regions of air-blood barriers (between arrows). vz = vesicular zone of capillary endothelium; az = avesicular zone; e = erythrocyte; s = surfactant. Original magnification, ×9300. Inset: Special affinity of plasmalemmal vesicles for gold-conjugates serum albumin. The particles appear in a single row adsorbed on vesicle membrane (arrow) and are absent on plasma membrane (pm). l = lumen. Original magnification, ×87,000.*

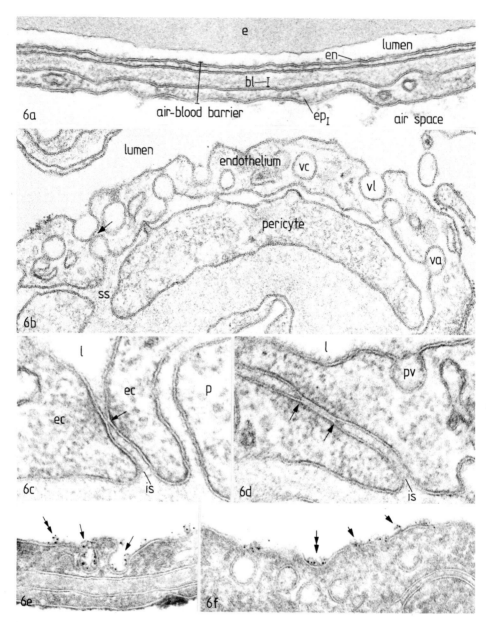

Figure 6.a-f: *Electron micrographs illustrating characteristic features and properties of the alveolar capillary endothelium.* **a**: *The thin avesicular zone of the endothelium (en) is usually adjacent to the thin type I epithelial cell (ep$_I$). The two basal laminae are fused (bl); the three constituents form the air-blood barrier. e = erythrocyte.* **b**: *The vesicular zone of the endothelial cell is characteristically provided with numerous plasmalemmal vesicles open on the luminal front (vl), on the albuminal front (va), or apparently free in the cytoplasm (vc). Two vesicles open on opposite fronts are almost completely fused to form a transendothelial channel (arrow). ss = subendothelial space.* **c and d**: *Tight junctions between two capillary endothelial cells (ec), appearing in cross-section as a point of close contact between the outer leaflets of the adjoining membranes (**c**, arrow), or as complete fusion (over a distance of ~120 nm) of the two outer*

location of these open junctions cannot be reliably identified in the lung; they may belong to the small postcapillary (pericytic) venules as demonstrated in other microvascular units in which sequential segments (arterioles, capillaries, and venules) could be easily recognized.[36,38]

The daily normal turnover rate of endothelial cells was estimated at about 1% of their total number,[6] but their capacity to divide seems to be much higher as suggested by the extent of their recovery from an injury. After oxygen injury, ~50% of the total pulmonary cells that actively synthesize DNA (8%) are endothelial cells.[3]

Endothelial cells are polarized, having one front toward the blood and the other toward the interstitial spaces. Very little is known about the chemistry and the particulars (if any) of each endothelial surface. The luminal membrane has a carbohydrate-rich glycocalyx which represents the terminal moieties of glycoproteins and/or glycolipids embedded in the lipid bilayer of plasmalemma. In addition, an adsorbed layer of plasma proteins is present in vivo on this surface on which fibrinogen and albumin have been detected immunocytochemically.[1] A special, locally restricted affinity of the endothelium for albumin is indicated by the preferential binding of the gold-labeled albumin to the plasmalemmal vesicles in situ after washing out the endogenous plasma (including its albumin) (Fig. 5, inset) (M. Simionescu et al., unpublished observations). Conversely, there is no affinity for gold particles which, instead of albumin, were stabilized with polyethyleneglycol. In addition, the endothelial plasma membrane is the bearer of the acidic sites (see below).

Because of its position in the circulation, it was hypothesized and thereafter proved that the lung is actively involved in removing harmful vasoactive substances and in the activation of some circulating hormones before they reach the systemic circulation.[47]

It was experimentally demonstrated that during one passage through the lung, the endothelium is capable of removing 80−90% of 5-hydroxytryptamine by a Na^+-dependent mechanism[20] of converting angiotensin I to angiotensin II,[27] and of inactivating bradykinin,[9] whereas histamine and angiotensin II pass freely.

Recently, a number of enzymes were identified on the luminal front, which is continuously exposed to circulating molecule-laden plasma. Thus, kininase II or angiotensin I converting enzyme (ACE) has been located cytochemically on or near the luminal membrane as well as in plasmalemmal vesicles open to the vascular lumen.[30] The same applies to 5'-nucleotidase, ATPase,[31] and lipoprotein lipase which hydrolyses circulating long chain triacylglycerols.[11] Cultured endothelial cells isolated mainly from the pulmonary artery synthesize and release into the culture medium a number of substances such as ACE, fibronectin, factor VIII antigen, prostaglandins. These activities may be shared by the alveolar capillary endothelium as well.

An eloquent example of biological equilibrium is that performed by the lung ACE. This is capable of converting angiotensin I to angiotensin II (the most

---

leaflets of the corresponding membranes (**d**, arrows). l = capillary lumen; is = intercellular space; p = pericyte; pv = plasmalemmal vesicle. **e and f**: Binding of gold-conjugated low density lipoproteins to endothelial surface (hamster lung). The LDL particles (~250 nm) can be seen in large number in plasmalemmal vesicles (arrow), on coated pits (double arrow), and on plasmalemma proper (arrowhead). Original magnifications: **a**, ×93,000; **b**, ×97,000; **c, d**, ×160,000; **e, f**, ×93,000.

potent hypertensive) and of degrading bradykinin (a hypotensive), thus manipulating simultaneously the amount of these potent antagonistic substances allowed to enter the systemic circulation. Unlike other vascular beds, the lung vasculature is the only place where angiotensin II is not inactivated.[9] In injured lung, removal of vasoactive substances is drastically altered.[17]

Most of these metabolic functions are also present in other vascular beds but not with the same intensity; this may be due either to the particularly large endothelial surface available in the lung or to an enhanced activity at this level.

Cholesterol is particularly important for the lung because it is utilized both for membrane biogenesis as well as a component of the surfactant; in the latter, cholesterol is a most abundant (8–14%) lipidic constituent second only to dipalmitoylphosphatidyl choline (DPC) (~55% of total lipids).[4]

Lung receptors for low density lipoproteins (LDL) (the main cholesterol carrier in many species) and high density lipoproteins (HDL) have been demonstrated using radiolabeled lipoproteins.[19,28] The rate of LDL uptake is significantly greater than that of HDL and appears to be a saturable, concentration-dependent process with a maximum at 20–30 minutes of perfusion. The process of binding and internalization was visualized using LDL coupled to colloidal gold[28] and mordanting tissue specimens with tannic acid during their preparation for electron microscopy.[41] Gold-labeled LDL bound to coated pits, and plasmalemma proper and labeled heavily plasmalemmal vesicles open on the blood front (Fig. 6e,f) or are apparently internalized. In vivo experiments with radiolabeled and gold-labeled LDL suggest that the endothelium of alveolar capillaries express LDL receptors as demonstrated for the endothelium of arteries[48] and microvessels.[42]

Epithelium

The lining of the alveolar space is of endodermal origin and is organized as a continuous layer made of thin squamous type I epithelial cells[23] interspersed with smaller cuboidal, type II epithelial cells (Fig. 4). Although these two cell types are almost equal in number, the alveolar surface area occupied by each type is greatly in favor of type I cells (~95%).[51]

Type I epithelial cells are very broad, flattened, and highly branching cells with few organelles and some vesicles possibly involved in transport. These cells are fragile and easily altered by a number of factors including infusion of histamine, epinephrine, and angiotensin.[13] Type I cells seem to have relatively low metabolic needs, being primarily organized to offer a thin barrier for gas diffusion. As other epithelia, they have a basal lamina (basement membrane) which is fused with the basal lamina of the corresponding avesicular zone of the endothelial cells. As such, over the major part of the alveolus, the gases diffuse across two highly attenuated cell layers, endothelium and epithelium and their fused basal laminae: this is the *air-blood barrier proper* (Fig. 6a) of 0.2–0.5 μm thick (large species variation).

The tight junctions between epithelial cells are quite strongly organized so as to provide a good barrier to fluid diffusion from the air space to the interstitia or back.[10,32] Together with the endothelial tight junctions, the epithelial junctions play an important role in sealing off the capillary and alveolar compartments and in keeping the alveolar interstitia free of excess water or proteins.

Type I epithelial cells do not divide and thus do not regenerate; in trauma of the alveolar lining, type II cells divide and replace the damaged epithelium.

Type II epithelial cells are intercalated and linked by tight junctions with type I epithelial cells. They have a typical structure of a polarized secretory cell: basal nucleus, apical microvilli, well-developed Golgi complex, endoplasmic reticulum, multivesicular bodies, and an impressive number of membrane-bound secretory vesicles termed *multilamellar bodies* (MLB) (Fig. 7). The MLB secretory product is continuously exocytosed into the alveolar space where the lamellae seem to unravel, and in glutaraldehyde-fixed tissues, appear as a lattice-like network (Fig. 7b,c) termed *tubular myelin*.[52] These structures are well preserved in specimens treated with tannic acid after osmication.[21,35] Actin filaments are considered to participate in the intracytoplasmic movement of lamellar bodies in their way to become adjacent to the apical surface and discharge their content.[45] The MLB product is part of, or is the whole *surfactant* molecule, a material present on the epithelial surface that opposes and reduces the surface tension produced in alveoli at the air-liquid interface, thus preventing alveolar collapse. In chemical composition, the alveolar surfactant is a mixture of phospholipids (~75%) complexed with a protein, and some carbohydrates. About half of the total lipids are represented by dipalmitoylphosphatidyl choline, an amphipathic molecule, and 8–14% is cholesterol.[4] Studies on lung homogenate have shown that both isolated lamellar bodies and tubular myelin have surface tension-lowering properties and a lipid composition similar to that of the surfactant. The protein content, which is different, may be added after extrusion of the lipids into the air space.[15,54]

Surfactant molecules have a short half-life (~4 h) and the information produced thus far suggests that type II cells are responsible for the continuous production of the surfactant or part of it. Isolated type II cells are capable of incorporating large amounts of [^{14}C]-palmitate or [^{14}C]-glucose and of synthesizing DPC as well as phosphatidyl glycerol, a highly saturated surfactant-associated phospholipid.[43] Endogenous synthesis of cholesterol destined for surfactant depends on and is regulated by the available plasma lipoproteins as a source of exogenous cholesterol. The lung secretes ~20% of its total cholesterol as a surfactant constituent.[19] When available, low density lipoproteins are taken up in large amount by lung parenchyma as shown by experiments with radio-labeled exogenous LDL.[19,28]

Type II epithelial cells are particularly important in the normal functioning of the lung as the generator of surfactant, the deficiency of which is lethal both in premature infants and in adults (respiratory distress syndrome). Since in development, the secretory type II cells appear late in gestation (~6 months in humans), the alveoli of the premature lung cannot be maintained open, and the respiratory function cannot be fulfilled. In addition, the phospholipid component of the surfactant has an antibacterial activity, particularly efficient against several gram-positive bacteria.[5]

Interstitia

The alveolar wall, lined by epithelial cells on both sides, is occupied by connective tissue components: fibroblasts, fibers (collagen and elastin), ground substance, and interstitial fluid. A large fraction (~40%) of the interstitia is occupied by special contractile interstitial cells, which have long cytoplasmic

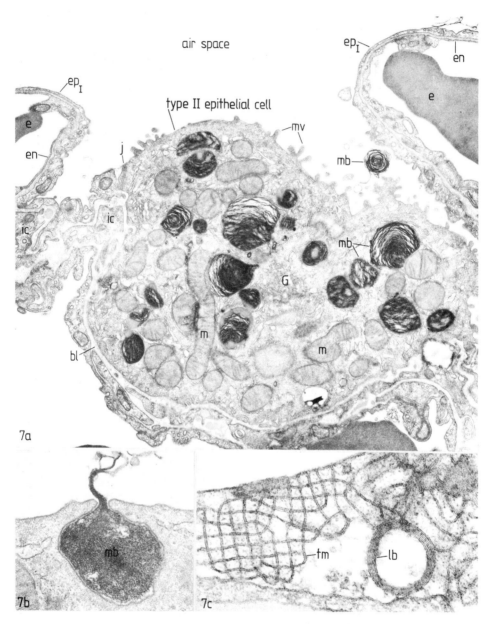

air space

ep$_I$

en

e

ep$_I$

e

en

type II epithelial cell

mv

ic

j

mb

ic

mb

G

m

m

bl

7a

mb

7b

tm

lb

7c

Figure 7.a-c: *Type II epithelial cell as a part of the epithelium lining the alveolus. This large cuboidal cell is linked by a tight junction (j) to the neighboring type I epithelial cell (ep$_I$); the latter is in close apposition to capillary endothelium (en). The type II cell has characteristic apical microvilli (mv), numerous mitochondria (m) and multilamellar bodies (mb), and a developed Golgi complex (G). Within the interstitium, part of two interstitial cells (ic) can be identified. e = erythrocyte.* **a,** *original magnification, ×20,000;* **b:** *Exocytosis of the content of a multilamellar body (mb). Original magnification, ×40,000;* **c:** *Unravelling of the lamellae of an extruded lamellar body (lb) to form tubular myelin (tm). Original magnification, ×90,000.*

extensions anchored upon the epithelial basal lamina.[22] These cells possess characteristic actin and myosin filaments in the cytoplasm and within their cytoplasmic extensions. By their contractile properties, the interstitial cells are likely to be involved in the mechanical autoregulation of the alveolus. This consists of the control and adjustment of (1) the ventilation/perfusion (V/Q) at the alveolar level,[22] and/or (2) the compliance and volume of the interstitia.[50] Unlike in other organs, the pulmonary interstitium is reduced to a bare minimum over the air-blood barrier per se, where only the fused basal laminae of endothelium and epithelium are present (Fig. 6a). Fibroblasts, contractile interstitial cells, pericytes (located next to endothelial cells), and smooth muscle cells (found at the tip of the alveolus) are permanent residents of the alveolar wall interstitia. In addition, a number of migratory cells such as macrophages and mast cells are encountered.

Collagen fibers (5–20% of the total lung proteins) and elastin bundles are quite abundantly scattered in the alveolar wall and at the tip of the alveolus (Fig. 8); together with smooth muscle cells, they participate in maintaining the shape of the alveolus. In normal lung, type I and III *collagens* (most abundant) have been detected in the extracellular matrix, whereas types IV and V were localized in the endothelial basal lamina.[24]

Laminin has been identified by immunocytochemistry in the epithelial and endothelial basal laminae, whereas *fibronectin* was found free in the interstitia and on the surface of collagen bundles.[14]

All the stromal components (cells and fibers) contribute to the formation of a solid but highly adjustable framework for maintaining the delicate lung structure.

Alveolar Macrophages

Since atmospheric air often carries bacteria, particles, and dust, a large population of macrophages (~1 per 3 alveoli) that are enzymatically well equipped to perform phagocytosis patrol the alveolar space within and above the lining layer of surfactant (Fig. 9). They originate from blood monocytes, ~15% of which leave the circulation in a steady-state condition to become lung macrophages;[2] the great majority of them populate the alveolar space, and only a few remain in the tissue. There is no clear evidence how the circulating monocytes reach the alveolar space.

Macrophages are large cells (~25 μm diameter) with a large nucleus, a well-developed Golgi complex, numerous mitochondria, and especially lysosomes (up to 100 per cell) rich in proteolytic and hydrolytic enzymes (collagenase, elastase, lysozymes, phospholipases, etc.). Because of their peculiar location in direct contact with the atmospheric air, the alveolar macrophages depend on aerobic metabolism.

Similar to other macrophages, they synthesize a large spectrum of products including fibronectin, which may be important as a nonimmune opsonin for promotion of binding and uptake of microorganisms or particles from the alveolar space.[49]

Normally, macrophages do not divide in the alveoli; their turnover time is ~27 days. For the upper airways, there are a number of additional defense mechanisms, e.g., lymphatic vessels and lymphocytes, and the mucus layer that is moved over the epithelia by the beating cilia toward larger airways. At the

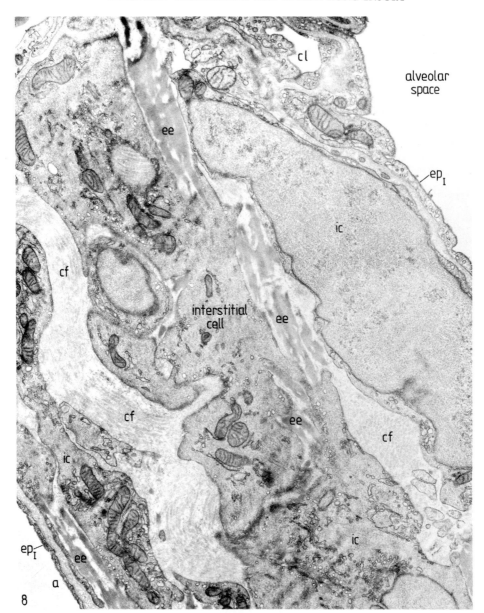

Figure 8: *In the relatively thick portions of an alveolar septum, the interstitium contains one or more layers of interstitial cells (ic) interspersed among bundles of elastic elements (ee), collagen fibers (cf) embedded in ground substance. ep$_I$ = type I epithelial cell; cl = capillary lumen. Original magnification, ×17,000.*

level of the alveolar-capillary unit, macrophages represent the main line of defense against microorganisms or particles (dust) and possibly for removing denatured surfactant.[26]

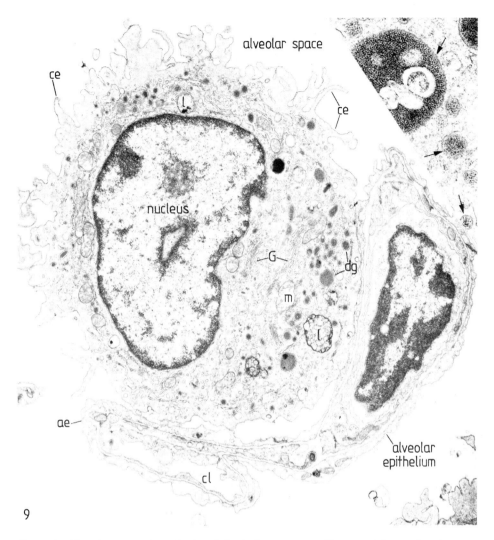

Figure 9: *Alveolar macrophage (rat lung) displaying numerous filament-rich cytoplasmic extensions (ce), a well-developed Golgi complex (G), dense membrane-bound granules (dg), and relatively large lysosomes (l) containing lipid inclusions. The cell is closely attached to the alveolar epithelium (ae). cl = capillary lumen. Original magnification, ×11,000. Inset: Cationized ferritin injected intratracheally is massively endocytosed by the alveolar macrophages (arrows). Original magnification, ×66,000.*

Cell Surface Charge of the Alveolar-Capillary Unit

Endothelial Lining

The surface charge of a cell is an effective contributor to the interaction with other cells, molecules, or macromolecular complexes, as well as for the uptake and transport of different molecules into or through the cell. There is a general agreement that, like other cells, the endothelial and blood cells have a net negative surface charge; thus, in normal conditions, they repel each other, a condition that insures blood fluidity at the blood-endothelial interface. Since most plasma proteins are negatively charged, the question arose of how they can cross the endothelium that has a similarly charged surface. To map the minute distribution pattern of anionic sites, of the endothelial luminal plasmalemma, cationic ferritin (CF) (pI 8.4, M_r 440,000, and molecular diameter ~11 nm) was perfused in situ in mice blood-free lung vasculature. At different time intervals (5 to 20 min), unbound CF was washed out and the tissue processed for electron microscopic examination.[34] On the endothelial surface of alveolar capillaries, CF was inhomogeneously distributed defining well-differentiated microdomains. In the vesicular zone, the endothelial plasma membrane was almost continuously marked except for the membrane and diaphragms (when present) of plasmalemmal vesicles and of rarely found transendothelial channels (Fig. 10, inset). Plasmalemma decoration stopped abruptly at the level of intercellular junctions. In the avesicular zone, the plasmalemma was not (or rarely) decorated by CF, indicating either a low density of CF-accessible anionic sites or the presence of very weak acidic residues of high pK_a values at this level. The existence of microdomains of different charge and/or charge density suggests the possibility of an adaptation of the two zones to different functions. One can speculate that along the avesicular zone, with low density of anionic sites, the red blood cells may be less repelled and their movement may be slowed down, a condition that would facilitate the gas exchange. In the vesicular zone, the vesicles may represent, as in other capillaries,[39] a preferential pathway for transport of anionic proteins by transcytosis. Moreover, the difference in charge between the plasmalemma and the vesicles may generate a concentration gradient of plasma proteins over the latter, a condition that may ease the diffusion of molecules into vesicles. The size, shape, and charge of plasma molecules are other important parameters that have to be taken into account when considering the transendothelial transport of water-soluble macromolecules.

Epithelial Lining

To analyze the distribution of anionic sites on the alveolar epithelium, CF was introduced intratracheally with or without previous washing of the alveolar content; after 5 to 20 minutes, the unbound CF was removed and the lung processed for electron microscopy.[34] A marked difference was found in the epithelium decoration by CF: type I cells were very little or not labeled, whereas neighboring type II cells were heavily marked by two to three tightly packed rows that followed the luminal contour (including the microvilli) up to the level of the junction with type I epithelial cells (Fig. 11). CF labeled rapidly (3 min) the membranes of the multilamellar bodies open to the cell surface (Fig. 11, inset), as well as the extruded lamellar bodies, which appeared decorated in a concentric fashion. This latter pattern may be induced by the polycationic probe since incubation in vitro of multilamellar vesicles with CF forms similar structures composed of alternating sheaths of bilayer and CF.[29] CF may form bridges between adjacent membrane surfaces. In cultured type II cells, it was demonstrated that the apical domain is negatively charged.[25] Alveolar macrophages were moderately labeled by CF that was bound to the plasmalemma, but a more intense endocytosis has taken place (Fig. 9, inset).

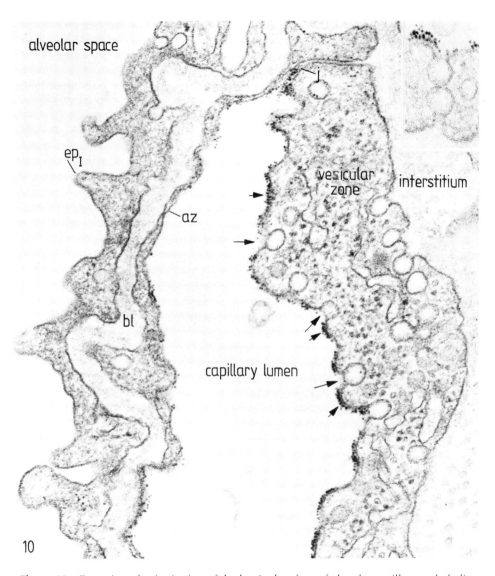

Figure 10: *Detection of anionic sites of the luminal surface of alveolar capillary endothelium after perfusion of cationized ferritin (pI 8.4) (mouse lung). CF distribution has two distinct patterns. Over the vesicular zone of the endothelium, CF binds almost continuously on the plasma membrane (arrowheads) but fails to decorate the plasmalemmal vesicles and their diaphragms (arrows), and transendothelial channels (inset). On the opposite avesicular zone of the endothelium (az), CF binding is very scarce or absent; the decoration stops at the level of the intercellular junction (j). ep_I = type I epithelial cell; bl = basal lamina. Original magnification, ×78,000.*

When epithelial lining is purposely or accidentally damaged, CF has access to the basal lamina and interstitia. In such cases, CF is bound in small clusters (40–70 nm in diameter) at regular intervals (~80–100 nm apart center-to-center) to the basal lamina and in a highly regular pattern to collagen fibers,

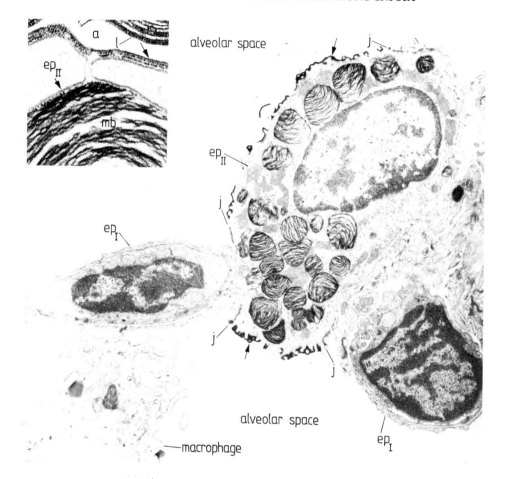

Figure 11: *Detection of the anionic sites on the surface of alveolar epithelium by intratracheal administration of cationized ferritin (CF) (pI 8.4). After 3 minutes, CF (arrows) binds heavily to the plasma membrane of the type II epithelial cell (ep$_{II}$) (which in this case corresponds to two alveolar spaces). CF labeling stops abruptly at the level of the junction (j) with the neighboring type I epithelial cells (ep$_I$), on the membrane of which there is little or no CF binding. Original magnification, ×72,000. Inset: On the plasmalemma of type II epithelial cell, CF decoration occurs in multiple closely packed rows (arrows). A multilamellar body (mb) open through a short neck to the alveolar space (a) contains CF particles on its outermost lamella (arrowhead). Some lamellae (l) in the alveolar space are cross-bridged by CF. Original magnification, ×94,000.*

which are connected in phase (Fig. 12). The anionic sites of the alveolar basal lamina, as detected with CF and Ruthenium red,[46] may be an additional sieve in the transport of anionic proteins. These acidic sites are contributed primarily by heparin sulfate proteoglycans.[46] The regular distribution of acidic sites along the collagen fibrils may be important in the periodicity and the bundling of the whole fiber.

The preferential distribution of anionic sites on the alveolar epithelium and endothelium may have physiological relevance, which at present is not well understood. The air-blood barrier proper lacks or has few acidic sites on both the

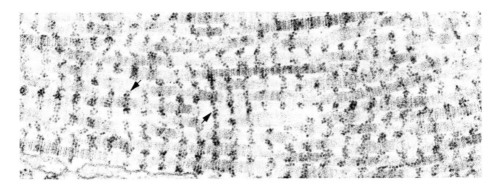

Figure 12: *Binding of cationized ferritin (arrows) to collagen fibers in the interstitia of the alveolar septum. Original magnification, ×87,000.*

epithelium and the endothelium. On the contrary, the neighboring type II cell luminal membrane is strongly anionic.

Internalization of Polycationic Ligands by Type II Epithelial Cells

At 1 to 3 minutes after intratracheal perfusion, the cationic ferritin can be found adsorbed to the luminal plasmalemma, microvilli, and the pits at their base. At 10 to 20 minutes, CF introduced both in vivo and in situ in the alveolar space begins to label internalized uncoated vesicles and coated vesicles (Fig. 13a). At 60 to 80 minutes, CF appears in multivesicular bodies (Fig. 13b) and in structures that resemble forming, young multilamellar bodies (Fig. 13c). After 3 hours and longer, all newly formed multilamellar bodies contain CF (Fig. 13d). Occasionally, 80 minutes after CF administration, the probe is found in the Golgi cisternae (Fig. 13e).

The internalization of CF after binding to the luminal plasmalemma suggests that recycling of membrane domains may occur. According to the information accumulated in recent years, it has become clear that many cells reutilize the membranes used in different transport processes.[8] Since CF binds electrostatically to the plasmalemma, it represents a suitable membrane marker to follow the route taken by domains of the apical plasmalemma inside the cell.

Type II cells perform continuously at their apical pole exocytosis that implies fusion of the membrane of the secretory granule (MLB) with the plasmalemma followed by discharge of its contents. Tracking the CF-labeled structures at different intervals suggests that in type II cells, retrieval of domains of the apical membrane may follow two alternative routes: (1) from the luminal plasmalemma via uncoated and coated vesicles to multivesicular bodies and to young forming lamellar bodies; or (2) from the luminal plasmalemma probably via another pool of vesicles to the Golgi complex. The second route is only rarely encountered in these cells. These pathways may represent both retrieval of domains of the apical membrane and a route of recovery of some surfactant constituents (yet CF is not a suitable marker for surfactant molecules) from the alveolar space back into the type II cells to be reutilized as recently suggested by an experiment using ^{32}P-labeled surfactant[18] and cationized ferritin.[53]

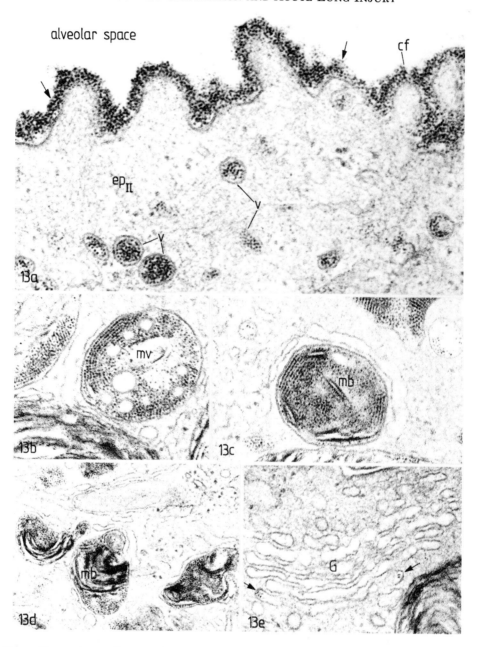

Figure 13.a-e: *Internalization of cationized ferritin (CF) pl 8.4 from the alveolar space into the type II epithelial cell (ep_{II}).* **a**: *20 min after CF intratracheal administration, the ligand labels in multiple, packed rows the apical plasma membrane (arrows), as well as vesicles (v) found in various stages of internalization.* **b and c**: *60–80 min after CF administration, multivesicular bodies (mv) and young multilamellar bodies (mb) become studded with CF particles.* **d**: *At 3 h, CF is present in the matrix of all forming lamellar bodies (mb).* **e**: *At 80 min, occasionally, CF (arrows) appears in the cisternae of the Golgi complex (G) (arrows). Original magnifications:* **a**, *×92,000;* **b, c**, *×86,000;* **d**, *×62,000;* **e**, *×74,000.*

Monosaccharides of the Cell Surface of the Alveolar-Capillary Unit

Glycoconjugates of the epithelial and endothelial cell membranes were identified using lectins of well-established specificity for some monosaccharide residues. The lectins used were wheat germ agglutinin (WGA) (recognizes β-N-acetylglucosaminyl and sialyl residues), lotus tetragonolobus lectin (for α-L-fucosyl), and peanut agglutinin (for β-D-galactosyl). Lectins were conjugated to horseradish peroxidase and their presence was detected indirectly via a peroxidatic reaction. All the monosaccharide moieties so detected were present on both endothelial and epithelial plasma membranes as well as in plasmalemmal vesicles (Fig. 14). The absence of CF-detectable anionic sites on the avesicular zone of the endothelium and the presence of WGA-labeling on the same surface suggest that the latter binds in this region, especially to the β-N-acetylglucosaminyl residues of glycoconjugates (M. Simionescu, unpublished observations). Concanavalin A does not bind to the alveolar epithelial cells.[7] The relatively high concentration of glycoconjugates on both endothelium and epithelium may impart a certain degree of selectivity in the recognition of proteins present in the plasma, interstitial fluid, and alveolar space. They may also play a role in growth, adhesion, and cell-to-cell interaction.

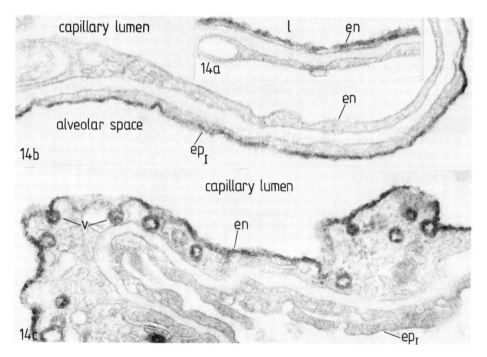

Figure 14.a-c: *Binding of peroxidase-conjugated wheat germ agglutinin to epithelial type I cells (ep$_I$) and endothelial cells (en). Intravascularly perfused conjugate decorates the luminal surface of capillary endothelium as a discrete, rather continuous reaction product in its avesicular zone (a) as well as in the vesicular zone where the labeling also appears on plasmalemmal vesicles (v) (c). When the conjugate was injected intratracheally, it marked almost homogeneously the luminal aspect of the alveolar type I epithelial cells (b) and type II epithelial cell (not shown). Original magnifications:* **a, b**, ×90,000; **c**, ×69,000.

Concluding Remarks

Through evolution, the lung has been adapted so that in the adult mammals, at the level of the alveolar-capillary unit, few metabolically sophisticated cells form a simple but highly efficient structure. This can be compared to Brancusi's sculptures, which are simply perfect because they are reduced to the essence. The design of the alveolar-capillary unit has been reduced to its essence: large alveolar spaces in which air can diffuse freely, and extensive vascular spaces in which the whole blood is slowly pumped. Both spaces are lined by continuous layers of cells that, together with the alveolar macrophages, which insure the lung sterility, establish the proper microenvironment for efficient multiple activites as known at present: exchange of gases, adjustment of the blood composition, monitoring of some plasma constituents, and addition of important hormones to the blood.

Acknowledgments

The excellent technical assistance of Stefania Tancov, M. Misici, V. G. Ionescu, and M. Mazilu is gratefully acknowledged. I also thank A. Radu for scanning electron microscopy. This chapter is based in part on work supported by the Ministry of Education, Romania, the National Institutes of Health grant HL-26343, and by funds made available through the 1978 International Artur and Louise Lucian Award given to Nicolae Simionescu and Maya Simionescu.

REFERENCES

1. Bignon, J., Chahinian, P., Feldmann, G., et al.: Ultrastructural immunoperoxidase demonstration of autologous albumin in the alveolar capillary membrane and in the alveolar lining material in normal rats. *J. Cell Biol.* 64:503–509, 1975.
2. Bluseé Van Oud Alblas, A. and Van Furth, R.: The origin, kinetics and characteristics of pulmonary macrophages in the normal steady state. *J. Exp. Med.* 149:1504–1518, 1979.
3. Bowden, D.H. and Adamson, I.Y.R.: Endothelial regeneration as a marker of the differential vascular responses in oxygen-induced pulmonary edema. *Lab. Invest.* 30:350–357, 1974.
4. Clements, J.A. and King, R.J.: Composition of the surface active material. In *The Biochemical Basis of Pulmonary Function.* Crystal, R.G., ed. New York, Marcel Dekker, 1976, vol. 2, p. 363–388.
5. Coonrod, J.D. and Yoneda, K.: Detection and partial characterization of antibacterial factor(s) in alveolar lining material of rats. *J. Clin. Invest.* 71:129–141, 1983.
6. Crystal, R.G.: The cell population of the normal lung. In *Lung Cells in Disease.* Bouhuys, A., ed. Amsterdam, North-Holland Biomedical Press, 1976, p. 17–38.
7. Dixon, M.T. and Jersild, R.A., Jr.: Influence of maternal diabetes on lectin binding to the surface of alveolar epithelial cells. Proceedings, 22nd Annual Meeting, *Am. Soc. Cell Biol.* 198:110a.
8. Farquhar, M.G.: Multiple pathways of exocytosis, endocytosis and membrane recycling: Validation of a Golgi route. *Fed. Proc.* 42:2407–2413, 1983.
9. Ferrreira, S.H. and Vane, J.R.: Half-lives of peptides and amines in the circulation. *Nature* 215:1237, 1976.
10. Fishman, A.P. and Pietra, G.G.: Hemodynamic pulmonary edema. In *Pulmonary Edema, Clinical Physiology Series.* Fishman, A.P. and Renkin, E.M., eds. Bethesda, MD, American Physiological Society, 1979, p. 79–96.
11. Gal, S., Basset, D.J.P., Hamosh, M, and Hamosh, P.: Triacylglycerol hydrolysis in the isolated perfused rat lung. *Biochim. Biophys. Acta* 713:222–229, 1982.

12. Gehr, P., Bachofen, M., and Weibel, E.R.: The normal human lung: Ultrastructure and morphometric estimation of diffusion capacity. *Respir. Physiol.* 32:121, 1978.
13. Gil, J. and McNiff, J.M.: Early cell alterations induced by histamine and epinephrine in rabbit lung. *Am. J. Physiol. (Cell Physiol.* 15) 246:C69–C76, 1984.
14. Gil, J. and Martinez-Hernandez, A.: The connective tissue of the rat lung. *J. Histochem. Cytochem.* 32:230–238, 1984.
15. Gil, J. and Reiss, O.K.: Isolation and characterization of lamellar bodies and tubular myelin from rat lung homogenates. *J. Cell Biol.* 58:152–171, 1973.
16. Gil, J. and Silage, D.A.: Morphometry of pinocytotic vesicles in the capillary endothelium of rabbit lungs using automated equipment. *Circ. Res.* 47:384–391, 1980.
17. Gillis, C.N. and Catravas, J.D.: Altered removal of vasoactive substances in the injured lung. In *Mechanisms of Lung Microvascular Injury.* Malik, A. B., and Staub, N. C., eds. New York, Annals of the New York Academy of Sciences, 1982, p. 458–474.
18. Hallman, M., Epstein, B.L., and Gluck, L.: Analysis of labeling and clearance of lung surfactant phospholipids in rabbit. *J. Clin. Invest.* 68:742–751, 1981.
19. Hass, M.A. and Longmore, W.J.: Regulation of lung surfactant cholesterol metabolism by serum lipoprotein. *Lipids* 15:401–406, 1980.
20. Junod, A.F.: The metabolic function of the pulmonary endothelium: Its clinical relevance. In *The Cells of the Alveolar Unit.* Favez, G., Junod, A., and Leuenberger, P., eds. Bern, Hans Huber Publishers, 1983, p. 116–123.
21. Kalina, M. and Pease, D.C.: The preservation of ultrastructure in saturated phosphatidyl cholines by tannic acid in model systems and type II pneumocytes. *J. Cell Biol.* 74:726–741, 1977.
22. Kapanci, Y., Assimacopoulos, A., Irle, C., et al.: Contractile interstitial cells in pulmonary alveolar septa: A possible regulator of ventilation/perfusion ratio? *J. Cell Biol.* 60:375–392, 1974.
23. Low, F.N.: Electron microscopy of the rat lung. *Anat. Rec.* 113:438, 1952.
24. Madri, J.A. and Furthmayr, H.: Collagen polymorphism in the lung. *Human Pathol.* 11(4):353–366, 1980.
25. Mason, R.J., Williams, M.C., Widdicombe, J.H., et al.: Transepithelial transport by pulmonary alveolar type II cells in primary culture. *J. Cell Biol.* 91:415a, 1981.
26. Nichols, B.A.: Normal rabbit alveolar macrophages. I. The phagocytosis of tubular myelin. *J. Exp. Med.* 144:906–919, 1976.
27. Ng, K.K.F. and Vane, J. R.: The conversion of angiotensin I to angiotensin II. *Nature* 216:762–766, 1967.
28. Nistor, A. and Simionescu, M.: Uptake of low density lipoproteins by the hamster lung perfused in situ. *Proceedings, The International Congress on Cell Biology,* 1984, Tokyo, Japan (In press, Abstr.).
29. Roifman, C.M., Eytan, G.D., and Iancu, T.C.: Ferritin-phospholipid interaction: A model system for intralysosomal ferritin segregation in iron-overloaded hepatocytes. *J. Ultrastr. Res.* 79:307–313, 1982.
30. Ryan, J.W., Ryan, U.S., and Schultz, D.R.: Subcellular localization of pulmonary angiotensin-converting enzyme. *Biochem. J.* 146:497–499, 1975.
31. Ryan, J.W. and Smith, U.: Metabolism of adenosine-5'-monophosphate during circulation through the lungs. *Trans. Assoc. Am. Physicians* 84:297–306, 1971.
32. Schneeberger, E.E.: Barrier function of intercellular junctions in adult and fetal lungs. In *Pulmonary Edema* (Clinical Physiology series). Fishman, A.P. and Renkin, E.M., eds. Bethesda, MD, American Physiological Society, 1979, p. 21–37.
33. Schneeberger, E.E. and Karnovsky, M.J.: The ultrastructural basis of alveolar-capillary membrane permeability to peroxidase used as a tracer. *J. Cell Biol.* 37:781–793, 1968.
34. Simionescu, D. and Simionescu, M.: Differentiated distribution of the cell surface charge on the alveolar capillary unit. Characteristic paucity of anionic sites on the air-blood barrier. *Microvasc. Res.* 25:85–100, 1983.
35. Simionescu, M.: Ultrastructural organization of the alveolar capillary unit. In

Metabolic Activities of the Lung. Ciba Found. Symposium 78 (new series), Excerpta Medica, 1980, p. 11–36.

36. Simionescu, M.: Transendothelial movement of large molecules in the microvasculature. In *Pulmonary Edema, Clinical Physiology Series.* Fishman, A.P. and Renkin, E.M., eds. Bethesda, MD, American Physiological Society, 1979, p. 39–52.

37. Simionescu, M.: Structural and functional differentiation of microvascular endothelium. In *Blood Cells and Vessel Walls: Functional Interactions.* Ciba Found. Symposium 71, Excerpta Medica, 1980, p. 39–60.

38. Simionescu, M., Simionescu, N., and Palade, G.E.: Segmental differentiations of cell junctions in the vascular endothelium. The microvasculature. *J. Cell Biol.* 67: 863–885, 1975.

39. Simionescu, N., Simionescu, M., and Palade, G.E.: Differentiated microdomains on the luminal surface of the capillary endothelium. I. Preferential distribution of anionic sites. *J. Cell Biol.* 90:605–613, 1981.

40. Simionescu, N.: The microvascular endothelium: Segmental differentiations, transcytosis, selective distribution of anionic sites. In *Advances in Inflammation Research.* Weissmann, G., Samuelson, B., and Paoletti, R., eds. New York, Raven Press, 1979, p. 64–70.

41. Simionescu, N. and Simionescu, M.: Galloylglucoses of low molecular weight as mordant in electron microscopy. I. Procedure and evidence for mordanting effect. *J. Cell Biol.* 70:608–621, 1976.

42. Simionescu, N. and Simionescu, M.: Interactions of endogenous lipoproteins with capillary endothelium in spontaneously hyperlipoproteinemic rats. *Microvasc. Res.* 1985 (In press).

43. Smith, F.B. and Kikkawa, Y.: The type II epithelial cells of the lung. V. Synthesis of phosphatidyl glycerol in isolated type II cells and pulmonary alveolar macrophages. *Lab. Invest.* 40:172–177, 1979.

44. Taylor, C.R., Maloiy, G.M.O., and Weibel, E.R.: Design of the mammalian respiratory system. III. Scaling maximum aerobic capacity to body mass: Wild and domestic mammals. *Respir. Physiol.* 44:25–37, 1981.

45. Tsilibary, E.C. and Williams, M.C.: Actin and secretion of surfactant. *J. Histochem. Cytochem.* 31:1298–1304, 1983.

46. Vaccaro, C.A. and Brody, J.S.: Structural features of alveolar wall basement membrane in the adult rat lung. *J. Cell Biol.* 91:427–437, 1981.

47. Vane, J.R.: The release and fate of vasoactive hormones in the circulation. *Br. J. Pharmacol.* 35:209–242, 1969.

48. Vasile, E., Simionescu, M., and Simionescu, N.: Visualization of the binding, endocytosis and transcytosis of low density lipoproteins in the arterial endothelium, in situ. *J. Cell Biol.* 96:1677–1689, 1983.

49. Villiger, B., Kelley, D.G., Engleman, W., et al.: Human alveolar macrophage fibronectin synthesis, secretion and ultrastructural localization during gelatin-latex particles binding. *J. Cell Biol.* 90:711–720, 1981.

50. Weibel, E.R. and Bachofen, H.: Structural design of the alveolar septum and fluid exchange. In *Pulmonary Edema.* Fishman, A.P. and Renkin, E.M., eds. Bethesda, MD, American Physiological Society, 1979, p. 1–21.

51. Weibel, E.R., Gehr, P., Haies, D., et al.: The cell population of the normal lung. In *Lung Cells in Disease.* Bouhuys, A., ed. Amsterdam, Elsevier/North Holland Biomedical Press, 1976, p. 3–16.

52. Weibel, E.R., Kistler, G.S., and Toendury, G.: Stereologic electron microscope study of tubular myelin figures in alveolar fluids of rat lung. *Z. Zellforsch. Mikrosk. Anat.* 69: 418–427, 1966.

53. Williams, M.C.: A possible endocytic pathway for return of secreted surfactant to lamellar bodies. *J. Cell Biol.* 95(2):388, 1982 (Abstr.).

54. Young, S.L, Kremers, S.A., Apple, J.S., et al.: Rat lung surfactant kinetics: Biochemical and morphometric correlation. *J. Appl. Physiol.: Respir. Environ. Exercise Physiol.* 51:248–253, 1981.

CHAPTER 3

Pulmonary Endothelium and Processing of Plasma Solutes: Structure and Function

Una S. Ryan and
Jørgen Frøkjaer-Jensen

Introduction

Often, the lungs are considered exclusively in terms of gas exchange. However, the lungs have additional functions not necessarily related to gas exchange. One such activity is the ability to process selectively hormones, hormone precursors, and other excitatory substances as they pass through the lungs via the bloodstream so that some are inactivated or otherwise removed from the blood, a second group is allowed free passage, while yet a third group is activated, the active products of which pass into the systemic arterial circulation.[12,13,35,36,50,58]

Thus, as the lungs convert venous blood to arterial blood they also regulate the entry of hormonal substances into the systemic arterial circulation. Through this selective processing, products of specific reactions of the lungs can influence specific actions of tissues and organs at a distance.[30]

The processing of vasoactive substances by the lungs covers a broad range of types of chemical compounds, including polypeptides, biogenic amines, prostaglandins, and steroids. The range of substances processed might suggest little specificity. However, the lungs are capable of distinguishing within chemical groups of hormones. For example, norepinephrine is taken up by the lungs, but its methylated homolog, epinephrine, is not. Prostaglandins of the E and F series are quantitatively metabolized as they enter the pulmonary circulation, but prostacyclin and prostaglandins of the A series pass intact through the lungs. Similarly, angiotensin II is not metabolized during passage through the lungs, but its higher homolog and precursor, angiotensin I, is degraded to smaller polypeptides, including angiotensin II.[36] The apparent selectivity of the lungs in processing circulating hormones is all the more remarkable in that the lungs, once disrupted (e.g., by homogenization), can be shown to contain an abundance of enzymes capable of inactivating all of the hormones listed above. Thus, it is clear that within the intact lungs, the enzymes are partitioned so that some have access to hormones within the blood circulation while others do not.

From Said, S.I. (ed.): *The Pulmonary Circulation and Acute Lung Injury*. Mount Kisco, N.Y., Futura Publishing Co., Inc., 1985.

This partitioning of enzymes among different cells of the lungs and among different organelles of a given cell type is a major determinant of which hormones are metabolized and which are not, and of the ultimate disposition of the metabolic products, and therefore of the physiological outcome of the reactions.[35]

The first level of compartmentation in the lungs is the separation of the blood supply from the air supply. Quite clearly, circulating substances are unlikely to have access to enzymes beyond the first cellular layer lining the vessels—the endothelium.[42] Therefore, enzymes of cells of the airways, alveoli, or interstitial regions, even if they are able to act on plasma substrates in vitro, are not likely to do so under normal conditions and are likely to have other more physiologically important actions.

In this chapter we will describe functional and structural aspects of the interaction of solutes and colloids of plasma with pulmonary endothelial cells.

First let us consider the basic architecture and environment of the lungs. The structure and situation of the lungs within the circulatory system which make them well suited for gas exchange may well explain how the lungs are so efficient in processing some hormones. The lungs are situated between the right and left sides of the heart and receive the entire cardiac output. However, resistance to blood flow is low and the pressure required to move blood through the lungs is a small fraction of the pressure required in the systemic circulation.

Thus, the lungs are strategically situated within the circulation and have pressure and flow characteristics for the efficient oxygenation of blood in bulk. It is also apparent that the lungs are extremely well designed as a bulk filter and purifier, very much more so than are the spleen, liver, and kidneys, the organs most commonly considered as blood cleansers.

The Pulmonary Capillary Bed

The next level of compartmentation is within the pulmonary circulation and is governed by the flow characteristics and relative surface areas of the vessels. It has been estimated that the adult human lungs contain some 300,000,000 terminal airspaces (alveoli), each of which is supplied with upwards of 1,000 capillary segments. The air is separated from blood by a "membrane" having an average thickness of a micron (Fig. 1). The surface exposed to blood (the inside surface of the capillaries) is very likely larger than that exposed to air.

Based on estimates of a standing blood volume of approximately 110 ml in the pulmonary capillary bed versus approximately 300 ml in the capillaries in the rest of the body, it can be estimated that surface area of the pulmonary capillary bed amounts to approximately one-fourth of the total capillary surface area in the whole body (75 m^2 versus 200 m^2 assuming a capillary radius of 3 μ). In addition, since the blood flow through the pulmonary bed is more constant than in, for example, muscle microcirculation where perhaps as few as one-fourth of the capillaries are perfused at rest, even this calculation tends to underestimate the fraction of capillary surface area that is actually exposed to circulating substances in the lungs compared to the rest of the body. These figures emphasize the overwhelming significance of endothelial cells of the pulmonary microvasculation in providing a surface for interaction with blood-borne substrates.

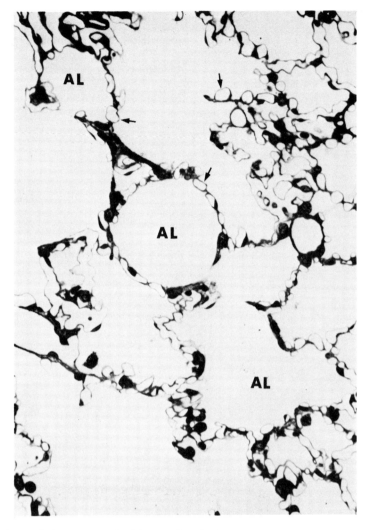

Figure 1: *Survey light micrograph of the capillary bed of a rat lung. The lung has been pumped free of blood with Krebs-Henseleit solution and fixed by vascular perfusion with glutaraldehyde. The air sacs or alveoli (AL) are surrounded by a network of capillaries. The alveolar-capillary wall (arrows) is extremely thin and its cellular components are not discernible. Original magnification, ×360.*

Taking, for example, the experimental data on the kinetics of disappearance of the polypeptide hormones, bradykinin and angiotensin I, it seemed inescapable that bradykinin was inactivated and angiotensin I was activated by enzymes on or very close to the innermost surface of the cells lining the blood vessels.[42] Considering the inverse relationship between the cross-sectional area and the velocity of flow,[20] we proposed that the degradations of bradykinin and angiotensin I would occur most efficiently in the capillary bed where slow flow allows time for interaction with the vast surface area of endothelium. Our hypothesis posed major problems, both conceptual and technical. The hypothesis implied some specificity of function of endothelial cells and prompted reconsideration of the structure and function of endothelial cells in the most basic terms.[62] Pulmonary endothelial cells, especially those of the alveolar capillary unit (Fig. 1) were not known to exist until lungs were examined by the electron microscope (Fig. 2), and it was tacitly assumed that these endothelial cells contain only that intracellular machinery needed to maintain the cells' vitality and integrity. Indeed, the most remarkable feature of the cell was its ability to assume an extensively flattened shape to facilitate the physical exchange of

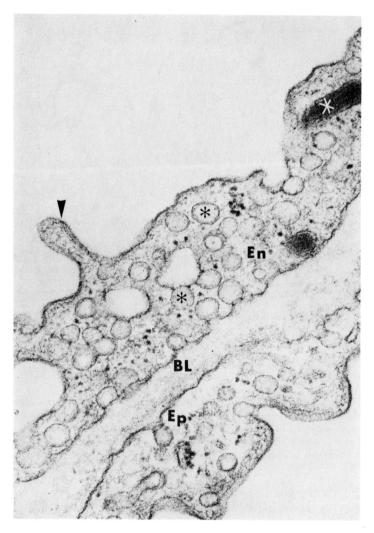

Figure 2: *Electron micrograph of a portion of the alveolar capillary unit showing that it is composed of three layers: endothelium (E), basement membranes (BL), and epithelium (EP). The endothelium is of the continuous type and contains large numbers of caveolae intracellulares (*), some of which are fused in pairs or groups. The profile of an endothelial projection is seen (arrowhead) at the left of the field. A Weibel-Palade body (white asterisk) is shown in the endothelial cell. Original magnification, ×95,000.*

gases. Even at the level of electron microscopy, endothelial cells are among the least impressive (in terms of structural complexity and morphological features) of all of the various cell types of the lungs. One might well ask where the cell could accommodate enzymes capable of degrading bradykinin and angiotensin I as they pass through the lungs. However, a large number of studies have now shown that these cells are capable of conducting an extensive range of metabolic activities, including specific protein synthesis.[12,13,35,36,50,58] Furthermore, when one examines these cells not by cross-section but by grazing section in areas near the nucleus, it is evident that not only is the machinery available for synthesis of cellular products but it is also well developed.[39]

The picture emerging is that of a highly complex cell important to the overall functioning of the lungs. Without question, its extremely flattened shape facilitates the exchange of gases; yet even in terms of gas exchange, it is likely that endothelial cells play more than a passive role. Indeed, it now appears that they contain carbonic anhydrase,[56] an enzyme that not only participates in maintaining the pH of arterial blood but also facilitates CO_2 excretion through the breakdown of bicarbonate.[5,11]

The major technical hurdle lies in gaining access to capillary endothelial cells in order to directly test their ability to metabolize bradykinin and angiotensin I. This problem was solved by two different approaches: immunocytochemical localization at the electron microscope level and endothelial cell culture.

Immunocytochemistry

When pure angiotensin converting enzyme (E.C. 3.4.15.1, also known as kininase II) became available,[10] we prepared antibodies to angiotensin converting enzyme and have bound to the antibodies an enzymatically active substance, microperoxidase.[25,57] Microperoxidase is capable of catalyzing the degradation of hydrogen peroxide. The degradation can effect a secondary oxidation of diaminobenzidine. The oxidized form of diaminobenzidine is insoluble and electron-dense. The specificity of the reaction of the antibody with its antigen and the electron density of the product provide the features required for the localization of angiotensin converting enzyme by electron microscopy (EM).

Lung tissue was incubated with the antibody-microperoxidase conjugate, and then the tissue was incubated with hydrogen peroxide and diaminobenzidine. The results are shown in Figure 3c. The luminal surface of the pulmonary endothelial cells was found to react with the antibody-microperoxidase reagent as expected.[52,57] The reaction product was most abundant on the cells of the capillaries and venules. Subsequently, the technique was used to localize other endothelial enzymes of interest such as carboxypeptidase N (Fig. 3d)[47,51] and carbonic anhydrase (Fig. 3e).[56]

The emerging picture is that of an enzyme anchored to the surface of the endothelial cells of the smallest blood vessels of the lungs. These cells are continuously washed with blood containing bradykinin and angiotensin I. Thus, the enzyme, in solid phase, is perfused with its substrates in a continuously flowing liquid phase. The enzyme occurs in greatest abundance at the level of the capillary bed, where one cubic centimeter of blood may occupy about 10 miles of capillary length. The effective layer of hormone-carrying plasma may be less than 1 micron. Blood, at the level of the capillaries, may not flow as a homoge-

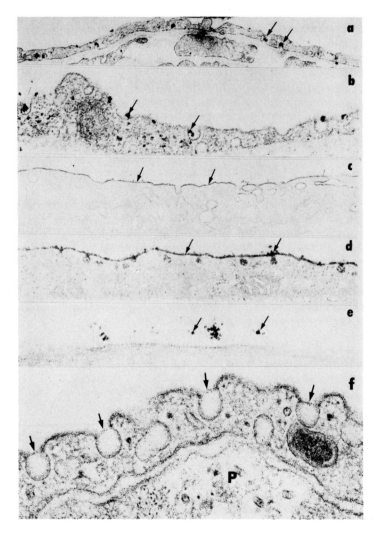

Figure 3: *Localization of endothelial enzymes by immunocytochemistry at the electron micro-scope level. **a** Shows cytochemical localization of ATPase in endothelial caveolae; **b** shows sites of 5'-nucleotidase in caveolae facing the vascular lumen; **c** shows immunocytochemical localization of angiotensin converting enzyme (ACE) on the luminal plasma membrane and associated caveolae; **d** shows immunocytochemical localization of carboxypeptidase N, and the distribution is similar to that of ACE (c); **e** shows localization of carbonic anhydrase where the antibodies were conjugated to ferritin. The enzyme is located on the plasma membrane but the ferritin marker is excluded by a layer approximately 100 Å thick. This layer may correspond to the glycocalyx (Fig. 13); **f** shows unreacted capillary endothelial cell. In this section, many caveolae are shown opening directly to the capillary lumen. The luminal stoma is usually spanned by a thin diaphragm composed of a single lamella (arrow). Part of a pericyte (P) is shown inside the basal lamina of the endothelial cell. Original magnifications: (a) ×36,000; (b) ×67,000; (c) ×36,000; (d) ×36,000; (e) ×178,000; (f) ×112,500.*

neous mixture, but may pass through the narrow vessels so that the plasma is divided into minute aliquots separated by red blood cells and perhaps mixed by endothelial projections.[64] Rapid hydrolysis of the hormones followed by rapid release of the metabolic products would tend to lessen the possibility of reaction product inhibition of the enzyme.

Since the endothelium of the pulmonary capillaries is of the continuous type, the cells being linked by junctions, processing by enzymes situated on the luminal surface not only provides ready access for hormones in the blood but also provides a means for the rapid return of hydrolysis products such as angiotensin II to the circulation. Again the exact cellular disposition of the enzyme determines the physiological outcome of the reactions.

Endothelial Cell Culture

If the enzymes that metabolize bradykinin and angiotensin I exist on the surface of endothelial cells, then the plasma membrane fraction of the lungs should account fully for the inactivation of bradykinin and the conversion of angiotensin I to angiotensin II. Such was found to be the case.[29] However, starting with a homogenate of whole lung tissue, one cannot know what proportion of the plasma membrane fraction is derived from endothelial cells and what proportion from other cell types of the lungs.

We then stripped a pure monolayer of endothelial cells (Hautchen preparation) from the main stem pulmonary artery.[63] These cells, like the plasma membrane fraction of lung homogenate, were capable of degrading bradykinin and of converting angiotensin I to angiotensin II.[28] However, the reactions were relatively slow, perhaps owing to the fact that the surface area of the cells collected in this way was but a small fraction of the surface area of the pulmonary capillary bed. One might also question whether endothelial cells of a large artery, such as the main stem pulmonary artery, are identical with capillary endothelial cells. Morphological differences can be detected by electron microscopy. Nevertheless these studies show that endothelial cells alone are capable of metabolizing bradykinin and angiotensin I to yield the same products as do intact lungs and emphasize the need to develop means for the isolation and culture of pure lines of pulmonary endothelial cells.

Early success at the culture of pulmonary endothelial cells[39,57] used modifications of methods developed for obtaining endothelial cells from umbilical veins.[19,22] We were able to isolate endothelial cells from pulmonary artery by rinsing the inside of the vessel with collagenase. Pure lines of endothelial cells were obtained by differential attachment and reattachment procedures using trypsin-EDTA mixtures.[39] Subsequent subculture of the lines was achieved with trypsin-EDTA.[39] These cultures of pulmonary artery endothelial cells proved to be extremely useful in helping to establish that ACE is a surface enzyme[39,52,57] and that the cells not only possess ACE but synthesize it as well.[39] In addition, once pure cultures became available, they could be used to investigate other properties of endothelial cells such as factor VIII antigen, carbonic anhydrase,[56] α_2-macroglobulin[39] and the production of prostaglandins,[5,6,34,43] and could be made available to other investigators (American Type Culture Collection, CCL 207 and CCL 209). However, it became apparent that traditional methods for harvesting and passaging endothelial cells using proteolytic enzymes tend to yield cultures that lack certain surface components.[44] Most particularly, surface enzymes such as angiotensin converting enzyme and carboxypeptidase N,[46] receptors, and junctional proteins are removed or damaged.[37,38,41,44] These findings indicate that one cannot with confidence use cells that lack the differentiated characteristics of the cell type in situ for studies of the role of endothelial cells in metabolic functions of the lung. However, they also serve to confirm that surface enzymes and other surface properties of endothelium are not only accessible to circulating substances but are also vulnerable to attack by proteases arriving via the blood stream.[54]

Endothelial cells can now be propagated for many years and over a hundred passages in vitro by methods that avoid exposure to proteolytic enzymes at both the isolation step and at each subculture.[37,38,41] The cells are isolated from large pulmonary vessels by scraping with a scalpel. The cells can be seeded onto microcarriers and grown in roller bottles (Fig. 4). This method not only allows vast scale-up of the cultures and great economy of supplies and personnel time, but also provides a method for nonenzymatic passaging. The cell-covered bead suspension can be divided into two or more aliquots in new bottles, fresh beads and fresh medium are added, the cells colonize the new beads, and nonenzymatic transfer and scale-up are achieved. If the cells are desired on flasks or cover slips, the cell-covered beads can be seeded onto the flat surface and the cells "walk" off the beads. Similarly, naked beads seeded on top of confluent monolayers are colonized within a matter of hours and can then be introduced to roller bottles as before. The propensity of endothelial cells for migrating on and off microcarrier beads can be exploited for harvesting cells from the microvasculature, the level of the circulation where processing is likely to be most efficient.[51,55]

Microcarrier beads $30-40$ μ in diameter are pumped into the lungs of a small animal or lobe of a lung of a larger animal that has been perfused blood-free. The beads cannot traverse the capillary bed and are closely packed at the level of the precapillary arterioles.[55] Here, presumably loosened by cold and EDTA and aided by the tight fit of the beads in the microvessels, the cells adhere to the beads and can be recovered by pumping in a retrograde direction. The microcarriers with attached cells are seeded into flasks onto which they migrate to form monolayers. Subsequently, they can be seeded back onto microcarriers to yield large-scale cultures of microvascular cells that have never been exposed to enzymes. The process can be adapted to obtain endothelial cells from the postcapillary venules by setting up the perfusion in the reverse direction.[51]

At the cellular level there are many opportunities for compartmentalization of functions. One point made clearly evident by studies using endothelial cells in culture is that they possess enzymes capable of metabolizing or otherwise transporting a variety of oligopeptide hormones, nucleotides, biogenic amines, and prostaglandins.[31] Some of these enzymes are intracellular (e.g., in lysosomes) and may have relatively little to do with the processing of hormones in vivo.

Some of the intracellular enzymes must respond to signals received by surface receptors. Such is the case for enzymes involved in the synthesis of prostaglandins, e.g., in the receptor-mediated bradykinin stimulated release of PGI_2.[6,7] Bradykinin also stimulates adenyl and guanyl cyclase of pulmonary endothelial cells.[40] However, it is only those enzymes and receptors disposed on the surface that are likely to be important in interactions with substances in perfusing blood.

For the final portion of this chapter, we will concentrate on endothelial surface specializations at the interface of the blood with the vessel wall that may

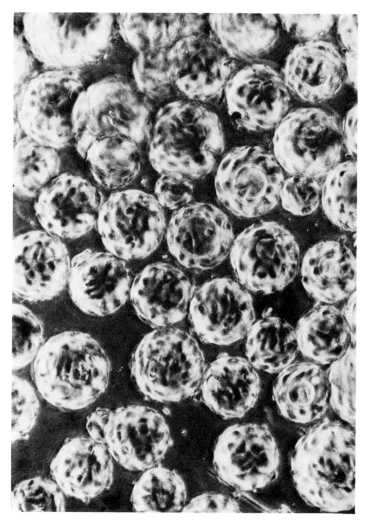

Figure 4: *Endothelial cells can be seeded onto microcarriers and grown in roller bottle cultures. The cells form a confluent monolayer on each bead. The microcarrier culture can be split into new bottles with addition of new beads and new growth medium and thus subcultured without treatment with trypsin/EDTA mixtures. In addition to yielding large scale cultures, microcarriers can be used to collect endothelial cells from the microvasculature of the lungs (see text). Original magnification, ×300.*

be important determinants of the physiological and pathophysiological outcomes of the interplay of blood-borne factors with endothelial cells.

Surface Specializations

Endothelial Projections

The pulmonary vessels are not cylinders having smooth interiors, but are, in fact, lined by endothelial cells covered with a profusion of finger-like projections that vastly expand surface area. The density and distribution of the projections is best appreciated by methods that allow examination of the luminal surface of vessels, such as scanning electron microscopy[64] or in surface replicas (Fig. 5). However, once their presence is accepted, projections can easily be seen in thin sections (e.g., Fig. 2). In addition to increasing surface area, the projections would have the effect of preventing blood cells from coming into direct contact with enzymes embedded in the plasma membranes of endothelial cells and would thereby provide a very thin layer of cell-free, hormone-laden plasma on the endothelial cells, an ideal situation for facilitating interactions

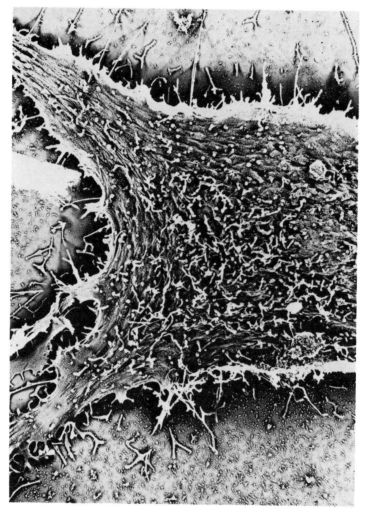

Figure 5: *Surface replica of the luminal surface of the pulmonary artery of a rabbit. The entire surface is covered with finger-like endothelial projections. The projections are 250−350 nm in diameter and 300−3000 nm in length. They increase surface area and may produce a flow of cell-free plasma over the endothelial surface, a condition likely to facilitate interactions with circulating substances. Original magnification, ×4,000.*

between solutes of plasma with endothelial surface structures (enzymes and receptors).[47-50] Because of their close spacing and their ability to reflect back on the cell surface, endothelial projections may aid in preventing unstirred layers. In addition, by acting in combination with the glycocalyx (see below), they may provide for a surface layer important in the discrimination of small molecules by endothelium.[24,48,49] It appears that endothelial projections are not permanent fixtures of the cell surface but appear to respond to cellular shape changes and changes in vessel tone, e.g., in cell division and in response to anaphylaxis.[46]

Caveolae

In addition to endothelial projections, the surface of endothelial cells is laden with small invaginations, caveolae, that open directly to the vascular lumen and thus extend surface area (Fig. 3f).[42,50,63] By virtue of the delicate diaphragm that covers the luminal stoma, the caveolae not only increase the surface area available for processing circulating substances but also provide a specialized microenvironment favoring interactions between blood-borne substrates and their cell-bound enzymes. Studies using immunocytochemical and cytochemical techniques at the electron microscope level have shown that caveolae are endowed with enzymes (Fig. 3). Some enzymes, such as ATPase and 5' nucleotidase, appear to reside specifically within caveolae.[26,61] Others, such as ACE and CPN, appear to be properties of plasma membrane including both caveolae and endothelial projections.[46,47,50,52,57] Carbonic anhydrase exhibits a patchy distribution on the endothelial surface,[56] while calmodulin, a specific binding protein, can be found in some, but not all, caveolae.[45] Caveolae, by numbers, position, structure, and enzymic properties, are well-suited to enhance the ability of endothelial cells, particularly those of the capillaries, to metabolize circulating hormones and other vasoactive substances. Clearly this role is most efficient if the entire endothelial vesicular system consists of invaginations of the plasmalemma,[2,17] a view that is substantiated by careful examination of and reconstruction from ultrathin serial sections.

In the past, however, the plasmalemmal "vesicles" in continuous capillary endothelium were thought to represent a specialized transcapillary transport device for macromolecules.[9,23,59,65] This hypothesis is based largely on the picture of the vesicular system derived from individual conventional EM thin sections (500–700 Å thick), with or without use of EM tracers. In such sections, the vesicular profiles appear in two forms, either as surface connected caveolae with apparently different degrees of opening to the surface, or as cytoplasmic entities with no apparent communication with the cell exterior. Connections between individual vesicular profiles are frequent (Fig. 2). Recently, the trancellular transport function of the vesicles has been seriously questioned since reconstructions of the three-dimensional organization of the vesicular system by ultrathin serial sectioning demonstrate that the picture of the plasmalemmal vesicular system as it appears in individual EM sections may be highly misleading.[3,14,15,16] In individual sections, 50–70% of the population of "vesicles" appear without connection to the surface, but reconstruction of the system from serial sections reveals that more than 99% of the vesicular units are, in fact, part of two sets of invaginations from the luminal and abluminal surfaces of the endothelial cells. It is the very act of sectioning the system that creates the many profiles of apparently free vesicles. Figure 6 shows a reconstruction of a segment from a frog muscle capillary based on 21 ultrathin (~140 Å) serial sections. Connections between the two sets of invaginations are very rare,[1,3,14–16] but might provide a diffusion pathway that could explain transcapillary exchange of macromolecules[4,15] and thus be the counterpart to the "large pore" system[21] in noninflamed capillaries. However, the abundance of vesicular invaginations, ending blind in the cytoplasm, suggests a more basic physiological role. Since a variety of cell types, e.g., mesothelial cells, pericytes, smooth muscle cells, and fibroblasts, possess vesicular invaginations a cell biological property common to several cells and not peculiar to endothelium must be considered.

The misleading picture of the vesicular system obtained by observation of conventional EM thin sections deserves some comments. In single sections of frog mesenteric and striated muscle capillaries, ~30% of the population of vesicular profiles open directly to the cell surface and ~70% appear "cytoplasmic." Ultrathin serial reconstruction of the very same capillaries, however, shows that ~70% of the population of vesicular units open directly to the surface. Only ~30% communicate indirectly via other vesicular units to the surface.[14,16] Hence, even in one plane, more than half of all vesicle intercommunications are lost in a conventional EM thin section. This is important since it illustrates that wherever fusions between individual smooth vesicles are common in the cytoplasm in single sections, it is probable that all vesicles communicate with the cell exterior. The neck of a surface-connected caveola or the point of fusion between multivesicular units must be located exactly in the center of a conventional section to appear as a communication on the screen. This is illustrated in Figure 7. Any degree of opening from fully closed to fully open is then simply a result of hitting the neck on or off center. This is clearly illustrated in the series of ultrathin sections in Figures 8 and 11.

Realizing the pitfalls inherent in individual sections is crucial in EM tracer studies where the localization of tracers in "luminal," "cytoplasmic," and "abluminal" vesicular profiles is used to investigate the role of the vesicular

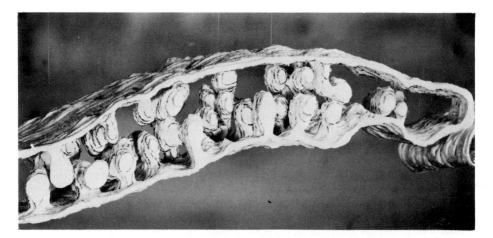

Figure 6: *Photograph of a model of a segment of a frog striated muscle capillary reconstructed from 21 ultrathin (~140 Å) serial sections. Lumen facing down.*

Projection

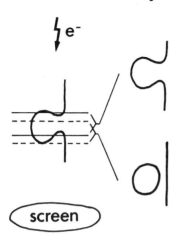

Figure 7: *Schematic representation of a single caveola sectioned with and without the midportion of the opening included in conventional EM thin sections (~500 Å thick). When the section contains the midportion, the projection (image) of an open vesicle is produced. When the section contains only part of the vesicle, apparently free profiles may be produced. (Reproduced with permission.[15])*

system in transcapillary exchange.[4,23] It is clear that such classification of vesicular profiles is spurious.

It is essential that the thickness of the individual sections in a series be dramatically reduced to yield a precise picture of the three-dimensional organization of the vesicular system. This is illustrated in Figures 9 and 10. Since vesicular units in the invaginations are often closely located and often span the entire cytoplasm (Fig. 6), it is essential to distinguish two closely located but noncommunicating vesicular units from two fused units. This is possible only when the thickness of the sections approaches a thickness comparable to two unit membranes (~150Å). Two nonconnecting vesicular units then end and start as electron-dense spots without membrane in the midsection, while the membrane remains distinct and the vesicle interior is electron-lucent in the midsection between connecting vesicles. Figure 11 shows an actual example of the two situations.

The plasmalemmal vesicular system is not a rigid permanent system, but one that may change during various conditions. In pulmonary capillaries of fetal lambs, the numerical density of vesicular profiles was reported to increase tenfold during gestation,[59] and the numerical density of "vesicles" was found to double in lung capillaries and in type I epithelial cells of isolated, perfused dog lungs after acute, severe edema formation.[9] Similarly, acute hypertension has been found to increase the number of vesicular profiles in mammalian brain capillaries.[65] It is most likely that these situations reflect an increase in plasmalemmal invaginations from the cell surfaces, which in individual conventional EM thin sections is observed as an increase in numerical density of vesicular profiles. Freeze-fracture analysis of endothelial cells in culture shows that the change in the vesicular system may occur within seconds.[18] In confluent monolayers of endothelial cells cultured from calf pulmonary artery, the vesicular openings (stomata) are frequently seen to occur in hexagonally packed patches or bands in certain areas (Fig. 12). Other areas may almost lack stomata. The same ordered pattern of vesicle openings can be seen in surface replicas of endothelial cells from guinea pig pulmonary artery fixed in situ (Fig. 13). When

Projection on screen

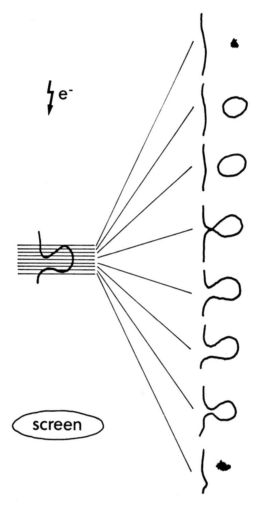

Figure 8: *Tracing of the membrane projections in seven consecutive untrathin (~140 Å) serial sections of a single surface-connected vesicle in frog muscle capillary endothelium. The vesicle first appears as a small electron-dense spot in a section that contains only the top of the vesicle. This spot changes into vesicle profiles that grow in size until a maximum is reached when the vesicle is cut in the midportion. Then, in the following sections, the vesicle profile decreases and finally disappears in the form of an electron-dense spot. The opening to the surface or to another vesicle with which it may be fused is typically seen on two or three of the midsections. (Reproduced with permission.[15])*

confluent monolayers are treated with trypsin and EDTA for 30 seconds, the cells separate from each other, and round up and detach from the growth surface. Cells fixed in this condition lose *all* of the unevenly distributed but highly ordered patterns in the stomata from the cell surface. In contrast, multi-

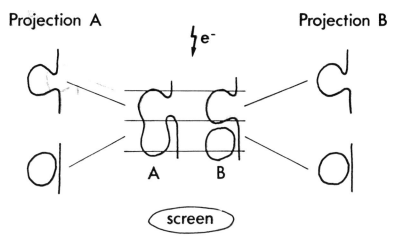

Figure 9: *Schematic representation illustrating the lack of resolution of vesicle interconnections by conventional (~500 Å thick) serial sectioning. The projections of two fused units (A) cannot be distinguished from two closely located but unconnected vesicular units (B). (Reproduced with permission.[15])*

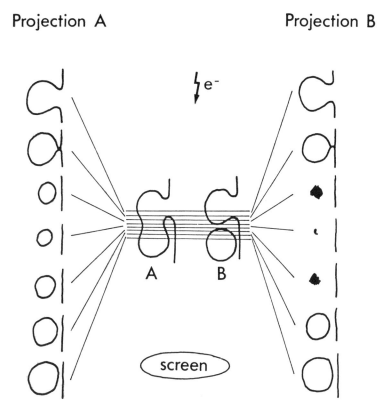

Figure 10: *Schematic representation illustrating the resolution of vesicle interconnections by ultrathin (~140 Å thick) serial sectioning. Two mutually fused units (A) can now be clearly distinguished from two closely located but nonconnecting vesicular units (B) by differences in the series of projections. (Reproduced with permission.[15])*

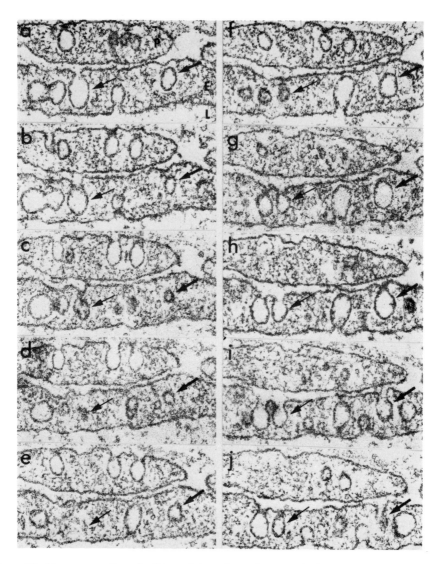

Figure 11: *Ten consecutive ultrathin serial sections of a part of a frog muscle capillary. Note how it is possible to distinguish between two closely located but nonconnecting vesicles (thin arrow) and two mutually fused vesicles (wide arrow) from the pattern of appearance and disappearance of the vesicular profiles in consecutive sections. P = pericyte; L = lumen; E = endothelium. Original magnification, ×67,000. (Reproduced with permission.[15])*

vesicle clusters become a prominent feature within the cytoplasm (Fig. 14). The few remaining openings become more randomly distributed on the surface. This indicates that the cellular rounding-up in response to trypsin/EDTA treatment is accompanied by infolding of the surface membrane areas, which contain the highly ordered patches and bands of stomata. It is still to be determined whether the multivesicle clusters all remain connected to the surface via the reduced number of surface openings or if they are truly internalized. In either case, the

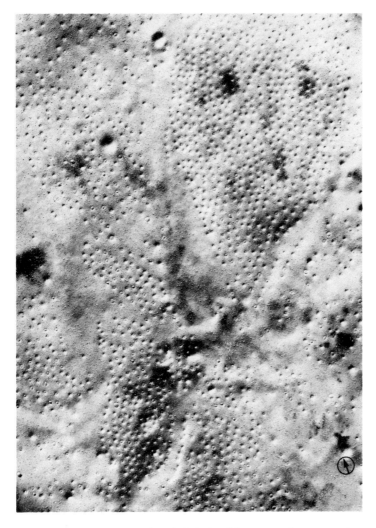

Figure 12: *Replica of a freeze-fractured endothelial cell from a confluent monolayer culture of a pulmonary artery endothelium. The P-face of the cell surface facing the flask is exposed. The openings of the caveolae are organized in patches of closely packed hexagonal arrays. The circled arrow indicates the direction of shadowing. Original magnification, ×26,500.*

observation shows that the organization of the plasmalemmal vesicular system can undergo rapid changes. The infolding/internalization of the membrane may simply serve to preserve plasma membrane during changes in cell shape or may be a mechanism to protect enzymes and receptors located in the plasma membrane during a cellular response to injury.

Glycocalyx

Focusing at a level smaller than that of projections and caveolae, we have recently found that the surface of normal endothelial cells in monolayer culture

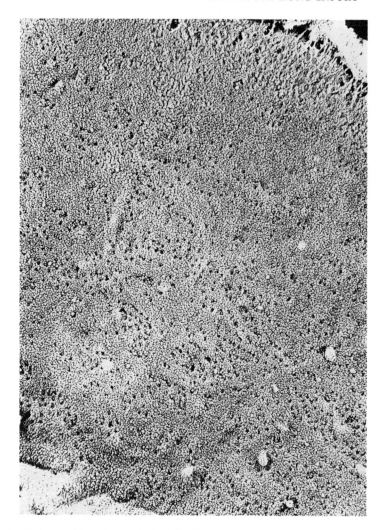

Figure 13: *Surface replica of an endothelial cell from guinea pig pulmonary artery, fixed in situ and rotary shadowed with platinum and carbon. As in cultured endothelial cells (Fig. 12), the openings of the caveolae are organized in bands and patches. The entire surface is covered with an orderly carpetwork or glycocalyx. Original magnification, ×28,000.*

contains not only enzymes, receptors, and transport proteins, but it is covered by a glycocalyx seen in surface replicas to consist of a regular carpetwork of extracellular materials synthesized by the cells themselves.[47–50] In vivo, this layer may also contain adsorbed plasma proteins and is the counterpart of the ruthenium red staining layer endothelial fuzz. Under normal conditions the glycocalyx may serve to provide a molecular sieve regulating access of circulating substrates to endothelial enzymes and may act as a size and charge barrier for small solutes and macromolecules.[48,60] In addition, it may correspond to the pericellular domain capable of discriminating between small macromole-

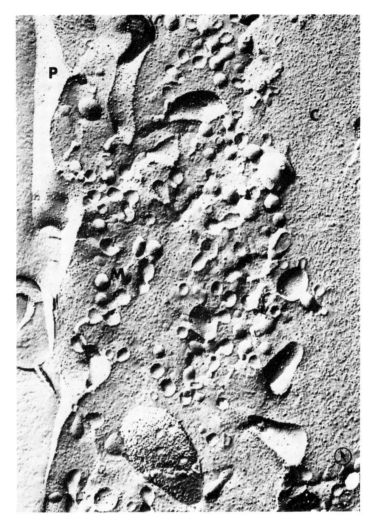

Figure 14: *Replica of a freeze-fractured endothelial cell, rounded up by treatment of a confluent monolayer culture with trypsin and EDTA. Multivesicle clusters (M) become numerous in the cytoplasm. P = P face of the surface membrane; C = cytoplasm; M = multivesicle cluster. The circled arrow indicates the direction of shadowing. Original magnification, ×67,000.*

cules such as sugars in Novikof hepatoma cells.[24] However, surface replicas of the glycocalyx indicate that it becomes disarrayed when endothelial cells are exposed to antibodies to endothelial surface enzymes in the presence of complement.[46,50,51] The same conditions that cause injury to the endothelial glycocalyx (viral infection, neutrophil proteases, and exposure to endothelial antibodies in the presence of complement) also cause unmasking of latent receptors (Fc and C3b) on the endothelial surface.[54] These receptors are not expressed in the absence of injury.[53] These data suggest that the glycocalyx also serves to mask latent receptors on the endothelial surface. Clq, the immunoglobulin-binding subunit of the first component of complement, binds to normal uninjured endothelial cells, so that after binding of Clq, the endothelial cells become reactive with IgG-coated red cells, suggesting that binding is via the collagenous portion of the molecule.[47] The collagenous tail of Clq is highly reactive with fibronectin, a component of the endothelial glycocalyx. Binding of Clq to the endothelial glycocalyx provides a means by which Clq-bearing soluble immune complexes can bind to the surface of endothelium and a means by which the Fc segment of many classes of immune globulins and their complexes may bind to endothelium. Each of the above provide conditions sufficient to stimulate attack of the complement system on microvessels and to attract activated neutrophils directly to the surface of endothelium. These may be the first events that lead to extensive microvascular occlusion and damage in inflammatory reactions such as aggregate anaphylaxis.[46]

Thus the glycocalyx may play a role in facilitating or limiting access of substrates to surface enzymes, in discriminating between substances allowed to traverse endothelium, and may also play a role in reactions of endothelium in the inflammatory response.

Future Directions

The capacity to inactivate bradykinin and to activate angiotensin I through a single enzyme system is not limited to the vascular bed of the lungs. However, no other vascular bed of the mammalian body processes as much blood and no other vascular bed empties into the systemic arterial circulation. The inactivation of a substance that tends to lower blood pressure coupled with the activation of a substance that tends to raise blood pressure suggests a role of the lungs in maintaining blood pressure.[32] Considering the ability of angiotensin II to stimulate the release of aldosterone, a sodium-retaining steroid of the adrenal cortex, the possibility arises of a pulmonary influence on salt and water balance.[33]

Although the "endocrine" functions of the lungs are not due to specific internal secretions of the lungs, the effects are much the same: a specific biologically active product, angiotensin II, is released into the general circulation where it can contribute to the overall functioning of the body.

It should be emphasized, however, that the lungs do have biologically active secretions that enter the general circulation. One of the clearest examples is that of the prostaglandins and their precursors. Synthesis and release of PGI_2 from the pulmonary endothelial cells can be triggered by the circulating hormone, bradykinin. Suffice it to say that in both instances it is the strategic positioning of the relevant enzymes and receptors on the luminal surface of an intact layer of endothelial cells that underlies the functions of pulmonary endothelium in controlling the quality (hormonal content and antithrombogenicity) of arterial blood.

It will be important for future studies to examine to what extent modulation of endothelial surface structures—projections, caveolae, glycocalyx, enzymes, receptors, and transport molecules—affect the overall functioning of endothelium as a tissue and the overall functioning of the lungs in maintaining the quality of the internal milieu.

Acknowledgments

It is a pleasure to acknowledge grants from the NIH (HL 21568), the Council for Tobacco Research, Inc., USA. J. Frøkjaer-Jensen holds an established Niels Bohr investigatorship sponsored by Egmont H. Petersens Foundation, under the Danish Academy of Sciences and Letters.

REFERENCES

1. Bundgaard, M. and Frøkjaer-Jensen, J.: Functional aspects of the ultrastructure of terminal blood vessels: A quantitative study on consecutive segments of the frog mesenteric microvasculature. *Microvasc. Res.* 23:1–30, 1982.
2. Bundgaard, M., Frøkjaer-Jensen, J., and Crone, C.: Endothelial plasmalemmal vesicles as elements in a system of branching invaginations from the cell surface. *Proc. Natl. Acad. Sci.* 76:6439–6442, 1979.
3. Bundgaard, M., Hagman, P., and Crone, C.: The three-dimensional organization of plasmalemmal vesicular profiles in the endothelium of rat heart capillaries. *Microvasc. Res.* 25:358–368, 1983.
4. Clough, G.: The dependence of vesicular transport on various physiological parameters. *Prog. Appl. Microcirc.* 1:35–50, 1983.
5. Crandall, E.D. and O'Brasky, J.: Direct evidence for participation of rat lung carbonic anhydrase in CO_2 reactions. *J. Clin. Invest.* 9:618–622, 1978.
6. Crutchley, D.J., Ryan, J.W., Ryan, U.S., et al.: Bradykinin-induced release of prostacyclin and thromboxanes from bovine pulmonary artery endothelial cells. Studies with lower homologs and calcuim antagonists. *Biochim. Biophys. Acta* 751:99–107, 1983.
7. Crutchley, D.J., Ryan, J.W., Ryan, U.S., et al.: Effects of bradykinin and its homologs on the metabolism of arachidonate by endothelial cells. *Adv. Exp. Med. Biol.* 156A:527–532, 1983.
8. Curry, F.E. and Michel, C.C.: A fiber matrix model of capillary permeability. *Microvasc. Res.* 20:96–99, 1980.
9. Defouw, D.O. and Chinard, F.P.: Variations in cellular attenuation and vesicle numerical densities in capillary endothelium and type I epithelium of isolated, perfused dog lungs after acute severe edema formation. *Microvasc. Res.* 26:15–26, 1983.
10. Dorer, F.E., Kahn, J.R., Lentz, K.E., et al.: Purification and properties of angiotensin-converting enzyme from hog lung. *Circ. Res.* 31:358–365, 1972.
11. Effros, R.M.: Pulmonary carbonic anhydrase and the release of carbon dioxide from the blood. *Trans. Assoc. Am. Physicians* 91:186–196, 1978.
12. Fishman, A.P. and Pietra, G.G.: Handling of bioactive materials by the lung (part 1). *N. Engl. J. Med.* 291:884–890, 1974.
13. Fishman, A.P. and Pietra, G.G.: Handling of bioactive materials by the lung (part 2). *N. Engl. J. Med.* 291:953–959, 1974.
14. Frøkjaer-Jensen, J.: Three-dimensional organization of plasmalemmal vesicles in endothelial cells. An analysis by serial sectioning of frog mesenteric capillaries. *J. Ultrastruc. Res.* 73:9–20, 1980.
15. Frøkjaer-Jensen, J.: The plasmalemmal vesicular system in capillary endothelium. Conventional electron microscopic (EM) thin sections compared with the picture arising from ultrathin (~140Å) serial-sectioning. *Prog. Appl. Microcirc.* 1:17–34, 1983.
16. Frøkjaer-Jensen, J.: The plasmalemmal vesicular system in striated muscle capillaries and in pericytes. *Tissue Cell.* 16:31–42, 1984.

17. Frøkjaer-Jensen, J. and Bundgaard, M.: Sessile vesicle "clusters" in frog mesenteric capillaries. A new concept of vesicular organization in the endothelial cell. *Microvasc. Res.* 18:297, 1979 (Abstr.).

18. Frøkjaer-Jensen, J. and Ryan, U.S.: Reorganization of the plasmalemmal vesicular system during shape changes of endothelial cells in culture. *Proceedings from the 2nd World Congress for Microcirculation.* Oxford, England, 1984.

19. Gimbrone, M.A., Cotran, R.S., and Folkman, J.: Human vascular endothelial cells in culture. *J. Cell Biol.* 60:673–684, 1974.

20. Green, H.D.: *Circulation: Physical Principles.* In *Medical Physics* series, Vol. 1, Glasser, O., ed. Chicago, Year Book Publishers, 1944, pp. 208–232.

21. Grotte, G.: Passage of dextran molecules across the blood lymph barrier. *Acta Chir. Scand.* (Suppl.) 221:1–84, 1956.

22. Jaffe, E.A., Nachman, R.L., Becker, C.G., et al.: Culture of human endothelial cells derived from umbilical veins. *J. Clin. Invest.* 52:2745–2756, 1973.

23. Palade, G.E., Simionescu, M., and Simionescu, N.: Structural aspects of the permeability of the microvascular endothelium. *Acta Physiol. Scand.* (Suppl.) 463:11–32, 1979.

24. Polefka, T.G., Garrick, R.A., Redwood, W.R., et al.: Solute excluded volumes near the Novikoff cell surface. *Am. J. Physiol.* 247: *Cell Physiol.* 16:C350–C356, 1984.

25. Ryan, J.W., Day, A.R., Ryan, U.S., et al.: Localization of angiotensin converting enzyme (kininase II). I. Preparation of antibody-heme-octapeptide conjugates. *Tissue Cell* 8:111–124, 1976.

26. Ryan, J.W. and Smith, U.: Metabolism of adenosine 5'-monophosphate during circulation through the lungs. *Trans. Assoc. Am. Physicians* 84:297–306, 1971.

27. Ryan, J.W. and Smith, U.: A rapid, simple method for isolating pinocytotic vesicles and plasma membrane of lung. *Biochim. et Biophys. Acta* 249:177–180, 1971.

28. Ryan, J.W. and Smith, U.: The metabolism of angiotensin I by endothelial cells. In *Protides of the Biological Fluids.* Peeters, H., ed. Oxford, England, Pergamon Press, 1973, pp. 379–384.

29. Ryan, J.W., Smith, U., and Niemeyer, R.S.: Angiotensin I: Metabolism by plasma membrane of lung. *Science* 176:64–66, 1972.

30. Ryan, J.W. and Ryan, U.S.: Is the lung a para-endocrine organ? *Am. J. Med.* 63:595–603, 1977.

31. Ryan, J.W. and Ryan, U.S.: Pulmonary endothelial cells. *Fed. Proc.* 36:2683–2691, 1977.

32. Ryan, J.W. and Ryan, U.S.: Humoral control of arterial blood pressure: A role for the lung? *Cardiovasc. Med.* 3:531–552, 1978.

33. Ryan, J.W. and Ryan, U.S.: Biochemical and morphological aspects of the actions and inactivation of kinins and angiotensins. In *Enzymatic Release of Vasoactive Peptides.* Gross, F., Vogel, H.G., eds. New York, Raven Press, 1980, pp. 259–274.

34. Ryan, J.W., Ryan, U.S., Habliston, D.H., et al.: Synthesis of prostaglandins by pulmonary endothelial cells. *Trans. Assoc. Am. Physicians* 91:343–350, 1978.

35. Ryan, U.S.: Structural bases for metabolic activity. *Ann. Rev. Physiol.* 44:223–239, 1982.

36. Ryan, U.S.: Processing of angiotensin and other peptides by the lungs. In *Handbook of Physiology.* Fishman, A.P., Fisher, A.B., eds. Bethesda, MD., American Physiological Society, 1984.

37. Ryan, U.S.: Isolation and culture of pulmonary endothelial cells. New York, *Environmental Health Perspectives*, 56:103–114, 1984.

38. Ryan, U.S.: Culture of pulmonary endothelial cells on microcarriers. In *Biology of the Endothelial Cell.* Jaffe, E.A., ed. The Netherlands, Martinus Nijhoff, 1984.

39. Ryan, U.S., Clements, E., Habliston, D., et al.: Isolation and culture of pulmonary endothelial cells. *Tissue Cell* 10:535–554, 1978.

40. Ryan, U.S., Lehotay, D.C., and Ryan, J.W.: Effects of bradykinin on pulmonary endothelial cells in culture. *Adv. Exp. Med. Biol.* 156B:767–774, 1983.

41. Ryan, U.S., Mortara, M., and Whitaker, C.: Methods for microcarrier culture and

bovine pulmonary artery endothelial cells, avoiding the use of enzymes. *Tissue Cell* 12:619–635, 1980.

42. Ryan, U.S. and Ryan, J.W.: Correlations between the fine structure of the alveolar-capillary unit and its metabolic activities. Chapter 7 in *Metabolic Functions of the Lung.* Bakhle, Y.S., Vane, J.R., eds. Vol. 4 of *Lung Biology in Health and Disease.* Lenfant, C., series ed. New York, Mercel Dekker, 1977, pp. 197–232.

43. Ryan, U.S. and Ryan, J.W.: Vasoactive substances and the lungs: Cellular mechanisms. In *The Microembolism Syndrome.* Salden, T., ed. Stockholm, Almqvist and Wiksell, Inc., 1979, pp. 213–221.

44. Ryan, U.S. and Ryan, J.W.: Vital and functional activities of endothelial cells. In *Pathobiology of the Endothelial Cell.* In *Pathobiology of the Endothelial Cell.* Nossel, H. L., Vogel, H. J., eds. New York, Academic Press, 1982, pp. 455–469.

45. Ryan, U.S. and Ryan, J.W.: Kinins, endothelial cells and calmodulin. *Adv. Exp. Med. Biol.* 156A:671–679, 1983.

46. Ryan, U.S. and Ryan, J.W.: Endothelial cells and inflammation. In *Clinics in Laboratory Medicine.* Ward, P.A., ed. Philadelphia, W. B. Saunders, 1983, pp. 577–599.

47. Ryan, U.S. and Ryan, J.W.: Surface properties of pulmonary endothelial cells. In *Surface Phenomena in Hemorrheology: Their Theoretical, Experimental and Clinical Aspects. Ann. N.Y. Acad. Sci.* 416:441–456, 1983.

48. Ryan, U.S. and Ryan, J.W.: The ultrastructural basis of endothelial cell surface functions. *Biorheology* 21:155–170, 1984.

49. Ryan, U.S. and Ryan, J.W.: The endothelial cell surface. *Biorheology* 21:39–56, 1984.

50. Ryan, U.S. and Ryan, J.W.: Cell biology of pulmonary endothelium. *Circulation* 70:III-46–III-62, 1984.

51. Ryan, U.S. and Ryan, J.W.: Inflammatory mediators, contraction and endothelial cells. In *Progress in Microcirculation Research,* II. Courtice, F.C., Garlick, D.G., and Perry, M.A., eds. Sydney, Australia, Committee in Postgraduate Medical Education, University of New South Wales, 1984.

52. Ryan, U.S., Ryan, J.W., Chiu, A.: Kinase II (angiotensin converting enzyme) and endothelial cells in culture. In *Kinins, Pharmacodynamics and Biological Roles.* Sicuteri, F., Bock, W., and Haberland, G.L., eds. New York, Plenum Press, 1976.

53. Ryan, U.S., Schultz, D.R., Del Vecchio, P., et al.: Endothelial cells of bovine pulmonary artery lack receptors for C3b and for the Fc portion of immunoglobulin G. *Science* 208:748–749, 1980.

54. Ryan, U.S., Schultz, D.R., and Ryan, J.W.: Fc and C3b receptors on pulmonary endothelial cells: Induction by injury. *Science* 214:557–558, 1981.

55. Ryan, U.S., White, L., Lopez, M., et al.: Use of microcarriers to isolate and culture pulmonary microvascular endothelium. *Tissue Cell* 14:597–606, 1982.

56. Ryan, U.S., Whitney, P.L., and Ryan, J.W.: Localization of carbonic anhydrase on pulmonary endothelial cells. *J. Appl. Physiol.* 53:914–919, 1982.

57. Ryan, U.S., Ryan, J.W., Whitaker, C., et al.: Localization of angiotensin converting enzyme (Kininase II). II. Immunocytochemistry and immunofluorescence. *Tissue Cell* 8:125–146, 1976.

58. Said, S.I.: The lung in relation to vasoactive hormones. *Fed. Proc.* 32:1972–1975, 1973.

59. Schneeberger, E.E.: Plasmalemmal vesicles in pulmonary capillary endothelium of developing fetal lamb lungs. *Microvasc. Res.* 25:40–55, 1983.

60. Simionescu, M., Simionescu, N., Silbert, J.E., et al.: Differentiated microdomains on the luminal surface of the capillary endothelium. II. Partial characterization of their anionic sites. *J. Cell Biol.* 90:614–621, 1981.

61. Smith, U. and Ryan, J.W.: Pinocytotic vesicles of the pulmonary endothelial cell. *Chest* 59:12S–15S, 1971.

62. Smith, U. and Ryan, J.W.: Electron microscopy of endothelial and epithelial compo-

nents of the lungs: Correlations of structure and function. *Fed. Proc.* 32:1957–1966, 1973.
63. Smith, U. and Ryan, J.W.: Electron microscopy of endothelial cells collected on cellulose acetate paper. *Tissue Cell* 5:333–336, 1973.
64. Smith, U., Ryan, J.W., Michie, D.D., et al.: Endothelial projections as revealed by scanning electron microscopy. *Science* 173:925–927, 1971.
65. Westergaard, E., van Deurs, B., and Brondsted, H.E.: Increased vesicular transfer of horseradish peroxidase across cerebral endothelium, evoked by acute hypertension. *Acta Neuropathol.* 35:141–152, 1977.

CHAPTER 4

Analysis of Autonomic Responses in the Pulmonary Vascular Bed

Albert L. Hyman, Howard L. Lippton,
Louis J. Ignarro, Keith S. Wood, Dennis B. McNamara,
and Philip J. Kadowitz

Introduction

The autonomic innervation of the pulmonary vascular bed has been studied extensively in recent years.[20,37,49,52,84] Studies in the cat and the dog from this laboratory using 6-hydroxydopamine to differentiate adrenergic and cholinergic terminals indicate that the pulmonary vascular bed is innervated by both the sympathetic and parasympathetic systems.[49,52] A periarterial plexus of nerves in the walls of pulmonary arteries extends into the lung to innervate small arteries possessing even a single layer of smooth muscle cells. Adrenergic nerves appear to surround all pulmonary arteries and extend into the tunica media of the large arteries, whereas cholinergic nerves are present in medium- and small-sized pulmonary arteries only.[52] However, the function of adrenergic and cholinergic nerve terminals in the pulmonary vascular bed is uncertain. Stimulation of the adrenergic nerves increases pulmonary vascular resistance and decreases pulmonary vascular compliance.[12,45,47,48] Since these responses are inhibited by alpha receptor and neuronal blocking agents, it appears the response to adrenergic nerve stimulation is the result of activation of alpha-adrenergic receptors by neuronally released norepinephrine.[46,48,49] The existence of postsynaptic alpha-1 and alpha-2 adrenergic receptor subtypes that, when stimulated, produce a pressor response in the systemic circulation has been reported recently.[17,57,80] However, the relative contribution of alpha receptor subtype(s) mediating the adrenergic vasoconstrictor response in the lung of the intact animal remains unclear.

Although adrenergic nerve stimulation increases pulmonary vascular resistance, isoproterenol has been shown to decrease pulmonary vascular resistance, suggesting that beta-adrenergic receptors are present in the pulmonary vascular bed.[38,67,76] Beta-adrenergically mediated vasodilation can be elicited by administration of isoproterenol or epinephrine as well as by norepinephrine when pulmonary vascular tone is elevated by hypoxia and acidemia; however, the actions of neuronally released norepinephrine on beta receptors in

From Said, S.I. (ed.): *The Pulmonary Circulation and Acute Lung Injury.* Mount Kisco, N.Y., Futura Publishing Co., Inc., 1985.

the pulmonary circulation are uncertain.[38,67,76] It has been reported that sympathetic nerve stimulation elicits vasodilation in the skeletal muscle, liver, spleen, adipose tissue, and in isolated facial vein of the rabbit.[27,28,65,66,85] The concepts that beta-adrenergic receptors in blood vessels are innervated and that neuronally released norepinephrine can elicit vasodilation by stimulating beta-2 receptors have been challenged recently.[36,71] Vasodepressor responses in the pulmonary circulation may be mediated by the parasympathetic system since decreases in pulmonary arterial pressure, although small and inconsistent, have been observed in response to vagosympathetic nerve stimulation in the dog.[10] In addition to the uncertainty of responses to vagal stimulation, there is disagreement on responses to acetylcholine in the pulmonary vascular bed. Both pressor and depressor responses to acetylcholine have been reported. Moreover, the relaxation of isolated arterial smooth muscle by muscarinic receptor agonists, including the cholinergic transmitter, is dependent on the presence of undamaged endothelium whereas contraction is the major response with damaged endothelium.[22] In addition to muscarinic receptor agonists, vascular smooth muscle relaxation elicited by bradykinin, divalent cation ionophore such as A23187, and a variety of vasodepressor substances appears to be dependent on an intact endothelial cell layer.[6,15,22,68] Furthermore, it has been proposed that acetylcholine-elicited relaxation of vascular smooth muscle is attributed to the release of an endothelium-derived lipooxygenase product of arachidonic acid metabolism that interacts with smooth muscle to increase cyclic GMP formation.[22,23] Moreover, these data are consistent with the hypothesis that activation of guanylate cyclase and subsequent accumulation of cyclic GMP are associated with relaxation of vascular smooth muscle by muscarinic agonists, including acetylcholine, as well as a variety of nitrogen oxide-containing vasodilators such as nitroglycerin and sodium nitroprusside.[43,44] It has also been suggested that the pulmonary vasodilator response to acetylcholine is secondary to its actions on the systemic vascular bed.[60] The variability in response to acetylcholine may depend on species, experimental preparation, dose of acetylcholine, and the initial level of tone in the pulmonary vascular bed.[13,38,60,70] Thus, there appears to be a paucity of data describing pulmonary vascular responses to sympathetic and parasympathetic nerve stimulation and an understanding as to the physiologic or pathophysiologic role since the presence of these autonomic neurons remains unclear. The mechanism by which both the cholinergic and adrenergic transmitters produce a vascular response is uncertain. In addition, the contribution of endothelium in pulmonary vascular responses is currently an enigmatic one, and the involvement of cyclic nucleotides as mediators in these vascular responses has recently been scrutinized.[43]

The present experiments were undertaken to investigate the actions of catecholamines and acetylcholine as well as vagal and sympathetic nerve stimulation on the pulmonary vascular bed of the intact-chest cat. The actions of acetylcholine on isolated bovine intrapulmonary arterial rings with and without endothelium were investigated in the present experiments and the association of these effects on isolated smooth muscle to changes in cyclic nucleotide levels was determined as well.

Methods

For studies on the actions of acetylcholine and vagal stimulation on the feline pulmonary vascular bed, adult cats of either sex weighing 2.3–3.7 kg were anesthetized with chloralose/urethane, 50–500 mg/kg IV, whereas sodium pentobarbital was used for studies on the actions of catecholamines and sympathetic nerve stimulation. The animal was strapped in the supine position to a Philip's fluoroscopic table. Supplemental doses of anesthetic were given as needed to maintain a uniform level of anesthesia. The trachea was intubated with a cuffed pediatric endotracheal tube, and the animals spontaneously breathed room air or room air enriched with 100% O_2. Systemic arterial pressure was measured from a catheter in the femoral artery, and systemic injections of drugs were made through a catheter in the femoral vein.

For perfusion of the left lower lobe, a specially designed 6F triple-lumen catheter was passed under fluoroscopic guidance from an external jugular vein into the arterial branch to that lobe. After the animals had been heparinized, 1,000 U/kg IV, and the lobar artery was isolated by distension of the balloon cuff on the catheter, the lobe was perfused by way of the catheter lumen immediately beyond the balloon cuff. The lobe was perfused with blood withdrawn from the femoral artery or vein, and no systematic difference in response to vagal stimulation and acetylcholine was observed when the lobe was perfused with femoral arterial or venous blood. In experiments in which airflow to the left lower lobe was interrupted, the lobe was perfused with arterial blood to lessen the effects of hypoxia. The lobe was perfused by means of a Harvard model 1210 peristaltic pump, and the perfusion rate was adjusted so that lobar arterial perfusion pressure approximated mean pressure in the main pulmonary artery and was thereafter not changed during an experiment. Flow rates to the lobe averaged 46 ± 0.7 ml/min. These procedures have been described recently.[40] Left arterial pressure was measured by means of a specially designed 5F or 6F double-lumen catheter placed transseptally into the lobar vein draining the left lower lobe. The catheter tip was positioned in the vein so that the pressure port at the distal lumen was approximately 1 cm into the lobar vein, and the second catheter port was at the venoatrial junction. When necessary, blood could be withdrawn or infused through this second catheter lumen to maintain left atrial pressure constant, and in various experiments left atrial pressure ranged between 2.5 and 4.5 mmHg. All vascular pressures were measured with Statham transducers zeroed at right atrial level, and mean pressures obtained by electronic averaging were recorded on an Electronics for Medicine recorder model DR-12.

In these experiments, responses to vagal stimulation and acetylcholine or catecholamines and sympathetic nerve stimulation were investigated when lobar vascular resistance was at resting level and when lobar resistance was elevated by infusions of the prostaglandin endoperoxide analog (15S)hydroxyl-11α,9α(epoxymethano)-prosta-5Z,13E dienoic acid or 15-methyl $PGF_{2\alpha}$ (Upjohn). The endoperoxide analog or 15-methyl $PGF_{2\alpha}$ was dissolved in 100% ethanol at a concentration of 5 mg/ml, and working solutions were prepared frequently. These substances were infused into the lobar artery with a variable-speed Harvard infusion pump model 945 at rates that increased lobar arterial pressure by approximately 200% and were 40–180 ng/min for the endoperoxide analog and 120–360 ng/min for 15-methyl $PGF_{2\alpha}$. The increase in lobar arterial pressure during infusion of the endoperoxide analog or 15-methyl $PGF_{2\alpha}$ was well maintained, and lobar arterial pressure returned to the control value 5–10 minutes after infusions were terminated.

In these experiments, a bipolar pacing catheter was positioned in the right ventricle under fluoroscopic guidance, and the bradycardia and/or sinus arrest that occurred during vagal stimulation was eliminated by means of a Medtronic model 5880A demand pacemaker.

The adrenergic blocking agents used in these studies were phenoxybenzamine (Dibenzyline, Smith, Kline and French) and propranolol (Ayerst, Sigma), phentolamine, Regitine; metoprolol, Lopressor (CIBA-Geigy); sotalol (Mead, Johnson) and practolol (Ayerst). Atropine and hexamethonium (Sigma) were used to block muscarinic and nicotinic (ganglionic) receptors, and cocaine (Mallinckrodt) was employed to block uptake of norepinephrine and tyramine. All blocking agents, with the exception of phenoxybenzamine, were dissolved in 0.9% NaCl solution and were injected slowly over a 2 to 5 minute period into the femoral vein. Phenoxybenzamine was dissolved in a vehicle of ethanol 10%, propylene glycol 40%, and 0.9% NaCl, 50% at a concentration of 10 mg/ml and was injected into the femoral vein over a 5 minute period. Under basal conditions, the alpha blocking agents produced only small $1-2$ mmHg decreases in lobar arterial pressure, whereas propranolol increased lobar arterial pressure by $1-4$ mmHg. Practolol, sotalol, and metoprolol had small, inconsistent effects on lobar arterial pressure.

In experiments where adrenergic neuronal blockade was employed, the animals were treated with 6-hydroxydopamine (Sigma), 100 mg/kg per day IP, for 3 days and were catheterized on days $4-6$. Reserpine (CIBA-Geigy) was given 1 mg/kg IM, and the animals were catheterized on day 2 or day 3.

Drugs used in the study were norepinephrine, 1-norepinephrine, quinacrine, methylene blue, epinephrine, 1-epinephrine, insoproterenol, 1-isoproterenol, acetylcholine, tyramine, and phenylephrine (all from Sigma), nitroglycerin (Parke Davis), UK14304 (Pfizer), and angiotensin II amide (CIBA-Geigy). These substances were dissolved in 0.9% NaCl or Krebs buffer and solutions were prepared on a frequent basis and, when appropriate, stored in a freezer. Prostaglandins (PG) E_1 and $F_{2\alpha}$ (Upjohn) were dissolved in 100% ethanol and stored in a freezer. On the day of use, working solutions were prepared in 0.9% NaCl. These agonists were either infused with a Harvard infusion pump model 945 or injected into the perfused lobar artery. For stimulation of the sympathetic nerves, the thorax was opened in the third interspace and a shielded Palmer electrode was placed around the left stellate ganglia. The nerve was stimulated with square wave pulses 2 msec in duration at stimulus frequencies of 3, 10, and 30 cycles/sec with a Grass model SD9 stimulator for 15 to 30 second periods. For vagal stimulation, the left cervical vagosympathetic nerve was approached through a midline incision on the ventral side in the midcervical region of the neck. The nerve was ligated, and a shielded Palmer electrode was placed around the distal portion of the ligated nerve. The nerve was stimulated with square wave 5 msec duration pulses at supramaximal voltage $(8-12$ V) for $60-90$ seconds with a Grass model SD9 stimulator.

Blood gases and pH were measured with an Instrumentation Laboratory model micro 13 blood gas analyzer. Arterial PO_2, PCO_2, and pH averaged 86 ± 3, 42 ± 2 mmHg, and 7.42 ± 0.02, respectively, in the control period, and were maintained in the physiological range. When necessary, acidosis was corrected by infusion of sodium bicarbonate solution. The preparation of bovine intrapulmonary rings has been described previously.[34] Briefly, bovine lungs were obtained from a nearby slaughterhouse and maintained in ice-cold, buffered (pH 7.4) salt solution during transportation and isolation of intrapulmonary arteries. The dorsal and ventral surfaces of each lobe were carefully dissected to expose the main intralobar artery. The second and third major arterial branches were exposed, isolated, and cleaned of loosely adhering connective tissue. These arteries possessed an undamaged endothelial layer, as assessed by the potent relaxant effect of acetylcholine on precontracted ring preparations. Endothelium was damaged in certain arteries by the following procedures. Glass rods were inserted into the intrapulmonary arterial branches and kept in place during the dissection and cleaning of the vessels. In addition, a hard cotton swab was inserted into the vessels and moved back and forth for about 1 minute. Rings prepared from these vessels contracted in response to acetylcholine. Intrapulmonary arteries ranged in diameter from 4 to 6 mm. Each artery was rapidly cut into 8 to 12 rings (3–4 mm wide), mounted by means of two L-shaped nichrome wires in drop-away chambers (Metro Scientific Inc., Farmingdale, NY) containing Krebs bicarbonate buffer (37°C) gassed with 95% O_2-5% CO_2.

Tension (6 g) was adjusted to the optimal length for isometric contractions. After 2 hours of equilibration, arterial rings were exposed to a depolarizing potassium solution. When contractile responses plateaued, rings were rinsed with Krebs buffer and allowed to return to baseline tension (30–45 min). Submaximal tone was then elicited by exposing rings to 10^{-5}M phenylephrine and rings were rinsed after peak contractions were attained. After equilibration (45 min), submaximal tone was again elicited with 10^{-5}M phenylephrine. Tone ranged from 3 to 5 g and was maintained for the period of time during which relaxants were subsequently tested. At peak contractions to phenylephrine, acetylcholine or other relaxants were added to the bathing medium. In other experiments, antagonists were added at various times before eliciting submaximal contractions with phenylephrine. Data are expressed as percentage of relaxation, which signifies the percentage of decrease in phenylephrine-induced submaximal tone.

All cyclic nucleotide determinations were made on arterial rings that had been equilibrated under 6 g of tension, depolarized with potassium, and submaximally contracted by phenylephrine before initiating any given protocol with contractile or relaxant agents. Frozen rings were homogenized, extracted, and assayed for cyclic GMP and cyclic AMP as described previously.[32]

All hemodynamic data represent peak changes and are expressed in absolute values. Perfusion pressures in the various experimental groups are illustrated in Tables I–VI. Data from studies using isolated intrapulmonary arterial rings are expressed as percentage of relaxation, which signifies the percentage of decrease in phenylephrine-induced submaximal tone. Data are expressed as mean ± SE and were analyzed by the methods of Snedecor and Cochran[77] for paired and group comparison. A p value of less than 0.05 was used as the criterion for statistical significance.

Results

Effects of Norepinephrine

Pulmonary vascular responses to norepinephrine were investigated in the intact-chest cat under conditions of controlled blood flow. In these experiments, the effects of norepinephrine infusions and adrenergic receptor blocking agents were studied under basal conditions and when pulmonary vascular tone had been elevated by infusion of a prostaglandin endoperoxide analog or 15-methyl $PGF_{2\alpha}$. Under resting conditions, intralobar infusions of norepinephrine at rates of 0.5, 1, 2, and 10 μg/kg per minute increased lobar arterial pressure in a dose-dependent fashion while lobar venous outflow pressure was maintained constant (Fig. 1). In 11 of the animals, the effects of propranolol, a beta receptor blocking agent, on the pressor response to norepinephrine in the pulmonary vascular bed were investigated; these data are also presented in Figure 1. After administration of propranolol, 2mg/kg IV, the increases in lobar arterial pressure in response to norepinephrine infusions at 0.5–10 μg/kg per minute were greatly enhanced (p < 0.01 at each infusion rate when compared to corresponding control). The dose-response curve for norepinephrine was shifted to the left and the threshold dose was decreased after administration of the beta receptor blocking agent (Fig. 1). In eight of the animals, the effects of phenoxybenzamine, an alpha receptor blocking agent, were studied, and in these experiments, the increases in lobar arterial pressure in response to norepinephrine

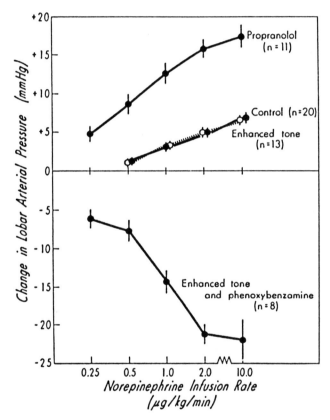

Figure 1: *Dose-response relationships comparing the effects of intrapulmonary infusions of norepinephrine on lobar arterial pressure under control conditions, when pulmonary vascular tone was enhanced, after administration of propranolol, 2 mg/kg IV and when pulmonary vascular tone was enhanced after administration of phenoxybenzamine, 5 mg/kg. n indicates number of cats in each experimental series. Increases in lobar arterial pressure in response to norepinephrine infusions, 1–10 μg/kg per minute, are significant in both control and enhanced tone animals. The increases in lobar arterial pressure in response to norepinephrine in cats receiving propranolol as well as the decreases in lobar arterial pressure in those with enhanced tone and phenoxybenzamine are significantly different from the increases in lobar arterial pressure under control conditions.*

infusions at 0.5 and 10 μg/kg per minute were blocked completely after administration of phenoxybenzamine, 5 mg/kg IV.

The effects of norepinephrine infusions on the pulmonary vascular bed were also investigated in this group of cats when pulmonary vascular tone was elevated by infusion of the endoperoxide analog. In 13 animals, lobar arterial pressure was increased from 13 ± 1 to 39 ± 2 mmHg by infusion of the endoperoxide analog; however, increases in lobar arterial pressure in response to norepinephrine infusions, 0.5–10 μg/kg per minute, were not significantly different when pulmonary vascular tone was at resting levels or when tone had been enhanced by infusion of the endoperoxide analog (Fig. 1). However, when lobar arterial pressure was increased from 13 ± 1 to 42 ± 2 mmHg in eight cats treated with phenoxybenzamine, 5 mg/kg IV, the pressor response to norepinephrine was reversed and infusions of norepinephrine at 0.25–10 μg/kg IV caused significant dose-dependent decreases in lobar arterial pressure (Fig. 1). The reductions in lobar arterial pressure in response to norepinephrine in animals treated with phenoxybenzamine were similar when lobar vascular resistance was enhanced by the endoperoxide analog or by 15-methyl $PGF_{2\alpha}$. In four of the eight animals in which phenoxybenzamine was administered and lobar vascular tone was enhanced, the effect of propranolol on the depressor responses to norepinephrine was investigated. In these four animals treated with phenoxybenzamine, 5 mg/kg IV, and propranolol, 2 mg/kg IV, lobar arterial pressure was increased by the endoperoxide analog, but infusion of norepinephrine, 10 μg/kg per minute, had little if any effect in that lobar arterial pressure decreased from 40 ± 2 to 39 ± 3 mmHg (p < 0.05).

Influence of Propranolol

The enhanced response to norepinephrine after administration of propranolol could result from blockade of beta-adrenergic receptors or other actions of the drug. To examine these possibilities, the effects of propranolol on responses to phenylephrine and tyramine were investigated. Intralobar infusions of phenylephrine, an agent that acts on alpha receptors, at 1 to 3 μg/kg per minute, increased lobar arterial pressure in a dose-dependent manner (Fig. 2). The increases in lobar arterial pressure in response to phenylephrine were not changed after administration of propranolol, 2 mg/kg IV, but were blocked after injection of phenoxybenzamine, 5 mg/kg IV (Fig. 2). In another group of animals, the effects of propranolol on responses to tyramine, an indirectly acting agent, were investigated, and these data are presented in Table I. Intralobar injections of tyramine caused dose-related increases in lobar arterial pressure. The increases in lobar arterial pressure in response to tyramine were enhanced after administration of propranolol, 2 mg/kg IV, but were blocked after administration of cocaine, 5 mg/kg IV (Table I). This dose of cocaine also enhanced the pressor response of intrapulmonary injections of norepinephrine.

Effects of Epinephrine

The effects of epinephrine on the pulmonary vascular bed were also investigated in another group of cats using a similar experimental protocol. Under resting conditions, intralobar infusion of epinephrine at 1 μg/kg per minute had

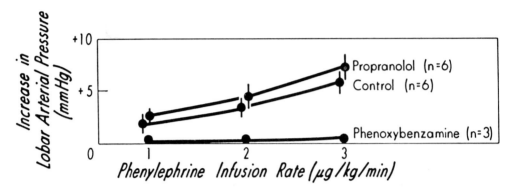

Figure 2: *Dose-response relationships illustrating the effects of intrapulmonary infusions of phenylephrine on lobar arterial pressure under control conditions, after administration of propranolol, 2 mg/kg IV, or after administration of phenoxybenzamine, 5 mg/kg IV. n indicates number of cats in each series. Propranolol had no significant effect on responses to phenylephrine, whereas responses to this alpha receptor agonist were decreased significantly by phenoxybenzamine.*

Table I
Influence of Propranolol and Cocaine on Responses to
Tyramine in the Lobar Vascular Bed

| | Lobar arterial pressure (mmHg) | | |
	Control	Propranolol	Propranolol and cocaine
Control	13 ± 1	18 ± 1	
Tyramine, 50 μg	16 ± 1*	24 ± 1*	
Control	13 ± 1	18 ± 1	20 ± 1
Tyramine, 100 μg	17 ± 1*	25 ± 1*	20 ± 1
Control	13 ± 1	18 ± 2	19 ± 1
Tyramine, 200 μg	17 ± 1*	25 ± 1*	19 ± 0

Results expressed as mean ± SE.
*$P < 0.05$ when compared to corresponding control.

no significant effect on lobar arterial pressure; however, when the infusion rate was increased to 2 μg/kg per minute, there was a small (3.5 ± 0.8 mmHg) but statistically significant ($p < 0.05$) reduction in lobar arterial pressure (Fig. 3). After administration of propranolol, 2 mg/kg IV, in four animals, intralobar infusions of epinephrine at 1–10 μg/kg per minute caused significant dose-related increases in lobar arterial pressure (Fig. 3). When lobar arterial pressure was increased from 14 ± 1 to 45 ± 3 mmHg by infusion of the endoperoxide analog, intralobar infusions of epinephrine at rates of 0.125–2.0 μg/kg per minute caused significant dose-dependent decreases in lobar arterial pressure (Fig. 3). When lobar vascular tone was enhanced in the presence of phenoxybenzamine, intralobar infusions of epinephrine at rates of 0.03–0.125 μg/kg per minute produced marked dose-dependent decreases in lobar arterial pressure that were not different from responses to isoproterenol when tone was enhanced (Fig. 3).

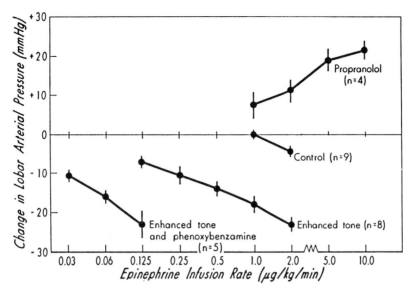

Figure 3: *Dose-response curves comparing the effects of intrapulmonary infusions of epinephrine on lobar arterial pressure under control conditions, after administration of propranolol, 2 mg/kg IV, and when tone was enhanced in animals treated with phenoxybenzamine. Under control conditions, epinephrine infusion at 2 μg/kg per minute caused a small but significant reduction in lobar arterial pressure. After propranolol administration, epinephrine infusions at rates of 1–10 μg/kg per minute caused significant increases in lobar arterial pressure. Decreases in lobar arterial pressure in the enhanced tone and enhanced tone and phenoxybenzamine series were significant. n indicates number of animals.*

Effects of Isoproterenol

In a fourth series of experiments, intralobar infusions of isoproterenol, a beta agonist, at 62 and 125 ng/kg per minute caused small but statistically significant reductions in lobar arterial pressure when lobar vascular resistance was at basal levels (Fig. 4). When lobar arterial pressure was increased from 14 ± 1 to 46 ± 2 mmHg by infusion of the endoperoxide analog, intralobar infusions of isoproterenol at rates of 12–125 ng/kg per minute caused marked dose-dependent decreases in lobar arterial pressure (Fig. 4). In addition, when lobar vascular resistance was elevated by the endoperoxide analog, decreases in lobar arterial pressure in response to intrapulmonary infusions of isoproterenol at 62 and 125 ng/kg per minute were almost completely blocked after administration of propranolol, 2 mg/kg IV (Fig. 4). In contrast, when lobar vascular tone was enhanced by the endoperoxide analog, the decreases in lobar arterial pressure in response to isoproterenol infusions at 25–125 ng/kg per minute were decreased significantly but not blocked after metoprolol, 2 mg/kg IV (n=4), or practolol, 4 mg/kg IV (n=4). The extent of beta-1 blockade was evaluated by comparing the increase in heart rate in response to isoproterenol before and after administration of metoprolol or practolol. In the control period, injection of isoproterenol, 3 μg IV, increased heart rate from 172 ± 6 to 205 ± 5 beats/min. After administration of metoprolol, 2 mg/kg IV (n=4), or practolol, 4 mg/kg IV (n=4), injection of isoproterenol, 3 μg/kg IV, increased heart rate from 142 ± 6 to 147 ± 6 beats/min.

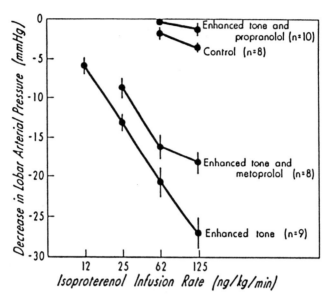

Figure 4: *Dose-response curves for isoproterenol comparing decreases in lobar arterial pressure under control conditions, when tone was enhanced, when tone was enhanced in cats treated with metoprolol, 2 mg/kg IV, or practolol, 4 mg/kg IV, and when tone was enhanced in those treated with propranolol, 2 mg/kg IV. Under control conditions, isoproterenol produced small but significant reductions in lobar arterial pressure. When tone was enhanced, responses to isoproterenol were greatly increased. Under enhanced tone conditions, metoprolol or practolol produced significant reductions in response to isoproterenol. After propranolol, responses to isoproterenol were abolished when tone was enhanced. n indicates number of animals.*

The increase in heart rate in response to isoproterenol was decreased significantly after adminstration of metoprolol or practolol (p < 0.05, paired comparison).

Effects of Sympathetic Nerve Stimulation

In the last series of experiments, the effects of neuronally released norepinephrine and adrenergic blocking agents were investigated in the feline pulmonary vascular bed. Under resting conditions, stimulation of the sympathetic nerves at 3, 10 and 30 cycles/sec caused significant frequency-related increases in lobar arterial pressure while lobar venous outflow pressure was held constant (Fig. 5). In 13 of the cats, the effects of phenoxybenzamine on responses to nerve stimulation and bolus injections of norepinephrine were investigated, and these data are shown in Figure 5. Under resting conditions, responses to the 1 μg dose of norepinephrine and nerve stimulation at 3 and 10 cycles/sec were completely blocked after phenoxybenzamine, 5 mg/kg IV, whereas responses to nerve stimulation at 30 cycles/sec and norepinephrine at 3 μg were reversed (Fig. 5). In additional experiments under resting conditions, responses to norepinephrine were enhanced after administration of beta receptor blocking agents, whereas the beta-blocking agents had no significant effect on the response to

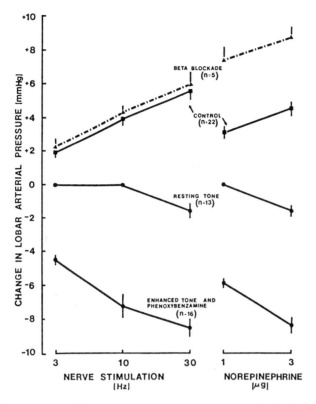

Figure 5: *Frequency- and dose-response curves for nerve stimulation and norepinephrine under control conditions, after administration of propranolol, 2 mg/kg IV, or sotalol, 4 mg/kg IV (beta blockade), after administration of phenoxybenzamine, 5 mg/kg IV, and after administration of phenoxybenzamine, 5 mg/kg IV, in animals in which tone was enhanced. Under control conditions nerve stimulation and norepinephrine injections caused significant increases in lobar arterial pressure. Responses to nerve stimulation and norepinephrine were abolished or reversed after administration of phenoxybenzamine under control (resting tone) conditions. Responses to norepinephrine but not to nerve stimulation were increased significantly after administration of the β blockers. After tone was enhanced in cats treated with phenoxybenzamine, nerve stimulation and norepinephrine caused significant decreases in lobar arterial pressure.*

sympathetic nerve stimulation (Fig. 5). In these experiments, both propranolol, 2 mg/kg IV (n=1), and sotalol, 4 mg/kg IV (n=4), an agent that may have fewer membrane effects than propranolol, were used. In 16 of the animals, the effects of nerve stimulation and norepinephrine were investigated when lobar vascular tone was enhanced after administration of phenoxybenzamine, 5 mg/kg IV. When lobar arterial pressure was increased from 15 ± 2 to 39 ± 2 mmHg by intrapulmonary infusion of the endoperoxide analog or 15-methyl $PGF_{2\alpha}$ in animals treated with this alpha blocking agent, stimulation of the sympathetic nerves at 3, 10, and 30 cycles/sec and intralobar injections of norepinephrine at 1 and 3 μg caused significant frequency- and dose-dependent decreases in lobar arterial pressure (Fig. 5). In four of the 16 cats, the decrease in lobar arterial pressure in response to nerve stimulation at 30 cycles/sec was blocked after administration of propranolol, 2mg/kg IV (control -9 ± 2 mmHg, after propranolol -1 ± 1 mmHg, p < 0.05). In four other cats with enhanced tone and alpha receptor blockade, the decrease in lobar arterial pressure in response to nerve stimulation at 30 cycles/sec was not modified after administration of atropine, 1 mg/kg IV (control -8 ± 1 mmHg, after atropine $-8 \pm$ mmHg). In four other experiments, the effects of phentolamine and atropine on responses to nerve stimulation were investigated, and these data are presented in Table II. Responses to nerve stimulation at 3, 10, and 30 cycles/sec were reversed after administration of phentolamine, 2.5 mg/kg IV, when tone was enhanced by intrapulmonary infusion of the endoperoxide analog (Table II). The vasodilator responses to nerve stimulation were not modified after administration of atropine, 1 mg/kg IV (Table II).

The specificity of the blocking effects of phentolamine and propranolol were investigated in four other animals, and these data are summarized in Table III.

Table II
Influence of Phentolamine and Atropine on Responses to Sympathetic Nerve Stimulation When Lobar Vascular Resistance was Elevated by an Endoperoxide Analog

	Lobar arterial pressure (mmHg)	
	Phentolamine	Phentolamine and atropine
Control	42 ± 1	43 ± 1
3 cycles/sec	$38 \pm 1^*$	$39 \pm 1^*$
Control	43 ± 1	43 ± 1
10 cycles/sec	$33 \pm 1^*$	$33 \pm 1^*$
Control	43 ± 2	44 ± 2
30 cycles/sec	$32 \pm 1^*$	$33 \pm 1^*$

n = 4
Results are expressed as mean ± SE.
*P < 0.05 when compared to corresponding control.

Table III
Effects of Phentolamine and Propranolol on Responses to Pressor and Depressor Substances in the Feline Pulmonary Vascular Bed

	Lobar arterial pressure (mmHg) under conditions			
	Control	Phentolamine (2.5 mg/kg, IV)	Phentolamine and enhanced tone	Propranolol and enhanced tone (2 mg/kg, IV)
Control	10 ± 1	10 ± 1		
Angiotensin II, 1 μg	$15 \pm 1^*$	$15 \pm 2^*$		
Control	10 ± 2	11 ± 1		
PGF$_2$, 0.03 μg	$20 \pm 2^*$	$20 \pm 2^*$		
Control			28 ± 2	30 ± 2
PGE$_1$, 0.03 μg			$19 \pm 2^*$	$21 \pm 1^*$
Control			28 ± 2	32 ± 2
Nitroglycerin, 3 μg			$19 \pm 2^*$	$23 \pm 1^*$

n = 4
Results expressed as mean ± SE.
*P < 0.05 when compared to corresponding control.

Phentolamine, 2.5 mg/kg IV, was without significant effect on increases in lobar arterial pressure in response to angiotensin II or $PGF_{2\alpha}$ (Table III). In addition, phentolamine was without significant effect on decreases in lobar arterial pressure in response to PGE_1 or nitroglycerin when lobar vascular resistance was elevated by the endoperoxide analog (Table III). In these same experiments, propranolol, 2 mg/kg IV, was without significant effect on decreases in lobar arterial pressure in response to PGE_1 or nitroglycerin when lobar vascular resistance was elevated by the endoperoxide analog (Table III).

The effects of bolus injections of phenylephrine, an alpha-1 receptor agonist, and UK14304, an alpha-2 receptor agonist, were investigated in pilot experiments using cats, and these data are summarized in Table IV. Under baseline conditions, intralobar administration of phenylephrine, 1–30 μg, or UK14304, 30–300 μg, increased lobar arterial pressure in a dose-related fashion whereas left arterial pressure remained unchanged (Table IV). Although UK14304 and phenylephrine possessed vasoconstrictor activity in the lobar vascular bed, prolonged and marked systemic hypotension was observed only following the intralobar injections of UK14304.

Pulmonary Vascular Responses to Vagal Stimulation and Acetylcholine

Pulmonary vascular responses to vagal stimulation and acetylcholine were investigated in the intact-chest cat under conditions of controlled pulmonary blood flow. Under baseline (resting tone) conditions in nine cats, stimulation of the left midcervical vagus at stimulus frequencies of 4, 8, and 16 Hz caused small (1 ± 0, 2 ± 1, $3 + 1$ mmHg, respectively) but statistically significant increases in lobar arterial pressure when left atrial pressure was maintained constant. In three of these animals, the effects of alpha receptor blockade on the pressor response to vagal stimulation under baseline conditions was investigated. Vagal stimulation increased lobar arterial pressure 1 ± 0, 2 ± 1, and 3 ± 1 mmHg at 4, 8, and 16 Hz under baseline conditions, whereas no measurable rise was observed at these stimulus frequencies after administration of phen-

---

Table IV
Effects of Intralobar Injections of Phenylephrine and UK14304 on Lobar Arterial Pressure Under Conditions of Resting Tone

	Increase in lobar arterial pressure (mmHg)
Phenylephrine (μg ia) n = 9	
1	3.0 ± 1.0
3	5.2 ± 1.2
10	7.6 ± 1.2
30	9.0 ± 1.0
UK14304 (μg ia) n = 8	
30	2.2 ± 0.3
100	5.0 ± 1.0
300	8.3 ± 1.4

Results expressed as mean ± SE.
n = number of cats.

oxybenzamine, 5 mg/kg IV. In contrast to the effects of vagal stimulation, intralobar injections of acetylcholine in eight of the cats in doses of 0.5 and 1.0 μg caused small (1 ± 0 mmHg) but statistically significant decreases in lobar arterial pressure under baseline conditions.

Since the magnitude of vasodilator responses in the lung is dependent on the existing level of vasoconstrictor tone, which is minimal under baseline conditions ($FIO_2 = 0.21$),[40,41] responses to vagal stimulation and acetylcholine were also investigated when lobar vascular tone was elevated. Intralobar infusion of U46619, a stable prostaglandin endoperoxide analog (n=9), or 15-methyl $PGF_{2\alpha}$ (n=3), increased lobar arterial pressure from 12 ± 1 to 36 ± 2 mmHg in the 12 animals. The increases in lobar arterial pressure in response to the prostaglandin analogs were well maintained during the infusion period. Under enhanced tone conditions in the group of 12 animals, vagal stimulation at 4, 8, and 16 Hz caused small (1 ± 0, 2 ± 1, 4 ± 1 mmHg, respectively) statistically significant decreases in lobar arterial pressure. In four of these animals, the effects of beta receptor blockade on the decrease in lobar arterial pressure in response to vagal stimulation were also investigated. Decreases in lobar arterial pressure at stimulus frequencies of 8 to 16 Hz were -2 ± 1 and -4 ± 1 mmHg before and -2 ± 1 and -4 ± 1 mmHg after administration of propranolol, 1 mg/kg IV. However, in eight of the animals, atropine, 1 mg/kg IV, significantly attenuated the decreases in lobar arterial pressure in response to vagal stimulation at 8 and 16 Hz, which were -1 ± 0 and -4 ± 1 mmHg before and 0 and -2 ± 0 mmHg after atropine.

Under conditions of enhanced vascular tone, intralobar injections of acetylcholine, $0.05-1.0$ μg, in eight animals caused significant dose-related decreases in lobar arterial pressure. Pressure decreased 19, 27, 45, and 48% at 0.05, 0.1, 0.5 and 1.0 μg doses, respectively. Responses to acetylcholine were rapid in onset and lobar arterial pressure returned to control values $1-3$ minutes after the injection. Lobar arterial pressure decreased -6 ± 1, -8 ± 1, -11 ± 1, and -13 ± 2 mmHg at the $0.05-1.0$ μg doses of acetylcholine under enhanced tone conditions, and these decreases in pressure were reduced to a similar extent as observed in 6-hydroxydopamine-treated animals after administration of atropine in Table V.

Influence of Adrenergic Neuronal Blockade and Hexamethonium

It has been reported that the vagus is a mixed nerve containing efferent fibers from both parasympathetic and sympathetic divisions of the autonomic nervous system.[24] Therefore, responses to vagal stimulation were investigated in animals treated with 6-hydroxydopamine, an agent that interferes with the capacity of adrenergic nerves to store catecholamines.[53] For these experiments, the animals were treated with 6-hydroxydopamine, 100 mg/kg IP, for 3 days and were catheterized on days $4-6$. In six animals treated with 6-hydroxydopamine, vagal stimulation at 4, 8, 16 Hz elicited small but statistically significant decreases in lobar arterial pressure of 1 ± 0, 2 ± 1, 2 ± 0 mmHg, respectively. In these animals, as in control animals, intralobar injections of acetylcholine caused small (1 ± 0, 2 ± 0 mmHg, respectively) but significant decreases in lobar arterial pressure at the 0.5 and 1.0 μg doses. However, when lobar arterial pressure was increased from 13 ± 1 to 34 ± 2 mmHg in 12 animals by intralobar infusion of U46619 (n=9), or 15-methyl $PGF_{2\alpha}$ (n=3), vagal stimulation at

Table V
Effect of Atropine on Responses to Vagal Stimulation and Acetylcholine*

	Lobar arterial pressure (mmHg)	
	Control	Atropine
Vagal stimulation		
Control	34 ± 2	35 ± 2
2 Hz	31 ± 2†	35 ± 2
Control	34 ± 1	46 ± 2
4 Hz	28 ± 1†	45 ± 3
Control	33 ± 2	34 ± 2
8 Hz	25 ± 2†	32 ± 2
Control	30 ± 1	44 ± 2
16 Hz	20 ± 2†	41 ± 1†
Acetylcholine		
Control	34 ± 2	45 ± 2
0.1 μg	25 ± 1†	45 ± 1
Control	27 ± 1	35 ± 1
0.5 μg	14 ± 2†	34 ± 1
Control	30 ± 2	38 ± 3
1.0 μg	15 ± 1†	36 ± 1†

n = 7
*When lobar vascular resistance was elevated by U46619 in 6-hydroxydopamine-treated cats.
†P < 0.05, compared with corresponding control.

2–16 Hz caused marked frequency-dependent decreases in lobar arterial pressure. The responses were slow in onset, reaching a steady state 30–60 seconds after onset of stimulation, and the decreases in lobar arterial pressure were well maintained during nerve stimulation for periods up to 90 seconds. Lobar arterial pressure decreased 12, 18, 25, and 38% at frequencies of 2, 4, 8, and 16 Hz, respectively, and pressure returned to control level over a 1 to 3 minute period after vagal stimulation was terminated. When lobar vascular resistance was elevated by infusion of U46619 (n=5) or 15-methyl $PGF_{2\alpha}$ (n=3), intralobar injections of acetylcholine (0.05, 0.1, 0.5, and 1.0 μg) caused significant dose-related reductions in lobar arterial pressure of 7 ± 1, 9 ± 1, 12 ± 1, 13 ± 1 mmHg, respectively. These responses were not significantly different from those observed in eight control animals when lobar vascular resistance was elevated to comparable levels by infusion of U46619.

In three of the 6-hydroxydopamine-treated animals, the effects of beta receptor blockade on the decreases in lobar arterial pressure in response to vagal stimulation were studied. The decreases in lobar arterial pressure at 8 and 16 Hz (-8 ± 1 and -11 ± 1 mmHg, respectively) in 6-hydroxydopamine-treated animals under enhanced tone conditions were not significantly different (-7 ± 1 and -11 ± 2 mmHg) after administration of propranolol, 1 mg/kg IV. However, the decreases in lobar arterial pressure in response to vagal stimulation and to acetylcholine in 6-hydroxydopamine-treated animals were blocked after administration of atroprine, 1 mg/kg IV (Table V). This table also shows the absolute values for lobar arterial pressure in these experiments, and these values were representative of all experiments in which responses were obtained under enhanced tone conditions. In other experiments, the effect of ganglionic blockade on responses to vagal stimulation and acetylcholine were investigated in 6-hydroxydopamine-treated animals, and these data are summarized in Table VI. In these experiments in five animals, when lobar vascular resistance was elevated by infusion of U46619, the reductions in lobar arterial pressure in response to vagal stimulation were blocked after administration of hexamethonium, 5 mg/kg IV. However, decreases in lobar arterial pressure in response to acetylcholine injections were not modified by the ganglionic blocking agent (Table VI).

The functional extent of depletion of catecholamines from adrenergic nerves was assessed by comparing responses to tyramine, an indirectly acting sympathomimetic agent, in control animals and in animals treated with 6-hydroxydopamine. In control animals (n=5), intralobar injections of tyramine, 200μg, increased lobar arterial and systemic arterial pressures 5 ± 1 and 24 ± 4 mmHg, respectively. In 6-hydroxydopamine-treated animals (n=4), this dose of tyramine increased lobar arterial and systemic arterial pressure 1 ± 0 and 4 ± 1 mmHg, respectively. The increases in lobar arterial and systemic arterial pressures were significantly less in 6-hydroxydopamine-treated animals, compared with controls. The effect of treatment with 6-hydroxydopamine was further investigated by comparing responses to norepinephrine in control animals (n=6) and in cats treated with the adrenergic neuronal blocking agent, 100 mg/kg IP, for 3 days and studied on days 4−6. In control animals, intralobar infusion of norepinephrine, 0.25 μg/kg per minute for 2−3 minutes, increased lobar arterial pressure from 12 ± 1 to 16 ± 1 mmHg. In animals treated with 6-hydroxydopamine (n=4), a similar increase in lobar arterial pressure (10 ± 1 to 13 ± 1 mmHg) was observed at a norepinephrine infusion rate of 0.025 μg/kg per minute, which was one-tenth the control rate.

Table VI
Effect of Hexamethonium on Responses to Vagal Stimulation and Acetylcholine*

	Lobar arterial pressure (mmHg)	
	Control	Hexamethonium
Vagal stimulation		
Control	38 ± 2	39 ± 1
4 Hz	33 ± 1†	38 ± 2
Control	39 ± 1	39 ± 2
8 Hz	31 ± 1†	38 ± 2
Acetylcholine		
Control	39 ± 1	40 ± 1
0.05 μg	34 ± 1†	35 ± 1†
Control	40 ± 1	40 ± 1
0.1 μg	31 ± 1†	32 ± 1†

n = 5
*When lobar vascular resistance was elevated by U46619 in 6-hydroxydopamine-treated cats.
†P < 0.05, compared with corresponding control.

In addition to experiments with 6-hydroxydopamine, the effects of a second adrenergic neuronal blocking agent were investigated in another group of five cats. These animals were treated with reserpine, 1 mg/kg IM, and the animals were catheterized on day 2 or 3. In these animals, vagal stimulation at 8 and 16 Hz and acetylcholine injections at the 1 μg dose caused small but significant decreases in lobar arterial pressure. However, when lobar vascular resistance was increased by infusion of U46619, vagal stimulation at 4–16 Hz and acetyl-choline injections, 0.1–1.0 μg, caused significant frequency- and dose-dependent decreases in lobar arterial pressure (Table VII). Although decreases in lobar arterial pressure in response to intralobar injections of acetylcholine were similar in animals treated with 6-hydroxydopamine or reserpine, responses to vagal stimulation were significantly smaller at 4, 8, and 16 Hz in reserpine-treated animals (Table VII).

Effect of Physostigmine

If responses to vagal stimulation are the result of release of acetylcholine from cholinergic terminals, then these responses should be enhanced by physo-stigmine, a cholinesterase inhibitor. In another group of cats treated with 6-hydroxydopamine, decreases in lobar arterial pressure in response to vagal stimulation at 1 and 2 Hz (n=5), and to acetylcholine at 0.5 and 1 μg (n=5), were enhanced significantly to 2 ± 0, 3 ± 1 mmHg and 2 ± 0, 3 ± 1 mmHg, respectively, after administration of physostigmine, 1 mg/kg IV. Furthermore, when lobar vascular resistance was elevated by infusion of U46619, the

Table VII
Lobar Vascular Responses to Vagal Stimulation and
Acetylcholine in Animals Treated with Reserpine*

	Lobar arterial pressure (mmHg)	
	Basal tone	Enhanced tone
Vagal stimulation		
Control		37 ± 1
4 Hz		34 ± 1†
Control	12 ± 1	39 ± 2
8 Hz	11 ± 0	34 ± 2†
Control	12 ± 0	38 ± 1
16 Hz	10 ± 0†	31 ± 2†
Acetylcholine		
Control		37 ± 2
0.1 μg		29 ± 2†
Control		35 ± 2
0.5 μg		24 ± 2†
Control	11 ± 1	40 ± 2
1.0 μg	10 ± 1	28 ± 2†

n = 5
*When lobar vascular resistance was at resting levels and when lobar vascular resistance was elevated by U46619.
†$P < 0.05$, compared with corresponding control.

frequency-response curve for vagal stimulation was shifted to the left by physostigmine and the threshold frequency for stimulation decreased from 2 Hz to 0.25 Hz. The dose-response curve for acetylcholine was also shifted to the left by the cholinesterase inhibitor and the threshold dose was reduced.

Influence of Systemic Hypotension and Bronchial Obstruction

Although bradycardia and systemic hypotension in response to vagal stimulation were minimized by ventricular pacing, using an electrode catheter in the right ventricle, aortic pressure decreased from 130 ± 5 to 115 ± 6 mmHg in control animals and from 105 ± 4 to 95 ± 5 mmHg in 6-hydroxydopamine-treated animals. Moreover, a decrease in systemic arterial pressure could change lobar arterial pressure by altering bronchopulmonary shunt flow.[11] Therefore, the effects of vagal stimulation were compared when aortic pressure was at normal levels and when pressure was reduced during a period of ventricular fibrillation. In four animals treated with 6-hydroxydopamine, a short period of high-frequency stimulation of the right ventricular free wall by way of an electrode catheter induced ventricular fibrillation, during which time aortic pressure decreased from 110 ± 6 to 50 ± 7 mmHg. The reduction in aortic pressure had no significant effect on lobar arterial pressure (control 35 ± 2 and 34 ± 2 during fibrillation) or on the response to vagal stimulation at 16 Hz (control -10 ± 1, during fibrillation -9 ± 2 mmHg). The period of ventricular fibrillation was $2-3$ minutes, and normal sinus rhythm was reestablished by direct current defibrillation.

Vagal stimulation increases bronchomotor tone.[11] Therefore, the contribution of changes in bronchomotor tone to the response to vagal stimulation was investigated in four cats treated with 6-hydroxydopamine in which the left lower lobe bronchus was obstructed by inflation of a 5F balloon catheter. The decreases in lobar arterial pressure in response to vagal stimulation at 4 and 8 Hz and to acetylcholine at 0.5 and 1.0 μg were not significantly different during normal ventilation, or when the left lower lobe bronchus was obstructed, blocking airflow (Table VIII).

Responses During Alveolar Hypoxia

The effects of vagal stimulation were also investigated in another group of cats treated with 6-hydroxydopamine when lobar arterial pressure was increased by ventilatory hypoxia. A record from an experiment is shown in Figure 6 and summary data are presented in Table IX. Ventilation with 10% O_2 in N_2 caused a significant increase in lobar arterial pressure without altering left atrial pressure (Table IX). When lobar arterial pressure was increased by ventilation with 10% O_2, vagal stimulation caused a significant reduction in lobar arterial pressure without altering left atrial pressure (Table IX).

Results from Studies in Isolated Intrapulmonary Vessels

Relaxant responses to acetylcholine. Isolated rings rather than the more conventional helical strip preparations were used in these experiments because

Table VIII
**Effect of Obstruction of the Left Lower Lobe Bronchus on
Responses to Vagal Stimulation and Acetylcholine***

	Lobar arterial pressure (mmHg)	
	Control	Bronchus obstructed
Vagal stimulation		
Control	34 ± 2	36 ± 2
4 Hz	27 ± 2†	30 ± 1†
Control	39 ± 1	37 ± 2
8 Hz	28 ± 1†	29 ± 1†
Acetylcholine		
Control	36 ± 3	35 ± 2
0.05 μg	28 ± 3†	30 ± 1†
Control	41 ± 1	39 ± 1
0.1 μg	32 ± 2†	29 ± 3†

n = 4
*When lobar vascular resistance was elevated by U46619.
†$P < 0.05$, compared with corresponding control.

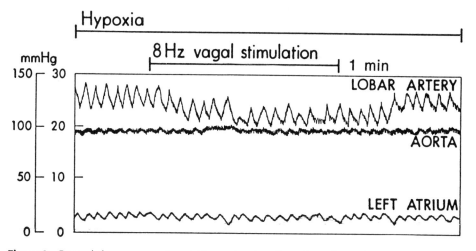

Figure 6: *Records from an experiment illustrating the effect of vagal stimulation at 8 Hz on lobar arterial pressure when lobar vascular resistance had been increased by ventilation with 10% O_2 in nitrogen. When the F_{IO_2} was decreased from 0.21 to 0.10, lobar arterial pressure was increased from 18 to 28 mmHg in this animal.*

rings were more consistently isolated with an intact or functioning endothelium, as assessed by reproducible relaxations in response to acetylcholine. The most consistent submaximal contractions to phenylephrine and relaxations to acetylcholine were obtained when arterial rings were first depolarized with potassium and then submaximally contracted with phenylephrine, as described under *Methods.* Acetylcholine produced a concentration-dependent relaxation of phenylephrine-precontracted arterial rings and this response was antagonized

Table IX
Effect of Vagal Stimulation on the Pulmonary Vascular Bed*

	Pressure (mmHg)		
	Lobar artery	Left atrium	Aorta
Control	13 ± 1	2 ± 0	110 ± 7
Hypoxia	17 ± 1†	2 ± 0	96 ± 4†
Vagal stimulation (4 Hz)	15 ± 1	3 ± 1	87 ± 2†
Control	14 ± 2	3 ± 1	113 ± 7
Hypoxia	21 ± 1†	3 ± 0	109 ± 7
Vagal stimulation (8 Hz)	16 ± 1	3 ± 1	100 ± 5

n = 11
*When pulmonary vascular tone is increased by ventilatory hypoxia in 6-hydroxydopamine-treated animals.
†$P < 0.05$ when compared to control.

by atropine (Fig. 7). Although acetylcholine also relaxed rings that were pre-contracted with 30 mM KCl, acetylcholine was tenfold more potent when phenylephrine was used to precontract the rings. A 10 μM concentration of quinacrine partially antagonized acetylcholine-elicited relaxation without affecting the contractile response to phenylephrine (Fig. 7). Higher concentrations (20–50 μM) of quinacrine, however, markedly depressed or abolished contractions to phenylephrine and were not employed in this study. Methylene blue enhanced contractile responses to phenylephrine and markedly antagonized relaxant responses to acetylcholine (Fig. 7).

Contractile responses to acetylcholine. Isolated rings prepared with a damaged endothelium contracted in response to acetylcholine (Fig. 8). Acetylcholine further contracted arterial rings that had been submaximally precontracted by phenylephrine. Contractile responses to acetylcholine were antagonized by atropine and enhanced by methylene blue. Quinacrine, at a concentration (10 μM) that depressed relaxant responses to acetylcholine (Fig. 8), also depressed contractile responses to acetylcholine (Fig. 8).

Effects of acetylcholine on arterial accumulation of cyclic GMP and cyclic AMP. In all of the present experiments, cyclic nucleotide determinations were made in arterial ring preparations that had been previously equilibrated under 6 g of tension, depolarized with potassium, and submaximally precontracted with phenylephrine. In addition, changes in isometric force were recorded until the time of freeze-clamping. The reason for this is that a considerable number of initial experiments in which arterial rings were incubated in the absence of tension, whether or not depolarization or contraction was induced, yielded inconsistent and highly variable values for cyclic nucleotide levels.

Acetylcholine elicited time-dependent (Fig. 9) and concentration-dependent (Fig. 10) increases in arterial cyclic GMP accumulation that correlated well with the development of relaxation. The onset of cyclic GMP accumulation (5 sec) preceded the onset of relaxation (15 sec). Furthermore, peak levels of cyclic GMP that occurred at 30 seconds preceded peak relaxant responses to acetylcholine. At 60 seconds after addition of 10^{-6}M acetylcholine, cyclic GMP levels were elevated 15-fold to 331 ± 21 pmol/g of tissue (Table X). At this time point (60 sec), acetylcholine elicited 75% to 80% of relaxation, which is less than

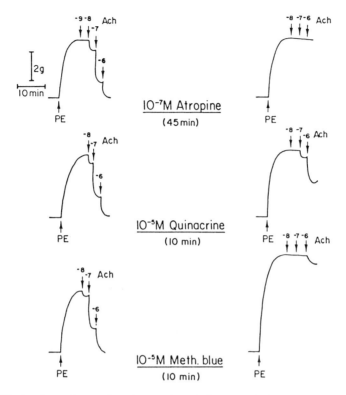

Figure 7: *Effects of atropine, quinacrine, and methylene (Meth) blue on relaxation of bovine intrapulmonary arterial rings elicited by acetylcholine (Ach). Arterial rings were isolated with an intact endothelium. After the induction of submaximal contractions with $10^{-5}M$ phenylephrine (PE), Ach was added in cumulatively increasing concentrations. The numbers corresponding to Ach concentrations are illustrated as exponents to the base power 10. Ring preparations were washed and allowed to equilibrate for 45 to 60 minutes after obtaining the tracings shown on the left-hand side of the figure. Atropine, quinacrine, and methylene blue were then added to bath chambers for the periods of time indicated and rings were contracted with PE followed by the addition of Ach. All concentrations are expressed as final bath concentrations.*

that for maximal relaxation by $10^{-6}M$ acetylcholine (Fig. 7) because maximal responses take about 120 seconds to develop. Concentration-dependent responses to acetylcholine appear to be relatively flat, which suggests that multiple endothelial-dependent mechanisms are involved in the regulation of the contractile state mediated by muscarinic receptors. Atropine and methylene blue markedly inhibited both relaxation and cyclic GMP accumulation caused by acetylcholine (Table X). Quinacrine caused a highly significant antagonism of relaxation without altering cyclic GMP accumulation in response to acetylcholine (Table X). Quinacrine at concentrations of 50 to 100 μM markedly inhibited cyclic GMP accumulation elicited by acetylcholine, but effects on relaxation could not be assessed because such high concentrations of quinacrine markedly depressed phenylephrine-induced precontractions.

Resting levels of cyclic AMP in arterial rings were 331 ± 16 pmol/g of tissue or about 15 times greater than those of cyclic GMP (not shown). Cyclic AMP

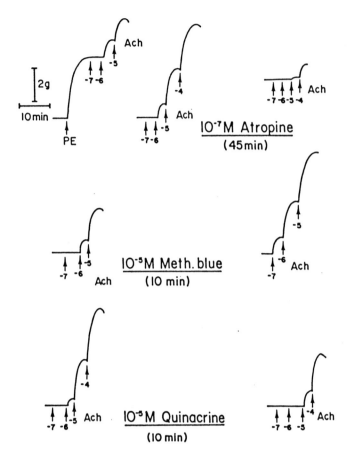

Figure 8: *Effects of atropine, quinacrine, and methylene (Meth) blue on contraction of bovine intrapulmonary arterial rings elicited by acetylcholine (Ach). Arterial rings were prepared with a damaged endothelium. The upper left-hand tracing illustrates contractions to Ach after the induction of submaximal contraction with $10^{-5}M$ phenylephrine (PE). All other tracings illustrate responses to cumulatively increasing concentrations of Ach in the absence of precontraction with PE. The numbers corresponding to Ach concentrations are illustrated as exponents to the base power 10. Ring preparations were washed and allowed to equilibrate for 45 to 60 minutes after obtaining the tracings shown on the left-hand side of the figure. Atropine, methylene blue, and quinacrine were than added to bath chambers for the periods of time indicated before the additions of Ach. All concentrations are expressed as final bath concentrations.*

levels remained relatively constant at times when both cyclic GMP levels and relaxation were increasing in response to acetylcholine (not shown).

Cyclic GMP levels were determined also in intrapulmonary arterial rings that had been prepared with a damaged endothelium. Resting cyclic GMP levels were 26 ± 1 pmol/g of tissue and were unaltered by phenylephrine (Table XI). Acetylcholine elevated cyclic GMP after 60 seconds by approximately six fold to 153 ± 12 pmol/g of tissue, and also elicited a contractile response. Atropine abolished both responses to acetylcholine, whereas methylene blue markedly

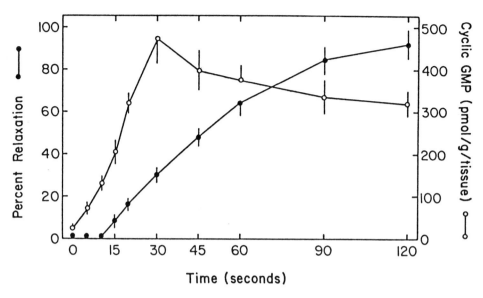

Figure 9: *Time course of cyclic GMP accumulation and relaxation in bovine intrapulmonary arterial rings elicited by acetylcholine. Arterial rings were isolated with an intact endothelium and were submaximally contracted with $10^{-5}M$ phenylephrine before exposure to acetylcholine ($10^{-6}M$). Rings were freeze-clamped at the times indicated. Values represent the mean ± SE, using six to 12 arterial rings isolated from three to six separate animals. Relaxation and cyclic GMP levels were determined in the same arterial rings. Relaxation is expressed as the percentage of decrease in phenylephrine-induced tone.*

Table X
Effects of Atropine, Quinacrine, and Methylene Blue on Relaxation and Cyclic GMP Accumulation in Bovine Intrapulmonary Arterial Rings Elicited by Acetylcholine (Ach)

Test agents	N	% Relaxation	Cyclic GMP
			pmol/g tissue
None	6		22 ± 3
PE, $10^{-5}M$	6		23 ± 4
PE + Ach, $10^{-6}M$	8	78 ± 6	331 ± 21
PE + Ach + atropine, $10^{-7}M$	6	3 ± 1*	36 ± 3*
PE + Ach + quinacrine, $10^{-5}M$	8	31 ± 3*	347 ± 28
PE + Ach + methylene blue, $10^{-5}M$	6	6 ± 1*	42 ± 5*

Arterial rings were isolated with an intact endothelium and, with one exception (None), were submaximally contracted with phenylephrine (PE). Atropine was added to bath chambers 45 min before PE, whereas 10 min was used for quinacrine and methylene blue. Rings exposed to Ach were freeze-clamped after 60 sec. Rings exposed only to PE were freeze-clamped 60 sec after peak contractions were attained. Unexposed rings (None) were freeze-clamped 45 to 60 min after initial submaximal contractions to PE and re-equilibration after washing. Relaxation and cyclic GMP levels were determined in the same arterial rings. Relaxation is expressed as the percentage of decrease in PE-induced tone. Results are expressed as the mean ± S.E. N = number of arterial rings from three to four separate animals.
*Significantly different (p < 0.05) from values obtained in response to PE plus Ach.

Table XI
Effects of Atropine, Quinacrine, and Methylene Blue on Contraction and Cyclic GMP Accumulation in Bovine Intrapulmonary Arterial Rings Elicited by Acetylcholine (Ach)

Test agents	N	Contraction	Cyclic GMP
		g tension	pmol/g tissue
None	10		26 ± 1
PE, 10^{-5}M	4	1.9 ± 0.3	27 ± 3
Ach, 10^{-5}M	10	1.7 ± 0.2	153 ± 12
Ach + atropine, 10^{-7}M	8	0.1 ± 0.03*	37 ± 2*
Ach + quinacrine, 10^{-5}M	7	0.5 ± 0.08*	148 ± 15
Ach + methylene blue, 10^{-5}M	8	3.5 ± 0.4*	34 ± 2*

Arterial rings were isolated with a damaged endothelium. Rings were exposed to atropine for 45 min and to quinacrine or methylene blue for 10 min before addition of Ach. Unexposed rings (none) were freeze-clamped 45 to 60 min after initial submaximal contractions to phenylephrine (PE) and re-equilibration after washing. Rings exposed to Ach or PE were freeze-clamped after 60 sec. Contraction and cyclic GMP levels were determined in the same arterial rings. Contraction is expressed as grams of tension developed. Results are expressed as the mean ± SE. N = number of arterial ring preparations from three to five separate animals.
*Significantly different (p < 0.05) from values obtained in response to Ach alone.

inhibited cyclic GMP accumulation and enhanced the contractile response to acetylcholine (Table XI). Quinacrine depressed contractions to acetylcholine and failed to alter arterial cyclic GMP accumulation (Table XI). Methylene blue (10^{-5}M) by itself lowered resting levels of cyclic GMP from 26 ± 1 to 14 ± 1 pmol/g of tissue. Similarly, in arterial rings possessing a functional endothelium, methylene blue (10^{-5}M) lowered the resting levels of cyclic GMP from 25 ± 3 to 11 ± 2 pmol/g of tissue.

Discussion

Results of the present study show that stimulation of the sympathetic nerves to the lung and norepinephrine administration increase lobar arterial pressure in the cat. Inasmuch as lobar blood flow and lobar venous outflow pressure were maintained constant, the increases in lobar arterial pressure indicate that nerve stimulation and norepinephrine increase pulmonary lobar vascular resistance. The increases in lobar arterial pressure in response to norepinephrine and nerve stimulation were dose- and frequency-dependent and these responses were blocked after administration of alpha receptor blocking agents. These data indiciate that the feline pulmonary vascular bed is functionally innervated by the sympathetic nervous system and that under basal conditions both exogenously administered and neuronally released norepinephrine cause vasoconstriction by stimulating alpha receptors. These results are similar to those of previous studies on the canine pulmonary vascular bed.[12,49,46] However, the present experiments extend the work of previous studies by showing that, when pulmonary vascular tone was elevated in animals treated with alpha receptor blocking agents, adrenergic nerve stimulation caused frequency-dependent decreases in lobar arterial pressure that were not blocked by atropine. The atropine-resistant neurogenically induced vasodilator responses were well maintained during the period of stimulation, and these responses

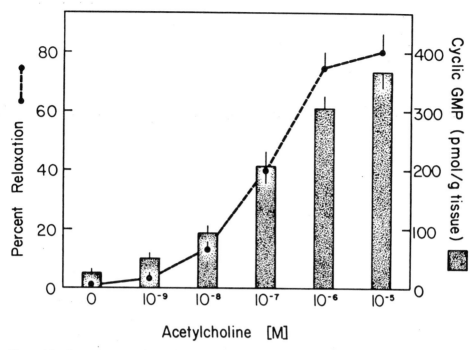

Figure 10: *Concentration-dependent cyclic GMP accumulation and relaxation in bovine intra-pulmonary arterial rings elicited by acetylcholine. Arterial rings were isloated with an intact endothelium and were submaximally contracted with $10^{-5}M$ phenylephrine before exposure to acetylcholine. All rings were freeze-clamped at exactly 60 seconds after the addition of acetylcholine to bath chambers. Values represent the mean ± SE, using six to 10 arterial rings isolated from three to five separate animals. Relaxation and cyclic GMP levels were determined in the same arterial rings. Relaxation is expressed as the percentage of decrease in phenylephrine-induced tone.*

were of greater magnitude than were the increases in lobar arterial pressure observed under basal conditions. Norepinephrine also caused dose-dependent decreases in lobar arterial pressure after alpha receptor blockade when pulmonary vascular tone was elevated. The vasodilator responses to norepinephrine and nerve stimulation were blocked by propranolol, a beta receptor blocking agent. These data indicate that the adrenergic transmitter acts on both alpha- and beta-adrenergic receptors and when pulmonary vascular tone is elevated and alpha receptors are masked, norepinephrine causes vasodilation in the pulmonary vascular bed. The present data for the pulmonary vascular bed are in agreement with previous studies in skeletal muscle, liver, spleen, and adipose tissue and in isolated facial vein of the rabbit and support the hypothesis that norepinephrine liberated from sympathetic nerves can act on beta-2 receptors in blood vessels.[27,28,61,62,65,85] However, other investigators have not been able to elicit vasodilator responses to adrenergic stimulation in a variety of organ systems.[14,24,69,71]

The hypotheses that vascular beta (beta-2) receptors are innervated and that neuronally released norepinephrine elicits vasodilation have been challenged recently.[71] These investigators were unable to confirm the classic studies in which nerve stimulation caused atropine-insensitive vasodilation in skeletal muscle.[85] In these studies, responses to adrenergic stimulation were reversed after intraarterial administration of dibozane, a substance that is poorly soluble at neutral pH, whereas responses to nerve stimulation were not reversed by phentolamine. However, when dibozane was administered IV at a dose of 10 mg/kg, vasodilator responses to nerve stimulation were blocked by atropine.[71] Moreover, results of the present study show that neuronally released norepinephrine can cause vasodilation and indicate that beta-2 receptors in the pulmonary vascular bed are innervated. In the present study, responses to nerve stimulation were reversed by phenoxybenzamine or phentolamine in doses that did not significantly alter responses to $PGF_{2\alpha}$, angiotensin II, PGE_1, or nitroglycerin in the pulmonary vascular bed. In addition, vasodilator responses to nerve stimulation were not modified by doses of atropine that reduced responses to acetylcholine in the feline pulmonary vascular bed (unpublished observations). These data suggest that reversal of the response to nerve stimulation was not dependent on the type of alpha blocker employed and did not involve a cholinergic mechanism. The reasons for the difference in results in the present study and in those of other investigators[71] are uncertain but may suggest differences in nerve terminal-adrenergic receptor relationships in the skeletal muscle and the pulmonary vascular beds. The hypothesis that the feline pulmonary vascular bed is well supplied with beta receptors is suggested by the observation that isoproterenol, a potent beta agonist, had marked vasodilator activity when pulmonary vascular tone was elevated. Moreover, the observation that vasodilator responses to isoproterenol were only partially decreased by metoprolol or practolol but were almost completely blocked by propranolol suggests that the vascular beta receptors in the lung are of the beta-2 type, as previously suggested.[56] Although metoprolol or practolol had only a small effect on the pulmonary vasodilator response to isoproterenol, these agents almost completely blocked the increases in heart rate in response to isoproterenol, confirming the cardioselective nature of these antagonists.[21,58]

It has been reported that vasoconstriction tone in the feline pulmonary vascular bed is minimal under resting conditions and that vasodilator responses to prostaglandins and nitroglycerin are dependent on the existing level of tone in the bed.[40] Vasodilation in response to beta receptor activation is caused by relaxation of basal tone, and variations in response to beta agonists may result from variations in the level of existing tone.[28] The present studies with isoproterenol are consistent with the results of studies in the hepatic bed and support the concept that responses to beta agonists are dependent on the existing level of vasoconstrictor tone.[4,28]

Epinephrine stimulates both alpha and beta receptors, and its potency on beta receptors is between that of norepinephrine and isoproterenol.[22] Reports in the literature on the pulmonary vascular effects of epinephrine vary with the study.[35,67] Results of the present study show that in the cat with an intact chest that epinephrine infusions produced modest decreases in pulmonary vascular resistance. Moreover, these decreases were greatly enhanced when pulmonary vascular tone was elevated. In addition, when tone was elevated and alpha receptors were blocked, epinephrine had potent vasodilator activity. Moreover, vasodilator responses to epinephrine after alpha blockade were nearly equal to vasodilator responses to isoproterenol when vasoconstrictor tone was elevated. These results indicate that epinephrine has good beta receptor stimulating activity in the feline pulmonary vascular bed but suggests that this activity is dependent on the existing level of tone in the bed. These data support our hypothesis that the feline pulmonary vascular bed is well supplied with beta receptors. The present data are in agreement with results of a recent study on skeletal muscle in regard to the relative potency of isoproterenol, epinephrine, and norepinephrine in stimulating vascular bed receptors.[71] Although epinephrine had no apparent vasoconstrictor activity when infused at rates of 1 or 2 μg/kg per minute, these concentrations caused significant vasoconstriction when beta receptors were blocked with propranolol. In addition, vasoconstrictor responses to norepinephrine were increased greatly after beta-adrenergic blockade. These data suggest that in the feline pulmonary vascular bed, epinephrine and norepinephrine act on both alpha and beta receptors and that the resulting response is the algebraic summation of these two opposing actions. Therefore, when beta receptors are blocked, both catecholamines have potent alpha-stimulating activity.

The possibility that propranolol was enhancing pressor responses to norepinephrine and epinephrine by a mechanism other than beta receptor blockade was investigated by evaluating the effects of the antagonist on responses to phenylephrine, tyramine, $PGF_{2\alpha}$, and angiotensin II. Since phenylephrine is a selective alpha receptor agonist, propranolol would not be expected to enhance the response to this agent.[19] The present studies show that propranolol in doses that blocked vasodilator responses to isoproterenol and enhanced vasoconstrictor responses to norepinephrine was without significant effect on the pressor response to phenylephrine infusion. Tyramine is an indirectly acting amine that must be taken up by the adrenergic nerves in order to displace norepinephrine.[81] However, in doses that blocked beta receptors in the feline pulmonary vascular bed, propranolol enhanced the pressor response to tyramine. In addition, propranolol did not modify pressor responses to $PGF_{2\alpha}$ and angiotensin II, which are nonadrenergic agonists. These data suggest that propranolol does not enhance pressor responses to norepinephrine or epinephrine by blocking uptake of these substances into adrenergic nerves or by a nonspecific effect on vascular smooth muscle. Although propranolol did not block responses to tyramine, the effects of this indirectly acting substance are inhibited by cocaine, an agent that blocks neuronal uptake.[79] The doses of cocaine that blocked responses to tyramine enhanced responses to norepinephrine, suggestng that neuronal uptake may be an important mechanism for terminating the actions of catecholamines in the pulmonary vascular bed. In addition, the observation that tyramine causes an indirectly mediated pressor response supports our hypothesis that the feline pulmonary vascular bed is innervated by the adrenergic nervous system. The enhanced pressor response to norepinephrine and the significant vasoconstrictor response to epinephrine after propranolol provide further support for the hypothesis that these catecholamines act on both alpha and beta receptors in the feline pulmonary vascular bed.

Although responses to sympathetic nerve stimulation were reversed after alpha receptors were blocked and tone was elevated, these responses were not enhanced after administration of beta blocking agents. Thus, in the same group of cats in which pressor responses to exogenously administered norepinephrine were augmented, responses to nerve stimulation were not modified. The explanation for the inability to enhance neurogenic responses is uncertain; however, it is possible that the beta blocking agents may have a depressant action on the processes by which norepinephrine is liberated by stimulation of the sympathetic nerves. Neither sotalol nor propranolol enhanced the response to nerve stimulation, and since sotalol has little, if any, "membrane stabilizing activity," the depressant action is probably not nonspecific.[21] The inability of the beta blockers to enhance responses to nerve stimulation, whereas these agents enhanced responses to tyramine and norepinephrine in the present study, suggests a very specific action on the neurogenic release process for norepinephrine in the adrenergic terminal. It has been reported that activation of presynaptic beta receptors enhances neuronal release of norepinephrine and that beta blocking agents such as sotalol decrease the release of the adrenergic transmitter.[1,86] It is, therefore, possible that the beta blocking agents may block presynaptic receptors and decrease the release of norepinephrine in response to nerve stimulation. This action would oppose the effects of blockade of vascular beta-2 receptors.

Results of the present study indicate that the feline pulmonary vascular bed is innervated by the sympathetic nervous system and that alpha- and beta-2 adrenergic receptors are present. In addition, these results suggest that neuronally released and blood-borne norepinephrine can act on beta receptors, but vasodilator responses are dependent on the existing level of vasoconstrictor tone in the bed.

Recent studies have indicated that in addition to postsynaptic alpha-1 adrenoceptors, postsynaptic alpha-2 receptors which produce a pressor response when activated exist as well.[17,57,80] Results from previous experiments have demonstrated the presence of both alpha receptor subtypes at the effector sites of vascular smooth muscle of the systemic circulation. Results from the present study demonstrate that in the intact animal, selective alpha-1 and alpha-2 receptor agonists produce a pressor response in the pulmonary vascular bed. Phenylephrine as an alpha-1 receptor agonist, when compared to UK14304, an alpha-2 agonist, has $20-30$ times greater pressor activity in the feline pulmonary vascular bed. It has been shown in isolated rabbit pulmonary arterial strips that postsynaptic alpha-1 adrenoceptors which mediate a contractile response and not alpha-2 receptors are present in vascular smooth muscle from the lung.[78] In contrast, results from the present study demonstrate that in the intact animal, substances that selectively activate alpha-1 or alpha-2 adrenoceptors may produce a pressor response in the pulmonary vascular bed of the cat. Additional experiments are necessary to characterize fully the nature of responses due to activation of alpha receptor subtypes and to determine which population of alpha receptor subtypes has an intra- and/or extrasynaptic location in the feline pulmonary vascular bed.

Results of the present investigation in the intact-chest cat also show that, under normal resting conditions, electrical stimulation of the peripheral segment of the vagus nerve in the midcervical region increases lobar arterial pressure. However, when vasoconstrictor tone in the pulmonary vascular bed was increased by several mechanisms, the pressor response was reversed and a depressor response was unmasked. The pressor response under baseline conditions was blocked by phenoxybenzamine, whereas the depressor response under enhanced tone conditions was blocked by atropine. These data suggest that in the cat, in the cervical region, the vagus is composed of efferent fibers from both sympathetic and parasympathetic divisions of the autonomic nervous system, as has been reported previously in the dog.[10] Since efferent fibers from both sympathetic and parasympathetic systems are represented in the cervical vagus, the effects of 6-hydroxydopamine, an agent that destroys the integrity of adrenergic terminals, on responses to vagal stimulation were investigated.[53] Treatment with 6-hydroxydopamine markedly inhibited pressor responses to tyramine and enhanced pressor responses to norepinephrine in the systemic and lobar vascular beds, suggesting that the neuronal blocking agent depleted adrenergic terminals of norepinephrine and inhibited uptake of adrenergic transmitter.[49,75,82] After treatment with 6-hydroxydopamine, stimulation of efferent vagal fibers decreased lobar arterial pressure, and responses to vagal stimulation were greatly enhanced when vasoconstrictor tone was increased to a high steady level during infusion of 15-methyl $PGF_{2\alpha}$ or U46619, a stable prostaglandin endoperoxide analog whose actions may mimic those of thromboxane A_2.[8] Since lobar blood flow and left atrial pressure were maintained constant, the reductions in lobar arterial pressure in response to vagal stimulation suggest that pulmonary lobar vascular resistance is decreased. The reductions in lobar arterial pressure in response to vagal stimulation were not modified by propranolol, suggesting that the vasodilator response is not mediated in part through activation of beta receptors by neuronally released norepinephrine.[41] When vasoconstrictor tone was enhanced during infusion of U46619 or 15-methyl $PGF_{2\alpha}$, intralobar infusions of acetylcholine decreased lobar arterial pressure and the response was not altered by treatment with 6-hydroxydopamine. However, decreases in lobar arterial pressure in response to vagal stimulation and acetylcholine in 6-hydroxydopamine-treated animals with enhanced tone were blocked by atropine, a muscarinic receptor-blocking agent. In contrast to experiments with atropine, responses to vagal stimulation and to acetylcholine in 6-hydroxydopamine-treated animals with enhanced tone were greatly increased by physostigmine, a cholinesterase inhibitor. These data suggest that vagal stimulation decreases lobar arterial pressure by releasing acetylcholine, which acts on muscarinic receptors in the pulmonary vascular bed. Vasodilator responses to vagal stimulation were blocked after treatment with hexamethonium, a ganglionic blocking agent, whereas responses to acetylcholine were not affected after ganglionic blockade. These data indicate that the decreases in lobar arterial pressure in response to vagal stimulation are due to activation of preganglionic cholinergic neurons.

In a recently published study, it has been shown that small- and medium-size intrapulmonary arteries in the cat have cholinergic terminals.[52] However, the effects of cholinergic (vagosympathetic) nerve stimulation are uncertain, since reports in the literature show modest increases, modest decreases, a biphasic response, or no change in pulmonary vascular resistance.[10,11] It has been shown in a perfused dog lung preparation that stimulation of the cervical vagosympathetic trunk increased pulmonary arterial pressure in two animals, decreased pulmonary arterial pressure in six, and elicited a biphasic response in two animals.[10] The decreases in pressure in response to vagal stimulation were small (1−4 mmHg) and were blocked by atropine.[10] However, these investigators concluded from their results that a final decision as to the existence of atropine-sensitive pulmonary vasodilator fibers must await further studies, including experiments designed to ensure that the pulmonary arterial pressure changes are not secondary to alterations in the transfer of blood from the bronchial (systemic) to the pulmonary circulation.[10] Results of the present investigation extend the work of these investigators by demonstrating that efferent vagal stimulation caused larger than previously recognized, consistent, stimulus-related decreases in lobar vascular resistance in intact-chest animals after treatment with 6-hydroxydopamine when vasoconstrictor tone was increased. The dilator responses were blocked by atropine and enhanced by physostigmine, and similar responses were elicited by intralobar injections of acetylcholine, suggesting that they were cholinergic in nature.

The contribution of the bronchial circulation to the response to vagal stimulation was minimal in these experiments, since transfer of blood from the lobar vascular bed to the systemic vascular bed would not occur when systemic arterial pressure was maintained at normal levels by cardiac pacing. In addition, experiments showing that responses to vagal stimulation and to acetylcholine were similar when systemic arterial pressure was decreased to levels approximately equal to or lower than lobar arterial pressure during a period of ventricular fibrillation suggests that alterations in bronchial blood flow contribute little, if anything, to the lobar vascular response to vagal stimulation or acetylcholine. In addition, a marked reduction in systemic arterial pressure had no significant effect on lobar arterial pressure, suggesting that changes in bronchial flow, which is less than 5% of pulmonary flow, had no measurable effect on lobar hemodynamics in the cat. Similar observations have been made in the intact-chest dog.[39,48]

It has been reported that vagal stimulation can increase bronchomotor tone, and it is possible that changes in bronchomotor tone could influence the vascular response to vagal stimulation.[9–12] To assess the contribution of changes in bronchomotor tone and lung volume on responses to vagal stimulation and acetylcholine, we compared responses during normal ventilation and when airflow to the left lower lobe was interrupted by inflation of a balloon catheter positioned in the left lower lobe bronchus. Since responses to vagal stimulation and to acetylcholine were not altered during the period of bronchial occlusion, these experiments suggest that changes in bronchomotor tone and lung volume contribute little, if anything, to the response of the pulmonary lobar vascular bed to vagal stimulation or acetylcholine. The data showing that responses to vagal stimulation occur independent of changes in bronchopulmonary shunt flow, bronchomotor tone, or lung volume, along with the recent demonstration of the presence of numerous cholinergic terminals in intrapulmonary arteries, suggest that vagal stimulation dilates the pulmonary vascular bed by releasing acetylcholine from postganglionic cholinergic terminals. The transmitter then acts on muscarinic receptors in pulmonary vessels.[52]

The results of the present study indicate that the vagus in the midcervical region in the cat carries efferent fibers innervating lung vessels, which have adrenergic and cholinergic terminals, and that, in order to demonstrate a vasodilator response to vagal stimulation, it is necessary to interfere with the integrity of the adrenergic nerves and to enhance vasoconstrictor tone, since the pulmonary vascular bed has little, if any, vasoconstrictor tone under resting conditions.[40,41,50] The physiological significance of the cholinergic dilator system is uncertain at resting tone (FIO_2 0.21) conditions. However, when vasoconstrictor tone is elevated by ventilatory hypoxia (FIO_2 0.10), the present data show that this neurogenic system could produce significant vasodilation. In addition to hypoxic vasoconstriction, pulmonary vascular resistance is increased by prostaglandins and thromboxane A_2 in a number of pulmonary disorders, including endotoxin shock and embolism.[5,16,83] The present data suggest that, in pathophysiological states in which tone is elevated by $PGF_{2\alpha}$ or thromboxane A_2, the neurogenic cholinergic vasodilator system could produce marked unloading of the right ventricle, since the actions of U46619 closely mimic those of thromboxane A_2.[8]

In all previously discussed experiments in which a vasodilator response to vagal stimulation was described, 6-hydroxydopamine was used to destroy the integrity of adrenergic terminals. To determine whether the vasodilator response to vagal stimulation could be demonstrated when adrenergic neuronal activity is inhibited with another neuronal blocking agent, the effects of reserpine were investigated. Reserpine also impairs adrenergic transmission by depleting nerve terminal stores of norepinephrine.[42,85] In animals pretreated with reserpine, vagal stimulation and intralobar acetylcholine injections caused significant decreases in lobar arterial pressure, and these responses were greatly enhanced when lobar vascular resistance was increased to a high steady level with U46619. When lobar vascular resistance was increased by the thromboxane analog, U46619, decreases in lobar arterial pressure in response to vagal stimulation and acetylcholine became frequency- and dose-dependent. However, in reserpine-pretreated animals, decreases in lobar arterial pressure in response to vagal stimulation were significantly smaller than in 6-hydroxydopamine-treated animals when lobar vascular resistance was increased to comparable levels during infusion of U46619. The explanation for the difference in magnitude of response to vagal stimulation in 6-hydroxydopamine and reserpine-pretreated animals is uncertain. However, responses to acetylcholine were similar in both groups of animals, suggesting that the difference may be related to the extent of adrenergic neuronal blockade achieved with the two agents in these experiments.

Results of the present study demonstrate that efferent vagal stimulation can elicit both vasoconstrictor and vasodilator responses in the feline pulmonary vascular bed. Moreover, when the integrity of the adrenergic nerves to the lung was destroyed and vasoconstrictor tone was elevated, vagal stimulation caused marked frequency-dependent decreases in pulmonary vascular resistance. Injections of acetylcholine also dilated the pulmonary vascular bed, and responses to vagal stimulation and acetylcholine were blocked by atropine and enhanced by physostigmine. Vasodilator responses to vagal stimulation were not dependent on changes in bronchomotor tone and lung volume, or changes in aortic pressure and bronchopulmonary shunt flow. The present studies indicate that stimulation of cholinergic fibers in the vagus releases acetylcholine, which acts on muscarinic receptors to dilate the pulmonary vascular bed. Studies with hexamethonium, a ganglionic blocking agent, suggest that the feline pulmonary vascular bed is well supplied with functional cholinergic terminals whose preganglionic fibers travel in the cervical vagus. The ability of acetylcholine to dilate pulmonary vessels may be dependent on the integrity of the endothelial cell layer and changes in the concentration of intracellular cyclic GMP.[55]

The observations in this study indicate clearly that acetylcholine-elicited relaxation of phenylephrine-precontracted rings of bovine intrapulmonary artery possessing an unrubbed intimal surface is accompanied by increases in arterial cyclic GMP but not cyclic AMP levels. Acetylcholine produced a time- and concentration-dependent accumulation of arterial cyclic GMP, which correlated well with relaxation. Moveover, the findings that both atropine and methylene blue inhibited not only relaxation but also arterial cyclic GMP accumulation are consistent with the close association of elevated cyclic GMP levels and intrapulmonary arterial relaxation.

The inhibition by atropine of the increase in cyclic GMP levels in response to acetylcholine provides evidence in support of a link between muscarinic receptors and cyclic GMP accumulation. We have previously demonstrated that methylene blue inhibits (1) the activity of soluble guanylate cyclase prepared from vascular smooth muscle,[29,30,33] (2) vascular cyclic GMP accumulation elicited by nitrogen oxide-containing vasodilators,[32,44] and (3) vascular smooth muscle relaxation caused by the above vasodilators.[29,30,31,44] Similarly, in the present study the inhibitory effect of methylene blue on acetylcholine-stimulated cyclic GMP accumulation is likely the result of the inhibition of guanylate cyclase activity. These observations point to a muscarinic receptor-mediated increase in arterial cyclic GMP formation by acetylcholine.

Acetylcholine elevates cyclic GMP levels in a variety of tissues including smooth muscle in a calcium-dependent manner.[25,55,72] The inability of many investigators to demonstrate significant activation of soluble or particulate guanylate cyclase by acetylcholine and related agents indicates that the stimulation of tissue cyclic GMP formation occurs by an indirect mechanism. Elevated intracellular concentrations of calcium probably do not directly stimulate cyclic GMP formation because micromolar concentrations of calcium markedly inhibit soluble guanylate cyclase activity.[31] Furchgott et al.[23] have forwarded the hypothesis that acetylcholine-mediated arterial relaxation is caused indirectly by the formation of a lipoxygenase metabolite or arachidonic acid in endothelial cells, which interacts with the adjacent smooth muscle to cause relaxation. The latter view was based on the observations that atropine, quinacrine (a phospholipase A_2 inhibitor), and ETYA (an inhibitor of both cyclooxygenase and lipoxygenase) antagonized the relaxant effect of acetylcholine, whereas indomethacin (a cyclooxygenase inhibitor) did not.

Several observations, however, appear to be inconsistent with a mediator effect of an endothelium-derived lipoxygenase metabolite of arachidonic acid on intrapulmonary arterial cyclic GMP accumulation caused by acetylcholine. At concentrations that antagonized relaxation by acetylcholine, quinacrine failed to inhibit arterial cyclic GMP accumulation. In addition, endothelium-damaged intrapulmonary arterial rings that contracted to acetylcholine also displayed a marked accumulation of cyclic GMP and the latter response was unaltered by quinacrine, whereas contraction was partially inhibited. Quinacrine is a nonspecific agent and possesses multiple actions. For example, quinacrine has been reported to inhibit guanylate cyclase activity and interfere with certain direct effects of added cyclic GMP on specific cellular functions.[26] Moreover, a recent study showed that quinacrine was less effective than indomethacin or meclofenamate in inhibiting phospholipase A_2 activity in rat aorta.[78] Nonspecific effects were evident also in the present study. Concentrations of quinacrine (20–50 µM) just in excess of those (5–10 µM) that inhibited relaxation by acetylcholine also markedly inhibited arterial contractions to phenylephrine and KCl. Even low concentrations (2–10 µM) of quinacrine inhibited arterial contraction elicited by acetylcholine. The observations that atropine and methylene blue nearly abolished relaxation and cyclic GMP accumulation whereas quinacrine partially inhibited only relaxation in response to acetylcholine suggest that the latter is a nonspecific effect of quinacrine.

Definitive conclusions cannot be drawn until selective inhibitors of lipoxygenase and phospholipase A_2 become available for study. In addition, a lipoxygenase metabolite must be identified and demonstrated to stimulate cyclic GMP accumulation and cause relaxation of endothelium-damaged vessels. It may not be as important to show that such a metabolite directly activates guanylate cyclase because this activation, if it occurs, may be an indirect effect. In view of our findings that concentrations of quinacrine that inhibited acetylcholine-elicited relaxation failed to influence cyclic GMP accumulation, it is conceivable also that an endothelium-derived factor other than an arachidonic acid metabolite could be responsible for the stimulation of arterial cyclic GMP accumulation in bovine intrapulmonary artery. Moreover, an endothelium-derived factor is not obligatory for acetylcholine-mediated increases in cyclic GMP formation because acetylcholine markedly increased cyclic GMP levels in endothelium-damaged arteries which contracted in response to acetylcholine.

The observations that both arterial cyclic GMP accumulation and relaxation elicited by acetylcholine were antagonized by atropine are consistent with the possibility that cyclic GMP mediates muscarinic receptor-linked relaxation of intrapulmonary arterial smooth muscle. Additional evidence for this view derives from the findings that methylene blue, an inhibitor of vascular soluble guanylate cyclase[29,30,33] inhibited both cyclic GMP accumulation and relaxation caused by acetylcholine. More definitive conclusions regarding a "mediator" role of cyclic GMP in acetylcholine-elicited vascular smooth muscle relaxation, however, awaits further experimentation.

Acetylcholine is well known to contract certain endothelium-damaged arterial segments. Earlier reports indicated that vascular cyclic GMP accumulation accompanied arterial contraction caused by acetylcholine.[2,7,16,72] Similarly, in the present study, acetylcholine contracted endothelium-damaged rings of intrapulmonary artery and stimulated the arterial accumulation of cyclic GMP. Atropine nearly abolished both responses, suggesting that muscarinic receptors in vascular smooth muscle are linked to cyclic GMP formation. On the other hand, methylene blue abolished the increase in cyclic GMP levels but potentiated the contractions elicited by acetylcholine. The latter observations are similar to those recently reported by Kukovetz et al.[54,55] These findings indicate clearly that methylene blue is not a muscarinic receptor antagonist because this agent enhanced contractions to acetylcholine while abolishing cyclic GMP accumulation. Methylene blue also enhanced contractile responses to phenylephrine. Moreover, methylene blue significantly lowered resting arterial levels of cyclic GMP. These observations suggest that maintaining low arterial concentrations of intracellular cyclic GMP, a known vascular smooth muscle relaxant,[64,73] could result in enhanced contractile responses.

The findings that acetylcholine increases cyclic GMP levels in both endothelium-intact and endothelium-damaged intrapulmonary artery, whereas the former undergoes relaxation and the latter undergoes contraction, could be taken as evidence to dissociate arterial relaxation from cyclic GMP accumulation. However, several explanations of these seemingly divergent observations are possible. In the absence of a functioning endothelium, muscarinic receptor activation may elicit a more pronounced increase in calcium ion concentrations in vascular smooth muscle, resulting in a contractile response that overrides any potential relaxant response attributable to the concomitant accumulation of cyclic GMP. In addition, although acetylcholine-mediated increases in tissue cyclic GMP levels are a calcium-dependent process,[25,55,72] this calcium effect is most likely indirect because elevated concentrations of calcium directly inhibit guanylate cyclase activity.[31] In the presence of an intact endothelium, the mechanism by which acetylcholine causes relaxation instead of contraction may be attributed to the generation of an unknown endothelium-derived relaxing factor which stimulates cyclic GMP formation without appreciably elevating intracellular calcium ion concentrations. Indeed, it is more reasonable to suspect that calcium concentrations would be lowered. In this regard, it is noteworthy that nitrogen oxide-containing vasodilators stimulate cyclic GMP formation by a calcium-independent mechanism,[51,74] and these vasodilators as well as cyclic GMP appear to relax vascular smooth muscle in a calcium-independent manner.[59] In a recent report, Lincoln[59] showed that reducing the concentration of calcium in vascular smooth muscle results in the enhancement of relaxation by sodium nitroprusside and 8-bromo-cyclic GMP. Alternative explanations are not ruled out, including the possibility that the apparently close association between acetylcholine-elicited cyclic GMP accumulation and relaxation is merely fortuitous. Clearly, additional experiments are essential to establish directly that cyclic GMP mediates relaxation. Attention should now be focused, perhaps, on biochemical events linking cyclic GMP to relaxation, assuming that such a link exists.

In summary, responses to vagal stimulation, acetylcholine, catecholamines, and sympathetic nerve stimulation were investigated in the feline pulmonary vascular bed under conditions of controlled pulmonary blood flow and constant left atrial pressure. Under baseline conditions, electrical stimulation of vagal efferent fibers, sympathetic nerve stimulation, and norepinephrine increased lobar arterial pressure in a frequency- and dose-related fashion, whereas, acetylcholine produced modest decreases in lobar arterial pressure. When pulmonary tone was enhanced, vagal stimulation produced a depressor response. The pressor response to vagal stimulation under baseline conditions and the depressor response under enhanced tone conditions were blocked by phenoxybenzamine and atropine. When pulmonary vascular tone is enhanced and alpha receptors blocked, norepinephrine and sympathetic nerve stimulation caused dose- and frequency-dependent decreases in pulmonary vascular resistance. The decreases in pulmonary vascular resistance in response to norepinephrine and sympathetic nerve stimulation were not altered by atropine but were blocked with propranolol. Under conditions of enhanced tone, selective beta-1 receptor atagonists had little effect on vasodilator responses to isoproterenol, whereas responses to this substance were blocked by propranolol. These data suggest that, in the cat, the vagus is composed of efferent fibers from both the sympathetic and parasympathetic systems. Furthermore, these results suggest the presence of alpha- and beta-2 adrenoreceptors in the feline pulmonary vascular bed and that both types of adrenergic receptors are innervated by the sympathetic nervous system.[63] Selective alpha-1 and alpha-2 receptor agonists produced dose-related increases in lobar arterial pressure under baseline conditions, suggesting the presence of both alpha-1 and aphpa-2 receptor subtypes which, when activated, may produce a vasoconstrictor response in the pulmonary vascular bed.

After chemical sympathectomy with 6-hydroxydopamine, vagal stimulation and acetylcholine caused frequency- and dose-related decreases in lobar arterial pressure when pulmonary vascular resistance was actively enhanced. Depressor responses to vagal stimulation and acetylcholine in 6-hydroxydopamine-treated animals were blocked by atropine and enhanced by physostigmine. Decreases in lobar arterial pressure in response to vagal stimulation in 6-hydroxydopamine-treated animals with enhanced tone were blocked by hexamethonium, whereas responses to injected acetylcholine were not altered by the ganglionic blocking agent. Decreases in lobar arterial pressure in response to vagal stimulation and acetylcholine were similar when the lung was ventilated and when the left lower lobe bronchus was obstructed. The present data also suggest that the feline pulmonary vascular bed is functionally innervated by cholinergic nerves and that vagal stimulation has the potential to dilate the pulmonary vascular bed when vasomotor tone is enhanced.

The present study also provides some evidence that muscarinic receptor stimulation is linked both to arterial cyclic GMP accumulation and relaxation. In contrast, vascular smooth muscle contraction is readily dissociated from acetylcholine-stimulated cyclic GMP accumulation. Consistent with the observations of others, muscarinic receptor-mediated relaxation of arterial smooth muscle is dependent on the presence of a functioning endothelium.[6,15,22,23] Moreover, the good correlation between cyclic GMP accumulation and relaxation elicited by either acetylcholine or nitrogen oxide-containing vasodilators is consistent with the hypothesis that cyclic GMP mediates vascular smooth muscle relaxation.[3,29,32,43,44,54] Muscarinic receptor-mediated stimulation of cyclic GMP formation and relaxation of bovine intrapulmonary artery appear to be dependent on an endothelium-derived factor, as originally proposed for other arterial beds by Furchgott and co-workers.[22,23] However, the nature of this endothelium-derived factor remains unknown. Resolution of this problem necessitates the isolation and unequivocal identification of this factor.

Acknowledgments

The authors wish to express our appreciation to Ms. Janice Ignarro for the excellent editorial assistance. The authors' research presented in this publication was supported in part by NIH grants HL11802, HL15580, HL18070, AM17692, HL29456, and HL27713.

REFERENCES

1. Adler-Graschinsky, E. and Langer, S.Z.: Possible role of a β-adrenoreceptor in the regulation of noradrenaline release by nerve stimulation through a positive feedback mechanism. *Br. J. Pharmacol.* 53:43–50, 1975.
2. Andersson, R., Nilsson, K., Wikberg, J., et al.: Cyclic nucleotides and the contraction of smooth muscle. *Adv. Cyclic Nucleotide Res.* 5:491–518, 1975.
3. Axelsson, K.L., Wikberg, J.E.S., and Andersson, R.G.G.: Relationship between nitroglycerin, cyclic GMP and relaxation of vascular smooth muscle. *Life Sci.* 24: 1779–1786, 1979.
4. Bevan, J.A.: Some bases of differences in vascular responses to sympathetic activity. *Circ. Res.* 45:161–171, 1979.
5. Casey, L.C., Fletcher, J.R., Zmudka, M.I., et al.: Prevention of endotoxin-induced pulmonary hypertension in primates by the use of a selective thromboxane synthetase inhibitor, OKY–1581. *J. Pharmacol. Exp. Ther.* 222:441–446, 1982.
6. Chand, N. and Altura, B.M.: Acetylcholine and bradykinin relax intrapulmonary arteries by acting on endothelial cells: Role in lung vascular diseases. *Science* 213: 1376–1379, 1981.
7. Clyman, R.I., Sandler, J.A., Manganiello, V.C., et al: Guanosine 3′,5′-monophosphate and adenosine 3′,5′-monophosphate content of human umbilical artery. *J. Clin. Invest.* 55:1020–1025, 1975.
8. Coleman, R.A., Humphrey, P.P.A., Kennedy, I., et al.: Comparison of the actions of U–46619, a prostaglandin H_2 analog, with those of prostaglandin H_2 and thromboxane A_2 on some isolated smooth muscle preparations. *Br. J. Pharmacol.* 73: 773–778, 1981.

9. Daly, I.D. and Hebb, C.O.: Bronchomotor and pulmonary arterial pressure responses to nerve stimulation. *Q. J. Exp. Physiol.* 31:211–226, 1942.

10. Daly, I.D. and Hebb, C.O.: Pulmonary vasomotor fibers in the cervical vago-sympathetic nerve of the dog. *Q. J. Exp. Physiol.* 37:19–43, 1952.

11. Daly, I.D. and Hebb, C.O.: *Pulmonary and Bronchial Vascular Systems.* London, Edward Arnold Ltd., 1966.

12. Daly, I.D., Ramsay, D.J., and Waaler, B.A.: The site of action of nerves in the pulmonary vascular bed in the dog. *J. Physiol. (Lond.)* 209:317–339, 1970.

13. Dawes, G.S. and Mott, J.C.: The vascular tone of the foetal lung. *J. Physiol. (Lond.)* 146:465–477, 1962.

14. Dawes, P.M. and Faulkner, D.C.: The effect of propranolol on vascular responses to sympathetic nerve stimulation. *Br. J. Pharmacol.* 53:517–524, 1975.

15. De Mey, J.G., Claeys, M., and Vanhoutte, P.M.: Endothelium-dependent inhibitory effects of acetylcholine, adenosine triphosphate, thrombin and arachidonic acid in the canine femoral artery. *J. Pharmacol. Exp. Ther.* 222:166–173, 1982.

16. Demling, R., Gee, M., and Flynn, J.: Changes in lung vascular permeability and lung lymph prostaglandins after endotoxin in sheep. *Am. Rev. Respir. Dis.* 121:429–436, 1980.

17. Doeherty, J.R. and McGrath, J.C.: An examination of factors in influencing adrenergic transmission in the pithed rat, with special reference to noradrenaline uptake mechanisms and postjunctional α-adrenoceptors. *Naunyn-Schmiedeberg's Arch. Pharmacol.* 313:101–111, 1980.

18. Dunham, E.W., Haddox, M.K., and Goldberg, N.D.: Alteration of vein cyclic 3′,5′-nucleotide concentrations during changes in contractility. *Proc. Natl. Acad. Sci. USA* 71:815–819, 1974.

19. Eckstein, J.W. and Abbound, F.M.: Circulatory effects of sympathomimetic animals. *Am. Heart J.* 63:119–135, 1962.

20. Fillenz, M.: Innervation of pulmonary and bronchial blood vessels of the dog. *J. Anat.* 196:449–461, 1970.

21. Fishman, W.: Clinical pharmacology of the new beta-adrenergic blocking drugs. Part I. Pharmacodynamics and pharmacokinetic properties. *Am. Heart J.* 97: 663–670, 1979.

22. Furchgott, R.F. and Zawadzki, J.V.: The obligatory role of endothelial cells in the relaxation of arterial smooth muscle by acetylcholine. *Nature (Lond.)* 288:373–376, 1980.

23. Furchgott, R.F., Zawadzki, J.V., and Cherry, P.D.: Role of endothelium in the vasodilator response to acetylcholine. In *Vasodilation.* New York, Raven Press, pp. 49–66, 1981.

24. Glick, G., Epstein, S.E., Wechsler, A.S., et al.: Physiological differences between the effects of neuronally released and blood borne norepinephrine on beta adrenergic receptors in the arterial bed of the dog. *Circ. Res.* 21:217–227, 1967.

25. Goldberg, N.D. and Haddox, M.K.: Cyclic GMP metabolism and involvement in biological regulation. *Ann. Rev. Biochem.* 46:823–896, 1977.

26. Greenberg, R.N., Guerrant, R.L., Chang, B., et al.: Inhibition of Escherichia coli heat-stable enterotoxin effects on inteatinal guanylate cyclase and fluid secretion by quinacrine. *Biochem. Pharmacol.* 31:2005–2009, 1982.

27. Greenway, C.V., Lawson, A.E., and Stark, R.D.: Vascular responses of the spleen to nerve stimulation during normal and reduced blood flow. *J. Physiol. (Lond.)* 194: 421–433, 1968.

28. Greenway, C.V. and Lawson, A.E.: β-Adrenergic receptors in the hepatic arterial bed of the anesthetized cat. *Can. J. Physiol. Pharmacol.* 47:415–419, 1969.

29. Gruetter, C.A., Barry, B.K., McNamara, D.B., et al.: Relaxation of bovine coronary artery and activation of coronary arterial guanylate cyclase by nitric oxide, nitroprusside and carcinogenic nitrosoamine. *J. Cyclic Nucleotide Res.* 5:211–224, 1979.

30. Gruetter, C.A., Barry, B.K., McNamara, D.B., et al: Coronary arterial relaxation and guanylate cyclase activation by cigarette smoke, N'-nitrosonornicotine and nitric oxide. *J. Pharmacol. Exp. Ther.* 214:9–15, 1980.

31. Gruetter, D.Y., Gruetter, C.A., Barry, B.K., et al.: Activation of coronary arterial guanylate cyclase by nitric oxide, nitroprusside and nitrosoguanidine inhibition by calcium, lanthanum and other cations, enhancement by thiols. *Biochem. Pharmacol.* 29:2943–2950, 1980.

32. Gruetter, C.A., Gruetter, D.Y., Lyon, J.E., et al.: Relationship between cyclic GMP formation and relaxation of coronary arterial smooth muscle by glyceryl trinitrate, nitroprusside, nitrite and nitric oxide: Effects of methylene blue and methemoglobin. *J. Pharmacol. Exp. Ther.* 219:181–186, 1981.

33. Gruetter, C.A., Kadowitz, P.J., and Ignarro, L.J.: Methylene blue inhibits coronary arterial relaxation and guanylate cyclase activation by nitroglycerin, sodium nitrite and amyl nitrite. *Can. J. Physiol. Pharmacol.* 59:150–156, 1981.

34. Gruetter, C.A., McNamara, D.B., Hyman, A.L., et al.: Contractile effects of a PGH_2 analog and PGD_2 on intrapulmonary vessels. *Am. J. Physiol.* 234:H139–H145, 1978.

35. Hauge, A., Lunde, P.K.M., and Waaler, B.A.: Effect of prostaglandin E_1 and adrenaline on the pulmonary vascular resistance (PVR) in isolated rabbit lungs. *Life Sci.* 6:673–680, 1967.

36. Hawthorn, M.H. and Broadley, K.J.: Evidence from use of neuronal uptake inhibition that β_1 adrenoceptors, but not β_2 adrenoceptors, are innervated. *J. Pharm. Pharmacol.* 34:664–666, 1982.

37. Hebb, C.: Motor innervation of the pulmonary blood vessels of mammals. In *Pulmonary Circulation and Interstitial Space.* Chicago, University of Chicago Press, pp. 195–222, 1959.

38. Hyman, A.L.: The direct effects of vasoactive agents on pulmonary veins. Studies of responses to acetylcholine, serotonin, histamine and isoproterenol in intact dogs. *J. Pharmacol. Exp. Ther.* 168:96–105, 1969.

39. Hyman, A.L., Knight, D.S., Joiner, P.D., et al.: Bronchopulmonary arterial shunting without anatomic anastomosis in the dog. *Circ. Res.* 37:285–298, 1975.

40. Hyman, A.L. and Kadowitz, P.J.: Pulmonary vasodilator activity of prostacyclin (PGI_2) in the cat. *Circ. Res.* 45:404–409, 1979.

41. Hyman, A.L., Nandiwada, P., Knight, D.S., et al.: Pulmonary vasodilator responses to catecholamines and sympathetic nerve stimulation in the cat: Evidence that vascular beta-2 adrenoreceptors are innervated. *Circ. Res.* 48:407–415, 1981.

42. Iggo, A. and Vogt, M.: Preganglionic sympathetic activity in normal and in reserpine-treated cats. *Br. J. Pharmacol.* 150:114–133, 1960.

43. Ignarrro, L.J., Gruetter, C.A., Hyman, A.L., et al.: Molecular mechanisms of vasodilatation. *Dopamine Receptor Agonists.* New York, Plenum Press, 1983.

44. Ignarro, L.J., Lippton, H., Edwards, J.C., et al.: Mechanism of vascular smooth muscle relaxation by organic nitrates, nitrites, nitroprusside and nitric oxide: Evidence for the involvement of S-nitrosothiols as active intermediates. *J. Pharmacol. Exp. Ther.* 218:739–749, 1981.

45. Ingram, R.H., Szidon, J.F., Skalak, R., et al.: Effects of sympathetic nerve stimulation on the pulmonary arterial tree of the isolated lobe perfused in situ. *Circ. Res.* 22:801–815, 1968.

46. Kadowitz, P.J., Joiner, P.D., and Hyman, A.L.: Differential effects of phentolamine and bretylium on pulmonary vascular responses to norepinephrine and nerve stimulation. *Proc. Soc. Exp. Biol. Med.* 144:172–176, 1973.

47. Kadowitz, P.J. and Hyman, A.L.: Effect of sympathetic nerve stimulation on pulmonary vascular resistance in the dog. *Circ. Res.* 32:221–227, 1973.

48. Kadowitz, P.J., Joiner, P.D., and Hyman, A.L.: Influence of sympathetic stimulation and vasoactive substances on the canine pulmonary veins. *J. Clin. Invest.* 56:354–365, 1975.

49. Kadowitz, P.J., Knight, D.S., Hibbs, R.G., et al.: Influence of 5- and 6-hydroxydopamine on adrenergic transmission and nerve terminal morphology in the canine pulmonary vascular bed. *Circ. Res.* 39:191–199, 1976.
50. Kadowitz, P.J., Nandiwada, P., Gruetter, C.A., et al.: Pulmonary vasodilator responses to nitroprusside and nitroglycerin in the dog. *J. Clin. Invest.* 67:893–902, 1981.
51. Katsuki, S. and Murad, F.: Regulation of adenosine cyclic 3',5'-monophosphate and guanosine cyclic 3',5'-monophosphate levels and contractility in bovine tracheal smooth muscle. *Mol. Pharmacol.* 13:330–341, 1977.
52. Knight, D.S., Ellison, P.J., Hibbs, G.R., et al.: A light and electron microscopic study of the innervation of pulmonary arteries in the cat. *Anat. Rec.* 201:513–521, 1981.
53. Kostrzewa, R.M. and Jacobowitz, D.M.: Pharmacological actions of 6-hydroxydopamine. *Pharmacol. Rev.* 18:619–629, 1974.
54. Kukovetz, W.R., Holzmann, S., Wurm, A., et al.: Evidence for cyclic GMP-mediated relaxant effects of nitro-compounds in coronary smooth muscle. *Naunyn-Schmiedeberg's Arch. Pharmacol.* 310:129–138, 1979.
55. Kukovetz, W.R., Scholz, N., and Paietta, E.: Influence of extracellular Ca^{2+} on acetylcholine-induced changes in cyclic nucleotides and tone of smooth muscle. *Naunyn-Schmiedeberg's Arch. Pharmacol.* 294(R):13, 1976.
56. Lands, E.M., Arnold, A., McAuliff, J.P., et al.: Differentiation of receptor systems activated by sympathomimetic amines. *Nature (Lond.)* 214:597–598, 1967.
57. Langer, S.Z., Massingham, R., and Shepperson, N.B.: Presence of postsynaptic α_2-adrenoceptors of predominantly extrasynaptic location in the vascular smooth muscle of the dog hindlimb. *Clin. Sci.* 59:225s–228s, 1980.
58. Lertora, J.J.L., Mark, A.L., Johannsen, U.J., et al.: Selective beta-1 receptor blockade with oral practolol in man. *J. Clin. Invest.* 56:719–725, 1975.
59. Lincoln, T.M.: Effects of nitroprusside and 8-bromo-cyclic GMP on the contractile activity of the rat aorta. *J. Pharmacol. Exp. Ther.* 224:100–107, 1983.
60. Lock, J.E., Hamilton, F., Luide, H., et al.: Direct pulmonary vascular responses in the conscious newborn lamb. *Am. J. Physiol.* 48:188–196, 1980.
61. Lundvall, J. and Jarhult, J.: Beta adrenergic micro-vascular dilation evoked by sympathetic stimulation. *Acta Physiol. Scand.* 92:572–574, 1974.
62. Lundvall, J. and Jarhult, J.: Beta adrenergic dilator component of the sympathetic vascular response in skeletal muscle. Influence on the micro-circulation and on transcapillary exchange. *Acta Physiol. Scand.* 96:180–192, 1976.
63. Nandiwada, P.A., Hyman, A.L., and Kadowitz, P.J.: Pulmonary vasodilator responses to vagal stimulation and acetylcholine in the cat. *Circ. Res.* 53(1):86–95, 1983.
64. Napoli, S.A., Gruetter, C.A., Ignarro, L.J., et al.: Relaxation of bovine coronary arterial smooth muscle by cyclic GMP, cyclic AMP and analogs. *J. Pharmacol. Exp. Ther.* 212:469–473, 1980.
65. Ngai, S.H., Rosell, S., and Wallenberg, L.R.: Nervous regulation of blood flow in the subcutaneous adipose tissue in dogs. *Acta Physiol. Scand.* 68:397–403, 1966.
66. Pegram, B.L., Bevan, R.D., and Bevan, J.A.: Facial vein of the rabbit: Neurogenic vasodilation mediated by β-adrenergic receptors. *Circ. Res.* 39:854–860, 1976.
67. Porcelli, R.J. and Bergofsky, E.: Adrenergic receptors in pulmonary vasoconstrictor responses to gaseous and humoral agents. *J. Appl. Physiol.* 34:483–488, 1973.
68. Regoli, D., Mizrahi, J., D'Orleans-Juste, P., et al.: Effects of kinins on isolated blood vessels: Role of endothelium. *Can. J. Physiol. Pharmacol.* 60:1580–1583, 1982.
69. Rosell, S. and Belfrage, E.: Adrenergic receptors in adipose tissue and their relation to adrenergic innervation. *Nature (Lond.)* 253:738–739, 1975.
70. Rudolph, A.M. and Scarpelli, E.M.: Drug action on pulmonary circulation of unanesthetized dogs. *Am. J. Physiol.* 206:1201–1206, 1964.
71. Russell, M.P. and Moran, N.C.: Evidence for lack of innervation of β-2 adrenoreceptors in the blood vessels of the gracilis muscle of the dog. *Circ. Res.* 46:344–352, 1980.

72. Schultz, G., Hardman, J.G., Schultz, K., et al.: The importance of calcium ions for the regulation of guanosine 3',5'-cyclic monophosphate levels. *Proc. Natl. Acad. Sci. USA* 70:3889–3893, 1973.
73. Schultz, K.D., Bohme, E., Kreye, V.A.W., et al.: Relaxation of hormonally stimulated smooth muscular tissues by the 8-bromo derivative of cyclic GMP. *Naunyn-Schmiedeberg's Arch. Pharmacol.* 306:1–9, 1979.
74. Schultz, K.D., Schultz, K., and Schultz, G.: Sodium nitroprusside and other smooth muscle relaxants increase cyclic GMP levels in rat ductus deferens. *Nature (Lond.)* 265:750–751, 1977.
75. Shibata, S., Kuchii, M., and Kurahashi, K.: The supersensitivity of isolated rabbit atria and aortic strips produced by 6-hydroxydopamine. *Eur. J. Pharmacol.* 18:271–280, 1972.
76. Silvone, E.D., Inoue, T., and Grover, R.F.: Comparison of hypoxia, pH and sympathomimetic drugs on bovine pulmonary vasculature. *J. Appl. Physiol.* 24:355–365, 1968.
77. Snedecor, G.W. and Cochran, W.G.: *Statistical Methods*, 6th ed. Ames, Iowa: The Iowa State University Press, 1967.
78. Thakkar, J.K., Sperelakis, N., Pang, D., et al.: Characterization of phospholipase A_2 activity in rat aorta smooth muscle cells. *Biochim. Biophys. Acta* 750:134–140, 1983.
79. Tainter, M.L. and Chang, D.K.: The antagonism of the pressor action of tyramine by cocaine. *J. Pharmacol. Exp. Ther.* 30:193–207, 1927.
80. Timmermans, P.B.M.W.M. and Van Zwieten, P.A.: Vasoconstriction mediated via postsynaptic α_2-adrenoceptor stimulation. *Naunyn-Schmiedeberg's Arch. Pharmacol.* 313:17–20, 1980.
81. Trendelenburg, U., Muskus, A., Fleming, W.W., et al.: Modification by reserpine of the action of sympathomimetic amines. *J. Pharmacol. Exp. Ther.* 138:170–180, 1962.
82. Tucker, A.: Pulmonary and systemic vascular responses to vasoactive agents after chemical sympathectomy. *Proc. Soc. Exp. Biol. Med.* 163:534–539, 1980.
83. Utsunomiya, T., Krauz, M.M., Levine, L., et al.: Thromboxane mediation of cardiopulmonary effects of embolism. *J. Clin. Invest.* 70:361–368, 1982.
84. Verity, M.A. and Bevan, J.A.: Fine structural study of the terminal factor plexus: Neuromuscular relationships in the pulmonary artery. *J. Anat.* 103:49–63, 1968.
85. Viveros, O.H., Arqueros, L., Connet, R.J., et al.: Mechanism of secretion from the adrenal medulla. IV. The fate of the storage vesicles following insulin and reserpine administration. *Mol. Pharmacol.* 5:69–82, 1969.
86. Yamaguchi, N., DeChamplain, J., and Nadeau, R.A.: Regulation of norepinephrine release from cardiac sympathetic fibers in the dog by presynaptic α- and β-receptors. *Circ. Res.* 41:108–117, 1977.

CHAPTER 5

Lung Peptides and the Pulmonary Circulation

Richard D. Dey and
Sami I. Said

Introduction

A large number of biologically active peptides have been identified and characterized in recent years. Although many were originally isolated from brain or gastrointestinal tissues, their presence in other organs is now well recognized.[101] These peptides exert an important regulatory influence on neural, endocrine, cardiovascular, respiratory, and other systemic functions. The importance of peptides in biological systems is underscored by their wide presence not only in mammals but also in lower vertebrates, notably in amphibians and primitive invertebrates.[24] The occurrence of vasoactive peptides in the lung was documented during the late 1960s in three separate reports demonstrating that lung extracts contained preformed vasoactive peptides[100] and that the pulmonary circulation was capable of both activating[79] and degrading[29] circulating vasoactive peptides.

An increasing number of peptides have now been detected and measured by radioimmunoassay in extracts of lung tissue.[90,102,103,108] These peptides are either (a) synthesized, stored, and released by specific lung cells, or (b) circulating peptides that are enzymatically altered during transit through the pulmonary circulation. The first category includes adrenocorticotrophic hormone, bombesin and gastrin-releasing peptide, calcitonin, cholecystokinin, complement, eosinophil chemotactic peptides, neuropeptide Y, opioid peptides, peptide histidine isoleucine and peptide histidine methionine (PHI/PHM), somatostatin, substance P (SP), spasmogenic lung peptide, and vasoactive intestinal peptide (VIP). Peptides that are metabolized in the lung include bradykinin, which is inactivated, and angiotensin I, which is activated into angiotensin II, in pulmonary endothelium.

Localization of Lung Peptides

Immunocytochemical techniques reveal that, in the lung, VIP, PHI/PHM, SP, neuropeptide Y, and somatostatin occur primarily in nerves, while bombesin

From Said, S.I. (ed.): *The Pulmonary Circulation and Acute Lung Injury.* Mount Kisco, N.Y., Futura Publishing Co., Inc., 1985.

(or the bombesin-like peptide GRP) and calcitonin are present predominately in epithelial endocrine cells.[3,16,18,20,90,103] Judging from observations in other organs, however, the same peptides are likely to be found in both nerves and endocrine cells.[101] Eosinophil chemotactic peptides are stored in mast cells,[41] and angiotensin II is formed in endothelial cells. The localizations of other peptides have not been fully determined.

It should be noted that the demonstration by radioimmunoassay or immunohistochemistry of a given peptide immunoreactivity does not establish the presence of that particular peptide; only its isolation and chemical characterization does. Large variations in the content of certain peptides have been noted between fetal, neonatal, and adult lungs,[34] as well as between different species.[24,33] Results to date, however, suggest that among peptides in the lung, VIP and substance P are present in larger concentrations than all others.[90]

Autonomic Innervation of the Lung and Neuropeptides: The Peptidergic System of Nerves

Autonomic nerves supplying the lung were described by early pulmonary anatomists.[26,31,51,113] More recent neuroanatomical and neurophysiological studies of the lung usually include a thorough discussion of the contributions of adrenergic and cholinergic nerves to pulmonary innervation.[76,77,95] Our knowledge of peptide-containing nerves in the lung, however, has emerged within the past decade, especially during the past 5 years. As a result of this recent information, descriptions of autonomic and sensory nerves supplying pulmonary structures must be expanded to include peptidergic, as well as adrenergic and cholinergic, components of pulmonary innervation.

The lung is supplied by motor nerves that comprise the sympathetic and parasympathetic divisions of the autonomic nervous system and by sensory nerves that originate primarily from sensory ganglia of the vagus nerve, but may also arise from dorsal root ganglia. There is evidence that some peptides may occur in sympathetic nerve fibers, but the relationship of peptides to sympathetic nerves in the lung has not been fully examined. On the other hand, peptides are also present in both preganglionic and postganglionic nerve fibers of the parasympathetic nerves as well as in peripheral projections of sensory nerves.[62,64] Figure 1 outlines the possible distribution of sensory and parasympathetic innervation of the lung in relation to two well-established neural peptides, VIP and SP.

The sensory nerves, with nerve cell bodies located mainly in the vagal ganglia, especially the nodose ganglion, project axons into the lung that terminate on blood vessels, bronchi, cartilage, and other structures (Fig. 1). These fibers are in part responsible for the afferent limb of reflexes that carry impulses from irritant, stretch, and chemoreceptors in the lung to the central nervous system.[10,11,128] The parasympathetic system is composed of preganglionic neurons located in the brain stem (primarily the dorsal motor nucleus of cranial nerve X and the nucleus ambiguus) and postganglionic neurons arising from the intrapulmonary ganglia present in the adventitia and submucosa of the airways. The preganglionic nerve fibers project axons to the lung along the vagus nerve and terminate at the postganglionic neurons. The postganglionic axons innervate vascular and bronchial smooth muscle and bronchial glands. This general pattern of sensory and parasympathetic innervation is supported by

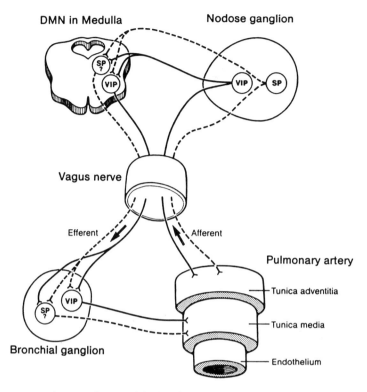

Figure 1: *Diagram showing the possible distribution of VIP- (solid lines) and SP- (dashed lines) containing nerves to the pulmonary vasculature. For description see text. Question marks in the SP-containing neurons of the dorsal motor nucleus (DMN) and bronchial ganglion indicate that the occurrence of this peptide has not been confirmed at these locations.*

recent neuroanatomical evidence using retrograde transport of horseradish peroxidase.[17,46,125]

Groups of sensory and motor nerve fibers within the lung travel together in bundles located in the adventitia of larger bronchi and blood vessels. Separate nerve fibers containing different neuropeptides may terminate in close proximity to one another in the same structure. As an example, Figure 2 demonstrates the close relationship between VIP- and SP-containing nerve terminals around the same pulmonary blood vessel.

Pulmonary Endocrine Cells and Neuroepithelial Bodies

The possible existence of endocrine and paracrine systems in the lung that regulate pulmonary function was originally proposed by Feyrter in 1938,[30] after observing "clear cells" (Helle Zellen system) located within the airway epithelium and elsewhere in the body. These are probably the same cells that were subsequently called Kultchitsky (or Argentaffin) cells.[4] The presence of dense-core secretory vesicles in pulmonary endocrine cells[14,28,52,53] and their ability to decarboxylate biogenic amine precursors to corresponding

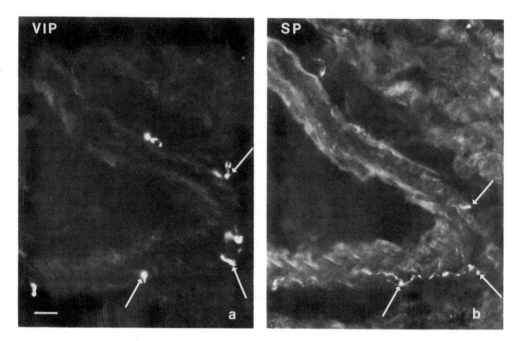

Figure 2: *Two adjacent serial sections of the same pulmonary artery in dog lung demonstrating nerve fibers containing VIP* **(a)** *or SP* **(b)**. *Several locations around the vessel (arrows) are innervated by both VIP- and SP-containing fibers. Scale = 10 μm.*

amines[14,21,22] suggested that these cells were also part of the APUD (amine precursor uptake and decarboxylation) system of peptide-producing endocrine cells described by Pearse in the 1960s.[86,87] Since then, four peptides have been demonstrated in lung endocrine cells: bombesin,[126] calcitonin,[3] leu-enkephalin,[16] and somatostatin.[18] Pulmonary endocrine cells occurring in clusters and called neuroepithelial bodies have been described by Lauweryns and found to contain the biogenic amine 5-hydroxytryptamine (5HT or sero-tonin).[18,21,22,52,53] Morphologic evidence that neuroepithelial bodies are innervated and that they release 5HT during hypoxia has led to the speculation that the liberated 5HT may mediate hypoxic vasoconstriction.[54]

Pulmonary Mast Cells

Mast cells in the lung are present in the adventitia of pulmonary blood vessels, in the submucosal loose connective tissue of bronchi, and within the airway epithelium. In addition to histamine, heparin, and a host of bioactive lipids and proteins, mast cells contain and release several peptides, including the eosinophilic chemotactic peptides.[58] Murine mast cells have also been shown to contain and release VIP together with the histamine.[15]

Pulmonary Endothelium

The formation of angiotensin II from angiotensin I and the inactivation of bradykinin take place in pulmonary endothelium, through the action of angiotensin-converting enzyme (kininase II) (see Chapter 3 of this book).

Brief Comments on Peptides that are Formed or Metabolized by the Lung

Adrenocorticotropic Hormone (ACTH)

This adenohypophyseal hormone, also found in the brain and in gastrointestinal organs, was reported present in extracts of human bronchial tumors and in nontumorous lung tissue from chronic smokers.[32,131] ACTH was later found in normal porcine lung.[9] In a recent immunocytochemical study of lung from human subjects, no ACTH-containing cells were observed in normal fetal, newborn, or adult lung, but such cells were present in lungs with chronic fibrotic disease.[121] Conditions that induce hyperplasia of pulmonary endocrine cells in culture, e.g., administration of the carcinogen nitrosamine, are associated with increased ACTH content in these cells.[60]

Angiotensin II

Angiotensin II, generated in pulmonary endothelium by activation of angiotensin I, is a potent constrictor of systemic vessels. Inhibition of angiotensin II generation (i.e., of angiotensin-converting enzyme activity) has been reported to reduce pulmonary arterial pressure and vascular resistance in man.[80] Angiotensin II also contracts tracheobronchial tree and gastrointestinal smooth muscle.[102,103] The possible regulatory significance of angiotensin II in the lung remains unknown.

Bombesin

Bombesin is a 14-residue peptide originally isolated from frog skin.[5] Bombesin-like immunoreactivity has been demonstrated in pulmonary endocrine cells (Fig. 3) and in extracts of human fetal lungs.[16,91,126] The 27-

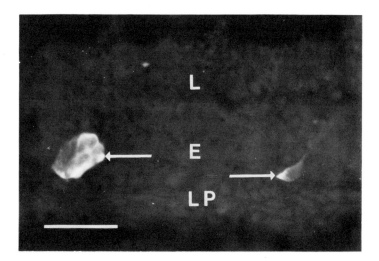

Figure 3: *Bombesin-immunoreactive cells (arrows) in the bronchial epithelium (E) from a human fetal lung. The cells occur both in groups (left) and as single cells (right). LP = lamina propria; L = bronchial lumen containing amorphous material. Scale = 50μm.*

residue gastrin-releasing peptide (GRP) may be the mammalian counterpart of bombesin.[72] Recent biochemical and immunocytochemical evidence indicates that the bombesin-like peptide in human fetal lung is more similar to porcine GRP than to amphibian bombesin.[91,121]

Bradykinin

Bradykinin may be formed in the lung through the action of activated kallikrein on tissue kininogens.[27] A potent systemic vasodilator and vaso-depressor, bradykinin contracts certain smooth muscles (e.g., those of airways, stomach, and gall bladder) and relaxes others (e.g., rat colon).[43,108] Brady-kinin also increases systemic (including bronchial) vascular permeability, but its ability to increase pulmonary microvascular permeability is unproven. Bradykinin stimulates prostaglandin biosynthesis and release by a number of organs and tissues, including the lung.The released prostaglandins may mediate or accentuate some actions of bradykinin, including its contractile effect on isolated guinea pig trachea.[103] Kinin-like substances have been detected in respiratory tract secretions of human subjects with asthma, hay fever, and bronchitis.[25] There is also evidence that bradykinin may be involved in eliciting pulmonary reflexes by stimulating afferent vagal C-fibers in the airways.[47]

Calcitonin

Calcitonin has been localized in human pulmonary endocrine cells.[3] The calcitonin-containing endocrine cells in hamster lungs undergo hyperplasia after exposure to the carcinogen diethylnitrosamine.[61] The possible role of calcitonin in mammalian lung function is unknown; interestingly, the lung is the major source of serum calcitonin in lizards.[92]

Cholecystokinin (CCK)

CCK-like immunoreactivity and biologic activity have been demonstrated in lung extracts.[90,103] CCK is a gastrointestinal and neural peptide that occurs in several different molecular forms. Its actions, exhibited by even the smaller molecular forms, include contraction of tracheobronchial, gastrointestinal, and other smooth muscle, and stimulation of pancreatic enzyme secretion.

Complement

Complement fragment C5 is normally present in primate alveoli. As discussed later, complement activation can be an important factor in the production of acute lung injury.

Eosinophil Chemotactic Peptides

This family of peptides, formerly called eosinophil chemotactic factor (ECF), includes: the ECF-A tetrapeptides with a molecular weight of 300 to

400, and the ECF-oligopeptides with a molecular weight from 1,300 to 2,500.[58] The larger ECF-oligopeptide has been extracted from lung tissues, but its localization in lung mast cells has not been demonstrated. However, ECF is also present in peritoneal mast cells,[7] suggesting a similar location in the lung.

Leukotrienes

These biologically active products of arachidonic acid, via the lipoxygenase system, are in fact peptido-lipids.[109] The best known leukotrienes (LTs) are: LTC_4 and LTD_4, which are capable of inducing high-permeability pulmonary edema, as well as bronchoconstriction and pulmonary vasoconstriction in experimental animals, and LTB_4, which is particularly potent in attracting and aggregating granulocytes.[104]

Neuropeptide Y

This 36-amino acid residue peptide was originally isolated from porcine intestine[118] and is structurally similar to avian, bovine, and porcine pancreatic polypeptide.[118] In the lung, neuropeptide Y is present in nerve fibers of the bronchial smooth muscle and of blood vessels.[123] These fibers may be of sympathetic origin because neuropeptide Y is also present in nerve cell bodies of the superior cervical ganglion, and because dopamine-β-hydroxylase, an enzyme that characterizes adrenergic nerve terminals, can be colocalized with neuropeptide Y in the same nerve terminals of the nasal mucosa.[123] This colocalization has not been confirmed in the lung. The action of neuropeptide Y on the pulmonary vasculature has not been investigated, but this peptide constricts pial and peripheral blood vessels.[69]

Opioid Peptides

Endogenous opioid peptides, first discovered in the mid-1970s, are now recognized to belong to one of three genetically distinct peptide families. The three biosynthetic precursors are: the beta-endorphin/ACTH precursor (or pro-opiomelanocortin); proenkephalin; and prodynorphin.[1] These peptide systems have characteristic localization in the brain and peripheral organs.[78] Leu-enkephalin immunoreactivity has been demonstrated in endocrine cells of normal human lungs.[16] Met-enkephalin has also been found in rat lung[39] and β-endorphin in porcine lung.[9] Another enkephalin, Met^5-enkephalin-Arg^6-Phe^7, has also been demonstrated in pulmonary neuroendocrine cells.[116,117] The pulmonary content of this peptide is relatively high and it is released from lung tissue by depolarizing concentrations of K^+ through a Ca^{++}-dependent mechanism.[117]

PHI and PHM

PHI-27, a 27-amino acid residue peptide that closely resembles VIP and was named for its N-terminal histidine and C-terminal isoleucine, was first isolated from porcine intestine.[119] The peptide PHM-27, almost identical to PHI-27 but with a C-terminal methionine, is considered the human counterpart of PHI.[40] Both VIP and PHM are synthesized from the same mRNA as a single precursor molecule called preproVIP.[40]

PHI immunoreactivity is present in the same autonomic neurons containing VIP immunoreactivity; some of these neurons also contain the cholinergic neurotransmitter, acetylcholine. In the lung, the distribution of these neurons includes bronchial and vascular smooth muscle and bronchial glands.[70] Radio-immunoassay results show immunoreactive VIP and PHI in normal tissues to be present in a molar ratio of about 2:1. Since VIP and PHM are present on the same gene in a 1:1 ratio, the greater-than-expected VIP tissue levels suggest that selective expression of VIP or PHI from the common precursor may be controlled by post-translational processing.[6,70] Like VIP, PHI relaxes bronchial and peripheral vascular smooth muscle, but is several times less potent than VIP.[70]

Somatostatin

This 14-amino acid residue peptide, first discovered as a hypothalamic growth hormone-inhibiting factor, has been localized in endocrine (D) cells in the pancreas and gastrointestinal tract, as well as in neurons in the central and peripheral nervous systems. Somatostatin inhibits the release and actions of numerous peptide hormones and neurotransmitters. Its role in the lung, where it is present in relatively low concentrations,[18,90] has not been explored.

Substance P (SP)

Unlike VIP, which has been associated primarily with efferent nerves, SP has received considerable attention as a possible neurotransmitter released from afferent nerve terminals.[81] SP was originally discovered in extracts of brain and intestine as the substance responsible for atropine-resistant peripheral vasodilation and gut contraction.[124] In the lung, SP-containing nerve fibers are located predominantly around airway and vascular smooth muscle (Fig. 2b) and close to and within the bronchial epithelium.[65,82,127]

Much of the SP in the lung is probably contained in sensory nerve fibers. Using horseradish peroxidase techniques, nerve fibers have been traced from the lung, through the vagus nerve, to primary sensory neurons in the nodose ganglion.[46,112] Although SP-containing nerve fibers have not been directly traced from the nodose ganglion to the lung, sensory neurons in this ganglion contain SP and could conceivably project to the lung.[62] The presence of SP in sensory nerve fibers of the lung is suggested by the finding that ligation of the vagus nerve in guinea pigs results in a more than 50% reduction in the amount of SP immunoreactivity in the ipsilateral lung, as measured by radioimmuno-assay.[120] Vagus nerve ligation also reduces the number of SP-positive nerve fibers in the trachea and main stem bronchi.[68] Further, the occurrence of SP-containing nerve fibers in mammalian lungs is almost completely abolished after treatment with capsaicin,[65,68,115] which causes selective degeneration of primary afferent neurons.[41,42] SP has not been observed in neuronal cell bodies of intrapulmonary ganglia.[68,127] However, in view of the common embryological origin of the lung and the upper gastrointestinal tract, and the presence of SP in nerve cell bodies of the myenteric and submucosal plexuses,[111,112] the possibility that some of the SP-containing nerve fibers in the lung originate from intrapulmonary ganglia should not be prematurely abandoned. We now have preliminary evidence supporting this possibility: Figure 4 shows two SP-reactive nerve cell bodies located in an intrapulmonary ganglion from cat lung (Dey and Said, unpublished).

Spasmogenic Lung Peptide

This peptide, extracted from the lung during the purification of VIP,[107] is distinct from other peptides with smooth muscle contracting activity. It dilates peripheral systemic vessels but contracts airway, pulmonary vascular, and other smooth muscle, including rat stomach and colon and guinea pig gall gladder. Spasmogenic lung peptide remains to be fully characterized.

Vasoactive Intestinal Peptide (VIP)

Athough VIP was first isolated and purified from extracts of porcine intestine,[106] biological activity of VIP was originally detected in lung extracts,[100,105] and its presence in the lung was later confirmed by radio-immunoassay.[107] In the vasculature of the lung, VIP is present in nerve fibers and nerve terminals around pulmonary arteries (Fig. 2a) and, to a lesser extent, pulmonary veins.[20,122]

Physiological studies indicate that VIP-containing fibers are motor nerves. Therefore, these fibers probably originate from nerve cell bodies located in intrapulmonary ganglia (Fig. 1). However, immunocytochemical studies have demonstrated that VIP-containing sensory nerve cell bodies are also present in

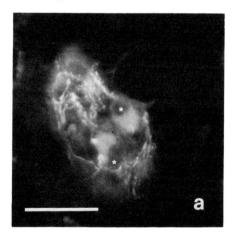
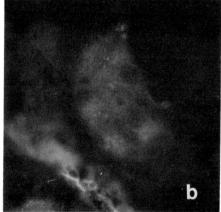

Figure 4: *Adjacent sections of a bronchial ganglion from cat lung. Two immunoreactive nerve cell bodies (*) are observed in the section incubated with antiserum to SP* **(a)**. *Specific fluorescence is not seen in the adjacent section incubated with the same antiserum absorbed with SP* **(b)**. *Scale = 25μm.*

the nodose ganglia and that VIP is transported peripherally in the vagus nerve.[62] Thus, the occurrence of VIP in the nodose ganglia and in pulmonary vagal fibers suggests a possibile sensory role for this peptide. The terminations of VIP-containing nerve fibers projecting to the lung from sensory neurons in the nodose ganglia have not been investigated. If present, their activation could conceivably affect pulmonary blood flow by reflex mechanisms.

In addition to its localization in nerve terminals, VIP is also present in mast cells of the lung and other tissues.[15]

Actions of Peptides in the Lung

Pulmonary Vascular Smooth Muscle

Among peptides occurring in the lung, angiotensin II, spasmogenic lung peptide, substance P and, to a lesser degree, bombesin, contract pulmonary vascular smooth muscle.[50,102-104,130] Although substance P may affect pulmonary vascular tone directly, the demonstrated sensory nature of substance P-containing nerve fibers in the lung suggests an involvement in pulmonary reflexes.[128] The direct effects of bombesin on pulmonary vascular tone are not impressive. Bombesin is a weak constrictor of pulmonary vascular smooth muscle strips in vitro,[108] and infusions of bombesin into lamb pulmonary artery have no measurable effect on pulmonary vascular resistance.[50]

VIP is the only peptide so far shown to relax pulmonary vessels. As a relaxant of cat or human pulmonary artery segments, VIP is many times as potent as prostacyclin.[37,99] VIP also exhibits pulmonary vasodilator activity in vivo in anesthetized cats, tending to reduce pulmonary arterial pressure while augmenting cardiac output.[74,104]

There is less information available on whether certain pulmonary peptides can also modify pulmonary vascular reactivity. Evidence for altered vascular reactivity (corresponding to airway reactivity) would include a shift of the concentration-response curve with a given pulmonary vasoconstrictor or vasodilator, upon addition of the peptide in question.

Bronchial Smooth Muscle

Bombesin, substance P, CCK, and the spasmogenic lung peptide are powerful constrictors of isolated guinea pig airways.[102-104] Substance P induces bronchoconstriction in other species as well.[35,63,65,82,115] On the other hand, VIP relaxes airway smooth muscle in several mammalian species in vitro and in vivo, and reduces or prevents the effect of bronchoconstrictor agents including histamine, prostaglandin $F_{2\alpha}$, and leukotriene D_4.[23,38] VIP also relaxes human bronchial segments in vitro and reduces airway constriction in asthmatic subjects when given as an aerosol.

Pulmonary Microvascular Permeability

Relatively little is known about the possible actions of various peptides of the lungs on pulmonary vascular endothelium. At present, it is known that *activated complement C5a* is capable of increasing pulmonary vascular permeability. This effect has been demonstrated in experimental models of acute lung injury where complement activation was induced by cobra venom or by IgG-containing immune complexes. The increased permeability promoted by activated complement is mediated in part by the participation of activated granulocytes and by the release of oxygen free radicals (see also Chapter 18 of this book).

The peptide-containing lipids, *leukotrienes,* especially LTC_4 and LTD_4, can also increase pulmonary microvascular permeability and thus induce pulmonary edema.[104]

It has been reported that *bradykinin,* together with hypoxia or prostaglandin E_2, can induce high-permeability pulmonary edema, though of a moderate degree.[85]

Whether any lung peptides may be able to protect pulmonary endothelium against increased permeability is at present unknown. Reports of such protection ascribed to prostaglandin E_1, prostacyclin, and β-adrenergic agonists suggest that a peptide such as VIP which, similar to these compounds, stimulates adenylate cyclase activity and dilates pulmonary vessels, may have a similar protective influence.

Bronchial Secretion

Both substance P and VIP have been reported to influence bronchial secretion. Substance P promotes glycoprotein secretion by canine airway mucosa,[2] by accelerating discharge, rather than synthesis, of mucus.[13,93] VIP stimulates tracheal submucosal gland secretion in the ferret,[88] but inhibits glycoconjugate secretion by explants of human airways.[12] Further, VIP also stimulates water and ion secretion by bronchial mucosa[42a] and by intestinal mucosa.[112a]

Peptide Receptors in the Pulmonary Vessels and Airways

Receptors for VIP have been detected in isolated rat lung membranes.[98] Autoradiographs of lung sections from dogs show specific binding of VIP in the smooth muscle layer of pulmonary arteries (Fig. 5), as well as in the bronchial epithelium and bronchial smooth muscle (Table I; Dey and Muntz, unpublished) and in the alveoli.[57] VIP receptors in lungs have also been demonstrated by an immunocytochemical technique based on the stimulation of cyclic AMP production that is triggered by VIP binding to its receptors.[55] The localization of stretch and irritant receptors in the bronchial epithelium and in bronchial and vascular smooth muscle parallels the distribution of substance P-containing nerve fibers in the lung. Stimulation of any of these receptors can dramatically affect cardiovascular and pulmonary function.[10,11,42]

Other peptide receptors have been shown to be present in the lung; these include PHI and opiate receptors.[110,129] A number of studies have demonstrated the occurrence of opiate receptors in extracts of lung tissue.[39,79,110] The 7-amino acid residue peptide, Met^5-enkephalin-Arg^6-Phe^7, has the highest affinity of several tested opioid substances.[117] The distribution of opiate receptors in relation to specific cell types in the lung has not been determined.

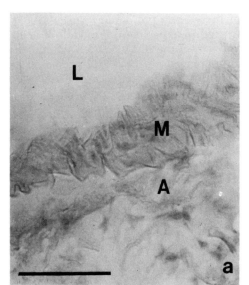
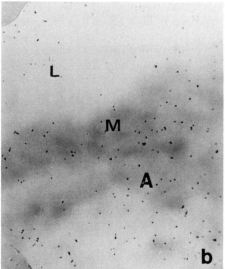

Figure 5: *Light micrographs of the same section of a dog pulmonary artery focusing on the tissue (a) or on the silver grains above the tissue (b). This section was incubated in I^{125}-labeled VIP (25 pmol) and then processed for autoradiography. The grains are preferentially distributed over the muscular (M) and adventitial (A) layers of the vessel wall. The number of grains over the same vessel in the adjacent section (not shown) was reduced by more than 50% after incubating in the same medium plus an excess of unlabeled VIP (See Table I). L = vessel lumen. Scale = 50μm.*

		Table I			
		Binding (grains/10 μm²)			
	n	**Total**	**Nonspecific**	**Specific**	**% Specific**
Blood Vessels	27	170	74	95	56
Epithelium	24	554	116	483	79
Bronchial Smooth Muscle	25	258	115	143	55

Receptor binding of I^{125}-labeled VIP determined by counting the number of grains over blood vessel walls, bronchial epithelium, and bronchial smooth muscle. The total binding represents the total grains/10μm² in a section incubated in 25 pmol of labeled VIP. Nonspecific binding was determined in the adjacent section incubated in the same medium plus excess cold VIP. Specific binding is then calculated by subtracting nonspecific from total binding, and % specific binding is calculated as the ratio of specific binding to total binding. Results from two sections (Dey and Muntz, unpublished).

Physiological Role of Lung Peptides in Relation to the Pulmonary Circulation

Pulmonary Vascular and Airway Smooth Muscle

The demonstration of certain vasoactive peptides (including VIP and substance P) within nerve fibers and nerve terminals innervating pulmonary vessels suggests the possibility that these neuropeptides may have a physiological influence on pulmonary vascular smooth muscle tone, either as direct neurotransmitters or as neuromodulators of other transmitters. Investigators of airway, gastrointestinal, and other smooth muscle have long recognized the existence of a component of relaxation that cannot be explained by either adrenergic or cholinergic transmission.[8,95,96] The existence of this nonadrenergic, noncholinergic component, considered the dominant relaxant influence in human airways, has never been explored in pulmonary vessels.

In order to investigate the possible importance of a nonadrenergic, noncholinergic relaxant (inhibitory) system in pulmonary vessels, we analyzed the responses of isolated strips of cat pulmonary artery to electrical field stimulation. The typical response was an initial, brief contraction, followed by a more sustained relaxation (the latter more evident if the resting tone has been raised by prostaglandin H_2 analog U-44069. The addition of phenoxybenzamine (α-adrenergic blockade) abolished the contraction. The addition of atropine (cholinergic muscarinic blockade) and propranolol (β-adrenergic blockade) moderately reduced the relaxation. Only tetrodotoxin (a neurotoxin) or lidocaine (local anesthetic) abolished or greatly attenuated the relaxation that is neither adrenergic nor cholinergic.[36]

The identity of the transmitter of nonadrenergic, noncholinergic relaxation of pulmonary vessels is at present unknown. One candidate transmitter for this system is VIP. It is the one pulmonary vasodilator neuropeptide known that is also present in nerves supplying pulmonary vessels, it has properties of a neurotransmitter or neuromodulator, and it is believed to be a likely transmitter of the same relaxant system in the airways, lower esophageal spincter, and other sites.[71] We are now investigating this possibility in field-stimulation experiments on isolated segments of cat and guinea pig pulmonary artery. In these experiments, atropine- and propranolol-resistant pulmonary arterial relaxation is correlated with VIP release, and the inhibition of this relaxation is attempted by the use of VIP antibodies.

Lung Development and Maturation

Recent observations suggest the possibility that bombesin may play a role in the development of the lung, including its vasculature. For instance, the number of bombesin-containing cells and the amount of bombesin-immunoreactivity measured chromatographically are higher in both fetal and neonatal lungs than in adult lungs.[34,126] In addition, there is a higher density of bombesin-immunoreactive cells in human newborns suffering from bronchopulmonary dysplasia than in newborns dying from nonpulmonary causes.[44] Abnormalities of the bombesin-containing endocrine cells may also be related to abnormal patterns of pulmonary vascular development associated with idiopathic pulmonary hypertension in the fetus and in the newborn.[90,94] Further, bombesin causes gastrin-cell hyperplasia in rats,[56] stimulates DNA synthesis and hyperplasia in cultured Swiss 3T3 cells,[98] and is consistently present in small-cell carcinoma of the lung where it may contribute to continued tumor growth.[75] Thus, the higher levels of bombesin in fetal lungs compared to adult lungs suggest that this peptide may help regulate normal growth and development in the fetal lung.

ACTH may play a direct role in lung maturation that is independent of cortisol-related effects. Thus, administration of ACTH increased pulmonary surfactant biosynthesis and improved lung compliance in hypophysectomized fetal sheep, while cortisol had no effect.[59]

The clinical observation that the incidence of respiratory distress syndrome is lower in infants of heroin-addicted mothers suggests a role for opioid peptides in lung maturation. Also, endorphin levels in amniotic fluid and fetal cord blood are increased during gestation.[132]

Factors regulating the biosynthesis, release, and metabolism of lung peptides are still largely unknown. The influence of hypoxia on angiotensin-converting enzyme activity—which governs the formation of angiotensin II and the breakdown of bradykinin—has been investigated, with conflicting results.[49,84,114]

Role of Lung Peptides in Acute Lung Injury

Pulmonary Microvascular Permeability

Of the different biologically active peptides present in the lung, only complement has been demonstrated unequivocally to participate in the mediation of increased pulmonary microvascular permeability.[102-104] This conclusion is based on the evidence that complement activation (C5a) leads to acute pulmonary edema, related to neutrophil aggregation and activation and the production of toxic oxygen metabolites (please refer to Chapter 18).

An extensive series of recent studies strongly supports the possibility that substance P released from sensory nerve terminals profoundly affects the permeability of blood vessels in the bronchial mucosa. Using Evans blue as a marker for vascular protein leakage, these studies have shown that either vagal nerve stimulation or mucosal injections of substance P increases vascular permeability and plasma extravasation in the tracheobronchial mucosa.[63,65] Furthermore, treating the tissue with a substance P-receptor antagonist reduced plasma extravasation significantly.[66] Also noteworthy is the finding that cigarette smoke-induced airway edema can be inhibited by applications of a substance P antagonist or by pretreatment with capsaicin.[67] Although these studies relate primarily to the capillary beds in the bronchial mucosa, a similar effect of substance P may exist in the pulmonary vessels. This possibility has not been investigated.

Pulmonary Vascular and Airway Constriction

Several peptides occurring in the lung have pulmonary vasoconstrictor and bronchoconstrictor properties (see above). The possible role of these peptides in mediating these changes in experimental or clinical conditions remains to be defined. Recently, Lundberg and co-workers showed that part of the contraction in bronchial smooth muscle observed during in vitro field stimulation is not affected by atropine, but is inhibited by a specific substance P-antagonist.[65,66] Furthermore, the increase in inflation pressure in the intact guinea pig lungs normally observed after intravenous substance P or after vagal nerve stimulation is blocked by prior treatment with the substance P-antagonist. In addition, capsaicin, a drug that depletes the substance P in nerve terminals, reduces the normal increase in inflation pressure after vagal nerve stimulation.[65,66] These results suggest that substance P may be released from nerve endings and act as a neurotransmitter mediating bronchial constriction.

Anaphylaxis and Acute Inflammation

Bradykinin is capable of increasing vascular permeability of systemic, but not pulmonary, vessels. When combined with hypoxia, however, bradykinin has been reported to induce moderate pulmonary edema.[85] The release of kallikreins and kallikrein precursors has been demonstrated in sensitized lungs following a challenge with appropriate antigens.[45] Recently, IgE-dependent release of a prekallikrein activating factor has been demonstrated in human lung fragments sensitized to ragweed pollen.[73] These findings suggest that kinins may be generated by lung tissues during IgE-mediated allergic responses through the production of a prekallikrein activator that converts inactive prekallikrein to an active kallikrein. Chemotactic peptides, including those attracting eosinophils and granulocytes, are among the mediators of anaphylaxis and acute inflammation.[19,48] The localization of VIP in mast cells suggests a possible role in modulating pulmonary vascular and airway tone during IgE-dependent immunological responses in the lung, such as immediate hypersensitivity, anaphylaxis, and allergic asthma.[58]

Systemic Shock

Enkephalins and endorphins participate in mediating the hypotension of endotoxemia and other forms of shock; opiate antagonists attenuate this hypotension.[1,83,89] Spasmogenic lung peptide and other peptides that constrict pulmonary vessels and airways may contribute to the pulmonary hypertension and airway constriction complicating acute lung injury.

Conclusion

A large number of peptide hormones and neurotransmitters have been discovered in normal and diseased lungs. Many of these peptides influence pulmonary vascular smooth muscle, tracheobronchial smooth muscle, pulmonary microvascular permcability, and the inflammatory response. Some of the lung peptides are localized in neurons, forming the peptidergic component of the autonomic nervous system; these peptides serve as neurotransmitters or neuromodulators. Other lung peptides are present mainly in endocrine cells or neuroepithelial bodies, and probably serve a local paracrine function. The localization of still other lung peptides remains uncertain. At least two peptides appear to have physiological roles in the regulation of pulmonary vascular (and bronchial) smooth muscle and possible other functions of the lung. Some lung peptides may also play a role in certain pulmonary vascular disorders, such as pulmonary edema and pulmonary hypertension. Exploration of the place of lung peptides in normal physiology and in lung disease is a major target of current and future research. An additional challenge for future research will be to understand how different lung peptides may interact together as well as with other, nonpeptide mediators in exerting their physiological and pathophysiological influence.

Acknowledgment

Supported in part by NIH research grant nos. HL30450 and HL31039, and by Veterans Administration medical research funds.

REFERENCES

1. Akil, H., Watson, S.J., Young, E., et al.: Endogenous opioids: Biology and function. *Ann. Rev. Neurosci.* 7:223-55, 1984.
2. Baker, A.P., Hillegass, L.M., Holden, D.A., et al.: Effects of kallidin, substance P, and other basic polypeptides on the production of respiratory macromolecules. *Am. Rev. Respir. Dis.* 115:811–817, 1977.
3. Becker, K.L., Monaghan, K.G., and Silva, O.L.: Immunocytochemical localization of calcitonin in Kulchitsky cells of human lung. *Arch. Pathol. Lab. Med.* 104: 196–198, 1980.
4. Bensch, K.G., Gordon, G.B., and Miller, L.R.: Studies on the bronchial counterpart of the Kulchitsky (Argentaffin) cell and innervation of bronchial glands. *J. Ultrastruct. Res.* 12:668–686, 1965.
5. Bertaccini, G.: Active polypeptides on nonmammalian origin. *Pharmacol. Rev.* 28:127–175, 1976.
6. Bishop, A.E., Polak, J.M., Yiangau, Y., et al.: The distribution of PHI and VIP in porcine gut and their co-localization to a proportion of intrinsic ganglion cells. *Peptides.* 5:255–259, 1984.
7. Bozwell, R.N., Austen, K.F., and Goetzl, E.J.: Intermediate molecular-weight eosinophil chemotactic factors in rat peritoneal mast cells: Immunologic release, granule association, and demonstration of structural heterogeneity. *J. Immunol.* 120:15–20, 1978.
8. Chesrown, S.E., Venugopalan, C.S., Gold, W.M., et al.: In vivo demonstration of nonadrenergic inhibitory innervation of the guinea pig trachea. *J. Clin. Invest.* 65:315–320, 1980.
9. Clements, J.A., Funder, J.W., Tracy, K., et al.: Adrenocorticotropin, β-endorphin, and β-lipotropin in normal thyroid and lung: Possible implications for ectopic hormone secretion. *Endocrinology.* 111:2097–2102, 1982.
10. Coleridge, H.M., Coleridge, J.C.G., and Kidd, C.: Role of the pulmonary arterial baroreceptors in the effects produced by capsaicin in the dog. *J. Physiol. (London)* 170:272–285, 1964.
11. Coleridge, H.M., Coleridge, J.C.G., Dangel, A., et al.: Impulses in slowly conducting vagal fibers from afferent endings in the veins, atria, and arteries of dogs and cats. *Circ. Res.* 33:87–97, 1973.
12. Coles, S.J., Said, S.I., and Reid, L.M.: Inhibition by VIP of glycoconjugate and lysozyme secretion by human airways in vitro. *Am. Rev. Respir. Dis.* 124:531–536, 1981.
13. Coles, S.J., Neill, K.H., and Reid, L.M.: Substance P and related peptides induce glycoprotein release by canine airway mucosa. *Fed. Proc.* 43:828, 1984.
14. Cutz, E., Chan, W., Wong, V., et al.: Ultrastructural and fluorescence histochemistry of endocrine (APUD-type) cells in tracheal mucosa of human and various animal species. *Cell. Tiss. Res.* 158:425–437, 1975.
15. Cutz, E., Chan, W., Track, N.S., et al.: Release of vasoactive intestinal polypeptide in mast cells by histamine liberators. *Nature* 275:661–662, 1978.
16. Cutz, E., Chan, W., and Track, N.S.: Bombesin, calcitonin, and leu-enkephalin immunoreactivity in endocrine cells of human lung. *Experientia* 37:765–767, 1981.

17. Dalsgaard, C.-J. and Lundberg, J.M.: Evidence for a spinal afferent innervation of the guinea pig lower respiratory tract as studied by the horseradish peroxidase technique. *Neurosci. Letters* 45:117−122, 1984.
18. Dayer, A.M., Rademakers, A., DeMey, J., and Will, J.A.: Serotonin, bombesin, and somatostatin-like immunoreactivity in neuroepithelial bodies (NEBs) of rhesus monkey fetal lung. *Fed. Proc.* 43:880, 1984.
19. Desai, U., Kruetzer, D.L., Showell, H., et al.: Acute inflammatory pulmonary reactions induced by chemotactic factors. *Am. J. Path.* 96:71, 1979.
20. Dey, R.D., Shannon, W.A., Jr., and Said, S.I.: Localization of VIP-immuno-reactive nerves in airways and pulmonary vessels of dogs, cats, and human subjects. *Cell Tiss. Res.* 220:231−238, 1981.
21. Dey, R.D., Echt, R., and Dinerstein, R.J.: Morphology, histochemistry, and distribution of serotonin-containing cells in tracheal epithelium of adult rabbit. *Anat. Rec.* 199:23−31, 1981.
22. Dey, R.D., Shannon, W.A., Jr., Hagler, H.K., et al.: Histochemical and ultrastructural characterization of serotonin-containing cells in rabbit tracheal epithelium. *J. Histochem. Cytochem.* 31:501−508, 1983.
23. Diamond, L., Szarek, J.L., Gillespie, M.N., et al.: In vivo bronchodilator activity of VIP in the cat. *Am. Rev. Respir. Dis.* 128:827−832, 1983.
24. Dockray, G.J.: Evolutionary relationships of the gut hormones. *Fed. Proc.* 38: 2295−2301, 1979.
25. Dolovitch, J., Back, N., and Arbesman, C.E.: Kinin-like activity in nasal secretions of allergic patients. *Int. Arch. Allergy Appl. Immunol.* 38:337−344, 1970.
26. Elftman, A.G.: The afferent and parasympathetic innervation of the lungs and trachea of the dog. *Am. J. Anat.* 72:1−27, 1943.
27. Erdös, E.G.: Kininases. In *Handbook of Experimental Pharmacology,* Vol. 25 (suppl.). Erdös, E.G., ed. Berlin, Springer-Verlag, 1979, pp.427−487.
28. Ericson, E., Håkanson, R., Larson, B., et al.: Fluorescence and electron microscopy of amine-storing enterochromaffin-like cells in tracheal epithelium of mouse. *Z. Zellforsch.* 124:532−545, 1972.
29. Ferreira, S.H. and Vane, J.R.: The disappearance of bradykinin and eledoisin in the circulation and vascular beds of the cat. *Br. J. Pharmacol. Chemother.* 30: 417−424, 1967.
30. Feyrter, F.: *Über Diffuse Endokrine Epitheliale Organe.* Leipzig, J.A. Barth, 1938.
31. Gaylor, J.B.: The intrinsic nervous mechanism of the human lung. *Brain* 57: 143−160, 1934.
32. Gerwitz, G. and Yalow, R.S.: Ectopic ACTH production in carcinoma of the lung. *J. Clin. Invest.* 53:1022−1032, 1974.
33. Ghatei, M.A., Sheppard, M.N., O'Shaughnessy, D.J., et al.: Regulatory peptides in the mammalian respiratory tract. *Endocrinology.* 111:1248−1254, 1982.
34. Ghatei, M.A., Sheppard, M.N., Henzen-Logman, S., et al.: Bombesin and vaso-active intestinal polypeptide in the developing lung: Marked changes in acute respiratory distress syndrome. *J. Clin. Endocrinol. Metab.* 57:1226−1232, 1983.
35. Grunstein, M.M., Tanaka, D.T., and Grunstein, J.S.: Mechanism of substance P induced bronchoconstriction in maturing rabbit. *J. Appl. Physiol.: Respir. Environ. Exercise Physiol.* 57:1238−1264, 1984.
36. Hamasaki, Y. and Said, S.I.: Evidence for a nonadrenergic, noncholinergic inhibitory nervous system in cat pulmonary artery. *Clin. Res.* 29:550A, 1981.
37. Hamasaki, Y., Mojarad, M., and Said, S.I.: Relaxant action of VIP on cat pulmonary artery: comparison with acetylcholine, isoproterenol, and PGE_1. *J. Appl. Physiol.: Respir. Environ. Exercise Physiol.* 54:1607−1611, 1983.
38. Hamasaki, Y., Saga, T., Mojarad, M., et al.: VIP counteracts leukotriene D_4-induced contractions of guinea pig trachea, lung and pulmonary artery. *Trans. Assoc. Am. Physicians* 96:406−411, 1983.
39. Hughes, J., Kosterlitz, H.W., and Smith, T.W.: The distribution of methionine-

enkephalin and leucine-enkephalin in the brain and peripheral tissues. *Br. J. Pharmacol.* 61:639–647, 1977.

40. Itoh, N., Obata, K., Yanihara, N., et al.: Human prepro-vasoactive intestinal polypeptide contains a novel PHI-27-like peptide, PHM-27. *Nature* 304:547–549, 1983.

41. Jancso, G., Kiraly, E., and Jancso-Gabor, A.: Pharmacologically induced selective degeneration of chemosensitive primary sensory neurones. *Nature* 270: 741–743, 1977.

42. Jancso, G. and Such, G.: Effects of capsaicin applied perineurally to the vagus nerve on cardiovascular and respiratory functions in the cat. *J. Physiol.* 341: 359–370, 1983.

42a. Nathanson, I., Widdicombe, J.H., and Barnes, P.J.: Effect of vasoactive intestinal peptide on ion transport across dog tracheal epithelium. *J. Appl. Physiol.: Respir. Environ. Exercise Physiol.* 55(6):1844–1848, 1983.

43. Johnson, A.R.: Effects of kinins on organ systems. In *Handbook of Experimental Pharmacology,* Vol. 25 (suppl.). Erdös, E.G., ed. Springer-Verlag, Berlin, 1979, pp. 357–399.

44. Johnson, D.E., Lock, J.E., Elde, R.P., et al.: Pulmonary neuroendocrine cells in hyaline membrane disease and bronchopulmonary dysplasia. *Pediatr. Res.* 16: 446–454, 1982.

45. Jonasson, O. and Becker, E.L.: Release of kallikrein from guinea pig lung during anaphylaxis. *J. Exp. Med.* 123:509–522, 1966.

46. Kalia, M. and Mesulam, M.-M.: Brainstem projections of sensory and motor components of the vagus complex in the cat. II. Laryngeal, tracheobronchial, pulmonary, cardiac, and gastrointestinal branches. *J. Comp. Neurol.* 193: 467–508, 1980.

47. Kaufman, M.P., Coleridge, H.M., Coleridge, J.C.G., et al.: Bradykinin stimulates afferent vagal C-fibers in intrapulmonary airways of dogs. *J. Appl. Physiol.: Respir. Environ. Exercise Physiol.* 48:511–517, 1980.

48. Kay, A.B. and Austen, K.F.: The IgE-mediated release of an eosinophil leukocyte chemotactic factor from human lung. *J. Immunol.* 107:899–902, 1971.

49. Krulewitz, A.H. and Fanburg, B.L.: The effect of oxygen tension on the in vivo production and release of angiotensin-converting enzyme by bovine pulmonary artery endothelial cells. *Am. Rev. Respir. Dis.* 130:866–869, 1984.

50. Kulik, T.J., Johnson, D.E., Elde, R.P., et al.: Pulmonary vascular effects of bombesin and gastrin-releasing peptide in conscious newborn lambs. *J. Appl. Physiol: Respir. Environ. Exercise Physiol.* 55:1093–1097, 1983.

51. Larsell, O. and Dow, R.S.: The innervation of the human lung. *Am. J. Anat.* 52:125–146, 1933.

52. Lauweryns, J.M., Coklaere, M., and Theunynck, P.: Serotonin-producing neuro-epithelial bodies in rabbit respiratory mucosa. *Science* 180:410–413, 1973.

53. Lauweryns, J.M., Coklaere, M., Theunynck, P., et al.: Neuroepithelial bodies in mammalian respiratory mucosa: Light optical, histochemical, and ultrastructural studies. *Chest* 65:22S-29S, 1974.

54. Lauweryns, J.M., Coklaere, M., Deleersnyder, M., et al.: Intrapulmonary neuro-epithelial bodies in newborn rabbits: Influence of hypoxia, hyperoxia, hypercapnia, nicotine, reserpine, L-DOPA, and 5-HTP. *Cell Tiss. Res.* 182:425–440, 1977.

55. Lazarus, S.C., Basbaum, C.B., Barnes, P.J., et al.: Mapping of vasoactive intestinal peptide (VIP) receptors using cyclic AMP (cAMP) immunocytochemistry. *Am. Rev. Respir. Dis.* 127(4) (part 2):274, 1983.

56. Lehy, T., Accary, J.P., LaBeille, D., et al.: Chronic administration of bombesin stimulates antral gastrin-cell proliferation in the rat. *Gastroenterology* 84:914–919, 1983.

57. Leroux, P., Vaudry, H., Fournier, A., et al.: Characterization and localization of vasoactive intestinal peptide receptors in the rat lung. *Endocrinology* 114: 1506–1512, 1984.

58. Lewis, R.A. and Austen, K.F.: Nonrespiratory functions of pulmonary cells: The mast cell. *Fed. Proc.* 36:2676–2683, 1977.

59. Liggins, G.C., Kitterman, J.A., Campos, G.A., et al.: Pulmonary maturation in the hypophysectomized ovine fetus: Differential responses to adrenocorticotropin and cortisol. *J. Dev. Physiol.* 3:1–14, 1981.

60. Linnoila, R.I., Nettesheim, R., and DiAugustine, R.P.: Lung endocrine-like cells in hamsters treated with diethylnitrosamine: Alterations in vivo and in cell culture. *Proc. Natl. Acad. Sci.* 78:5170–5174, 1981.

61. Linnoila, R.I., Becker, K.L., Silva, O.L., et al.: Calcitonin as a marker for diethylnitrosamine-induced pulmonary endocrine cell hyperplasia in hamsters. *Lab. Invest.* 51:39–45, 1984.

62. Lundberg, J.M., Hökfelt, T., Nilsson, G., et al.: Peptide neurons in the vagus, splanchnic, and sciatic nerves. *Acta Physiol. Scand.* 104:499–501, 1978.

63. Lundberg, J.M. and Saria, A.: Capsaicin-sensitive vagal neurons involved in control of vascular permeability in rat trachea. *Acta Physiol. Scand.* 115:521–523, 1982.

64. Lundberg, J.M., Hökfelt, T., Änggård, A., et al.: Organizational principles in the peripheral sympathetic nervous system: Subdivision by coexisting peptides (somatostatin-, avian pancreatic polypeptide-, vasoactive intestinal polypeptide-like immunoreactive materials). *Proc. Natl. Acad. Sci.* 79:1303–1307, 1982.

65. Lundberg, J.M., Brodin, E., and Saria, A.: Effects and distribution of vagal capsaicin-sensitive substance P neurons with special reference to the trachea and lungs. *Acta Physiol. Scand.* 119:243–252, 1983.

66. Lundberg, J.M., Saria, A., Brodin, E., et al.: A substance P antagonist inhibits vagally induced increase in vascular permeability and bronchial smooth muscle contraction in the guinea pig. *Proc. Natl. Acad. Sci.* 80:1120–1124, 1983.

67. Lundberg, J.M., Martling, C.-R., Saria, A., et al.: Cigarette smoke-induced airway edema due to activation of capsaicin-sensitive vagal afferents and substance P release. *Neuroscience* 10:1361–1368, 1983.

68. Lundberg, J.M., Hökfelt, T., Martling, C.-R., et al.: Substance P-immunoreactive sensory nerves in the lower respiratory tract of various mammals including man. *Cell Tiss. Res.* 235:251–261, 1984.

69. Lundberg, J.M. and Tatemoto, K.: Pancreatic polypeptide family (APP, BPP, NPY, and PYY) in relation to sympathetic constriction resistant to α-adreno-receptor blockade. *Acta Physiol. Scand.* 116:393–402, 1982.

70. Lundberg, J.M., Fahrenkrug, J., Hökfelt, T., et al.: Co-existence of peptide HI (PHI) and VIP in nerves regulating blood flow and bronchial smooth muscle tone in various mammals including man. *Peptides* 5:593–606, 1984.

71. Matsuzaki, Y., Hamasaki, Y., and Said, S.I.: Vasoactive intestinal peptide: A possible transmitter of nonadrenergic relaxation of guinea pig airways. *Science* 210:1252–1253, 1980.

72. McDonald, T.J., Jörnvall, H., Nilsson, G., et al.: Characterization of a gastrin-releasing peptide from porcine non-antral gastric tissue. *Biochem. Biophys. Res. Comm.* 90:227–233, 1979.

73. Meier, H.L., Kaplan, A.P., Lichtenstein, L.M., et al.: Anaphylactic release of a prekallikrein activator from human lung in vitro. *J. Clin. Invest.* 72:574–581, 1983.

74. Mojarad, M. and Said, S.I.: Vasoactive intestinal peptide (VIP) dilates pulmonary vessels in anesthetized cats. *Am. Rev. Respir. Dis.* 123:239, 1981.

75. Moody, T.W., Pert, C.B., Gazdar, A.F., et al.: High levels of intracellular bombesin characterize human small-cell lung carcinoma. *Science* 214:1246–1248, 1981.

76. Nadel, J.A. and Barnes, P.J.: Autonomic regulation of the airways. *Ann. Rev. Med.* 35:451–467, 1984.

77. Nagaishi, C.: *Functional Anatomy and Histology of the Lung.* Baltimore, University Park Press, 1972.

78. Neidle, A., Manigault, I., and Wajda, I.J.: Distribution of opiate-like substances in rat tissues. *Neurochem. Res.* 4:399–410, 1979.

79. Ng, K.K.F. and Vane, J.R.: The conversion of angiotensin I to angiotensin II. *Nature* 216:762–766, 1967.

80. Niarchos, A.P., Roberts, A.J., and Laragh, J.H.: Effects of the converting enzyme inhibitor (SQ 20881) on the pulmonary circulation in man. *Am. J. Med.* 67: 785–791, 1979.

81. Nicoll, R.A., Schenker, C., and Leeman, S.E.: Substance P as a transmitter candidate. *Ann. Rev. Neurosci.* 3:227–68, 1980.

82. Nilsson, G., Dahlberg, K., Brodin, E., et al.: Distribution and constrictor effect of substance P in guinea pig tracheobronchial tissue. In *Substance P*. von Euler, U.S., Pernow, B., eds. New York, Raven Press, 1977, pp. 75–81.

83. Olson, G.A., Olson, R.D., and Kastin, A.J.: Endogenous opiates: 1983. *Peptides.* 5:975–992, 1984.

84. Oparil, S., Winternitz, S., Gould, V., et al.: Effect of hypoxia on the conversion of angiotensin I to II in the isolated perfused rat lung. *Biochem. Pharmacol.* 31:1375–1379, 1982.

85. O'Brodovich, H.M., Stalcup, S.A., Pang, L.M., et al.: Bradykinin production and increased pulmonary endothelial permeability during acute respiratory failure in unanesthetized sheep. *J. Clin. Invest.* 67:512–522, 1981.

86. Pearse, A.G.E.: Common cytochemical and ultrastructural characteristics of cells producing polypeptide hormones (the APUD series) and their relevance to thyroid and ultimobranchial C cells and calcitonin. *Proc. Roy. Soc. B.* 170:71–80, 1968.

87. Pearse, A.G.E.: The cytochemistry and ultrastructure of polypeptide hormone-producing cells of the APUD series and the embryologic, physiologic, and pathologic implications of the concept. *J. Histochem. Cytochem.* 17:303–313, 1969.

88. Peatfield, A.D., Barnes, P.J., Bratcher, C., et al.: VIP stimulates tracheal submucosal gland secretion in ferret. *Am. Rev. Respir. Dis.* 128:89–93, 1983.

89. Peters, W.P., Johnson, M.W., Friedman, P.A., et al.: Pressor effect of naloxone in septic shock. *Lancet* I:529, 1980.

90. Polak, J.M. and Bloom, S.R.: Regulatory peptides: Localization and measurement. In *The Endocrine Lung in Health and Disease*. Becker, K.L., Gazdar, A., eds. Philadelphia, W.B. Saunders, 1984, pp. 300–327.

91. Price, J., Penman, E., Bourne, G.L., et al.: Characterization of bombesin-like immunoreactivity in human fetal lung. *Regul. Peptides* 7:315–322, 1983.

92. Ravazzola, M., Orci, L., Girgus, S.I., et al.: The lung is the major organ source of calcitonin in the lizard. *Cell Biol. Internatl. Rep.* 5:937–944, 1981.

93. Reid, L.M. and Coles, S.J.: The bronchial epithelium of humans. In *The Endocrine Lung In Health and Disease*. Becker, K.L., Gazdar, A.F., eds. Toronto, W.B. Saunders Co., 1984, pp. 56–78.

94. Rendas, A., Brown, E.R., Avery, M.E., et al.: Prematurity, hypoplasia of the pulmonary vascular bed, and hypertension: Fatal outcome in a ten-month-old infant. *Am. Rev. Respir. Dis.* 121:873–880, 1980.

95. Richardson, J.B.: Nerve supply to the lungs. *Am. Rev. Respir. Dis.* 119:785–802, 1979.

96. Richardson, J. and Beland, J.: Nonadrenergic inhibitory nervous system in human airways. *J. Appl. Physiol.* 41:764–771, 1976.

97. Robberecht, P., Chatelain, P., de Neef, P., et al.: Presence of vasoactive intestinal peptide receptors coupled to adenylate cyclase in rat lung membranes. *Biochem. Biophys. Acta* 678:76–82, 1981.

98. Rozengurt, E. and Sinnett-Smith, J.: Bombesin stimulation of DNA synthesis and cell division in cultures of Swiss 3T3 cells. *Proc. Natl. Acad. Sci.* 80:2936–2940, 1983.

99. Saga, T. and Said, S.I.: Vasoactive intestinal peptide relaxes isolated strips of

human bronchus, pulmonary artery, and lung parenchyma. *Trans. Assoc. Am. Physicians* (In press).

100. Said, S.I.: Vasoactive substances in the lung. In *Proceedings of the Tenth Aspen Emphysema Conference,* Aspen, Colorado, June 7–10, 1967. US Public Health Service Publication 1787, 1967, pp. 223–228.

101. Said, S.I.: Peptides common to the nervous system and the gastrointestinal tract. In *Frontiers in Neuroendocrinology,* Vol.6. Martin, L., Ganong, W.F., eds. New York, Raven Press, 1980, pp. 293–331.

102. Said, S.I.: Vasoactive peptides and the pulmonary circulation. *Ann. N.Y. Acad. Sci.* 384:207–212, 1982.

103. Said, S.I.: Peptide hormones and neurotransmitters of the lung. In *The Endocrine Lung in Health and Disease.* Becker, K.L., Gazdar, A., eds. Philadelphia, W.B. Saunders, 1984, pp. 267–275.

104. Said, S.I.: Peptides, endothelium and pulmonary vascular reactivity. *Chest* (In press).

105. Said, S.I. and Mutt, V.: Long acting vasodilator peptide from lung tissue. *Nature* 224:699–700, 1969.

106. Said, S.I. and Mutt, V.: Isolation from porcine intestinal wall of a vasoactive octacosapeptide related to secretin and to glucagon. *Eur. J. Biochem.* 28:199–204, 1972.

107. Said, S.I. and Mutt, V.: Relationship of spasmogenic and smooth muscle relaxant peptides from normal lung to other vasoactive compounds. *Nature* 265:84–86, 1977.

108. Said, S.I., Mutt, V., and Erdös, E.G.: The lung in relation to vasoactive poly-peptides. In *Ciba Foundation Symposium,* Vol. 78: *Metabolic Activities of the Lung.* 1980, pp. 217–237.

109. Samuelsson, B.: Leukotrienes: Mediators of immediate hypersensitivity reactions and inflammation. *Science.* 220:568–575, 1983.

110. Sapru, H.N., Gupta, S., and Krieger, A.J.: Opiate receptors in the rat lung: pharmacological evidence. *Fed. Proc.* 39:1017, 1980.

111. Schultzberg, M., Dreyfus, C.F., Gershon, M.D., et al.: VIP-, enkephalin-, substance P-, and somatostatin-like immunoreactivity in neurons intrinsic to the intestine: Immunohistochemical evidence from organotypic tissue cultures. *Brain Res.* 155:239–248, 1978.

112. Schultzberg, M., Hökfelt, T., Nilsson, G., et al.: Distribution of peptide- and catecholamine-containing neurons in the gastrointestinal tract of rat and guinea pig: Immunohistochemical studies with antisera to substance P, vasoactive intestinal polypeptide, enkephalins, somatostatin, gastrin/cholecystokinin, neurotensin, and dopamine-hydroxylase. *Neuroscience* 5:689–744, 1980.

112a. Schwartz, C.J., Kimberg, D.V., Sherrin, H.E., et al.: Vasoactive intestinal peptide (VIP): stimulation of adenylate cyclase and active electrolyte secretion in intestinal mucosa. *J. Clin. Invest.* 54:536–544, 1972.

113. Spencer, H. and Leof, D.: The innervation of the human lung. *J. Anat.* 98:599–609, 1964.

114. Stalcup, S.A., Lipset, J.S., Legant, P.M., et al.: Inhibition of converting enzyme activity by acute hypoxia in dogs. *J. Appl. Physiol.: Respir. Environ. Exercise Physiol.* 46:227–234, 1979.

115. Szolcsányi, J. and Bartho, L.: Capsaicin-sensitive noncholinergic excitatory innervation of the guinea pig tracheobronchial smooth muscle. *Neurosci. Letters* 35:247–251, 1982.

116. Tang, J., Panula, P., Chou, J., et al.: Polypeptides in lung: content and site of action. *Soc. Neurosci. Abst.* 8:14, 1982.

117. Tang, J., Chou, J., Zhang, A.Z., et al.: Met[5]-enkephalin-arg[6]-phe[7] and its receptor in lung. *Life Sci.* 32:2371–2377, 1983.

118. Tatemoto, K.: Neuropeptide Y: Complete amino acid sequence of the brain peptide. *Proc. Natl. Acad. Sci.* 79:5485–5489, 1982.
119. Tatemoto, K. and Mutt, V.: Isolation and characterization of the intestinal peptide porcine PHI (PHI-27), a new member of the glucagon-secretin family. *Proc. Natl. Acad. Sci.* 78:6603–6607, 1981.
120. Terenghi, G., McGregor, G.P., Bhuttacharji, S., et al.: Vagal origin of substance P-containing nerves in the guinea pig lung. *Neurosci. Letters* 36:229–236, 1983.
121. Tsutsumi, Y., Osamura, Y., Watanabe, K., et al.: Immuno-histochemical studies on gastrin-releasing peptide- and adrenocorticotropic hormone-containing cells in the human lung. *Lab Invest.* 48:623–632, 1983.
122. Uddman, R., Alumets, J., Densert, O., et al.: Occurrence and distribution of VIP nerves in the nasal mucosa and tracheobronchial wall. *Acta Otolaryngol.* 86: 443–448, 1978.
123. Uddman, R., Sundler, F., and Emson, P.: Occurrence and distribution of neuropeptide-Y-immunoreactive nerves in the respiratory tract and middle ear. *Cell Tissue Res.* 237:321–327, 1984.
124. von Euler, U.S. and Gaddum, J.H.: An unidentified depressor substance in certain tissue extracts. *J. Physiol.* 72:74–87, 1931.
125. Wallach, J.H., Rybichi, K.J., and Kaufman, M.P.: Anatomical localization of the cells of origin of efferent fibers in the superior laryngeal and recurrent laryngeal nerves of dogs. *Brain Res.* 261:307–311, 1983.
126. Wharton, J., Polak, J.M., Bloom, S.R., et al.: Bombesin-like immunoreactivity in the lung. *Nature* 273:769–770, 1978.
127. Wharton, J., Polak, J.M., Bloom, S.R., et al.: Substance P-like immunoreactive nerves in mammalian lung. *Invest. Cell Pathol.* 2:3–10, 1979.
128. Widdicombe, J.G.: Pulmonary and respiratory tract receptors. *J. Exp. Biol.* 100: 41–57, 1982.
129. Willette, R.N. and Sapru, H.N.: Pulmonary opiate receptor activation evokes a cardiorespiratory reflex. *Eur. J. Pharmacol.* 78:61–70, 1982.
130. Worthen, G.S., Tanaka, D.T., Gumbay, R.S., et al.: Substance P causes pulmonary vasoconstriction in rabbits. *Am. Rev. Respir. Dis.* 129:A337, 1984.
131. Yalow, R.S., Eastridge, C.E., Higgins, G., et al.: Plasma and tumor ACTH in carcinoma of the lung. *Cancer* 44:1789–1792, 1979.
132. Ballard, P.L.: Hormonal influences during fetal lung development. In *Ciba Foundation Symposium, vol. 78: Metabolic Activities of the Lung.* 1980, pp. 251–274.

CHAPTER 6

Leukotrienes, the Pulmonary Circulation, and Vascular Injury

Philip J. Kadowitz,
Dennis B. McNamara, and
Albert L. Hyman

Introduction

The leukotrienes are a family of biologically active substances formed from arachidonic acid via the 5-lipoxygenase pathway.[11] In the lipoxygenase pathway, which is alternative to the cyclooxygenase pathway, the substrate is converted to 5-hydroperoxyeicosatetraenoic acid, which is oxygenated to a labile epoxide intermediate named leukotriene (LT)A_4.[1-3] This labile epoxide intermediate, which is analogous to the pivotal prostaglandin (PG) endoperoxide intermediate PGH_2 in the cyclooxygenase pathway, can be transformed enzymatically to LTB_4, which has potent chemotactic activity.[1,2,10] LTA_4 can also be converted to LTC_4 by the addition of glutathione, and this leukotriene can be further metabolized to LTD_4 by a γ-glutamyl transpeptidase.[11,30,31]

It has been recently reported that LTC_4 and LTD_4 are major components of the slow reacting substance of anaphylaxis.[27,29,30] Since SRS-A is a contractile substance that is released by immunologic challenge from the lung, it has been hypothesized that SRS-A is an important mediator of symptoms in asthma and other immediate-type hypersensitivity reactions.[4,6,25] The effects of the leukotrienes on the lung are of considerable interest because of the postulated role as a mediator in asthma.[6] Leukotrienes C_4 and D_4 have potent contractile activity on preparations of airway and vascular smooth muscle from the lung.[7,8,12,19,26] These substances have significant bronchoconstrictor activity in a variety of species.[8,13,34] However, little has been written about the effects of the leukotrienes on the pulmonary vascular bed. In the monkey, the predominant response to injection of LTC_4 is a fall in pulmonary arterial pressure, whereas aerosol administration of LTC_4 caused a marked rise in pulmonary arterial pressure.[34] In the rat, injections of LTC_4 caused a dose-related fall in pulmonary arterial pressure.[18] In contrast to studies with LTC_4 in the rat and monkey, LTD_4 caused a marked increase in pulmonary vascular resistance in the newborn lamb when injected into the pulmonary artery.[39] However, less is

From Said, S.I. (ed.): *The Pulmonary Circulation and Acute Lung Injury.* Mount Kisco, N.Y., Futura Publishing Co., Inc., 1985.

known about responses to LTD_4 on the pulmonary vascular bed of the mature animal.[23] The purpose of this report is to describe and compare responses to LTD_4 in the pulmonary vascular bed of cat and sheep under conditions of controlled blood flow using recently described methods.[14,15,22] The effects of LTD_4 and of the primary prostaglandins are also compared in the pulmonary vascular bed of the cat.

Results

LTD_4 Responses in the Sheep

Pulmonary lobar vascular responses to LTD_4 in the intact-chest sheep were studied in 11 animals and these data are presented in Table I. Under constant flow conditions, intralobar injections of LTD_4 in doses of 0.1–1.0 μg caused significant dose-related increases in lobar arterial and small vein pressures without changing left atrial pressure. In the range of dose used in the present study in the sheep, LTD_4 had no significant effect on systemic arterial pressure. The increases in lobar arterial and small vein pressures were rapid in onset and mean vascular pressures returned to baseline value over a 0.5–4 minute period, depending on the dose of the leukotriene. The lobar arterial to small vein pressure gradient and the gradient from small vein to left atrium pressure increased significantly at all doses of LTD_4 studied (Table II).

Influence of Cyclooxygenase and Thromboxane Synthesis Inhibitors in the Sheep

In order to determine if pulmonary vascular responses to LTD_4 in the sheep were dependent on formation of products in the cyclooxygenase pathway, the effects of sodium meclofenamate, a cyclooxygenase inhibitor, and of OKY1581, a thromboxane synthesis inhibitor, were investigated. After administration of sodium meclofenamate in a dose of 2.5 mg/kg IV, the increases in lobar arterial pressure in response to LTD_4 were reduced markedly at each dose of the leukotriene studied. The thromboxane synthesis inhibitor, OKY1581, in doses

Table I
Influence of Intralobar Injections of Leukotriene D_4 (LTD_4) on Mean Vascular Pressures in the Sheep

| | Pressure (mmHg) | | | |
	Lobar artery	Small vein	Left atrium	Aorta
Control	15 ± 1	11 ± 1	5 ± 0	102 ± 4
LTD_4, 0.1 μg	26 ± 2*	15 ± 1*	5 ± 0	103 ± 4
Control	17 ± 1	12 ± 1	5 ± 1	100 ± 5
LTD_4, 0.3 μg	34 ± 2*	20 ± 2*	5 ± 1	100 ± 5
Control	15 ± 1	11 ± 1	5 ± 1	97 ± 5
LTD_4, 1 μg	39 ± 2*	22 ± 3*	5 ± 1	101 ± 4

n = 11

*$P < 0.05$ when compared to corresponding control, paired comparison.[35]

Table II
Influence of Intralobar Injections of Leukotriene D_4 (LTD_4)
on Mean Vascular Pressure Gradients in the Sheep Lung

	Pressure gradient (mmHg)		
	Lobar artery− left atrium	Lobar artery− small vein	Small vein− left atrium
Control	10 ± 1	4 ± 1	6 ± 3
LTD_4, 0.1 μg	21 ± 4*	11 ± 2*	10 ± 2*
Control	12 ± 1	5 ± 1	7 ± 2
LTD_4, 0.3 μg	29 ± 4*	14 ± 3*	15 ± 4*
Control	10 ± 2	4 ± 1	6 ± 3
LTD_4, 1 μg	34 ± 5*	17 ± 4*	17 ± 5*

n = 10−11
*$P < 0.05$ when compared to corresponding control, paired comparison.[35]

of 5−10 mg/kg IV, also significantly reduced the increases in lobar arterial pressure in response to the three doses of LTD_4. However, the inhibitory effects of the cyclooxygenase inhibitor on responses to LTD_4 were greater than were the inhibitory effects of the thromboxane synthesis inhibitor. Neither OKY1581 nor sodium meclofenamate had significant effect on pulmonary vascular or systemic arterial pressure in the sheep.

The effects of sodium meclofenamate and OKY1581 on pulmonary vascular responses to an agent whose actions mimic those of thromboxane A_2 were also investigated. U46619, an agent whose actions are similar to those of thromboxane A_2 on smooth muscle, caused dose-dependent increases in lobar arterial and small vein pressures without affecting left atrial or systemic arterial pressure. The increases in lobar arterial pressure in response to U46619 were not altered after administration of sodium meclofenamate, 2.5 mg/kg IV, or OKY1581, 5−10 mg/kg IV. In biochemical studies, the effects of OKY1581 on the metabolism of arachidonic acid and of the prostaglandin endoperoxide, PGH_2, by microsomal fractions from sheep lung were investigated using recently described methods.[33,36] The addition of 1-^{14}C-arachidonic acid (20 μM) to the microsomal fraction (200 μg protein) resulted in the formation of 6-keto-$PGF_{1\alpha}$, the stable breakdown product of PGI_2, 255 ± 21 picomoles and TxB_2, the stable breakdown product of TxA_2, 230 ± 19 picomoles per hour in the absence of the inhibitor. Prostaglandins $F_{2\alpha}$, E_2, and D_2 were also formed. However, when OKY1581 was added to the incubation medium in concentrations of 10^{-9}M or greater, the formation of TxB_2 was reduced to 37% of control at 10^{-7}M and 31% of control at 10^{-6}M. Moreover, the synthesis of 6-keto-$PGF_{1\alpha}$, was not decreased at concentrations of OKY1581 up to 10^{-6}M. The formation of $PGF_{2\alpha}$, PGE_2, and PGD_2 was not decreased by OKY1581 in concentrations up to 10^{-6}M.

The effects of OKY1581 on thromboxane synthesis were also studied in two sheep. In these animals, the lungs were removed after the animals were treated with OKY1581, 10 mg/kg IV. When thromboxane synthesis activity was compared in homogenates from the treated animals, it was found to be markedly depressed when compared to control animals.

The influence of OKY1581 on endoperoxide metabolism by sheep lung microsomal fraction was also investigated. In the absence of inhibitor, 166 ± 15 picomoles of 6-keto-$PGF_{1\alpha}$ and 161 ± 17 picomoles of TxB_2 were formed per 2 minute period when 10 µM PGH_2 was added to 200 µg microsomal protein. $PGF_{2\alpha}$, PGE_2, and PGD_2 were also formed from PGH_2. However, the addition of OKY1581 in concentrations of $10^{-9}M$ or higher reduced the formation of TxB_2. TxB_2 formation was reduced by more than 80% at the higher concentrations of the inhibitor. The formation of $PGF_{2\alpha}$, PGE_2, or PGD_2 was not reduced by OKY1581.

The effects of the cyclooxygenase and thromboxane synthesis inhibitors on lobar vascular responses to arachidonic acid were also investigated in the sheep. Intralobar injections of arachidonic acid in doses of 30 and 100 µg caused a significant dose-dependent increase in lobar arterial pressure without affecting left atrial pressure. The increases in lobar arterial pressure in response to arachidonic acid were also decreased significantly after administration of OKY1581, 5–10 mg/kg IV.

Effect of Ventilation on Responses to LTD₄ in the Sheep

The relationship between the effects of LTD_4 on ventilation and on the pulmonary vascular bed was studied in four sheep. In these experiments, responses to LTD_4 were obtained when the left lower lobe was ventilated and when lobar ventilation was arrested at end-expiration by inflating a balloon catheter in the left lower lobe bronchus. In these experiments, the left lower lobe was perfused with arterial blood to lessen the effects of hypoxia on the lung and 1–3 ml of a 2% lidocaine viscous solution was instilled into the lobar bronchus to prevent coughing. The correlation between the increases in lobar arterial pressure in response to intralobar injections of LTD_4, 0.1–1.0 µg when the lobe was ventilated and when lobar ventilation was arrested was very good. The correlation coefficient of the regression line was 0.90 (p < 0.05) with a slope of (0.83) that was not significantly different from the line of identity. These data indicate that responses to LTD_4 are similar when the lobe is ventilated and when ventilation is arrested. These results suggest that the effects of LTD_4 on vascular and airway smooth muscle in the lung occur independently.

Species and Response to LTD₄ in the Pulmonary Vascular Bed

In order to determine if responses to LTD_4 varied with species, the effects of LTD_4 on the pulmonary vascular bed were investigated in the intact-chest cat and these data are summarized in Table III. Intralobar injections of LTD_4 in doses of 0.3, 1, and 3 µg caused small but significant dose-related increases in lobar arterial pressure without affecting left atrial pressure. Systemic arterial pressure was increased significantly in response to intralobar injections of the 1 and 3 µg doses of LTD_4. Although lobar vascular responses to LTD_4 were modest in the cat, U46619 had marked vasoconstrictor activity (Table III). As described earlier, both LTD_4 and U46619 had marked vasoconstrictor activity in the sheep pulmonary vascular bed and the dose-response curves for both substances in this species were superimposable. However, in the cat, U46619 had far greater vasoconstrictor activity than did LTD_4. Dose-response curves for LTD_4 and U46619 are illustrated in Figure 1.

In other experiments in the sheep and in the cat, responses to LTD_4 were similar when the lung was perfused with blood or with low molecular weight

Table III
Influence of Intralobar Injections of Leukotriene D_4 (LTD_4) on U46619
on Mean Vascular Pressures in the Cat

| | Pressure(mmHg) | | |
	Lobar artery	Left atrium	Aorta
Control	14 ± 1	3 ± 1	110 ± 5
LTD_4, 0.3 μg	16 ± 1*	3 ± 1	113 ± 5
Control	13 ± 1	2 ± 1	110 ± 8
LTD_4, 1 μg	16 ± 1*	2 ± 1	119 ± 6*
Control	13 ± 1	3 ± 1	115 ± 10
LTD_4, 3 μg	21 ± 2*	3 ± 1	124 ± 11*
Control	14 ± 2	3 ± 1	130 ± 8
U46619, 0.003 μg	20 ± 3*	2 ± 1	133 ± 7
Control	12 ± 1	3 ± 1	124 ± 9
U46619, 0.01 μg	23 ± 3*	3 ± 1	130 ± 7
Control	11 ± 2	3 ± 1	118 ± 6
U46619, 0.03 μg	28 ± 4*	4 ± 2	124 ± 8

n = 6–9
*P < 0.05 when compared to corresponding control, paired comparison.[35]

dextran. The role of the cyclooxygenase pathway in the mediation of pulmonary vascular responses to LTD_4 was also investigated in the cat. Administration of indomethacin or sodium meclofenamate, 2.5 mg/kg IV, had no significant effect on pulmonary vasoconstrictor responses to U46619 or LTD_4 in the cat. The increases in systemic arterial pressure in response to the 1 and 3 μg doses of LTD_4 were not altered by the cyclooxygenase inhibitors. However, the cyclooxygenase inhibitors, in the doses employed, significantly reduced the increases in lobar arterial pressure in response to intralobar injections of arachidonic acid. The cyclooxygenase inhibitors had no significant effect on pulmonary vascular or systemic arterial pressure in the cat. The effects of the cyclooxygenase products of arachidonic acid are shown in Figure 2. It can be seen that all products in this pathway had far greater vasoconstrictor activity than did LTD_4 in the feline pulmonary vascular bed.

Discussion

Experiments in the intact-chest sheep demonstrate that intralobar injections of LTD_4 increase pulmonary lobar arterial pressure in a dose-related manner.[23] Since pulmonary blood flow was maintained constant and left atrial pressure was unchanged, the increase in pressure gradient across the lung lobe suggests that pulmonary lobar vascular resistance was increased by LTD_4.[23] The increases in lobar arterial pressure in response to LTD_4 were associated with dose-related increases in small intrapulmonary vein pressure. In addition to increasing lobar arterial and venous pressures, LTD_4 increased the pressure gradient from lobar artery to small vein. These experiments in the sheep suggest that LTD_4 increases pulmonary vascular resistance by constricting intrapulmonary veins and segments upstream to the small veins believed to be small arteries.[23] Results obtained in mature animals are consistent with re-

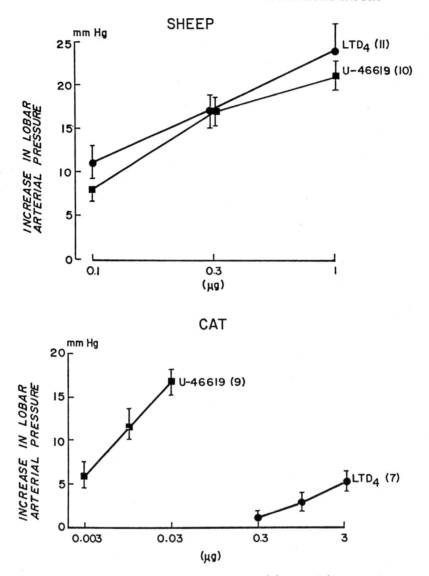

Figure 1: *Dose-response curves comparing increases in lobar arterial pressure in response to injections of LTD₄ and U46619 in the sheep and cat. n indicates number of sheep or cats.*

sults in the newborn lamb in which LTD_4 increased pulmonary and systemic vascular resistances and decreased cardiac output.[23,39] It has been reported that LTD_4 has potent coronary vasoconstrictor activity in the sheep that can be associated with left ventricular impairment.[28] However, in the sheep, LTD_4 had no significant effect on systemic arterial or left atrial pressures in the range of doses studied. The effects of LTD_4 on left atrial pressure in the newborn lamb were not measured so that the mechanism of the fall in cardiac output is uncertain.[39] The effects of LTD_4 on the systemic vascular resistance of the newborn lamb appear to be greater than those observed in the mature animal.

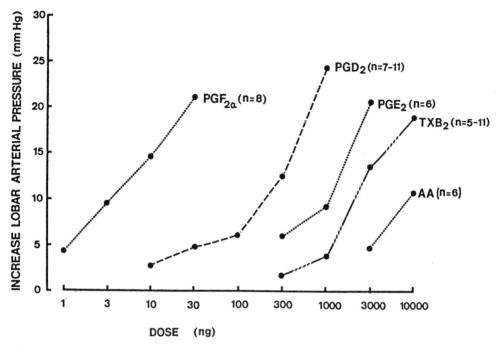

Figure 2: *Dose-response relationships comparing increases in lobar arterial pressure in response to injections of graded doses of PGF₂ₐ, PGD₂, PGE₂, thromboxane (Tx) B₂, and arachidonic acid (AA) in the cat. n indicates number of cats.*

In terms of relative pressor activity in the pulmonary vascular bed of the sheep, LTD_4 was very potent with activity paralleling that of U46619, a stable prostaglandin analog whose actions are thought to mimic those of thromboxane A_2.[5] Moreover, when compared to other vasoactive hormones whose effects have been studied in the sheep, LTD_4 is far more active than other arachidonic acid metabolites, alveolar hypoxia, or histamine, which acts over a similar portion of the pulmonary vascular bed and is released along with the leukotrienes in immediate hypersensitivity reactions.[4,14,22,24]

It has been reported that LTD_4 has potent contractile activity on isolated airway smooth muscle and lung parenchyma and that it increases bronchomotor tone.[7,8,13,19,26] However, in the intact-chest sheep, the effects of LTD_4 on the pulmonary vascular bed appear to be independent of alterations in ventilation or those that occur as a consequence of changes in bronchomotor tone or lung volume, since similar responses were obtained when the lobe was ventilated or when lobar ventilation was arrested by obstruction of bronchial airflow. In previous studies, responses to a number of vasoactive substances, including cyclooxygenase metabolites of arachidonic acid and histamine, were similar when the lobe was ventilated or lobar ventilation was arrested, suggesting that the actions of these vasoactive hormones on pulmonary vascular resistance appear to be independent of alterations in bronchomotor tone.[16,22] Both in the cat and in the sheep, pulmonary hypertensive responses to LTD_4 appear similar when the lung was perfused with blood or low molecular weight dextran.

Thus, responses to LTD_4 in both species are not dependent on the interaction with formed elements in blood.

In the sheep, pulmonary vasoconstrictor responses to LTD_4 were markedly attenuated after treatment with sodium meclofenamate, suggesting that responses to this lipoxygenase product are dependent on the formation of products in the cyclooxygenase pathway. In addition, vasoconstrictor responses to LTD_4 were decreased by OKY1581, a thromboxane synthesis inhibitor. These data suggest that a substantial portion of the pulmonary vasoconstrictor response to LTD_4 is due to the release of thromboxane A_2. The observation that meclofenamate had greater inhibitory effect on responses to LTD_4 than did OKY1581 suggests that pulmonary vasoconstrictor responses to this lipoxygenase metabolite are dependent on the formation of thromboxane A_2 and other cyclooxygenase products such as prostaglandins (PG) D_2 and $F_{2\alpha}$, which have substantial pressor activity in the pulmonary vascular bed.[21,24] It has been shown that injections of SRS-A or synthetic LTC_4 and LTD_4 cause the release of prostaglandins and TxA_2 from isolated guinea pig lung.[9,32] The results of the present experiments in the sheep are consistent with data obtained with isolated guinea pig parenchyma and on bronchoconstrictor responses in the guinea pig indicating that responses to LTD_4 are dependent on the release of TxA_2 and prostaglandins.[32,38]

A similar relationship between these inhibitors and responses to arachidonic acid was also observed in that there was a greater reduction in response to LTD_4 after treatment with meclofenamate than after OKY1581. These data confirm previous studies showing that pulmonary vasoconstrictor responses to arachidonic acid are due to formation of products in the cyclooxygenase pathway[16,17,37] and extend these findings by showing that a portion of the response is due to TxA_2 formation.

Although responses to LTD_4 and arachidonic acid were markedly reduced by meclofenamate, this cyclooxygenase inhibitor had no significant effect on pulmonary vasoconstrictor responses to U46619, an analog whose actions are thought to mimic those of thromboxane A_2.[5] These data indicate that sodium meclofenamate inhibited cyclooxygenase activity in the pulmonary vascular bed and that the cyclooxygenase inhibitor did not influence vascular responses to the thromboxane mimic. In addition, vasoconstrictor responses to U46619 were not altered by OKY1581 in doses that inhibited responses to LTD_4 and arachidonic acid. These results also suggest that the thromboxane synthesis inhibitor did not alter thromboxane receptor-mediated responses and that the effects of the inhibitor were due to inhibition of the formation of thromboxane A_2. These data also suggest thromboxane A_2 would have marked vasoconstrictor activity in the sheep pulmonary vascular bed if U46619 actually does mimic responses to this labile hormone.

The inhibition of thromboxane A_2 synthesis was also investigated in microsomal fractions from sheep lung using recently described methods.[33,36] The results of these studies show that OKY1581 inhibited the formation of TxA_2 as measured by formation of its stable breakdown product TxB_2. TxB_2 formation was inhibited over a wide range of concentration of OKY1581 when either arachidonic acid or the endoperoxide PGH_2 was employed as substrate. Although TxB_2 formation was decreased by OKY1581, PGI_2 formation as measured by the production of 6-keto-$PGF_{1\alpha}$ was not inhibited even at very high concentrations of the thromboxane synthesis inhibitor. Prostaglandins E_2, $F_{2\alpha}$, and D_2 were formed when PGH_2 or arachidonic acid was added to the microsomal fractions. It is not known if this prostaglandin synthesis was enzymatic; however, the amount of these substances formed was not decreased by OKY1581 and, in the case of PGE_2, was enhanced by the inhibitor. Since the total amount of product formed from arachidonic acid (6-keto-$PGF_{1\alpha}$, TxB_2, $PGF_{2\alpha}$, PGE_2, and PGD_2) was not decreased although TxB_2 formation was reduced, it is unlikely that OKY1581 had a significant inhibitory effect on sheep lung cyclooxygenase activity. These experiments suggest that effects of OKY1581 on responses to LTD_4 and arachidonic acid are due to inhibition of thromboxane synthetase activity and not to an effect on cyclooxygenase activity or on thromboxane receptor-mediated activity in the pulmonary vascular bed of the sheep. In other experiments in lung homogenates taken from sheep receiving OKY1581, 5–10 mg/kg IV, TxB_2 formation was greatly reduced.

The results of studies in the sheep demonstrate that LTD_4 has very potent vasoconstrictor activity in the pulmonary vascular bed of this species and that this activity is due for the most part to release of products in the cyclooxygenase pathway. However, the effects of LTD_4 in the pulmonary vascular bed of the sheep and the cat are different. In the cat, LTD_4 had only modest pressor activity equal to that of arachidonic acid and far less than that of $PGF_{2\alpha}$, PGD_2, or PGE_2 in that species.[21] Furthermore, in this species, cyclooxygenase blockers did not modify responses to this lipoxygenase product. Although the relative magnitude of responses to LTD_4 as well as the mechanism of action differ in the sheep and the cat, both species were extremely sensitive to the effects of U46619. Thus, there appears to be true species variation in the pulmonary vascular response to this lipoxygenase metabolite. This variation was not observed with U46619, which may operate via TxA_2 receptors in the pulmonary vascular bed. In addition to demonstrating marked species variation in the response to LTD_4, the present data may be interpreted to suggest that LTD_4 itself does not have potent vasoconstrictor activity in the lung when the cyclooxygenase system is blocked. Moreover, the remaining pressor activity of LTD_4 in the sheep after cyclooxygenase blockade and the pressor activity in the cat which were very similar suggest that the activity of this lipoxygenase metabolite is far less than that of products of the cyclooxygenase pathway such as TxA_2, $PGF_{2\alpha}$, or PGD_2.[20,21] The data from the present study suggest that it would be difficult to formulate a unified hypothesis on the role of LTD_4, a major component of SRS-A, on the pulmonary circulation since species variation is so marked. The present data, however, suggest that LTD_4 could have pronounced effects on lobar arterial and small vein pressures in the sheep. These effects on venous pressures could contribute to an increase in capillary pressure and may alter fluid balance in the sheep lung. These hydrostatic effects along with alterations in capillary permeability that could occur as a consequence of lung injury could result in pulmonary edema and marked abnormalities in gas exchange.

Summary

Pulmonary vascular responses to leukotriene (LT) D_4 were compared in the sheep and cat under conditions of controlled lobar blood flow. Intralobar injections of LTD_4 in the sheep caused dose-dependent increases in lobar arterial and small vein pressures without altering left atrial or systemic arterial pressure. LTD_4 was very potent in increasing pulmonary vascular resistance in the sheep with activity similar to U46619, a thromboxane (Tx) A_2 mimic. Pulmonary vascular responses to LTD_4 in the sheep were similar when the lung was ventilated and when lobar ventilation was arrested and when the lobe was perfused with blood or with dextran. Pulmonary vasoconstrictor responses to LTD_4 but not U46619 in the sheep were reduced by inhibitors of cyclooxygenase and thromboxane synthesis. In contrast, LTD_4 had modest pressor activity in the pulmonary vascular bed of the cat whereas U46619 had marked activity in this species. Responses to LTD_4 in the cat were not altered by cyclooxygenase inhibitors. It is concluded that LTD_4 has marked pulmonary vasoconstrictor activity in the sheep, increasing pulmonary vascular resistance by constricting intrapulmonary veins and upstream segments. In this species, responses to LTD_4 were indepdendent of changes in ventilation but were dependent on the formation of cyclooxygenase products including TxA_2. However, in the cat, LTD_4 had very weak pressor activity and this activity was not dependent on the integrity of the cyclooxygenase system. In this species, LTD_4 had far less vasoconstrictor activity than did prostaglandins E_2, $F_{2\alpha}$, or D_2. These studies indicate that there is considerable species difference in responses to LTD_4, a major component of the slow reacting substance of anaphylaxis, in the pulmonary vascular bed.

Acknowledgments

The authors thank Drs. Joshua Rokach and Barry M. Weichman for the LTD_4 used in the study and Ms. Alice Landry for help with the biochemical experiments. We also thank Ms. Janice Ignarro for help in preparing the manuscript. This work was supported by National Heart, Lung and Blood Institute Grants HL15580, HL18060, HL29456, HL11802, and HL29450.

REFERENCES

1. Borgeat, P. and Samuelsson, B.: Arachidonic acid in metabolism in polymorphonuclear leukocytes: Unstable intermediates in formation of dihydroxy acids. *Proc. Natl. Acad. Sci. USA* 76:3212–3217, 1979.
2. Borgeat, P. and Samuelsson, B.: Metabolism of arachidonic acid in polymorphonuclear leukocytes: Structural analysis of novel hydroxylated compounds. *J. Biol. Chem.* 254:7865–7869, 1979.
3. Borgeat, P., Hamberg, M., and Samuelsson, B.: Transformation of arachidonic acid and homo-γ-linolenic acid by rabbit polymorphonuclear leukocytes. Monohydroxy acids from novel lipoxygenases. *J. Biol. Chem.* 251:7816–7820, 1976.
4. Brocklehurst, W.E.: The release of histamine and formation of a slow-reacting substance during anaphylactic shock. *J. Physiol.* 151:416–435, 1960.
5. Coleman, R.A., Humphrey, P.P.A., Kennedy, I., et al.: Comparison of the actions of U46619, a prostaglandin H_2-analogue, with those of prostaglandin H_2 and thromboxane A_2 on some isolated smooth muscle preparations. *Br. J. Pharmacol.* 73: 773–778, 1981.
6. Dahlen, S.E., Hansson, G., Hedqvist, P., et al.: Allergic challenge of lung tissue from asthmatics elicits bronchial contraction that correlates with the release of leukotriene C_4, D_4, and E_4. *Proc. Natl. Acad. Sci. USA* 80:1712–1716, 1983.
7. Dahlen, S.E., Hedqvist, P., Hammarström, S., et al.: Leukotrienes are potent constrictors of human bronchi. *Nature* 288:484–486, 1980.

8. Drazen, J.M. Austen, K.F., Lewis, R.A., et al.: Comparative airway and vascular activities of leukotrienes C-1 and D in vivo and in vitro. *Proc. Natl. Acad. Sci. USA* 77:4354–4358, 1980.
9. Engineer, D.M., Morris, H.R., Piper, P.J., et al.: The release of prostaglandins and thromboxanes from guinea pig lung by slow-reacting substances of anaphylaxis and its inhibition. *Br. J. Pharmacol.* 64:211–218, 1978.
10. Ford-Hutchinson, A.W., Bray, M.A., Doig, M.V., et al.: Leukotriene B: A potent chemokinetic and aggregating substance released from polymorphonuclear leukocytes. *Nature* 286:264–265, 1980.
11. Hammarström, S.: Leukotrienes. *Ann. Rev. Biochem.* 52:355–377, 1983.
12. Hand, J.M., Will, J.A., and Buckner, C.K.: Effects of leukotrienes on isolated guinea pig pulmonary arteries. *Eur. J. Pharmacol.* 76:439–443, 1981.
13. Holroyde, M.D., Altounyan, R.E.C., Cole, M., et al.: Bronchoconstriction produced in man by leukotrienes C and D. *Lancet* II:17–18, 1981.
14. Hyman, A.L. and Kadowitz, P.J.: Effect of alveolar and perfusion hypoxia and hypercapnia on pulmonary vascular resistance in the lamb. *Am. J. Physiol.* 228:397–403, 1975.
15. Hyman, A.L. and Kadowitz, P.J.: Pulmonary vasodilator activity of prostacyclin (PGI_2) in the cat. *Circ. Res.* 45:404–409, 1979.
16. Hyman, A.L., Mathé, A.A., Leslie, C.A., et al.: Modification of pulmonary vascular responses to arachidonic acid by alterations in physiologic state. *J. Pharmacol. Exp. Ther.* 207:388–401, 1978.
17. Hyman, A.L., Spannhake, E.W., and Kadowitz, P.J.: Divergent responses to arachidonic acid in the feline pulmonary vascular bed. *Am. J. Physiol.* 239:H40–H46, 1980.
18. Iacopino, V.J., Fitzpatrick, T.M., Ramwell, P.W., et al.: Cardiovascular responses to leukotriene C_4 in the rat. *J. Pharmacol. Exp. Ther.* 227:244–247, 1983.
19. Jones, T.R., Davis, C., and Daniel, E.E.: Pharmacological study of the contractile activity of leukotrienes C_4 and D_4 on isolated human airway smooth muscle. *Can. J. Physiol. Pharmacol.* 60:638–643, 1982.
20. Kadowitz, P.J. and Hyman, A.L.: Influence of a prostaglandin endoperoxide analogue on the canine pulmonary vascular bed. *Circ. Res.* 40:282–287, 1977.
21. Kadowitz, P.J. and Hyman, A.L.: Comparative effects of thromboxane B_2 on the canine and feline pulmonary vascular bed. *J. Pharmacol. Exp. Ther.* 213:300–305, 1980.
22. Kadowitz, P.J. and Hyman, A.L.: Pulmonary vascular responses to histamine in sheep. *Am. J. Physiol.* 244:H423–H428, 1983.
23. Kadowitz, P.J. and Hyman, A.L.: Analysis of responses to leukotriene D_4 in the pulmonary vascular bed. *Circ. Res.* 55:707–717, 1984.
24. Kadowitz, P.J., Joiner, P.D., and Hyman, A.L.: Influence of prostaglandins E_1 and $F_{2\alpha}$ on pulmonary vascular resistance in the sheep. *Proc. Soc. Exp. Biol. Med.* 145:1258–1261, 1974.
25. Kellaway, C.H. and Trethewie, E.F.: The liberation of slow reacting smooth muscle-stimulating substances in anaphylaxis. *Q. J. Exp. Physiol.* 30:121–145, 1940.
26. Krell, R.D., Osborn, R., Vickery, L., et al.: Contraction of isolated airway smooth muscle by synthetic leukotrienes C_4 and D_4. *Prostaglandins* 22:387–409, 1981.
27. Lewis, R.A., Austen, K.F., Drazen, J.M., et al.: Slow-reacting substances of anaphylaxis: Identification of leukotrienes C and D from human and rat sources. *Proc. Natl. Acad. Sci. USA* 77:3710–3714, 1980.
28. Michelassi, F., Landa, L., Hill, R.D., et al.: Leukotriene D_4: A potent coronary artery vasoconstrictor associated with impaired ventricular contraction. *Science* 217:841–843, 1982.
29. Morris, H.R., Taylor, G.W., Piper, P.J., et al.: Structure of slow-reacting substance of anaphylaxis from guinea pig lung. *Nature* 285:104–108, 1980.
30. Murphy, R.C., Hammarström, S., and Samuelsson, B.: Leukotriene C: A slow-

reacting substance from murine mastocytoma cells. *Proc. Natl. Acad. Sci. USA* 76:4275–4279, 1979.

31. Orning, L., Hammarström, S., and Samuelsson, B.: Leukotriene D: A slow-reacting substance from rat basophilic leukemic cells. *Proc. Natl. Acad. Sci. USA* 77: 2014–2017, 1980.

32. Piper, P.J. and Samhoum, M.N.: The mechanism of action of leukotriene C_4 and D_4 in guinea pig isolated perfused lung and parenchymal strips of guinea pig. *Prostaglandins* 21:793–803, 1981.

33. She, H.S., McNamara, D.B., Spannhake, E.W., et al.: Metabolism of prostaglandin endoperoxide by microsomes from cat lung. *Prostaglandins* 21:531–541, 1981.

34. Smedegård, G., Hedqvist, P., Dahlen, S.E., et al.: Leukotriene C_4 affects pulmonary and cardiovascular dynamics in monkey. *Nature* 295:327–329, 1982.

35. Snedecor, C.W. and Cochran, W.G.: *Statistical Methods,* 6th Ed. Ames, Iowa, Iowa State University Press, 1967.

36. Spannhake, E.W., Colombo, J.L., Craigo, P.A., et al.: Evidence for modification of pulmonary cyclooxygenase activity by endotoxin in the dog. *J. Appl. Physiol.* 54: 191–198, 1983.

37. Spannhake, E.W., Hyman, A.L., and Kadowitz, P.J.: Dependency of the airway and pulmonary vascular effects of arachidonic acid upon route and rate of administration. *J. Pharmacol. Exp. Ther.* 212:584–590, 1980.

38. Weichman, B.M., Muccitelli, R.M., Osborn, R.R., et al.: In vitro and in vivo mechanisms of leukotriene-mediated bronchoconstriction in the guinea pig. *J. Pharmacol. Exp. Ther.* 222:202–208, 1982.

39. Yokochi, K., Olley, P.M., Sideris, E., et al.: Leukotriene D_4: A potent vasoconstrictor of the pulmonary and systemic circulations in the newborn lamb. In *Leukotrienes and Other Lipoxygenase Products.* New York, Raven Press, 1982, pp. 211–214.

III

Morphological and Pathophysiological Basis of Lung Injury

Patterns of Remodeling of the Pulmonary Circulation in Acute and Subacute Lung Injury

Rosemary Jones,
David Langleben, and
Lynne M. Reid

Introduction

Acute and subacute lung injury often results in pulmonary hypertension, with profound implications for lung function and survival. In particular, injury to the pulmonary microcirculation commonly causes structural remodeling of precapillary units, which leads to increase in pulmonary vascular resistance (PVR) and pulmonary artery pressure (PAP). Structural changes in upstream or proximal segments of pulmonary arteries then occur in response to increase in wall tension secondary to peripheral obstruction, and reflect, rather than cause, the rise in PAP. Right ventricular hypertrophy develops in response to increased PAP. Pulmonary hypertension also arises from obstruction to large arteries, or in response to a rise in venous pressure, caused by obstruction to large veins, or passively from a pressure rise in the left side of the heart, or by constriction of vein walls. Here we focus on the structural remodeling of pulmonary arteries that results from microvascular injury.

Structural remodeling of the walls of pulmonary preacinar and intraacinar arteries is a striking feature of normal lung growth.[108,109] In the postnatal period, a rapid reduction in the thickness of medial muscle occurs, mostly in preacinar arteries less than 300 μm in external diameter (ED), that contributes to the sharp fall in PVR in this period (Fig. 1). A less marked reduction in muscle also occurs in larger arteries. In the perinatal period, muscle is not normally present in the walls of intraacinar arteries.[108,109] As the lung grows, however, muscle appears increasingly in vessels within the acinus, although it is several years before it reaches the level of the alveolar duct, and only in the adult lung is it present in many vessels within the alveolar wall (i.e., 50%). As further lung growth occurs, the density of intraacinar arteries increases until the adult concentration of vessels is reached at about 8 years.

In response to many forms of injury, muscle rapidly appears in distal units of the pulmonary artery bed increasing the proportion of segments that are completely muscular.[108] This muscularization of the vessel wall occurs faster

From Said, S.I. (ed.): *The Pulmonary Circulation and Acute Lung Injury.* Mount Kisco, N.Y., Futura Publishing Co., Inc., 1985.

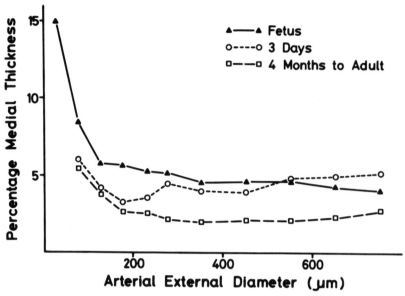

Figure 1: *Arterial medial thickness as percent of external diameter, in all size vessels, is thicker in the fetus than in the adult. By 3 days, increase in compliance of small arteries is apparent by a decrease in their wall thickness to adult levels. (From ref. 108 with permission.)*

than in the growing lung, i.e., within days.[49,67,86] Endothelial cell injury may result in obstruction and obliteration of distal vessels, another feature of structural remodeling. Each of these effects of injury contributes to the develoment of pulmonary hypertension, and each is the basis of a maintained rise in PAP. In the normal lung as well as in established pulmonary hypertension, pressure partly falls in response to vasodilatory agents (Fig. 2). While the response in the hypertensive bed is greater, there is also a larger component of pressure that is unresponsive and is maintained by structural remodeling.

We first describe the structure of the normal human pulmonary arterial bed as a basis for understanding the changes that occur in response to injury. General structural features that contribute to pulmonary hypertension, or represent adaptation to it, are described before the specific changes in disease. Rapid and extensive remodeling of the human pulmonary vasculature in acute and subacute lung injury is illustrated by reference to the changes found in the adult respiratory distress syndrome (ARDS). ARDS is a clinical condition of major importance and its experimental study is currently of great interest. Over a period of days to weeks, remodeling of pulmonary arteries, with development of pulmonary hypertension, occurs in many ARDS patients, unfavorably affecting prognosis. Finally, we discuss several animal models in which remodeling of the pulmonary vascular bed is produced by acute and subacute lung injury, and mention putative mechanisms and mediators.

Normal Pulmonary Vascular Structure and Its Modification in Hypertension

The structure of the normal pulmonary artery bed reflects its low resistance and pressure, contrasting with the highly muscular arrangement of vessels of

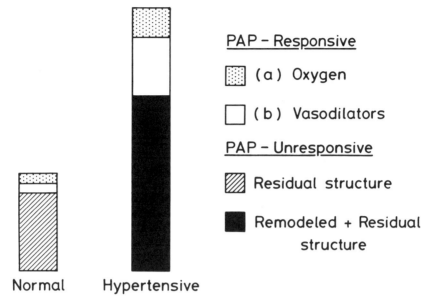

PAP – Responsive

(a) Oxygen

(b) Vasodilators

PAP – Unresponsive

Residual structure

Remodeled + Residual structure

Normal   Hypertensive

Figure 2: *Responsive and unresponsive components of pulmonary artery pressure (PAP) in the normal and hypertensive bed. In the hypertensive bed, the increase in PAP, which is unresponsive to the action of oxygen or other vasodilators, is maintained by pulmonary artery remodeling.*

the systemic circulation where pressure is normally about six times that of the pulmonary bed. Morphometric techniques allow the structural pattern of the normal pulmonary vascular bed to be established and the changes produced by injury to be assessed. The use of a technique that fully distends and recruits all patent pulmonary arteries is necessary for precise quantitation; to this end, we perfuse these vessels with a barium sulfate-gelatin mixture (at 60°C) at hypertensive pressure (100 cm H_2O). This fills pulmonary arteries greater than 15 μm in ED but the medium does not enter the capillaries, thereby identifying the pulmonary artery from the pulmonary venous bed. Radiography of the vasculature perfused in this way demonstrates both normal and abnormal filling patterns. The central-most area on the lung radiograph is occupied by the relatively few large conducting arteries; in distal lung regions, it is occupied by the many smaller distributing arteries. Pulmonary arteries greater than 160 μm in ED are discerned as separate lines on the radiograph while smaller ones appear as a fine background haze.[89]

Pulmonary Microcirculation

Normal Structure

Intraacinar arteries, capillaries, and veins together comprise the pulmonary microcirculation (Fig. 3). In the adult human lung, the acinus is about 1 cm in diameter. Acini occur at the distal ends of pulmonary airway and artery branches, most being present in the subpleural region.

Pulmonary Arteries: Where present in the pulmonary artery wall, smooth muscle maintains tone and achieves constriction. Along any one arterial path-

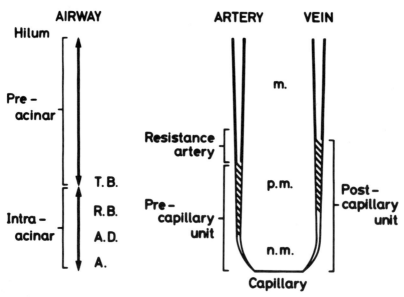

Figure 3: *Diagrammatic representation of a pulmonary vascular pathway (not to scale). The acinus is the respiratory unit of lung supplied by a respiratory bronchiolus (RB). In the adult human, muscular arteries are found in the most distal alveoli of the acinus, whereas in the human fetus muscular arteries are normally preacinar. (TB = terminal bronchiolus; AD = alveolar duct; A = alveolar wall; m = muscular; pm = partially muscular; nm = nonmuscular).* (From Reid and Meyrick, Ciba Foundation Symposium 78, 1980, p. 38, with permission.)

way from the lung hilum to the periphery, the thickness of the muscle layer decreases; and in many vessels it then forms an incomplete coat or spiral (Fig. 4) before ultimately disappearing from the vessel wall. In tissue sections, vessel profiles with a complete medial coat of muscle are termed *muscular*, while those with an incomplete coat are termed *partially muscular*, and those without medial muscle, *nonmuscular* (Fig. 5). Vessel size is assessed by measuring the ED (Fig. 5), and the thickness of the muscle coat is assessed by measuring the medial thickness (MT) (Fig. 5). From these two values, the percent medial thickness (%MT) is calculated ([2 × MT]/ ED × 100 for muscular arteries and MT/ED × 100 for partially muscular ones), the thickness of the muscle coat being related to vessel size.

It is important to note that in the normal lung the proportion of alveolar wall vessels that is nonmuscular varies between species. In the adult human lung, for example, muscle is present as a complete coat as far distally as the alveolar wall,[108] while in other species, e.g., the rat, muscle is seen only rarely in this region.[51] Along any arterial pathway the structure of the wall does not change at precisely the same lumen diameter or branch level within the lung,[20,106] and so vessels are landmarked by their accompanying airway to assess their position in the arterial branching pattern (Fig. 5). The density of pulmonary arteries (per mm^2) is related to the number of alveoli (per mm^2), this value being relatively independent of the degree of fixation. To analyze the microcirculation, therefore, we assess vessels by structural distribution related to arterial ED and to airway level. The %MT of muscular arteries that are

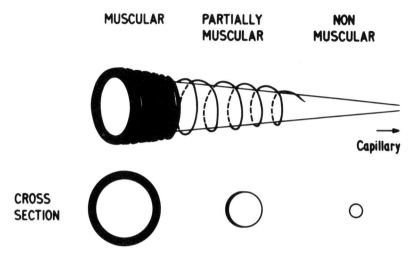

Figure 4: *Along any arterial pathway, the muscular coat gives way to a partially muscular structure while still in vessels larger than a capillary. The transition from one type to another does not always occur in arteries of the same size or at the same level in the branching pattern. To characterize the microcirculation, the "population" of arterial types must be analyzed. (From ref. 107 with permission.)*

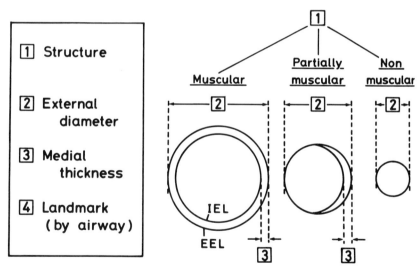

Figure 5: *Illustration of the way pulmonary arteries are measured and results recorded: (1) vessel structure is noted (as muscular, partially muscular, nonmuscular); (2) ED is measured (as the distance between the two edges of the external elastic lamina); (3) MT is measured (as the distance between the internal [iel] and external [eel] elastic lamina); (4) accompanying airway is recorded as a landmark (see text).*

immediately preacinar or proximal within the acinus is the greatest in the lung. These vessels, which are >200 and <500 μm in ED in the adult human lung, as well as having a more muscular wall, present a rapid reduction in lumen size and represent the resistance arteries.

In addition to the medial smooth muscle cell, several cell types comprise the vessel wall, namely the endothelial cells, pericyte[85,135] and intermediate cell[85] of the intima (Fig. 6), and the adventitial fibroblast. The various metabolic functions performed by the pulmonary endothelial cell are discussed in Chapter 1 of this volume. The pericyte and intermediate cell are found in the nonmuscular region of the vessel wall: the pericyte is present most distally, in the nonmuscular segment, and the intermediate cell in the nonmuscular region of the partially muscular segment.[85] While the pericyte shares the basement membrane of the endothelial cell, the intermediate cell (so-called because of its structure and position) lies within its own basement membrane abluminal to the endothelial cell. These cells play an important role in the development of new vascular smooth muscle in response to various stimuli (see next section) and so are termed *precursor smooth muscle cells*. This term also describes both these cells in 1 μm sections since the pericyte can be identified from the intermediate cell only by electron microscopy.

Pulmonary Capillaries and Veins: The pulmonary capillary bed forms a vast network of intercommunicating vessels; it contains most of the endothelial surface area within the lung and thus offers the greatest opportunity for interaction with the blood, both for respiratory and nonrespiratory functions. Latex casts of rat lung reveal two types of capillary tubules: sparse, long tubular capillaries that comprise both a thin subpleural layer and fill peribronchial spaces and, within the alveolus, tightly matted short tubules arranged in a spherical array.[35] The capillary wall consists of endothelial cells and basement membrane. In its thinnest region, the region of optimum gas exchange, the

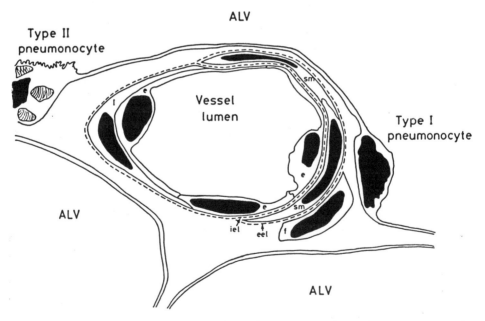

Figure 6: *Illustration of a partially muscular wall artery in rat lung, showing position of a precursor smooth muscle cell, in this case an intermediate cell: internal (iel) and external (eel) elastic laminae (broken lines), endothelial cell (e), intermediate cell (i), smooth muscle cell (sm), fibroblast (f).*

alveolar-capillary membrane consists only of the capillary wall covered by epithelial cells; in its thick regions, fibroblasts, myofibroblasts, migratory cells (leukocytes and macrophages) are present, as well as collagen fibers and fibrils, and elastin. The arrangement of pulmonary veins resembles that described here for arteries, there being first a nonmuscular segment with precursor cells, and then a spiral of muscle before the muscle coat becomes complete as vessel diameter increases.[47]

Changes in Pulmonary Hypertension

Structural remodeling of distal vessels is evident on the pulmonary arteriogram from a loss of background haze, i.e., a reduction in the density of filled arteries that are less than 160 µm in ED (see Figs. 13 and 23).

The size of the vessel lumen is reduced both by a decrease in ED and an increase in MT, this narrowing being indicated by an increase in the %MT. Even in the absence of an increased MT, a decrease in vessel ED will impede blood flow. The ED may be reduced by compression of the vessel wall by edema or fibrosis; each can occur within the vessel wall, the connective tissue septa, or the alveolus. The vessel lumen also narrows from constriction of medial or intimal cells. Swelling (i.e., intracellular edema with a reduction in the ratio of organelles to cytoplasm), hypertrophy, or hyperplasia of cells of the media and intima can also encroach on the vessel lumen. Partial block of the lumen by white blood cells, platelet or fibrin aggregates, or by recanalized thrombi will also reduce lumen size.

In the barium-injected lung, a decrease in the density of perfused pulmonary arteries leads to a reduced artery/alveolar density. Nonfilling indicates lumen block, functional closure, or vessel loss. Each of the features listed above as causing partial occlusion of the vessel lumen can cause complete occlusion. Functional closure probably results from encroachment on the lumen by wall structures. As injury continues, a cycle of cell proliferation, death, and necrosis can lead to loss of integrity of endothelium and fragmentation and resorption of the vessel wall. Fibrosis also obliterates a vessel. By light microscopy, vessel remnants are identified only by their persisting elastic lamina, although by electron microscopy other remnants of the wall are usually visible. For each of the above features of injury, within any one lung there is focal accentuation, the degree of increase in PVR reflecting all the changes.

While muscle increases in normally muscular regions by smooth muscle cell proliferation, muscle also develops in previously nonmuscular segments. The increased muscularization of the vessel wall thus both extends the length of the resistance segment and, by encroaching on the lumen of small vessels, increases resistance. Development of new muscle is established by the analysis of a population of pulmonary artery profiles in tissue sections. This identifies an increase in the mean medial thickness and the relative number of profiles with a muscular wall. Typically, a shift in distribution is demonstrated by an increase in the number of muscular and partially muscular profiles at the expense of nonmuscular ones.

How does new muscle arise in these previously nonmuscular artery segments? Stimulation of precursor smooth muscle cells, the pericyte and intermediate cell, leads to hypertrophy, with or without hyperplasia[85,88] and change in phenotype by these cells. Within each cell type filaments are formed; the pericyte forms a basement membrane, while the intermediate cell forms dense bodies and thus has the structural features of a smooth muscle cell. Eventually, a new internal elastic lamina is formed and the original elastic lamina becomes external in position; additional elastic laminae may also criss-cross the media, a feature not seen in normal muscular vessels.[17] Nonmuscular and partially muscular segments of the vessel wall thus become partially or fully muscular (Fig. 7).

Immunofluorescent techniques identify the contractile proteins within cells of the vessel wall. The smooth muscle cell contains muscle actin and muscle myosin, and the endothelial cell contains nonmuscle actin and non-

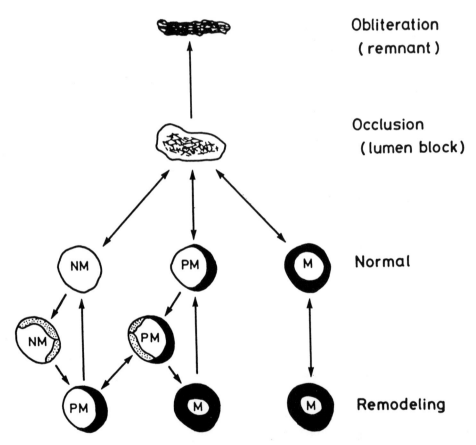

Figure 7: *Illustration depicting patterns of remodeling of the pulmonary artery wall. By hypertrophy, hyperplasia, and change in phenotype, precursor smooth muscle cells (stippled) develop into new smooth muscle (black) in previously nonmuscular segments, converting nonmuscular and partially muscular regions to partially muscular and muscular ones. Hypertrophy and hyperplasia of smooth muscle cells thicken the media. A thickened media also results from decrease in external diameter (not shown). Each of these changes is reversible. Occlusion of the vessel lumen is also reversible, but obliteration of the vessel is probably not.*

muscle myosin. The precursor cell is evidently a committed smooth muscle cell since it contains smooth muscle myosin.[82]

In contrast to the typical pattern of restriction and narrowing of the vessel lumen described here, some vessels dilate (Fig. 8). A region of partial or total vascular occlusion can increase blood flow to unaffected regions, and thus dilate vessel walls. The increased wall tension, or shearing stress, that results from this increase in flow can produce endothelial cell injury.[138] Dilatation can also result from increase in arterial wall compliance. Although the structural basis of vessel dilatation is not yet identified, it is likely that ulceration and destruction of the wall causes loss of endothelial and precursor cells, or can impair their function. This may prevent formation of new muscle that, if present, would buttress the wall against increased transmural pressure.

Regression of muscle occurs, being evident from the analysis of a population of pulmonary artery profiles, the shift being now from muscular and partially muscular to nonmuscular ones (Fig. 7). Presumably this also results from change in phenotype, although the features of regression are not yet established. During recovery, certainly the medial thickness of vessels can decrease and the external diameter increase. Restoration of patency to vessels is evident by an increase in haze on the arteriogram, and by an increase in the artery/alveolar density in tissue sections. As these structural features regress, PAP falls and right ventricular hypertrophy decreases.

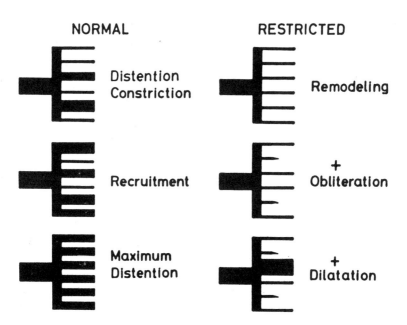

Figure 8: *In the normal pulmonary artery bed, there is both distention and constriction of vessels. The cross-sectional area of the bed is increased by recruitment of more vessels and by their distention until maximal distention is achieved. In the restricted bed, narrowing of the vessel lumen by mural remodeling and by obliterative loss of vessels can result in dilatation of other vessels.*

Preacinar Arteries

Normal Structure

All preacinar arteries in the human lung have a complete muscle coat as well as elastic laminae. At the hilum, the arteries are described as elastic, their medial muscle layer being included between an internal and external elastic lamina, with seven or more central laminae.[20,106] The central laminae then decrease, passing distally along the vessel wall. By the ninth airway generation (i.e., in arteries of about 2,000 μm in ED), the structure is described as muscular, there being now four or fewer central laminae.

A branch of the pulmonary artery accompanies each airway branch, and is called a conventional vessel. In addition to these, a number of extra or supernumerary arteries are found that do not accompany airway branches.[20,107] These are about three times as numerous as conventional artery branches, but have a smaller cross-sectional area. Therefore, at any level of an axial artery, supernumerary arteries comprise only about a quarter to a third of the potential cross-section area of the branch vessels.

Changes in Pulmonary Hypertension

Increase in transmural pressure, the result of distal vessel remodeling, almost certainly leads to remodeling of the walls of proximal vessels; however, direct injury of cells in the vessel wall in this region cannot be excluded.

On the pulmonary arteriogram there is a measurable reduction in the lumen of large arteries (see Figs. 13 and 23). As in pulmonary microcirculation, the cross-sectional area of preacinar arteries is reduced by a decrease in ED and by an increase in MT as muscle increases in existing segments of the pulmonary artery wall by cell proliferation. Unlike its effect in small arteries, constriction does not close the lumen of preacinar vessels, and only through occlusion by macrothrombi do these vessels become functionally nonpatent to blood flow.

In experimental studies, there is evidence of reversibility of the structural changes in preacinar arteries, namely lumen increase on pulmonary arteriograms, and a measurable increase in ED and decrease in MT in tissue sections. This is associated with a fall in PAP, but its contribution and that of the regression of changes within the microcirculation cannot be separately assessed.

Mediators of Pulmonary Artery Remodeling (Pathways of Action and Interaction)

The previous section describes the structural response of the pulmonary artery wall to injury. It is increasingly evident that changes in pulmonary vascular structure are effected and modulated by mediators of homeostatic processes that operate in the lung, and that these defense mechanisms also may cause cell injury, and so amplify the response. We briefly consider here the ones most relevant to pulmonary artery remodeling and their pathways of action and interaction.

Endothelial cell dysfunction increasingly appears to be a key event in the disturbance of homeostasis within pulmonary vessels. Its position makes it the cell most vulnerable to the action of toxic agents carried in the blood. Activation of cellular and humoral inflammatory pathways, the coagulation cascade, and arachidonic acid products each can cause or potentiate endothelial cell injury, and conversely, these processes can be activated by injured endothelial cells.

The inflammatory process activated by lung injury involves products of leukocytes,[133,137] macrophages,[9,62] mast cells, [93,132] complement,[40] kinins,[97] and immune complexes.[131] Leukocytes are recruited to the lung by chemotactic factors[16,22,28,96] and by complement activation.[40,56] The resultant generation of free radicals[23,61,80,137] augments injury. Lysosomal products also contribute to cell injury, and released phospholipase A_2[73] provides a substrate for prostanoid synthesis. Histamine released by mast cells and serotonin from platelets will alter vessel tone. Vascular tone is raised also by increased release of thromboxane[55] from activated platelets and by reduced release of prostacyclin from injured endothelial cells. Generation of leukotrienes increases vascular permeability and promotes leukocyte adherence to the vessel surface.[15]

The pulmonary endothelium participates in the coagulation process by producing the procoagulant factor VIII,[58,59] by releasing plasminogen activator,[77] which activates fibronolysis to maintain patency of pulmonary vessels, and by secreting prostacyclin, which inhibits platelet aggregation. Endothelial injury increases the release of factor VIII and diminishes plasminogen activator and prostacyclin production, reducing protection and so favoring hemostasis and thrombosis. In addition, platelet activation in the presence of damaged endothelium enhances thrombosis. Decreased endothelial cell function is also shown by decreased metabolism or production of vasoactive peptides (see Chapters 3 and 6).

Specific growth factors that stimulate cells of the vessel wall are now recognized. Platelet-derived growth factor (PDGF), released from alpha granules, stimulates growth of smooth muscle cells in vitro.[115] Serotonin can enhance the PDGF effect[10] and other growth factors are released by granulocytes.[37,76] Whether these agents act on medial smooth muscle or precursor smooth muscle cells in vivo has yet to be established, but they seem likely candidates, both in the normal circulation and in response to injury.

Adult Respiratory Distress Syndrome — Pulmonary Vascular Remodeling

ARDS (synonyms — acute respiratory failure, shock lung, Da Nang lung, wet lung syndrome, white lung syndrome, bypass lung, respirator lung, stiff lung syndrome) describes the sudden onset of respiratory distress (severe dyspnea) with hypoxemia and radiographic evidence of diffuse lung infiltrates and decreased lung compliance. Blaisdell and Lewis[4] document the historical events that led to the recognition of this syndrome in the mid-1960s, discuss its etiology and pathogenesis, and describe the typical pathological changes. While the primary injury may be to the lung (e.g., thoracic trauma or aspiration of gastric contents), ARDS may result from a variety of illnesses that do not cause a primary lung insult.[53,99] In ARDS patients, secondary injury to the lung may also occur, e.g., from treatment with a high FiO_2 (oxygen toxicity) or mechanical ventilation (barotrauma), from septicemia or endotoxemia, or even from release of the endogenous mediators associated with the inflammatory response, activation of the clotting cascade, or other homeostatic mechanisms.[39,100,114] The early hallmarks of lung injury are pulmonary endothelial damage, increased pulmonary capillary permeability, edema, and hemorrhage (Fig. 9). Within days of the onset of illness, diffuse pulmonary thromboemboli are often present[19,116] and disruption and destruction of the pulmonary capillary bed is extensive.[2,33,113] With advances in supportive respiratory care, increasingly more patients survive this early phase. Within 2–3 weeks there is organization of the alveolar wall and space, while in late-stage ARDS, alveolar wall and space fibrosis are typical.[42,102,122]

Relatively recent studies have established that within this time-course, lumen block (Fig. 10a and b) is frequent in large arteries[34] and that the structure of the pulmonary vascular bed is profoundly remodeled.[63,119,122,139] The structural changes form the basis of the increase in PAP and PVR (Fig. 11a and b) in ARDS patients.[140] While early in the disease vasodilators are effective, they are less so as it progresses and pulmonary vascular structure is altered. Remodeling of the pulmonary vasculature occurs despite the diverse causes of the lung injury (Figs. 12a and b, 13a–d). The degree of reduced filling evident on pulmonary arteriograms increases with the duration of illness (Figs. 14a–d). The range of lesions evident histologically and their timing (Fig. 15) indicate progressive injury to arteries, veins, and lymphatics.[122] As the illness progresses, the cross-sectional area of pulmonary intraacinar and preacinar arteries is further reduced (Fig. 16a and b). Recanalization of blocked vessels becomes evident (Fig. 17), as well as chronic vascular injury and attempts at

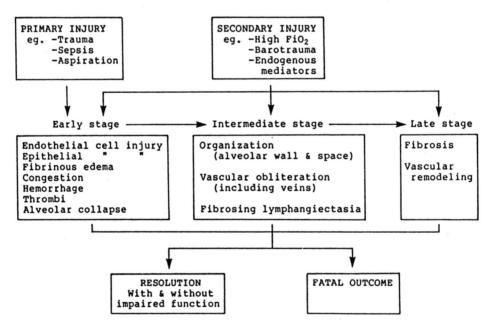

Figure 9: *Pathological changes typical of ARDS in the early (days 0–10), intermediate (days 10–20), and late (days 20–30+) stages. Only after recovery from late-stage ARDS is there resolution with impaired respiratory function.*

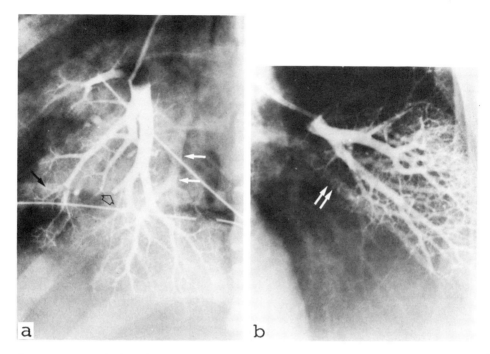

Figure 10: a: *Multiple pulmonary artery filling defects (PAFD) in a 19-year-old patient with severe ARDS from viral pneumonia, disseminated intravascular coagulopathy (DIC), and elevated PVR 48 h after endotracheal intubation. One of many PAFD is visible in an opacified segment of the right lower lobe (black arrow). A truncated occlusion in an adjacent artery is also present (open arrow). A draining vein is partially opacified (white arrows). Widespread pulmonary artery thrombosis was found in both lungs at 72 h postmortem after angiography.* **b:** *Normal angiogram in a 71-year-old patient who eventually recovered from mild ARDS secondary to sepsis, associated with elevated PVR and low cardiac output. Note the absence of PAFD, normal background opacification, and faint filling of a draining vein parallel to a segmental artery (arrows). (From ref. 34, with permission.)*

repair, indicated by the presence of duplicate basement membranes (Fig. 18). Vessel remnants are visible (Figs. 19a and b, 20a) in which extensive endothelial cell injury is evident (Fig. 20b). Dilatation and tortuosity of distal pulmonary arteries is demonstrated by arteriography (Fig. 21).

Animal Models of Acute and Subacute Lung Injury – Pulmonary Vascular Remodeling

We discuss here several agents that have been shown in experimental studies both to injure and stimulate cells of the pulmonary artery wall and to lead rapidly to structural remodeling, the development of pulmonary hypertension, and right ventricular hypertrophy. By careful dissection of cause and effect we will begin to understand the mechanism and mediators that trigger and modulate the processes that restructure the pulmonary vascular bed in

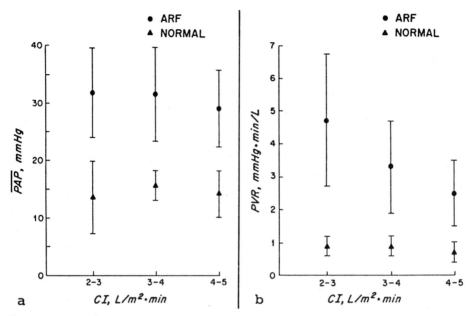

Figure 11: a: *Pulmonary artery pressure (PAP) and* **b:** *pulmonary vascular resistance (PVR) as a function of cardiac index (CI) for patients with ARF (adult respiratory failure); ARDS (●) and normal controls (▲). (From ref. 140 with permission.)*

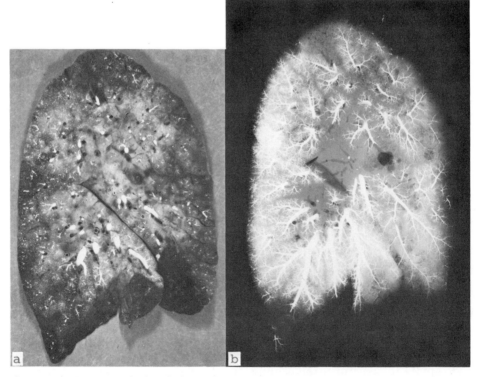

Figure 12: a: *One cm-thick right lung slice (× 0.4) in ARDS (15 days, drug overdose, aspiration). The arteries are injected with barium sulfate gelatin and appear white. Filled vessels are irregularly distributed, being greatly reduced in the center of the slice, as is evident by arteriography.* **b:** *Arteriogram (original magnification × 0.4) of the lung slice shown in* **a.** *Reduced filling of large arteries and decreased background haze is evident. (From ref. 63 with permission.)*

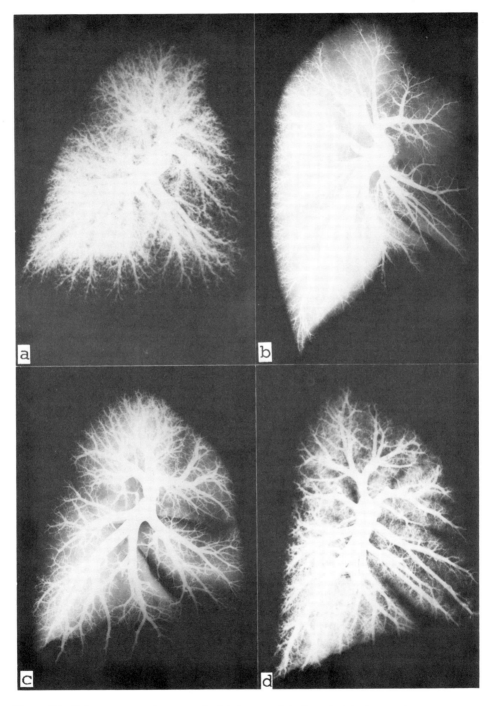

Figure 13: *Pulmonary arteriograms of adult human right lung (original magnification, ×0.4) contrasting even filling in the normal lung with the abnormal patchy filling in ARDS (note different etiology of ARDS):* **a:** *Normal (from ref. 106 with permission);* **b:** *15 days, drug overdose and aspiration (from ref. 63 with permission);* **c:** *18 days, pneumonoccal sepsis, bacterial pneumonia (from ref.63 with permission);* **d:** *27 days, multiple fractures, with lung contusion; fat emboli, septicemia (from ref. 119 with permission).*

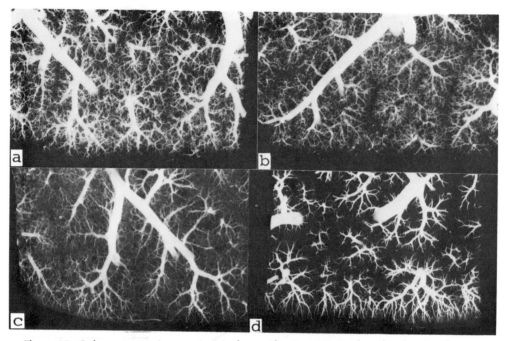

Figure 14: *Pulmonary arteriograms (original magnification, ×2.4); pleural surface is at bottom:* **a:** *Normal adult lung;* **b:** *Early ARDS (6 days, aspiration) showing reduced filling of small periacinar arteries and prominent, edematous interlobular septa.* **c:** *Intermediate stage ARDS (16 days, viral pneumonia) showing marked reduction of filled small vessels, and prominent interlobular septa;* **d:** *Intermediate stage ARDS (16 days, toxic inhalation) showing more extensive reduction of filled small arteries due to intimal obliteration. Stretching of subpleural branches of the pulmonary artery about dilated air spaces creates a "picket-fence" appearance. (From ref. 122 with permission.)*

VASCULAR LESIONS IN ARDS

THROMBOSIS ⟶

- - - - - - - - - - - - - - - - - ENDOTHELIAL INJURY ⟶

NECROTIZING VASCULITIS ⟶

LYMPHATIC THROMBOSIS ⟶

- - - - - -OBLITERATIVE INTIMAL SCLEROSIS ⟶
(INCLUDING VENOSCLEROSIS)

- - - - - -ARTERIAL MUSCULARIZATION ⟶

TORTUOSITY & DILATATION ⟶

DAYS 0   10   20   30
   EARLY   INTERMEDIATE   LATE

Figure 15: *Timing of pulmonary vascular injury and remodeling in ARDS.*

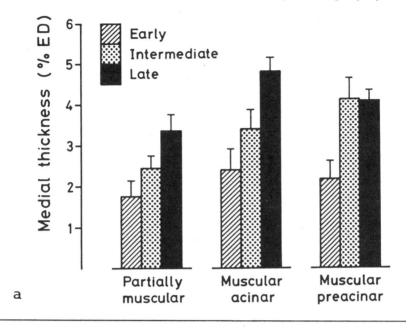

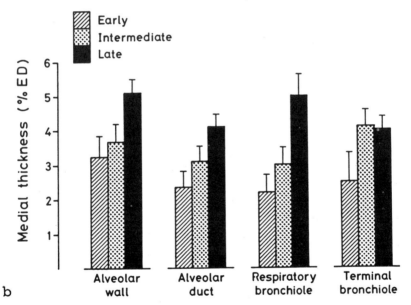

Figure 16: a: *Variation in % MT of partially muscular and muscular intraacinar arteries (mean ± SEM), and of muscular preacinar arteries in early, intermediate, and late stage ARDS.*
b: *Variation in % MT (mean ± SEM) of arteries associated with the alveolar wall, alveolar duct respiratory bronchiolus, and terminal bronchiolus in early, intermediate, and late stage ARDS. (From ref. 122 with permission.)*

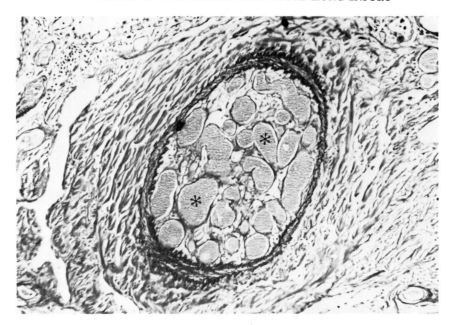

Figure 17: *Recanalized pulmonary artery (390 μm ED) in ARDS (27 days, trauma with lung contusion, fat emboli, and septicemia); patent areas of the vessel lumen are filled with barium-sulfate gelatin mixture (*). (4 μm section stained with elastic van Gieson, ×1,389). (From ref. 63 with permission.)*

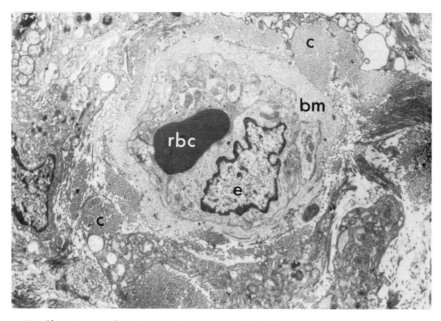

Figure 18: *Chronic vascular injury in late stage ARDS (25 days, aspiration): narrowing of capillary lumen by endothelial cell (e); red blood cell (rbc). Duplicate basement membranes (bm) are present and there is abundant perivascular collagen (c) (×5,264). (From ref. 122 with permission.)*

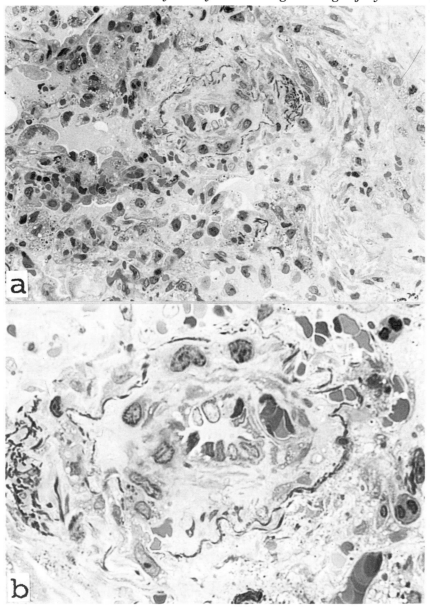

Figure 19: a: *Consolidated lung parenchyma in ARDS (same patient as in Fig. 13b) with a small vessel delineated by a single elastic lamina showing luminal narrowing (1 μm sections stained with toluidine blue, ×342).* **b:** *Higher magnification of vessel shown in* **a.** *(×547). (From ref. 63 with permission.)*

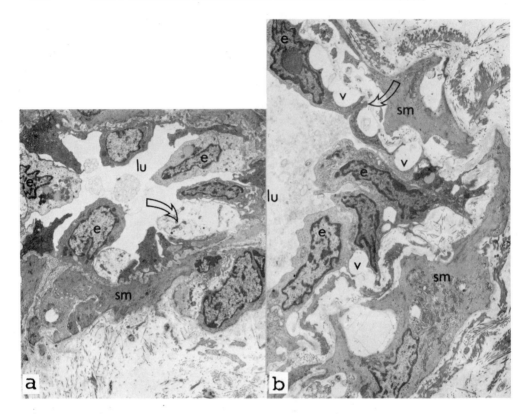

Figure 20: *Pulmonary vessels in ARDS (18 days, pneumonia and secondary Klebsiella bacteremia), biopsy tissue.* **a:** *Muscular vessel—vessel lumen (lu), hypertrophied endothelial cells (e) showing variation in density of cytoplasm, cell "ghost" (arrow) with outer membrane and lysed external contents, cellular debris, smooth muscle cells (sm) (original magnification, ×4,455).* **b:** *Muscular vessel—vessel lumen (lu), subendothelial vacuoles (v) forming pallisades (arrow) between endothelial cells (e) and basement membrane, smooth muscle cells (sm) (original magnification, ×4,455). (From ref. 63 with permission.)*

acute and subacute lung injury. At first glance the response seems stereotypic, but the various forms of injury produce patterns of remodeling that indicate different mechanisms operate, or at least vary, in their relative importance. In response to hyperoxia and monocrotaline, for example, the remodeling typically includes obliteration of small pulmonary arteries that is not seen in response to hypoxia or high flow, although all evoke hypertrophy that reduces the cross-sectional area of the pulmonary vascular bed by thickening vessel walls. The remodeling that results from both sepsis and endotoxin typically includes thinning of vessel walls and dilatation of the pulmonary vascular bed, and, in the case of endotoxin, lysis of vessel walls. All are known to stimulate precursor smooth muscle cells, except high flow (which has not been studied in the same detail). The nature, severity, and sequence of the mechanisms that operate in response to each ultimately determine the remodeling achieved. The speed of the structural changes in response to each emphasizes the lability of the various cell populations within the pulmonary artery wall.

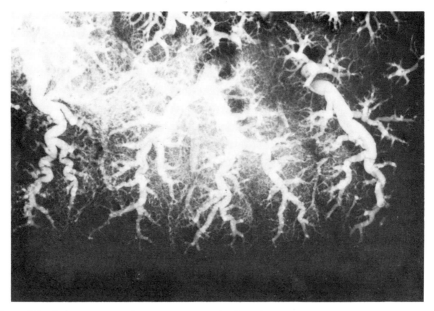

Figure 21: *Pulmonary arteriogram (×2.4) with pleural surface at bottom; late stage ARDS (28 days, bacterial pneumonia and sepsis), showing marked arterial tortuosity. (From ref. 63 with permission.)*

Oxygen Toxicity

It is well established that breathing high concentrations of oxygen at hyperbaric or normobaric pressure injures the lung. During ventilator therapy, most patients now receive as low an FiO_2 as is consistent with an adequate PaO_2, and since the introduction of mechanical ventilation, lower levels of oxygen can be used. The problem of treatment with very high levels of oxygen now exists only for patients with the degree of hypoxemia typical of severe ARDS.

The effects of hyperoxia on lung structure and function have been extensively reviewed.[8] Normobaric hyperoxia is associated with widespread alveolar wall injury, including cell edema, cell destruction (particulary of endothelial cells and type 1 pneumonocytes), and increase in the number of type 2 pneumonocytes; alveolar wall collapse, alveolar edema, and formation of hyaline membranes; increase in the number of leukocytes and nonspecific mononuclear cells in the alveolar wall, and alveolar macrophages; and interstitial and intra-alveolar fibrosis. Our recent studies have established that, in addition, the walls of pulmonary arteries are extensively remodeled, particularly those of the microcirculation and the resistance vessels, and that pulmonary hypertension and right ventricular hypertrophy develop.[64-67]

Experimental studies have established that the severity of pulmonary changes depends on the level of inspired oxygen. Cell necrosis results from intracellular generation of toxic free radicals (superoxide and hydroxyl) and their products (particularly hydrogen peroxide).[60] Generation of these metabolites above basal rates raises cellular levels of protective enzymes (such as superoxide dismutase, catalase, or glutathione reductase) and free radical scavengers (such as tocopherol or ascorbate).[60] These changes permit cell survival and adaptation to hyperoxic conditions. However, if the production of toxic products overwhelms the process of adaptation, the animal does not survive. Levels above 90% are usually fatal after 72 hours; oxygen levels >80% and <90% cause extensive lung injury, and adaptation, which allows survival as well as remodeling of the pulmonary vascular bed.[11-13,67]

After a few days of exposure to hyperoxia, edema diminishes as the integrity of the alveolar-capillary membrane is restored; there is cell hypertrophy, and cell hyperplasia, which changes the distribution of the various cell types.[68,134] After 4–7 days, the cells in the wall of small pulmonary arteries hypertrophy, including the endothelial cell, precursor smooth muscle cell (Fig. 22a and b), smooth muscle cell, and fibroblast. While the other cells also undergo hyperplasia, endothelial cell number first falls (i.e., after 2 days of exposure) returning to the normal value only after 28 days.[66] Both pericytes and intermediate cells contribute to the increased number of percursor cells, although intermediate cells are always more frequent. In this way, in response to hyperoxia a new baseline is set within the adapted lung as the alveolar-capillary membrane is stablilized and pulmonary vessels begin the process of remodeling (Fig. 22c).

By 7 days the cross-sectional area of the pulmonary vascular bed is strikingly reduced (Fig. 23a and b). Lumen diameter falls, by both a decrease in ED and an increase in MT, and the number of perfused arteries is reduced by one-third.[67] Muscle increases in previously muscular segments of vessel walls and appears in previously nonmuscular segments; PAP (Fig. 24) and PVR are increased. An additional and rapid rise in PAP occurs on return to breathing air (Fig. 24), perhaps the result of hypoxia caused by impaired diffusion across a thickened alveolar-capillary membrane, or by intraalveolar edema.

Each of the above changes is exacerbated by longer exposure, 28 days being the longest we have studied.[64] At this time, precursor smooth muscle cells form a complete layer in the intima (Fig. 25a and b) of about half of the partially muscular arteries and virtually all of the remaining nonmuscular ones.[66] The number of muscularized arteries associated with alveolar ducts doubles and the number associated with alveolar walls (Fig. 25c) increases threefold. The number of perfused vessels is less than half the normal value and many vessel remnants are apparent both by light and electron microscopy (Fig. 26a and b). Pulmonary artery pressure is twice normal.

Despite weaning from hyperoxia by a daily reduction in FiO_2, a return to breathing air after 28 days of exposure further remodels the pulmonary vascular bed.[64] In an 8-week period after weaning, there is both progressive and regressive modification to the walls of pulmonary arteries. In both preacinar and intraacinar regions, the thickness of medial muscle regresses in a time-dependent way, although never to normal levels. But in intraacinar regions, particularly after 2 weeks in air, medial muscle is now present in virtually all vessels. While the number of vessels with muscle decreases with time, even after 8 weeks many more are present than normal. After 8 weeks PAP is still above normal. Since the number of perfused vessels does not return to normal, it is likely that vessel obliteration, as well as increased muscle, contributes substantially. Evidently, normoxia represents a potent stimulus to the cells of pulmonary arteries remodeled by hyperoxia.

In addition to injury by the generation of free radicals, hyperoxia alters the balance of mediators in the lung. Short exposure (i.e., 2–3 days) increases levels

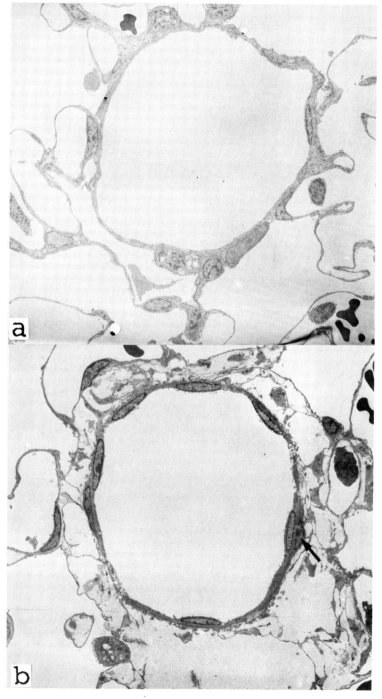

Figure 22.: a: *Normal rat pulmonary artery (ED 31μm), (original magnification, ×2,222).* **b:** *Rat pulmonary artery (ED 34μm) after 4 days at 87% O$_2$ showing edema, hydropic disruption/vacuolization of interstitium. A precursor smooth muscle cell (arrow) lies behind an endothelial cell. The increased number of endothelial cell nuclei suggests hyperplasia (original magnification, ×1,995). (From ref. 63 with permission.)*

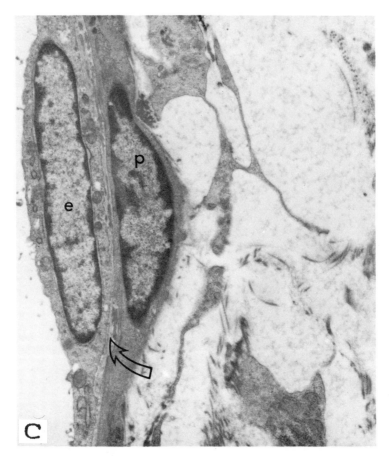

Figure 22c: *Higher magnification of b showing precursor smooth muscle cell (p) behind the basement membrane (arrow) of the endothelial cell (e), (×12,425) (from ref. 63 with permission).*

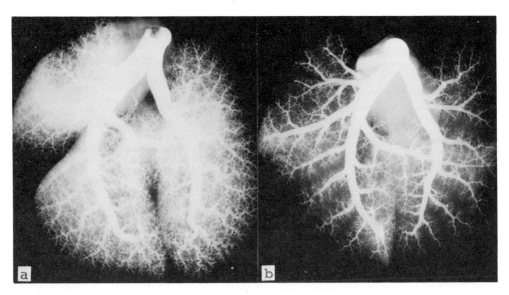

Figure 23: *Rat pulmonary arteriograms (× 2):* **a:** *normal;* **b:** *87% O$_2$ for 7 days. (From ref. 67 with permission.)*

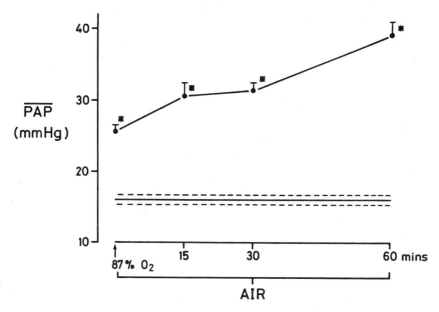

Figure 24: *Mean (± SEM) pulmonary artery pressure (PAP) showing basal value (17.0 + 0.7 mmHg) in rats, the increase after breathing 87% O_2 for 7 days (△ 9.8 mmHg, p < 0.01) and the further increase on return to air after 15 min (△14.3 mmHg, p < 0.01). After 60 min in air, PAP is significantly above the value at the end of exposure to oxygen (△ 21.3 mmHg, p < 0.01).*

of bradykinin and norepinephrine.[3] Clearance by endothelial cells of serotonin and norepinephrine is progressively depressed over 48 hours[5] and at 48 hours, prostaglandin dehydrogenase is inhibited, resulting in impaired prostaglandin catabolism by the lung.[123] After 2 weeks of hyperoxia, thromboxane (TxB_2) levels are unchanged while prostacyclin (6-keto-$PGF_{1\alpha}$) levels are greatly increased.[63] In the isolated lung, the increased levels of free radicals generated by hyperoxia evoke a pressor response,[36] and the vasoconstrictive response to hypoxia is diminished by preexposure to hyperoxia, possibly by the release of a vasodilator prostaglandin.[95] Conversely, in rats preexposed to hypoxia, survival in hyperoxia is increased, probably the result of an increase in superoxide dismutase.[117] Jenkinson[60] has recently discussed modification of hyperoxic lung injury by pharmacologic agents.

Monocrotaline

Monocrotaline is an inert pyrrolizidine alkaloid found in the shrub *Crotalaria spectabilis*.[69] Pulmonary hypertension develops in animals after ingestion of plant seeds or ingestion of alkaloid, or injection of the alkaloid or its metabolites.[7,38,43,48,69,83] After intake, monocrotaline passes to the liver where it is converted to an active pyrrole.[81] The pyrrole then passes to the lung, injuring the vasculature. Early pulmonary microvascular injury leads to later secondary arterial structural changes and pulmonary hypertension. Regardless of the method of administration, arterial remodeling is the common end-point,

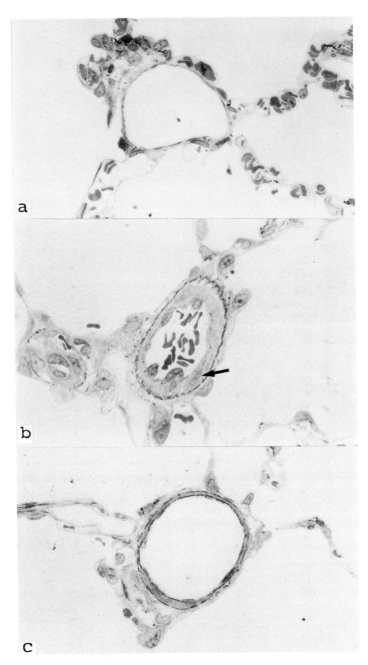

Figure 25: *Rat alveolar wall arteries (1μm sections stained with toluidine blue, ×860).* **a:** *normal vessel (ED 35 μm), (×860);* **b:** *vessel (28 μm ED) after breathing 87% O_2 with precursor smooth muscle cells (arrow) lie behind the endothelial cell layer.* **c:** *vessel (ED 36μm) after breathing 87% O_2 for 28 days; the wall of the vessel is fully muscularized, with well-defined internal and external elastic laminae. (From ref. 63 with permission.)*

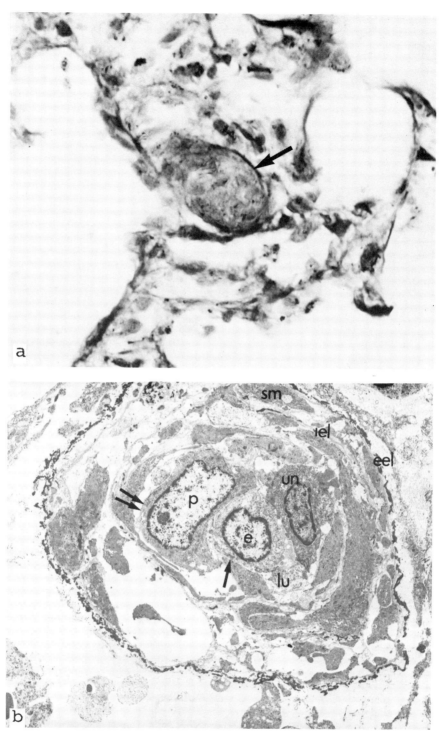

Figure 26: a: *Remnant of rat alveolar duct artery (arrow) after 87% O_2 for 28 days (4 μm section stained with elastic van Gieson, original magnification, ×781)* **b:** *Rat alveolar wall artery (ED 21μm) after 87% O_2 for 28 days: external elastic lamina (eel), fragments of an internal elastic lamina (iel) with a smooth muscle cell in between (sm). The vessel lumen (lu) is occluded by an endothelial cell (e) and an unidentified cell (un) that has well-developed endoplasmic reticulum. The basement membrane is partly visible (arrow). A precursor smooth muscle cell (p) lies external to basement membrane (original magnification ×4,725). (From ref. 65 with permission.)*

but the severity of injury varies with the method of administration and the dose of monocrotaline.[43,83] The injury usually progresses, leading to death. Recovery has been reported only in animals fed *C. spectabilis* seeds.[48]

Within hours after injection of monocrotaline, the pulmonary endothelium is swollen and damaged, and pulmonary edema forms.[101,121,125] Early transcapillary leakage of carbon and Thorotrast has been demonstrated.[101,125] Platelet-fibrin thrombi are also found early.[74,124] Over the next 1–4 weeks, at a rate dependent on whether monocrotaline is injected or ingested, progressive remodeling of small pulmonary arteries occurs.[30,48,70,83] Vessels with a lumen occluded by endothelial swelling, platelet-fibrin plugs, or cellular debris are increasingly found[48,75,83] (Fig. 27a, b, and c). Extension of muscle into previously nonmuscular segments and hypertrophy of muscle in previously muscular segments occurs.[48,83] These changes precede and directly lead to an increase in PVR, which is reflected as pulmonary hypertension, medial hypertrophy of larger proximal arteries, and right ventricular hypertrophy (RVH) (Fig. 28). Arteriography shows vessel narrowing and loss of background haze (Fig. 29). Hypoxia, polycythemia, or hemodynamically significant vasoconstriction are not detected, and therefore do not contribute to remodeling.[83]

In recent years, interest in the mediators of vascular remodeling from monocrotaline has increased. Clearly, there is a loss of protective homeostasis of the pulmonary microvascular environment. Endothelial function is deranged, with reduced angiotensin converting enzyme levels[70,90] and decreased uptake of norepinephrine and serotonin.[31,44] Although unstimulated release of prostacyclin (6-keto $PGF_{1\alpha}$) is increased in monocrotaline-treated lungs,[29,90] arachidonic acid infusion fails to cause the normal burst in 6-keto $PGF_{1\alpha}$ release.[29] Lungs treated with monocrotaline also demonstrate hyperreactive responses to vasoconstrictor agents. Angiotensin II, serotonin, and hypoxia all cause abnormally high vasopressor responses during the post-monocrotaline period.[45,110] Plasminogen activator activity is decreased by monocrotaline.[90]

Platelets contribute, in part, to remodeling of the vascular bed by monocrotaline. Prostacyclin infusion at the time of adminstration of monocrotaline diminishes thromboxane production and lung edema formation.[14] Induction of thrombocytopenia at the time of monocrotaline administration does not reduce RVH, but platelet depletion 4 or 7 days after monocrotaline does.[46] This suggests that there are discrete critical periods of injury, with early monocrotaline injury, and later activation of secondary processes (involving platelets), that lead to remodeling. We have provided additional evidence of two phases of structural changes by showing that methylprednisolone, a glucocorticoid, is more effective in preventing remodeling if given daily, starting 24 hours after a single dose of monocrotaline, than if administered as two boluses that cover only the time of monocrotaline injection.[75] Although the monocrotaline injury initiates the processes leading to remodeling, ultimately it is the loss of endothelial protection and later activation of secondary biological cascades that determine its degree and nature.

Figure 27 a–c: *Rat pulmonary arteries 21 days after a subcutaneous injection of monocrotaline (4 μm sections, stained with elastic van Gieson, original magnification ×984); all vessels are "occluded" and have a lumen filled with debris. The barium-gelatin mixture used did not perfuse these vessels, indicating that they are functionally not patent.*

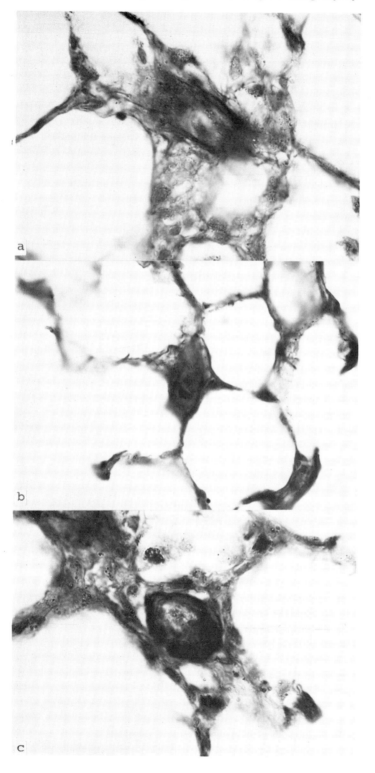

Figure 27a–c: *(See legend on previous page)*

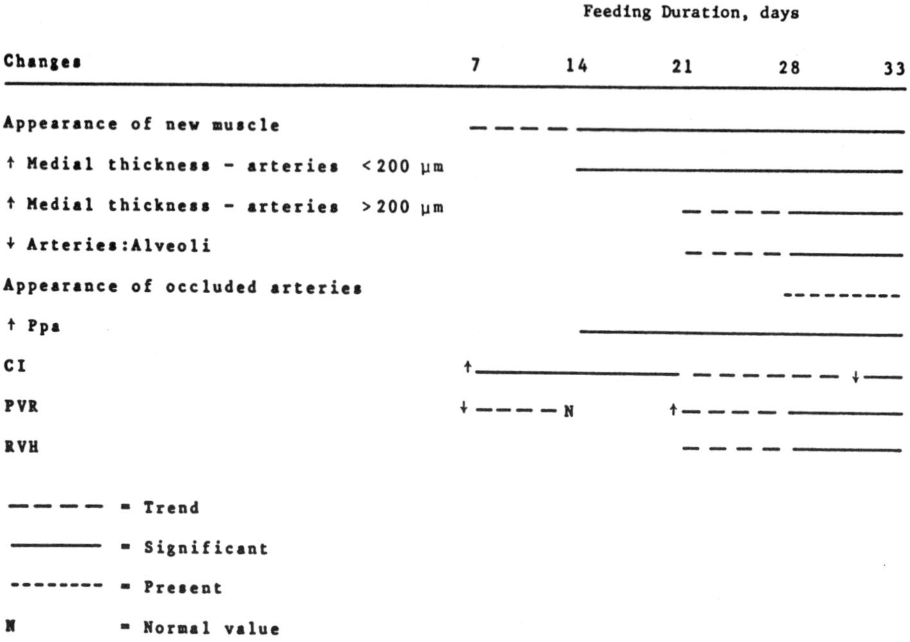

Changes	Feeding Duration, days				
	7	14	21	28	33
Appearance of new muscle	– – – – ————————————				
↑ Medial thickness – arteries <200 µm		————————————			
↑ Medial thickness – arteries >200 µm			– – – – ———————		
↓ Arteries:Alveoli			– – – – ———————		
Appearance of occluded arteries				- - - - - - - -	
↑ Ppa			————————————		
CI	↑————————————			– – – – – ↓—	
PVR	↓ – – – – N		↑ – – – – ———————		
RVH			– – – – ———————		

– – – – = Trend

————— = Significant

- - - - - - - - = Present

N = Normal value

Figure 28: *Timing of structural and hemodynamic changes, and right ventricular hypertrophy (RVH) in rats fed* Crotalaria spectabilis *for periods up to 33 days (Ppa = pulmonary artery pressure; CI = cardiac index; PVR = pulmonary vascular resistance). (From ref. 83 with permission.)*

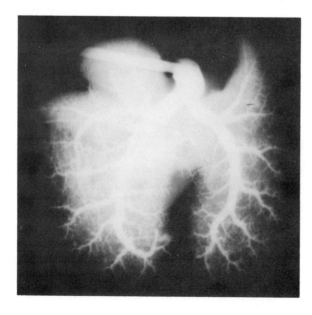

Figure 29: *Rat pulmonary arteriogram (×2) after 21 days of* Crotalaria spectabilis *feeding; the lumen of the axial pathway is reduced and there is a loss of background haze (compare with Fig. 23a). (From ref. 83 with permission.)*

Hypoxia

In man, as in many other species, the individual degree of vasoconstrictive response to hypoxia varies widely, from virtually no change in PAP to more than doubling. Acute exposure to hypoxia raises PAP by rapid and reversible constriction (Fig. 30). We have found that subacute exposure to hypoxia leads to a higher PAP than acute exposure, the result of persistent vasoconstriction and structural remodeling (Fig. 30). Polycythemia contributes in a major way to the increase in PVR and PAP caused by subacute exposure.[25]

From our studies we know that the acute pressor response persists throughout several weeks of exposure to hypoxia and begins to fall within 1 hour of return to air. After chronic exposure and return to air, acute exposure to hypoxia reestablishes the vasoconstrictive response, the degree of reactivity of the remodeled vascular bed being similar to that of the normal lung.

Within the first days of exposure to hypoxia, structural remodeling of the pulmonary vascular bed begins. Endothelial and precursor smooth muscle cell swelling, hypertrophy (Fig. 31), and hyperplasia occur, without cell death.[84] Large arteries are remodeled in a striking way, especially the adventitia,[87] with a reduced lumen evident on the pulmonary arteriogram (Fig. 32). Vessel remnants are not seen, suggesting that the reduction in artery/alveolar density

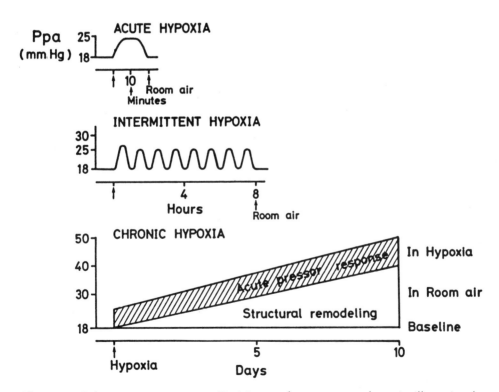

Figure 30: *Pulmonary artery pressure (Ppa) in rats after exposure to hypoxia, illustrating the rapidly reversible rise in Ppa after acute or intermittent hypoxia. After 10 days of hypoxia, the rise in Ppa is based mostly on structural remodeling, but a reversible acute pressor response persists.*

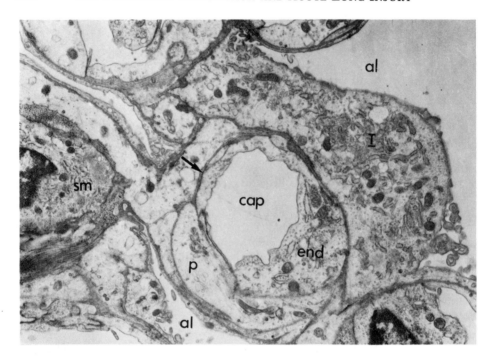

Figure 31: *Electron micrograph of an alveolar capillary (cap) in rat lung after 10 days of exposure to hypoxia. The endothelial cells (end) appear pale, swollen, and thickened. The associated pericyte (p) also appears pale and swollen. The intercellular space (arrow) is more electron dense than normal. al = Alveolus; I = type I pneumonocyte; sm = smooth muscle cell (original magnification, ×11,900). (From ref. 84 with permission.)*

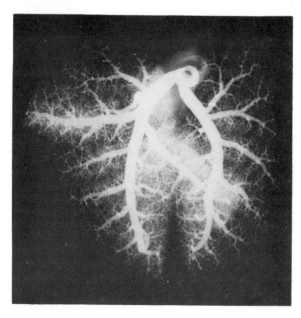

Figure 32: *Rat pulmonary arteriogram (×2) after 2 weeks of hypoxia (at 360 torr); the lumen of the axial pathway is reduced and there is a loss of background haze (compare with Fig. 23a).*

that occurs is probably the result of functional closure of vessels rather than vessel obliteration.[26] These structural changes contribute little to the early rise in PAP, but are the major cause of rise in pressure after longer exposure.[103] Young rats are more susceptible to hypoxia than adults, and adult males are more susceptible than adult females.[104] In polycythemic rats, the increase in PAP and PVR in response to hypoxia is greater than in rats in which the hematocrit is corrected (Fig. 33a and b).

The structural changes in large and small arteries and hemodynamic changes caused by hypoxia regress in air (Fig. 34a and b).[26,50] The hematocrit falls rapidly, correlating with an early fall in PVR; PAP is slower to fall and does not return to normal within 30 days.[26] In intraacinar arteries, muscle regresses, the greatest change occurring in distal vessels.

We find that some rats do not develop vasoconstriction in response to acute hypoxia, but structural changes are present in virtually all animals exposed to chronic hypoxia. In animals that do not respond to acute hypoxia, however, the

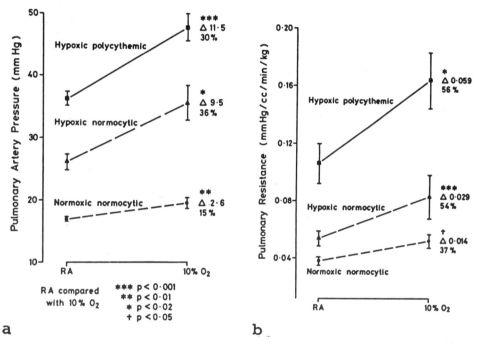

Figure 33: a: *Pulmonary arterial pressure (Ppa) in controls (n = 9, hypoxic-normocytic rats (n = 5) with hypoxia-induced structurally remodeled vascular beds, and hypoxic-polycythemic rats (n = 8). In room air (RA) Ppa is greater in hypoxic-polycythemic animals compared with controls and intermediate in hypoxic-normocytic animals. With acute hypoxic exposure (10% O_2), all groups showed an increase in Ppa with the greater rises, expressed both as absolute and as a percent rise above baseline, in hypoxic animals. Increases as a percent of baseline were similar in two hypoxic groups.* **b:** *Pulmonary arterial resistance (Rp) in three groups of rats in RA (room air) and 10% O_2. A high Rp is found in hypoxic animals (hypoxic-normocytic, n = 5; hypoxic-polycythemic, n = 8) than in controls (n = 9) whether measured in RA or 10% O_2 with greater increases, both absolute and as a percent above baseline, in the hypoxic group. Percent increases are similar in the two hypoxic groups. Levels of significance as in a). (From ref. 25 with permission.)*

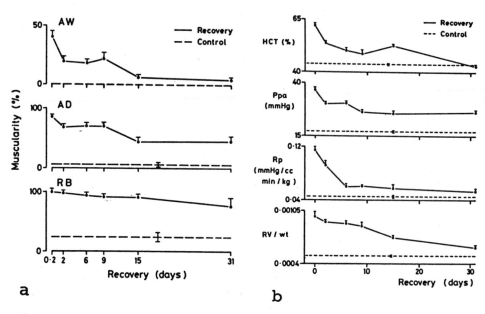

Figure 34: a: *Number (%) of rat intraacinar arteries associated with alveolar walls (AW), alveolar ducts (AD), and respiratory bronchioli (RB) that are muscularized (i.e., muscular or partially muscular) after exposure to hypoxia for 14 days and on return to air for periods up to 31 days. (From ref. 26 with permission.)* **b:** *Hematocrit (Hct), pulmonary artery pressure (Ppa), pulmonary vascular resistance (Rp), and right ventricular weight (RV/wt.) in rats after exposure to hypoxia for 14 days and on return to air for periods up to 31 days. (Modified from ref. 26 with permission.)*

degree of structural remodeling after subacute exposure has yet to be established. It may be that the structural remodeling component is dissociated from the acute vasoconstrictive response. Weir[136] has recently reviewed the mechanisms and mediators of the acute vasoconstrictive response to hypoxia.

Sepsis/Endotoxin

We have developed a model of subacute intraperitoneal sepsis in which there is reproducible bacteremia and a protracted course.[71] To produce an analog of clinical peritonitis, gelatin capsules containing a combined inoculum of *Escherichia coli* and *Bacteroides fragilis* are implanted. These organisms are the most common clinical aerobic and anaerobic isolates from human intraperitoneal infections.[1,120] Single implants on four or eight weekly occasions (intermittent sepsis) alter pulmonary artery structure more than continuous bacteremia of shorter duration, i.e., bacteremia produced by four implants within one week.

After four or eight implants, small intraperitoneal abscesses (1-2 mm in diameter) are present and the total number of leukocytes and relative number of neutrophils are greatly increased. While these changes increase with time, paradoxically, the animals appear less sick as the number of implants increases. Pulmonary hypertension does not develop in this model and gas exchange is unchanged despite extensive injury and remodeling both of alveolar walls and the walls of pulmonary arteries.

In contrast to the pattern of reduction in the cross-sectional area of the pulmonary vascular bed in the other models mentioned here, there is dilatation of small vessels, seen on the arteriogram as an increase in background haze (Fig. 35a and b), with some arteries near the pleura being dilated enough to be seen as

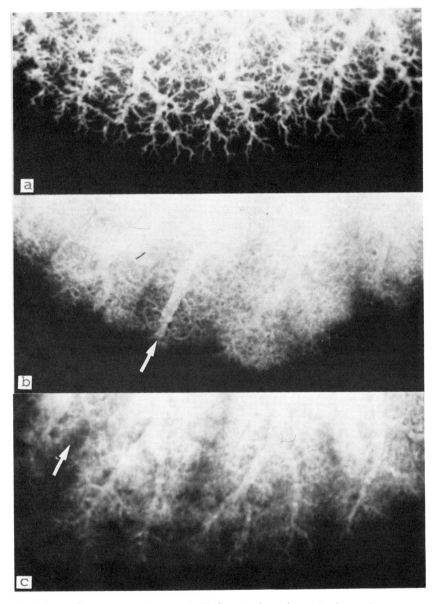

Figure 35: *Rat pulmonary arteriograms (×5) showing lateral anterior lung edge:* **a:** *normal;* **b:** *after 4 weeks of intermittent sepsis, large vessels are dilated (arrow) and filling of small intraacinar arteries increased;* **c:** *after 7 days continuous endotoxin filling of small intraacinar vessels is increased, patchy nonfilled regions are evident (arrow). (From ref. 63 with permission.)*

separate vessels. There is perivenular edema and progressive increase in the cellularity of the alveolar wall and alveolar space by neutrophils and nonspecific mononuclear cells (Fig. 36a, b, and c). In small intraacinar arteries, endothelial cells and precursor smooth muscle cells are hypertrophied (Figs. 37a and 38a). There is disruption of the interstitium (Fig. 39a). The walls of the capillaries are attenuated and many degranulated neutrophils are present within the lumen (Fig. 39b).

To analyze the effect of endotoxin, an important component of the sepsis model, we infused purified *E. coli* endotoxin lipopolysaccharide (LPS B4-0111). Continuous and intermittent infusion each produce vascular injury but the nature of the injury is different. Continuous administration of endotoxin for 7 days (300 μg daily) doubles the total number of circulating leukocytes and triples the relative number of neutrophils. There is thrombocytopenia until day 3, but thereafter the platelet count is normal; PAP is significantly increased and moderate right ventricular hypertrophy is present. The pattern on the pulmonary arteriogram (Fig. 35c) resembles that after sepsis, there being dilatation of small arteries, although patchy areas of nonfilling are more evident. There is medial thickening in intraacinar arteries and an increase in the number of muscularized arteries, changes consistent with the degree of pulmonary hypertension.

Intermittent infusion of endotoxin (as a bolus of 300 μg over 2–3 hours) produces similar changes in leukocyte count and proportion of neutrophils.

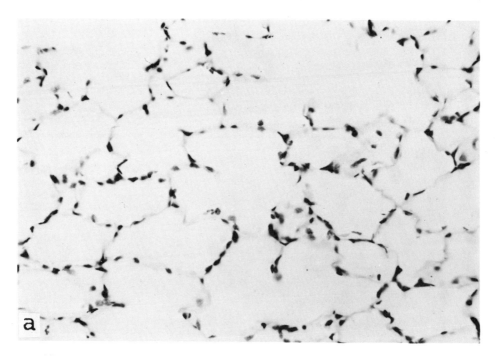

Figure 36: *Micrographs of rat lung:* **a:** *normal lung,* **b:** *after four implants of* E. coli *and B. fragilis at weekly intervals, and* **c:** *after eight implants (4 μm sections; stained with H & E, original magnification ×488). (From ref. 71 with permission.)*

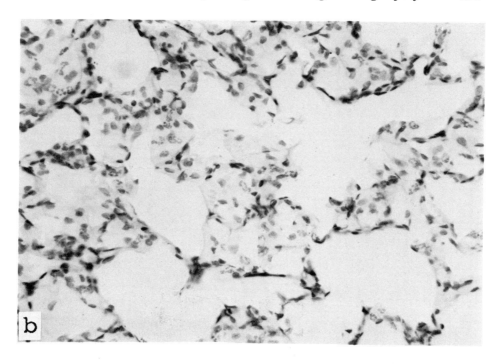

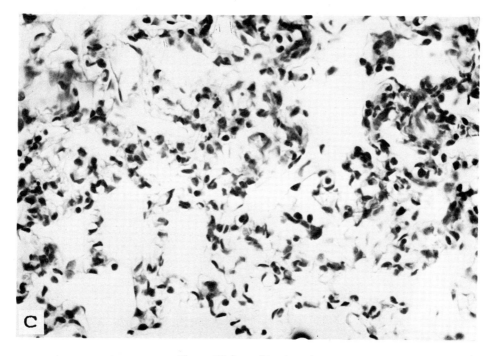

Figure 36 b,c: *(Continued)*

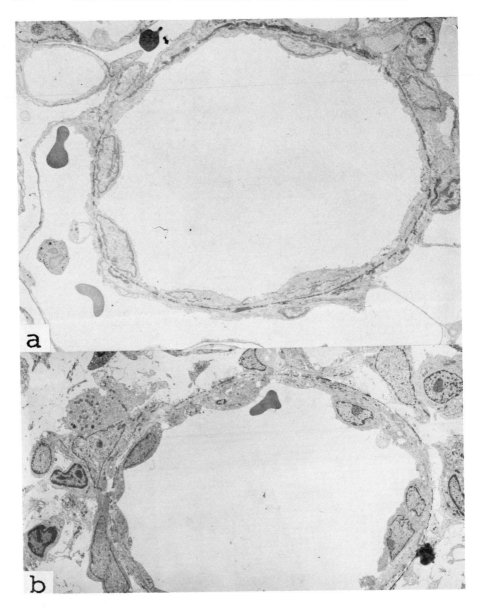

Figure 37: *Rat intraacinar arteries showing hypertrophied intimal layer including endothelial and precursor smooth muscle cells:* **a:** *after 4 intraabdominal implants of* E. coli *and* B. fragilis *at weekly intervals (ED 34 μm, ×2,756).* **b:** *after 4 bolus infusions of endotoxin at weekly intervals (ED 34μm, ×2,222). (From ref. 63 with permission.)*

Histological changes, however, are more severe than after continuous infusion: there is greater thickening of the alveolar wall and the alveolar space is more cellular. Hypertrophied endothelial cells and precursor smooth muscle cells are evident in intraacinar arteries (Figs. 37b and 38b). The walls of other vessels are

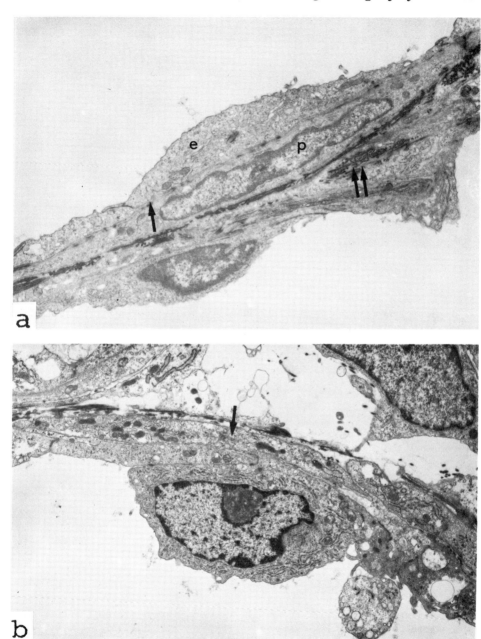

Figure 38: a: *Higher magnification of vessel shown in Fig. 37a. Precursor smooth muscle cell (p), endothelial cell (e), basement membrane (arrow), external elastic lamina (eel), elastin fragments (double arrows), endothelial cell process (×10,325).* **b:** *Higher magnification of vessel wall shown in Fig. 37b, subendothelial cell processes (arrow), (×10,325). (From ref. 63 with permission.)*

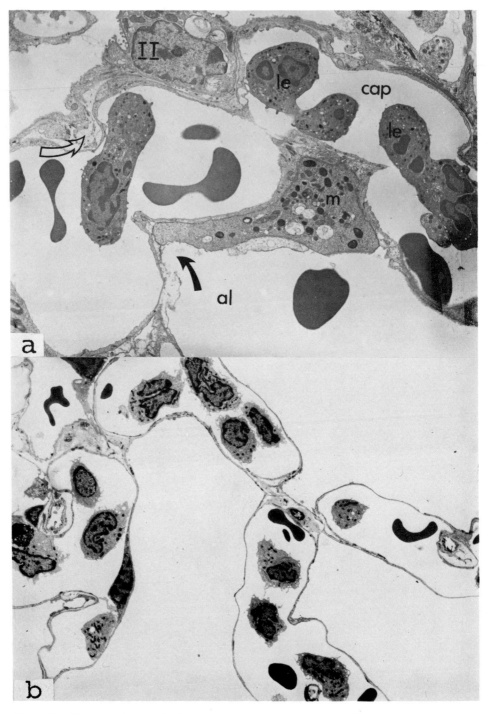

Figure 39: *Electron micrograph of rat alveolar wall:* **a:** *After four implants, showing interstitial edema (open arrow), migratory cell (m), type II pneumonocyte (II), alveolus (alv), leukocytes (1), fragmented cell process (solid arrow), capillary (cap) (×4725).* **b:** *after eight implants, showing relative extension of the air-blood barrier over the alveolar surface, with many degranulated leukocytes present within the vascular space (×2,222). (From ref. 71 with permission.)*

lysed (Fig. 40a and b). In the case of small arteries, this often leaves only the elastic laminae, with cell debris between (Fig. 40a).

Jacobs and Bone[57] have recently reviewed the mechanisms and mediators of lung injury in sepsis (see also Chapter 19 of this volume). The biological effects of endotoxin are reviewed by Morrison and Ulevitch.[91] The effect of endotoxin on the lung is complex, involving the inflammatory response, platelets and thromboxane, and complement.[32,98,118] Brigham[6] has discussed the effect of endotoxin on pulmonary microvascular permeability and vasoreactivity.

High Flow

The pulmonary bed, through recruitment of vessels, is easily able to accommodate a doubling or tripling of blood flow without the development of pulmonary hypertension.[41,78,130] If flow is maintained at high levels for prolonged periods, however, particularly at high pressure, pulmonary microvascular injury and remodeling may occur. The growing lung may be more susceptible to high flow injury than the adult lung.[52] Pulmonary artery disease and pulmonary hypertension is seen not only with congenital heart defects but is sometimes caused by palliative surgical procedures that produce systemic-to-pulmonary shunts.[94]

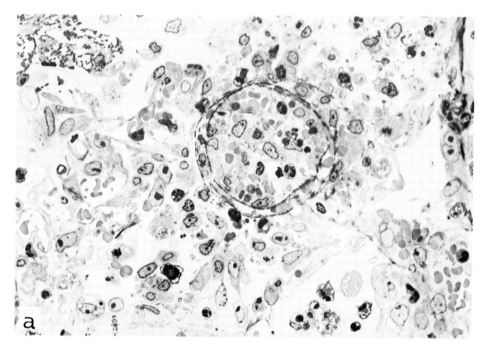

Figure 40 a: *Rat intraacinar pulmonary artery (ED 32 μm) after four bolus infusions of endotoxin at weekly intervals. The vessel is undergoing lysis with replacement of medial smooth muscle cells by nonspecific mononuclear cells. The vessel lumen is occluded by erythrocytes and leukocytes and cell debris (1 μm section stained with toluidine blue, original magnification, ×781). (From ref. 63 with permission.)*

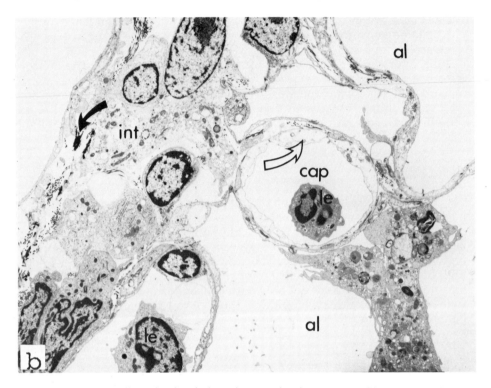

b: *Rat pulmonary capillary after four bolus infusions of endotoxin at weekly intervals. Alveolar space (al), capillary (cap), hydropic degeneration of endothelial cells (open arrow), elastin (solid arrow), interstitium (int), leukocytes (le), (original magnification, ×4,725). (From ref. 63 with permission.)*

Models of high flow can be produced by systemic-to-pulmonary artery shunts, or diversion of the normal pulmonary artery blood flow from one region of the lung to give excessive flow to another region. A reduction in the pulmonary bed available to blood flow is produced by pneumonectomy, lobectomy, application of a constricting band to a pulmonary artery, or by thrombotic, embolic, or obliterative obstruction of the vessel lumen. Patchy obliteration of arteries, such as that seen typically in the lungs of ARDS patients, or after hyperoxia or monocrotaline, results in diversion of blood flow to unaffected vessels, which may injure them.

A systemic-to-pulmonary artery shunt in growing animals results, after 5 weeks, in pulmonary hypertension,[111] which reverses 10 weeks after closure of the shunt[112] (Fig. 41). On insertion of the shunt, the pulmonary arterial bed remodels, resulting in reduction of the cross-sectional area (Fig. 42). Medial hypertrophy occurs in preacinar arteries with appearance of muscle in previously nonmuscular intraacinar vessels (Fig. 43a and b). Animals 4 weeks old develop greater muscularization than animals 8 weeks old. Only the older animals develop dilation of the main and branch pulmonary arteries[111] (Fig. 43a and b). Although hemodynamic recovery occurs 10 weeks after correction of the shunt and arterial diameter returns to normal, the increased muscularization of vessels persists.[112]

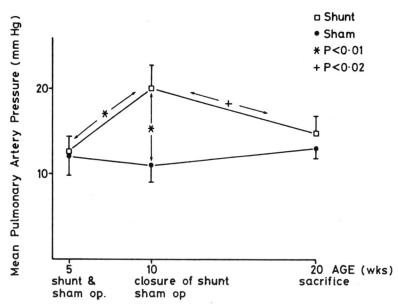

Figure 41: *Mean pulmonary artery pressure in the pig at 5, 10, and 20 weeks of age, after insertion of an aortic-pulmonary shunt, or after a sham procedure. In animals with shunts, pressure is elevated 5 weeks after opening the shunt (i.e., at 10 weeks of age) and has returned to the basal level 10 weeks after closure (i.e., at 20 weeks of age). (From ref. 112 with permission.)*

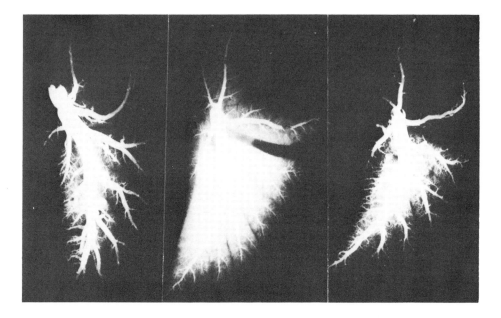

Figure 42: *Pig pulmonary arteriograms at 16 weeks of age. Center, normal (×0.58); left, shunt at 8 weeks (×0.47); right, shunt at 4 weeks, (×0.53). Dilation of the main vessels is evident after shunt insertion at 8 weeks of age. (From ref. 111 with permission.)*

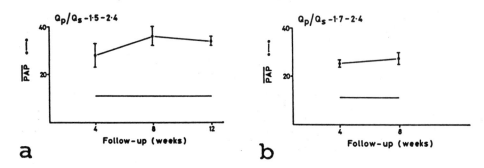

Figure 43: *Summary of structural and functional findings in the pig after insertion of an aortic-pulmonary shunt.* **a:** *Shunt at 4 weeks of age followed for 12 weeks;* **b:** *shunt at 8 weeks of age followed for 8 weeks. Greater muscularization of arteries occurs in the younger animals than in the older ones while dilatation of preacinar arteries occurs only in the latter. WT = wall thickness; Ext = distal extension of muscle along the peripheral arterial pathway; No = arterial number per unit area of lung tissue (square centimeters); PAP = mean pulmonary arterial pressure; Qp/Qs = pulmonary-to-systemic flow ratio; N = no change. (From ref. 111 with permission.)*

In adult animals, diversion of pulmonary blood flow by pneumonectomy results in arterial remodeling that is apparent 5 years later. The medial thickness of muscular vessels increases (Fig. 44) and, to a lesser extent, muscle develops in previously nonmuscular arteries[18] (Fig. 45). In this model, young animals are less susceptible to the effects of high flow, and while they develop right ventricular hypertrophy, vessel remodeling is minimal.

Left pulmonary artery banding causes, in both lungs, a slight rise in PAP and an increase in medial thickness of muscular arteries. Muscle also appears in previously nonmuscular vessels, but to a lesser degree than the increase in medial thickness. Arterial density is decreased.[105] In animals exposed to hypoxia, left pulmonary artery banding increases the extent of the muscularization of nonmuscular segments but does not affect the increased medial thickness or reduced arterial density seen in animals exposed to hypoxia alone (see Fig. 46 for summary of findings).

The mechanisms and mediators of high flow injury are not fully elucidated. Increased blood flow and pressure, particularly if the flow is pulsatile, lead to increased wall tension and shear stress on the endothelium.[21,24,27,92,127] The lung responds to high flow by increasing prostacyclin production,[128] and in experimental studies of systemic vessels, endothelial damage prevents the arterial dilation that otherwise occurs in response to high flow.[54] High flow also

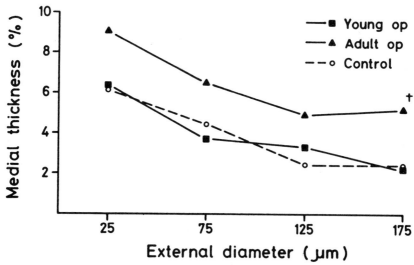

Figure 44: *The effect of contralateral pneumonectomy on pulmonary artery medial thickness in young (6–9 weeks) and older (52 weeks) dogs. Percent medial thickness (mean ± SEM) of intraacinar partially muscular and muscular arteries by external diameter. (From ref. 18 with permission.)*

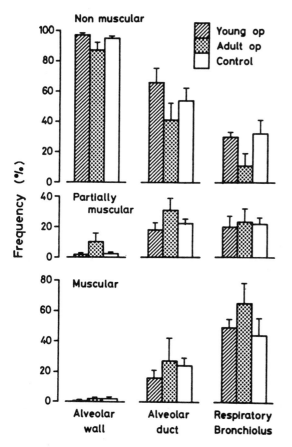

Figure 45: *The effect of contralateral pneumonectomy on pulmonary artery structure in young (6–9 weeks) and older (52 weeks) dogs. Percent frequency (mean ± SEM) of each of the three structural types of intraacinar artery at each of three airway levels. (From ref. 18 with permission.)*

Feature	Band	Hypoxia	Band + Hypoxia
P̄pa and Rp (R)	↑	↑↑	↑↑
RV/(LV + S)	↑	↑↑	↑↑
Lung volume (R)	↑	—	↑
(L)	↓	—	—
PA lumen diameter on			
Angiograms (R)	↑	↓	↑
(L)	—	↓	—
Extension (R)	↑	↑↑	↑↑↑
(L)	↑	↑↑	↑
Wall thickness (R)	↑	↑↑	↑↑↑
(L)	↑	↑↑	↑
Arterial concentration (R)	↓	↓↓	↓↓
(L)	↓	↓↓	↓↓
Arterial size (R)	—	—	—
(L)	↓	—	—

Figure 46: *The effect of banding of the left pulmonary artery, hypoxia or banding + hypoxia on lung and heart in the rat. R = right lung; L = left lung; Ppa = pulmonary artery pressure; Rp = pulmonary vascular resistance; RV/LV+S = ratio of weight of right ventricle to left ventricle plus septum; ↑ = increase; ↓ = decrease; - = no change. Number of arrows denotes severity of change. (From ref. 105 with permission.)*

enhances the pulmonary response to barbiturate vasoconstrictors.[79] Cultured endothelial cells increase factor VIII production[72] and realign their internal stress fibers in response to increased shear stresses.[138] With high flow, platelet consumption is increased, and elevation of PVR can be reduced by antiplatelet agents.[126] Medial hypertrophy may result from a direct response to stretch, or from platelet activation by damaged endothelium or by exposed underlying collagen, leading to release of muscle growth factors. The development of systems to study the effect of shear stress on cultured cells will lead to a better understanding of high flow vascular injury.[129]

Acknowledgments

We thank Mr. E. Quintinilla and Mr. T. Williams for the photographs and the diagrams. The studies reported here were supported by NHLBI ARF SCOR grant # 23591 and by the Canadian Heart Foundation. Dr. Langleben is a Research Fellow of the Canadian Heart Foundation.

REFERENCES

1. Altemeier, W.A., Culbertson, W.R., Fuller, W.P., et al.: Intra-abdominal abscess. *Am. J. Surg.* 125:70–79, 1973.
2. Bachofen, M. and Weibel, E.: Structural alterations of lung parenchyma in the adult respiratory distress syndrome. *Clin. Chest Med.* 3:35–56, 1982.

3. Batcha, K., Stalcup, S.A., Mellins, R.B., et al.: Hyperoxia alters concentrations of circulating vasoactive mediators and hemodynamics. *Circulation* 62 (Suppl. III): III-26, 1980 (Abstr.).

4. Blaisdell, F.W. and Lewis, F.R.: *Respiratory Distress Syndrome of Shock and Trauma: Post-Traumatic Respiratory Failure.* Major Problems of Clinical Surgery XXI. Philadelphia, W.B. Saunders, 1977.

5. Block, E.R. and Cannon, J.K.: Effect of oxygen exposure on lung clearance of amines. *Lung* 155:287–295, 1978.

6. Brigham, K.L.: Mechanisms of lung injury. *Clin. Chest Med.* 3:9–24, 1982.

7. Bruner, L.H., Hilliker, K.S., and Roth, R.A.: Pulmonary hypertension and ECG changes from monocrotaline pyrrole in the rat. *Am. J. Physiol.* 245:H300–306, 1983.

8. Clark, J.M. and Lambertsen, C.J.: Pulmonary oxygen toxicity: A review. *Pharmacol. Rev.* 23:37–133, 1981.

9. Cohen, A.B.: Potential adverse effects of lung macrophages and neutrophils. *Fed. Proc.* 38:2644–2647, 1979.

10. Coughlin, S.R., Moskowitz, M.A., Antoniades, H.N., et al.: Serotonin receptor-mediated stimulation of bovine smooth muscle cells, prostacyclin synthesis and its modulation by platelet-derived growth factor. *Proc. Natl. Acad. Sci.* 78:7134–7138, 1981.

11. Crapo, J.D., Barry, B.E., Foscue, H.A., et al.: Structural and biochemical changes in rat lungs occurring during exposures to lethal and adaptive doses of oxygen. *Am. Rev. Respir. Dis.* 122:123–143, 1980.

12. Crapo, J.D., Peters-Golden, M., Marsh-Salin, J., et al.: Pathologic changes in the lungs of oxygen-adapted rats. A morphometric analysis. *Lab. Invest.* 39:640–653, 1978.

13. Crapo, J.D. and Tierney, D.F.: Superoxide dismutase and pulmonary oxygen toxicity. *Am. J. Physiol.* 2256:1401–1407, 1974.

14. Czer, G. and Moser, K.M.: Prostacyclin prevents monocrotaline-induced pulmonary hypertension, edema formation, and thromboxane production in dogs. *Am. Rev. Respir. Dis.* 129:A334, 1984 (Abstr.).

15. Dahlen, S.-E., Bjork, J., Hedqvist, P., et al.: Leukotrienes promote plasma leakage and leukocyte adhesion in post-capillary venules: In vivo effects with relevance to the acute inflammatory response. *Proc. Natl. Acad. Sci.* 78:3887–3891, 1981.

16. Dauber, J.H. and Daniele, R.P.: Secretion of chemotaxins by guinea pig lung macrophages. *Exp. Lung Res.* 1:23–32, 1980.

17. Davies, P., Maddalo, F., and Reid, L.: The effects of chronic hypoxia on structure and reactivity of rat lung microvessels. *J. Appl. Physiol.* 1985 (In press).

18. Davies, P., McBride, J., Murray, G.F. et al.: Structural changes in the canine lung and pulmonary arteries after pneumonectomy. *J. Appl. Physiol.: Respir. Environ. Exercise Physiol.* 53:859–864, 1982.

19. Eeles, G.H. and Sevitt, S.: Microthrombosis in injured and burned patients. *J. Pathol. Bacterol.* 93:275–293, 1967.

20. Elliott, F.M. and Reid, L.: Some new facts about the pulmonary artery and its branching pattern. *Clin. Radiol.* 16:193–198, 1965.

21. Esterly, J.A., Glagov, S., and Ferguson, D.J.: Morphogenesis of intimal obliterative hyperplasia of small arteries in experimental pulmonary hypertension. *Am. J. Pathol.* 52:325–337, 1968.

22. Fantone, J.C., Kunkel, S.L., and Ward, P.A.: Chemotactic mediators in neutrophil-dependent lung injury. *Ann. Rev. Physiol.* 44:283–293, 1982.

23. Fantone, J.C. and Ward, P.A.: Role of oxygen-derived free radicals and metabolites in leukocyte-dependent inflammatory reactions. *Am. J. Pathol.* 107:397–418, 1982.

24. Ferguson, D.J. and Varco, R.L.: The relation of blood pressure and flow to the development and regression of experimentally induced pulmonary arteriosclerosis. *Circ. Res.* 3:152–158, 1955.

25. Fried, R., Meyrick, B., Rabinovitch, M., et al.: Polycythemia and the acute hypoxic response in awake rats following chronic hypoxia. *J. Appl. Physiol.* 55:1167–1172, 1983.

26. Fried, R. and Reid, L.: Early recovery from hypoxic pulmonary hypertension. *J. Appl. Physiol.* 57:1247–1253, 1984.

27. Fry, D.L.: Acute vascular endothelial changes associated with increased blood velocity gradients. *Circ. Res.* 22:165–197, 1968.

28. Gadek, J.E., Hunninghake, G.W., Zimmerman, R.L., et al.: Regulation of the release of alveolar macrophage-derived neutrophil chemotactic factor. *Am. Rev. Respir. Dis.* 121:723–733, 1980.

29. Ganey, P.E. and Roth, R.A.: Release of 6-keto-prostaglandin $F_{1\alpha}$ and thromboxane B_2 from isolated perfused lungs of monocrotaline pyrrole-treated rats. *Fed. Proc.* 43:808, 1984 (Abstr.).

30. Ghodsi, F. and Will, J.A.: Changes in pulmonary structure and function induced by monocrotaline intoxication. *Am. J. Physiol.* 240:H149, 1981.

31. Gillis, C.N., Huxtable, R.J., and Roth, R.A.: Effects of monocrotaline pretreatment of rats on removal of 5-hydroxytryptamine and noradrenaline by perfused lung. *Br. J. Pharmacol.* 63:435–443, 1978.

32. Goodman, M.L., Way, B.A., and Irwin, J.W.: The inflammatory response to endotoxin. *J. Pathol.* 128:7–14, 1979.

33. Greenberg, S.D., Schweppe, H.I., and Harness, M.: Shock lung: Disruption of alveolar capillary walls. *Tex. Med.* 72:45–54, 1976.

34. Greene, R., Zapol, W.M., Snider, M.T., et al.: Early bedside detection of pulmonary vascular occlusion during acute respiratory failure. *Am. Rev. Respir. Dis.* 124: 593–601, 1981.

35. Guntheroth, W.G., Luchtel, D.L., and Kawabori, I.: Pulmonary microcirculation: Tubules rather than sheet and post. *J. Appl. Physiol.* 53:510–515, 1982.

36. Gurtner, G.H., Knoblauch, A., Brennen, N., et al.: Pulmonary pressor response to hydroperoxides. *Am. Rev. Respir. Dis.* 123:246, 1981 (Abstr.).

37. Guyton, J.R. and Karnovsky, M.: Smooth muscle cell proliferation on the occluded rat carotid artery: Lack of requirement for luminal platelets. *Am. J. Pathol.* 94:585–602, 1979.

38. Hayashi Y., Hussa, J.F., Lalich, J.J.: Cor pulmonale in rats. *Lab. Invest.* 16: 875–881, 1967.

39. Hempel, F.G., Lenfant, C.J.M.: Current and future research on adult respiratory distress syndrome. *Semin. Respir. Med.* 2:165–172, 1981.

40. Henson, P.M., Larsen, G.L., Webster, R.O., et al.: Pulmonary microvascular alterations and injury induced by complement fragments: Synergistic effect of complement activation, neutrophil sequestration, and prostaglandins. *Ann. N.Y. Acad. Sci.* 384:287–300, 1982.

41. Hickam, J.B. and Cargill, W.H.: Effect of exercise on cardiac output and pulmonary arterial pressure in normal persons and in patients with cardiovascular disease and pulmonary emphysema. *J. Clin. Invest.* 27:10–23, 1948.

42. Hill, J.D., Ratliff, J.L., Lamy, M., et al.: Pulmonary pathology in acute respiratory insufficiency: Lung biopsy as a diagnostic tool. *J. Thorac. Cardiovasc. Surg.* 71: 64–69, 1976.

43. Hilliker, K.S., Bell, T.G., and Roth, R.A.: Pneumotoxicity and thrombocytopenia after single injection of monocrotaline. *Am. J. Physiol.* 242:H573–H579, 1972.

44. Hilliker, K.S., Garcia, C.M., and Roth, R.A.: Effects of monocrotaline and monocrotaline pyrrole on 5-hydroxytryptamine and paraquat uptake by lung slices. *Res. Comm. Chem. Pathol. Pharmacol.* 40:179–197, 1983.

45. Hilliker, K.S. and Roth, R.A.: Altered response to vasoconstrictor agents in lungs from rats with monocrotaline-pyrrole induced pulmonary hypertension. *Fed. Proc.* 42:303, 1983 (Abstr.).

46. Hilliker, K.S., Bell, T.G., Lorimer, D., et al.: Effects of thrombocytopenia on monocrotaline pyrrole-induced pulmonary hypertension. *Am. J. Physiol.* 246: H747–H753, 1984.

47. Hislop, A. and Reid, L.: Fetal and childhood development of the intra-pulmonary veins in man: Branching pattern and structure. *Thorax* 28:313–319, 1973.
48. Hislop, A. and Reid, L.: Arterial changes in Crotalaria spectabilis-induced pulmonary hypertension in rats. *Br. J. Exp. Pathol.* 55:153–163, 1974.
49. Hislop, A. and Reid, L.: New findings in pulmonary arteries of rats with hypoxia induced hypertension. *Br. J. Exp. Pathol.* 57:542–554, 1976.
50. Hislop, A. and Reid, L.: Changes in pulmonary arteries of the rat during recovery from hypoxia-induced pulmonary hypertension. *Br. J. Exp. Pathol.* 58:653–662, 1977.
51. Hislop, A. and Reid, L.: Normal structure and dimensions of the pulmonary arteries in the rat. *J. Anat.* 125:71–84, 1978.
52. Howe, A., Tsakiris, A.G., Rastelli, G.C., et al.: Experimental studies on the pathogenesis of pulmonary vascular obstructive disease. *J. Thorac. Cardiovasc. Surg.* 63:652–664, 1972.
53. Hudson, L.D.: Causes of the adult respiratory distress syndrome: Clinical recognition. *Clin. Chest Med.* 3:1956, 1982.
54. Hull, S.S., Romig, G.D., Sparks, H.V.: Flow-induced vasodilation of large arteries is dependent on endothelium. *Fed. Proc.* 43:900, 1984 (Abstr.).
55. Hyman, A.L., Mathe, A.A., Lippton, H.L., et al.: Prostaglandins and the Lung. *Med. Clin. N. Am.* 65:789–808, 1981.
56. Jacob, H.S., Graddock, P.R., Hammerschmidt, D.E., et al.: Complement-induced granulocyte aggregation. *New Engl. J. Med.* 302:789–794, 1980.
57. Jacobs, E.R. and Bone, R.C.: Mediators of septic lung injury. *Med. Clin. N. Am.* 67:701–715, 1983.
58. Jaffe, E.A., Hoyer, L.W., and Nachman, R.L.: Antihemophilic factor antigen. Localization in endothelial cells by immunofluorescence microscopy. *J. Clin. Invest.* 52:2757–2764, 1973.
59. Jaffe, E.A., Hoyer, W., Nachman, R.L.: Synthesis of von Willebrand factor by cultured human endothelial cells. *Proc. Natl. Acad. Sci. USA* 71:1906–1909, 1974.
60. Jenkinson, S.G.: Pulmonary oxygen toxicity. *Clin. Chest Med.* 3:109–119, 1982.
61. Johnson, K.J. and Ward, P.A.: Role of oxygen metabolites in immune complex injury of lung. *J. Immunol.* 126:2365–2369, 1981.
62. Johnston, R.B., Godzik, C.A., and Cohn, Z.A.: Increased superoxide anion production by immunologically and chemically elicited macrophages. *J. Exp. Med.* 148: 115–127, 1978.
63. Jones, R., Zapol, W.M., Tomashefski Jr., J.F., et al.: Pulmonary vascular pathology: Human and experimental studies. In *Acute Respiratory Failure*. Zapol, W.M., series ed. Volume entitled *Lung Biology in Health and Disease*. Lenfant, C., ed. New York, Marcel Dekker, Inc. (In press) 1984.
64. Jones, R., Zapol, W.M., and Reid, L.: Progressive and regressive structural changes in rat pulmonary arteries during recovery from prolonged hyperoxia. *Am. Rev. Respir. Dis.* 125:227, 1982.
65. Jones, R., Zapol, W.M., and Reid, L.: Pulmonary artery wall injury and remodeling by hyperoxia. *Chest* 83S: 40S-42S, 1983.
66. Jones, R., Zapol, W.M., and Reid, L.: Hyperoxia induces hypertrophy of intimal precursor smooth muscle cells in pulmonary arteries. *Fed. Proc.* 43: 884, 1984 (Abstr.).
67. Jones, R., Zapol, W.M., and Reid, L.: Pulmonary artery remodeling and pulmonary hypertension after exposure to hyperoxia for 7 days: A morphometric and hemodynamic study. *Am. J. Pathol.* 117: 273–285, 1984.
68. Kapanci, Y., Weibel, E.R., Kaplan, H.P., et al.: Pathogenesis and reversibility of the pulmonary lesions of oxygen toxicity in monkeys II. Ultrastructural and morphometric studies. *Lab. Invest.* 20:101–116, 1969.
69. Kay, J.M. and Heath, D.: *Crotalaria Spectabilis: The Pulmonary Hypertension Plant*. Springfield, Ill., Charles C. Thomas, 1969.
70. Kay, J.M., Keane, P.M., Suyama, K.L., et al.: Angiotensin-converting enzyme

activity and evolution of pulmonary vascular disease in rats with monocrotaline pulmonary hypertension. *Thorax* 37:88–96, 1982.

71. Kirton, O.C., Jones, R., Zapol, W.M., et al.: The development of a model of subacute lung injury after intra-abdominal infection. *Surgery* 96:384–394, 1984.

72. Koslow, A., Stromberg, R., Gritsman, H., et al.: Response of endothelial cells grown on microcarrier beads to shear stress. *Fed. Proc.* 43:783, 1984 (Abstr.).

73. Kunze, H. and Vogt, W.: Significance of phospholipase A_2 for prostaglandin formation. *Ann. N.Y. Acad. Sci.* 180:123–125, 1971.

74. Lalich, J.J., Johnson, W.D., Raczniak, T.J., et al.: Fibrin thrombosis in monocrotaline pyrrole induced cor pulmonale in rats. *Arch. Pathol. Lab. Med.* 101: 69–73, 1977.

75. Langleben, D. and Reid, L.M.: Effect of methylprednisolone in monocrotaline-induced pulmonary vascular disease and right ventricular hypertrophy. *Lab. Invest.* (In press) 1985.

76. Leibovich, S.J. and Ross, R.: A macrophage-dependent factor that stimulates the proliferation of fibroblasts in vitro. *Am. J. Pathol.* 84:501–514, 1976.

77. Levin, E.G. and Loskutoff, D.J.: Cultured bovine endothelial cells produce both urokinase and tissue-type plasminogen activators. *J. Cell Biol.* 94:631–636, 1982.

78. Levy, S.E. and Blalock, A.: Experimental observations on the effects of connecting by suture the left main pulmonary artery to the systemic circulation. *J. Thorac. Surg.* 8:525–530, 1939.

79. Linde, L.M., Goldberg, S.J., Takahashi, M., et al.: Pulmonary vasoreactivity in animals with relatively increased pulmonary blood flow. *Cardiovasc. Res.* 4: 99–104, 1970.

80. Marcus, A.J., Silk, S.T., Safier, L.B., et al.: Superoxide production and reducing activity of human platelets. *J. Clin. Invest.* 59:149–158, 1977.

81. Mattocks, A.R.: Toxicity of pyrrolizidine alkaloids. *Nature* 217:723–728, 1968.

82. Meyrick, B., Fujiwara, K., and Reid, L.: Smooth muscle cell myosin in precursor and mature smooth muscle cells in normal pulmonary arteries and the effect of hypoxia. *Exp. Lung Res.* 2:303–313, 1981.

83. Meyrick, B., Gamble, W., and Reid, L.: Development of Crotalaria pulmonary hypertension: Hemodynamic and structural study. *Am. J. Physiol.* 239:H692–H702, 1980.

84. Meyrick, B. and Reid, L.: The effect of continued hypoxia on rat pulmonary arterial circulation: An ultrastructural study. *Lab. Invest.* 38:188–200, 1978.

85. Meyrick, B. and Reid, L.: Ultrastructural features of the distended pulmonary arteries of the normal rat. *Anat. Rec.* 193:71–97, 1979.

86. Meyrick, B. and Reid, L.: Development of pulmonary arterial changes in rats fed Crotalaria spectabilis. *Am. J. Pathol.* 94:37–50, 1979.

87. Meyrick, B. and Reid, L.: Hypoxia-induced structural changes in the media and adventitia of rat hilar pulmonary artery and their regression. *Am. J. Pathol.* 100:151–179, 1980.

88. Meyrick, B. and Reid, L.: Pulmonary hypertension: Anatomic and physiologic correlates. *Clin. Chest Med.* 4:199–217, 1983.

89. Millard, J.: The development and electrocardiographic diagnosis of right ventricular hypertrophy in chronic lung diseases. M.D. thesis, University of London, 1965.

90. Molteni, A., Ward, W.F., Ts'ao, C., et al.: Monocrotaline-induced pulmonary injury in rats. *Fed. Proc.* 42:778, 1982 (Abstr.).

91. Morrison, D.C. and Ulevitch, R.J.: The effects of bacterial endotoxins on host mediation systems. *Am. J. Pathol.* 93:527–617, 1978.

92. Muller, W.H., Dammann, J.F., and Head, W.H.: Changes in the pulmonary vessels produced by experimental pulmonary hypertension. *Surgery* 34:363–375, 1953.

93. Newball, H.Y. and Lichtenstein, L.M.: Mast cells and basophils: Effector cells of inflammatory disorders in the lung. *Thorax* 36:721–725, 1981.

94. Newfield, E.A., Waldman, J.D., Paul, M.H., et al.: Pulmonary vascular disease after systemic-pulmonary arterial shunt operations. *Am. J. Cardiol.* 39:715–720, 1977.

95. Newman, J.H., McMurtry, I.F., and Reeves, J.T.: Blunted pulmonary pressor response to hypoxia in blood perfused, ventilated lungs isolated from oxygen-toxic rats: Possible role of prostaglandins. *Prostaglandins* 22:11–20, 1981.

96. Obrien, R.F., Seton, M.P., Makarski, J.S., et al.: Thiourea causes endothelial cells in tissue culture to produce neutrophil chemoattractant activity. *Am. Rev. Respir. Dis.* 130:103–109, 1984.

97. Obrodovitch, H.M., Stalcup, S.A., Pang, L.M., et al.:Bradykinin production and increased pulmonary endothelial permeability during acute respiratory failure in unanesthetized sheep. *J. Clin. Invest.* 67:514–522, 1981.

98. Parratt, J.R. and Sturgess, R.M.: The possible roles of histamine, 5-Hydroxy-tryptamine and prostaglandin $F_{2\alpha}$ as mediators of the acute pulmonary effects of endotoxin. *Br. J. Pharmacol.* 60:209–219, 1977.

99. Patten, M.T.: Etiology. In *Acute Respiratory Failure: Etiology and Treatment.* Hechtman, H.B., ed. Boca Raton, Florida, CRC Press, Inc., 1979, pp. 127–153.

100. Pingleton, S.K.: Complications associated with the adult respiratory distress syndrome. *Clin. Chest Med.* 3:143–155, 1982.

101. Plestina, R. and Stoner, H.B.: Pulmonary edema in rats given monocrotaline pyrrole. *J. Pathol.* 106:235–249, 1972.

102. Pratt, P.C., Vollmer, R.T., Shelburne, J.D., et al.: Pulmonary morphology in a multihospital collaborative extracorporeal membrane oxygenation project. I. Light microscopy. *Am. J. Pathol.* 95:191–214, 1979.

103. Rabinovitch, M., Gamble, W.J., Nadas, A.S., et al.: The rat pulmonary circulation after chronic hypoxia: Hemodynamic and structural features. *Am. J. Physiol.* 236:H818-H827, 1979.

104. Rabinovitch, M., Gamble, W.J., Miettinen, O.S., et al.: Age and sex influence on pulmonary hypertension of chronic hypoxia and on recovery. *Am. J. Physiol.* 240:H62–H72, 1981.

105. Rabinovitch, M., Konstam, M.A., Gamble, W.J., et al.: Changes in pulmonary blood flow affect vascular response to chronic hypoxia in rats. *Circ. Res.* 52: 432–441, 1983.

106. Reid, L.: The angiogram and pulmonary artery structure and branching (in the normal and with reference to disease). *Proc. R. Soc. Med.* 58:681–684, 1965.

107. Reid, L.: Structural and functional reappraisal of the pulmonary artery system. *Scientific Basis of Medicine, Annual Review.* London, The Athlone Press, 1968, pp. 289–307.

108. Reid, L.: The 1978 J. Burns Amberson Lecture. The pulmonary circulation: remodeling in growth and disease. *Am. Rev. Respir. Dis.* 119:531–546, 1979.

109. Reid, L.M.: Lung growth in health and disease (Tudor Edwards Memorial Lecture). *Br. J. Dis. Chest* 78:113–134, 1984.

110. Reinsel, C.N., Olson, J.W., Altiere, R.J., et al.: Monocrotaline provokes a transient increase in pulmonary vascular responsiveness in isolated buffer perfused rat lungs. *Fed. Proc.* 43:881, 1984.

111. Rendas, A., Lennox, S., and Reid, L.: Aorta-pulmonary shunts in growing pigs. *J. Thorac. Cardiovasc. Surg.* 77:109–118, 1979.

112. Rendas, A. and Reid, L.: Pulmonary vasculature of piglets after correction of aorta-pulmonary shunts. *J. Thorac. Cardiovasc.* 85:911–916, 1983.

113. Riede, U.N., Joachim, H., Hassenstein, J., et al.: The pulmonary air-blood barrier of human shock lungs (a clinical, ultrastructural and morphometric study). *Pathol. Res. Pract.* 162:41–72, 1978.

114. Rinaldo, J.E. and Rogers, R.M.: Adult respiratory distress syndrome changing concepts of lung injury and repair. *N. Engl. J. Med.* 306:900–909, 1982.

115. Ross, R., Glomset, J., Kariya, B., et al.: A platelet-dependent serum factor that stimulates the proliferation of arterial smooth muscle cells in vitro. *Proc. Natl. Acad. Sci. USA* 71:1207–1210, 1974.

116. Saldeen, T.: Trends in microvascular research: The microembolism syndrome. *Mircovasc. Res.* 11:227–259, 1976.

117. Sjostrom, K. and Crapo, J.D.: Structural and biochemical adaptive changes in rat lungs after exposure to hypoxia. *Lab. Invest.* 48:68–79, 1983.
118. Smith, M.E., Gunther, R., Gee, M., et al.: Leukocytes, platelets and thromboxane A₂ in endotoxin-induced lung injury. *Surgery* 90:102–107, 1981.
119. Snow, R.L., Davies, P., Pontoppidan, H., et al.: Pulmonary vascular remodeling in adult respiratory distress syndrome. *Am. Rev. Respir. Dis.* 126:887–892, 1982.
120. Stone, H.H., Kolb, L.D., and Gelebar, C.E.: Incidence and significance of intraperitoneal anaerobic bacteria. *Ann. Surg.* 181:705–715, 1975.
121. Sugita, T., Hyers, T.M., Dauber, I.M., et al.: Lung vessel leak precedes right ventricular hypertrophy in monocrotaline treated rats. *J. Appl. Physiol.* 54:371–374, 1983.
122. Tomashefski, J.F. Jr., Davies, P., Boggis, C., et al.: The pulmonary vascular lesions of the adult respiratory distress syndrome. *Am. J. Pathol.* 112:112–126, 1983.
123. Vader, C.R., Mathias, M.M., and Schatte, C.L.: Response of rat lung prostaglandin metabolism to normobaric hyperoxia. *Fed. Proc.* 38:1329, 1979 (Abstr.).
124. Valdivia, E., Hayashi, Y., Lalich, J.J., et al.: Capillary obstruction in experimental cor pulmonale. *Circulation* 32 (Suppl. 2):211, 1965 (Abstr.).
125. Valdivia, E., Sonnad, J., Hayashi, Y., et al.: Experimental interstitial pulmonary edema. *Angiology* 18:378, 1967.
126. Van Benthuysen, K.M., Dauber, I.M., Hyers, T.A., et al.: The role of platelets in hypertensive pulmonary vascular disease. *Fed. Proc.* 40:794, 1981 (Abstr.).
127. Van Benthuysen, K.M., Hammon, J.W., Mitchner, J.S., et al.: Electron microscopic alterations in experimental pulmonary hypertension. *J. Surg. Res.* 22:398–418, 1977.
128. Van Grondelle, A., Voelkel, N.F., Mathias, M., et al.: Lung prostacyclin production with change in shear stress and vascular distension. *Fed. Proc.* 41:1749, 1982 (Abstr.).
129. Van Grondelle, A., Moon, D.G., Kaplan, J.E., et al.: Apparatus to assess the influence of shear stress on cultured cells. *Fed. Proc.* 43:522, 1984 (Abstr.).
130. Von Euler, U.S. and Liljestrand, G.: Observations on the pulmonary arterial blood pressure in the cat. *Acta Physiol. Scand.* 12:301, 1946.
131. Ward, P.A.: Immune complex injury of the lung. *Am. J. Pathol.* 97:85–92, 1979.
132. Wasserman, S.I.: The lung mast cell: Its physiology and potential relevance to defense of the lung. In *Proceedings of the Symposium on Experimental Models for Pulmonary Research.* Environmental Protection Agency, EPA-5600/9-79-022, 1979, pp. 273–296.
133. Wedmore, C.V. and Williams, T.J.: Control of vascular permeability by polymorphonuclear leukocytes in inflammation. *Nature* 289:646–650, 1922.
134. Weibel, E.R.: The ultrastructure of the alveolar-capillary membrane or barrier. In *The Pulmonary Circulation and Interstitial Space,* Chicago, University of Chicago Press, 1969, pp. 9–27.
135. Weibel, E.R.: On pericytes, particularly their existence in lung capillaries. *Microvasc. Res.* 8:218–235, 1974.
136. Weir, E.K.: Acute hypoxic pulmonary hypertension. In *Pulmonary Hypertension.* Weir, E.K. and Reeves, J.T., eds. Mount Kisco, N.Y., Futura Publ. Co., 1984, pp. 251–289.
137. Weissman, G.: Leukocytes as secretory organs of inflammation. *Hospital Practice* 13:53–62, 1978.
138. White, G.E., Fujiwara, K., Shefton, E.J., et al.: Fluid shear stress influences cell shape and cytoskeletal organization in cultured vascular endothelium. *Fed. Proc.* 41:321, 1982 (Abstr.).
139. Zapol, W.M., Kobayashi, K., Snider, M.T., et al.: Vascular obstruction causes pulmonary hypertension in severe acute respiratory failure. *Chest* 71S:306S-307S, 1977.
140. Zapol, W.M. and Snider, M.T.: Pulmonary hypertension in severe acute respiratory failure. *N. Engl. J. Med.* 296:476–480, 1977.

CHAPTER 8

Sites of Leakage in Pulmonary Edema

Richard K. Albert

Introduction

In both normal permeability (hydrostatic or cardiogenic) and increased permeability (inflammatory) edema, fluid and protein move from the intravascular to the interstitial space, and subsequently into alveoli. Neither the site or sites of leakage, nor the actual pathways across the endothelial or epithelial barriers have been determined. This chapter will review the forces determining fluid and protein exchange across various segments of the pulmonary vascular endothelium. In addition, data suggesting that the bronchial circulation may be a site of leakage in pulmonary edema will be summarized, as will information pertaining to the site at which fluid and protein move from the interstitium across the epithelial barrier into the alveolar space.

Physiological Determinants of Fluid and Protein Movement

The rate of fluid and protein movement through a barrier relates to the surface area, fluid conductance, and protein sieving properties of the barrier, as well as to the hydrostatic and osmotic pressure gradients. Using the notation suggested by Staub[1,2] as applied to the pulmonary vascular endothelium,

$$Qf = Kf\left[(Pmv - Ppmv) - \sigma\left(\pi mv - \pi pmv\right)\right] \tag{1}$$

where Qf is the net rate of fluid flow; Kf is the apparent filtration coefficient or transvascular conductance of the endothelium per unit surface area; Pmv is the microvascular hydrostatic pressure; Ppmv is the perimicrovascular hydrostatic pressure; σ is the reflection coefficient or sieving tendency of the vessel wall for protein; and πmv and πpmv are the osmotic pressures inside and around the microvessels, respectively. The term *microvascular* was chosen to avoid implying that all fluid and protein exchange occurs across alveolar capillaries.[2] The

From Said, S.I. (ed.): *The Pulmonary Circulation and Acute Lung Injury.* Mount Kisco, N.Y., Futura Publishing Co., Inc., 1985.

results of studies that will be described below suggest that both pre- and postcapillary vessels are also capable of leakage. The Pmv in these vessels is clearly different from that found in the alveolar capillaries. In addition, the morphologic features of these pre- and postcapillary vessels suggest that they may also have a Kf different from that of the alveolar capillaries.

The term *perimicrovascular* was used to allow for the presence of different interstitial spaces having different Ppmv's.[2] A substantial body of information has demonstrated that the Ppmv's in the interstitial spaces surrounding these pre- and postcapillary vessels are different from those in the alveolar septal interstitium.

The bronchial circulation may also be an important site of fluid and protein exchange in some forms of pulmonary edema. The membrane characteristics of the driving pressures relating to these vessels may differ from those relating to any segment of the pulmonary circulation.

As written, equation [1] applies to fluid exchange between the vascular and interstitial spaces. The epithelial barrier also has a Kf and driving pressures different from those of the endothelial membrane. Since the Kf's, the Pmv's, and the Ppmv's of the alveolar capillaries, the pre- and postcapillary vessels, the various segments of bronchial circulation, and the epithelial barrier are all different, it is apparent that transvascular fluid and protein exchange in the lung cannot be accurately expressed using single estimates of these variables. Rather, these variables must be considered separately relative to each vascular bed, as well as for the epithelial segment or segments.

A Two-Compartment Model of the Pulmonary Vasculature

The pulmonary vessels and the interstitium immediately surrounding them can be divided into alveolar (A) and extraalveolar (EA) compartments based on how lung inflation affects the vessels within each compartment. Macklin[3] and subsequently Howell, Permutt, et al.[4] noted that when vascular pressure (Pvas) was low, and was kept constant relative to pleural pressure (Ppl), lung inflation compressed the alveolar vessels (AVs) and expanded the extraalveolar vessels (EAVs) (Fig. 1). Cuffs of edema are seen around these EAVs (both arteries and veins) early in the course of pulmonary edema.[5] However, the primary site of leakage is thought to be at the AV level in both hydrostatic and increased permeability edema.[1] The major support for this assumption is the observation that the "surface area per unit membrane thickness" of alveolar capillaries is 20–30 times greater than that of the small arteries and veins.[1] As a result of this assumption, estimates of the forces affecting fluid movement have been related almost exclusively to vessels in the alveolar compartment, despite the nonspecificity implied by the notation in equation [1], and the absence of histologic evidence of AV leakage.

Sites of Leakage

In the systemic circulation, arterial, venous, and capillary vessels are all thought to be capable of fluid and protein leakage.[6-8] The relative permeability of these vessels is thought to increase from the arterial to the venous end of the circulation.

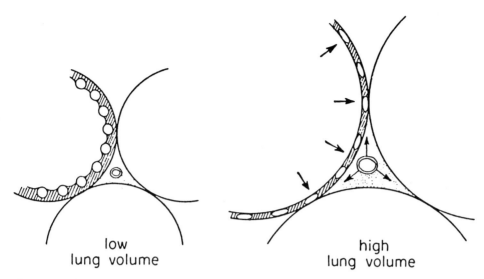

Figure 1: *Alveolar and extraalveolar vessels are distinguished by their response to lung inflation. When transpulmonary pressure and lung volume are increased and vascular pressures are kept constant relative to pleural pressure, alveolar vessels are compressed while extraalveolar vessels are expanded. (Used with permission from Albert, R.K.: Pulmonary edema. In Pulmonary Emergencies. Sahn, S.A., ed. New York, Churchill-Livingstone, 1982.)*

The results of studies examining the sites of leakage in the pulmonary circulation are conflicting. Electron microscopic examination of lungs with normal permeability edema has shown interstitial fluid widely separating the connective tissue fibrils in the thick side of the alveolar septum. Red blood cells have been present in the alveolar spaces and in the septal interstitium. However, the actual site of leakage has not been observed as both the vascular endothelium and alveolar epithelium seem to be intact, and no separation of intercellular junctions is apparent unless very high vascular pressures are used.[9–11]

Early studies of increased permeability edema described capillary endothelial injury and sometimes alveolar epithelial injury as well.[12] When various agents are used in animal models to create increased permeability edema, both endothelial and epithelial damage result. A carefully done study of the pathologic changes in patients with the adult respiratory distress syndrome (ARDS) associated with sepsis suggests that the alveolar epithelium has extensive defects very early in the process but that the microvascular endothelium and intercellular junctions are normal. Platelet-fibrin thrombi seem to cover the occasional endothelial defect. Because there was a large amount of interstitial fibrin seen in this investigation, temporary endothelial leaks were presumed to have existed.[13,14]

Bohm studied pulmonary edema induced in rats by alpha-naphthylthiourea (ANTU).[15] Colloidal carbon was injected into the circulation to mark the site of fluid leakage. While the carbon particles accumulated in both venules and capillaries, they were only thought to be outside the endothelial wall of the venules, perhaps trapped by the basement membrane. In a later paper, Bohm suggested that ANTU induced leakage from precapillary vessels as commonly as it caused venular leakage.[16] Other investigators studied ANTU-induced edema and found electron microscopic evidence of damage confined only to the AVs.[17,18] However, preliminary data of a recent study using dextran 70 as an electron microscopic marker showed that AVs, as well as nonmuscular arterial and venous EAVs, were sites of leakage after ANTU-induced damage.[19]

Hovig et al.[20] examined AVs and found no ultrastructural abnormalities despite marked edema induced by hypocalcemia. In lungs of dead rats, Whayne and Severinghaus[21] produced perivascular edema in response to pulmonary arterial hypertension after polystyrene beads were injected to prevent the hydrostatic stress from reaching the capillary vessels. They suggested that the leakage occurred across the arterial EAVs directly into the perivascular cuffs.

Iliff,[22] Smith et al.,[23] and Mitzner and Robotham[24] documented that fluid transudation occurred under zone I conditions (alveolar pressure (P_A) greater than either pulmonary arterial (Ppa) or venous (Ppv) pressure) from both arterial and venous EAVs in response to a hydrostatic stress. These three studies were performed in excised lungs with severed bronchial, lymphatic, and neural connections. Since the Kf for excised lungs may be higher than that estimated for an intact preparation,[25] we sought to determine if EAV leakage would occur in an in situ lung model.[26] Fluid accumulation was assessed using continuous weighing of lobes in anesthetized, open-chest dogs to determine a fluid filtration rate (FFR) as described by Hauge et al.[27] as well as by histologic examination of the lobes removed at the conclusion of the study. EAVs were isolated by compressing the AVs with P_A high enough above Pvas to stop completely pulmonary arterial to venous blood flow (stop-flow pressure). There was a significant increase in the FFR when Ppa or Ppv was raised to 1 cmH$_2$O below the stop-flow pressure (Fig. 2). Similar amounts of edema were observed whether Ppa and/or Ppv were increased. Because some AVs at the lung base could have remained open and leaked despite the zone I conditions, EAVs also were separated from AVs by embolizing enough 30 μm glass beads to stop perfusion when the upstream pressure (either Ppa or Ppv) measured from the bottom of the lobe was at least 10 cmH$_2$O above P_A. Results were similar (Fig. 3). Electron microscopic evaluation demonstrated interstitial edema in the experimental lobes. Edema was not present in control lobes with undistended EAVs at the same P_A. From these studies, we concluded that leakage from both arterial and venous EAVs could contribute to the edema seen in response to a hydrostatic stress.

Bo et al.[28] found that transvascular fluid filtration increased when excised rabbit lungs were inflated under zone III conditions (Ppa > Ppv > P_A). This change was attributed to either an increase in the surface area of exchange vessels, or a decrease in the Ppmv around either AVs or EAVs. Subsequently, several estimates and direct measurements of EA interstitial fluid pressure (Pxf) and total EA interstitial pressure (solid and fluid pressure, Px) have been made.[29–32] These are summarized in Figure 4. Two qualitative trends are consistently observed. First, Pxf becomes more negative relative to Ppl as the lung expands. Second, the reduction in Pxf is greater the lower the vascular pressure. These findings imply that (1) an EAV transmural pressure (Ptm) sufficiently high to cause fluid transudation might be produced by high lung volumes, particularly if vascular pressures are low, and (2) fluid leakage from EAVs should increase with increasing lung volume.

Using the same in situ, continuously weighed LLL, we investigated whether

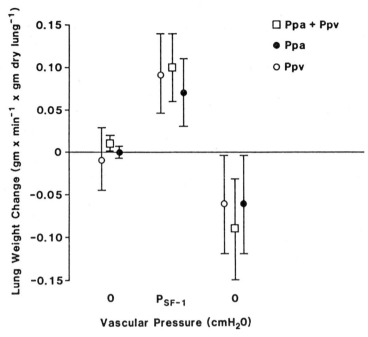

Figure 2: *Effect of pulmonary vascular pressure alteration on lung weight. Alveolar vessels compressed by alveolar pressure with vascular pressure never exceeding that at which flow from pulmonary artery to vein (or vein to artery) completely stopped (the stop-flow pressure, Psf).*

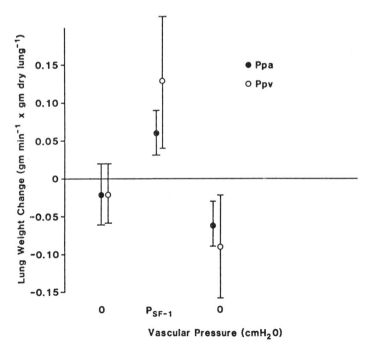

Figure 3: *Effect of pulmonary vascular pressure alteration on lung weight. Alveolar vessels prevented from seeing the hydrostatic stress by embolization of either the arterial or venous extraalveolar vessels.*

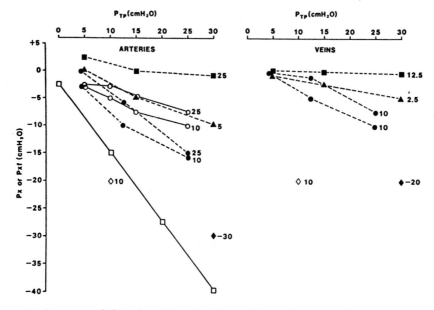

Figure 4: *Summary of data describing the effect of increasing transpulmonary pressure on extraalveolar interstitial fluid or total pressure. Vascular pressures are indicated to the right of the symbols. Solid squares are data from Smith and Mitzner.[31] Open circles are data from Goshy et al.[32] Solid triangles are data from Permutt et al.[35] Solid circles are data from Lai-Fook.[30] Solid diamonds are data from Howell et al.[4] Open squares are data from Inoue et al.[29] Open triangles are data from Benjamin et al.[34]*

the FFR would increase due to lung inflation in zone I when AVs were collapsed by the high P_A.[33] Pvas was kept at either 1 or 5 cmH$_2$O. Lung weight gain due to edema occurred with inflation of P_A above 10 cmH$_2$O (Fig. 5). Greater lung distension resulted in greater rates of weight gain. No difference was observed between the results seen with the two vascular pressures. This was predicted by the observation that the degree to which a change in Ptp reduces the EAV Pxf (and increases the EAV Ptm and leakage) is inversely related to the vascular pressure or volume.[4,29,34−36]

Transvascular fluid filtration could therefore increase, decrease, or remain constant in response to lung inflation depending upon (1) whether Pvas was kept constant relative to Ppl or to P_A, and (2) whether the increase in lung volume primarily affected AVs or EAVs. If vascular pressures are kept constant relative to Ppl, then lung inflation would affect AVs and EAVs in an opposite fashion, and the overall effect on transvascular fluid flux would depend upon the zonal conditions present. In zone I (when vascular pressures are less than P_A and AVs are collapsed), lung inflation would only affect EAVs, and would increase EAV Ptm and transvascular fluid filtration by decreasing the EA Pxf. In zones II and III (when both AVs and EAVs are filled), inflation would compress the AVs while distending the EAVs. The effect on EAVs would depend on the change in Ptp and the level of Pvas present.[4,28−39]

If vascular pressures are kept constant relative to P_A, lung inflation should only increase the EAV Ptm as Pxf would decrease, and the EA intravascular pressure would increase. AV Ptm would remain unchanged.[36] Under these

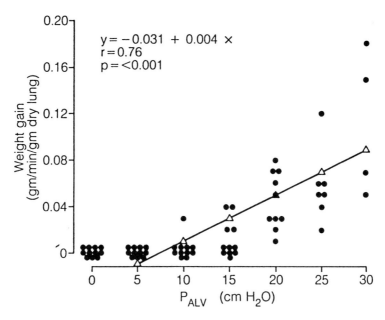

Figure 5: *Relation of lung weight gain to increasing alveolar pressure (P_{ALV}). Pulmonary arterial and venous pressures = 1 cmH$_2$O. Solid line and triangles represent calculated regression line using data from P_{ALV} of 5 through 30. (Used with permission from Albert et al.: Lung inflation can cause pulmonary edema in zone I of in situ dog lungs. J. Appl. Physiol.: Respir. Environ. Exercise Physiol. 49:815–819, 1980.)*

conditions, transvascular fluid filtration should increase with lung inflation.[28] A zone II situation will exist if flow is kept constant during the lung inflation. Ppa, and presumably the AV intravascular pressures, should remain unchanged relative to P_A, but Ppa would increase relative to Ppl and Pxf, increasing the EAV Ptm.

Alveolar Vessels

There are two types of AVs: those located in the corners of alveoli where adjacent septae join, and those located within the septae, between two alveolar spaces. Alveolar septal vessels are compressed throughout their length in zone I when P_A is greater than either Ppa or Ppv.[40] Corner vessels are partially exposed to P_A but may remain open in zone I,[41–43] secondary to the effects of surface tension and interdependence properties of the lung[42–45] (Fig. 6). With increasing lung inflation, corner vessels are drawn out of the corners as septae unfold and move out into the septum where they become compressed by P_A.[46] With this as background, another study examining fluid leakage in zone I lungs can be reviewed.

Nicolaysen and Hauge[47] increased Ptp either by increasing P_A or by decreasing Ppl and found different effects on the rate of transvascular fluid flux. Three experiments were performed. First, P_A was alternated between two levels while Ppl was held constant, Ppa was kept equal to Ppv, and both were

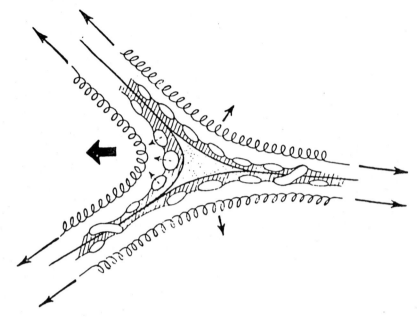

Figure 6: *Two types of alveolar vessels. Septal vessels lie in the flat portion of the septum where surface tension has little, if any, effect. Alveolar septal vessels are therefore subjected to most or all of the unopposed alveolar pressure. Alveolar corner vessels are partially protected from alveolar pressure due to surface tension in the curved portion providing a countering recoil pressure. Lung interdependence provides an additional force that would lower the perimicrovascular hydrostatic pressure around the corner vessels. (Used with permission from Albert, R.K.: Pulmonary edema. In* Pulmonary Emergencies. *Sahn, S.A., ed. New York, Churchill-Livingstone, 1982.)*

held constant relative to Ppl. In seven out of eight experiments, the rate of fluid leakage decreased with lung inflation. Under the conditions described, lung inflation should have increased the EAV Ptm by reducing EAV Pxf. This should have increased fluid leakage. Alveolar septal vessels should have been collapsed by the zone I conditions, and been unaffected by the increase in P_A. Lung inflation could have decreased the Pxf and consequently increased the Ptm of alveolar corner vessels, also increasing the rate of leakage. However, with lung inflation, some of these vessels should have been pulled away from the alveolar corner (where surface forces and lung interdependence produce the negative Pxf relative to P_A) out along the septum where they would become compressed by the increased P_A.[46] This should decrease fluid filtration. To explain a reduction in fluid filtration with lung inflation, either this latter effect would have to predominate, or the increase in P_A would have to raise the Pxf around corner vessels decreasing fluid leakage from those vessels more than it increased EAV leakage.

In the second experiment, Nicolaysen and Hauge increased P_A and Ppl an equal amount (no change in Ptp or lung volume). Ppa was kept equal to Ppv and both were at least 5 cmH$_2$O below P_A and held constant relative to atmospheric pressure. The rate of fluid leakage decreased at the higher P_A and Ppl. The formulation described above would predict these results as the increase in P_A

and Ppl should not have affected EAV Ptm as Ptp and lung volume did not change. Alveolar septal vessels also would be unaffected as they were collapsed under both conditions. The Ptm of alveolar corner vessels should have decreased somewhat as the intravascular pressure would have remained constant, the perivascular pressures generated by lung interdependence and recoil pressure would remain the same since Ptp and V_L did not change, but the increase in P_A would be partially transmitted to the interstitium in the corners, raising the corner vessel Pxf.

In the third experiment, Ppl was reduced while P_A was held constant, Ppa was kept equal to Ppv, and both were kept constant relative to P_A. With lung inflation, the rate of fluid leakage increased. This result would also be predicted by the above formulation as the increase in Ptp would have decreased EAV and corner vessel Pxf, increasing EAV and corner vessel Ptm. Again, AVs in the septum would be unaffected.

Nicolaysen and Hauge interpreted the reduction in fluid filtration seen when lung volume increased (experiment 1) as indicating that the relative contribution of EAVs to the transvascular fluid flux that occurs in zone I was small. From the positive correlation between the changes in P_A and fluid leakage seen in experiments 2 and 3, together with the demonstration that alveolar corner vessels remain open well into zone I, they suggested that these alveolar corner (or transition) vessels, rather than the EAVs, were the site of fluid leakage in zone I.

Relative Contribution of Extraalveolar Vessels to Edema

The relative contribution of EAVs to the edema produced by a hydrostatic stress has been assessed in three studies and in one preliminary report. Iliff used an excised dog lung and isolated the EAVs by varying P_A relative to Pvas.[22] She found that the arterial EAVs contributed 16% of the total fluid leakage and that the venous EAVs contributed 46%. Mitzner and Robotham also studied excised dog lungs and isolated the EAVs by varying P_A relative to Pvas.[24] They found the arterial and venous EAVs contributed 23% and 27%, respectively.

In the same in situ model used in the previous studies, we measured the FFR when Pvas was raised from -15 cmH$_2$O to P_A + lung height, a pressure selected to assure that all the vessels from the top to the bottom of the lobe would have vascular pressures greater than P_A. This hydrostatic stress was applied before and after isolating the arterial or venous EAVs from the AVs by embolizing $27-74$ μm polystyrene beads into either the pulmonary artery or vein.[48] To determine these FFRs in situ, it was necessary to interrupt the bronchial circulation. This was accomplished by embolizing $425-600$ μm glass beads into the intercostal arteries (from which the bronchial arteries arise in the dog) via the descending thoracic aorta. To determine whether bronchial arterial embolization increased pulmonary vascular permeability and artifactually caused EAV leakage, we compared the FFR for the entire pulmonary circulation before and after bronchial arterial embolization. No difference was observed. To determine whether the pulmonary arterial or venous emboli increased vascular permeability and artifactually caused EAV leakage, FFRs for the entire pulmonary circulation were determined before and after either pulmonary arterial or venous embolization. Again, no difference was observed. We then determined the relative contribution of EAVs by raising the vascular pressure upstream of the emboli. Leakage from the arterial and venous EAVs accounted for 41% and 32%, respectively, of the total transvascular fluid flux occurring after embolization (Fig. 7 a and b).

The study was performed at a P_A of 25 and 10 cmH$_2$O. At the lower P_A, a greater Pvas was needed to produce EAV leakage (Fig. 8 a and b). At a lower P_A, the EAV Pxf would be less negative, resulting in a lower EAV Ptm. A greater intravascular pressure would thus be needed to raise the EAV Ptm above the level required to cause transvascular fluid filtration.[49]

In both the studies of Iliff[22] and Mitzner and Robotham,[24] EAV leakage at one P_A was compared with the combined AV and EAV leakage at a lower P_A. As Mitzner and Robotham observed, this ignores any effect that changing P_A has on the back pressure for EAV fluid leakage, the EAV Pxf. Several studies have demonstrated that Pxf is markedly affected by P_A (Fig. 2).[29-32] Additionally, changes in P_A may also affect the relationship of the change in EA interstitial volume to the change in Pxf (the EA interstitial compliance).[50,51] In the estimates of the relative contribution of EAVs that we made, P_A was kept constant and therefore Pxf should have been constant except for any changes that occurred secondary to interstitial edema.

Iliff's estimation of EAV leakage was determined after a hydrostatic stress was applied for 30 minutes to 2 hours. While the amount of weight gain she observed was less than 20% of the original lung weight and no alveolar edema was seen, she may have underestimated the EAV contribution since the

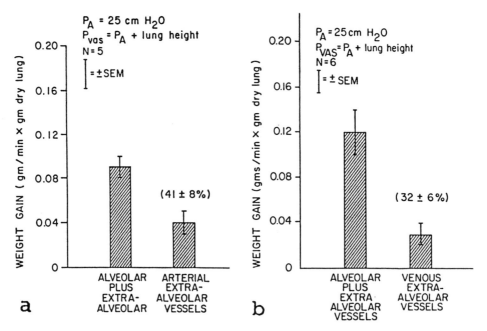

Figure 7: *Relative contribution of extraalveolar vessels to weight gain resulting from a zone III hydrostatic stress after embolization to restrict application of the stress to either the arterial (A) or venous (B) extraalveolar vessels. Alveolar pressure = 25 cmH$_2$O, vascular pressure = 25 + lung height. (Used with permission from Albert, R.K., et al.: Extraalveolar vessel contribution to hydrostatic pulmonary edema in in situ dog lungs. J. Appl. Physiol.: Respir. Environ. Exercise Physiol. 54:1010–1017, 1983.*

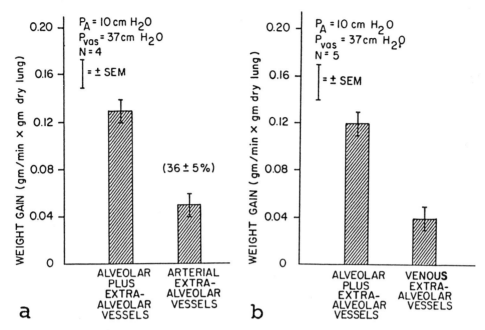

Figure 8: *Relative contribution of extraalveolar vessels to weight gain resulting from a zone III hydrostatic stress after embolization to restrict application of the stress to either the arterial (A) or venous (B) extraalveolar vessels. Alveolar pressure = 10 cmH$_2$O, vascular pressure = 37 cmH$_2$O. (Used with permission from Albert, R.K., et al.: Extra-alveolar vessel contribution to hydrostatic pulmonary edema in in situ dog lungs. J. Appl. Physiol.: Respir. Environ. Exercise Physiol. 54:1010–1017, 1983.*

edema-induced changes in interstitial hydrostatic and oncotic pressures were ignored.[22] Mitzner and Robotham's estimation in excised lungs was done after a 10-minute hydrostatic stress.[24] Apparently, a range of lung water contents up to alveolar edema was produced. In our study, the lungs were in situ and exposed to two to four hydrostatic stresses, each lasting 5 minutes. Between each stress, Pvas was returned to 0 cmH$_2$O to allow for fluid resorption, which occurred to a variable degree. The mean lung wet-to-dry ratio after all stresses, without correction for trapped blood, was 6.2 ± 0.4 (SD). The results from each of these studies would also underestimate the relative contribution of EAVs to the extent that Pxf increased (became less negative), or perimicrovascular osmotic pressure decreased with progressive edema. We may also have underestimated the EAV contribution because it was likely that some EAVs were located downstream of the emboli and thus were protected from the hydrostatic stress applied. We could have overestimated the EAV contribution if alveolar flooding increased the local P$_A$ or the interstitial hydrostatic pressure in the alveolar septum, and as a result, reduced the AV leakage we observed.

In all three of these studies, the relative contribution of arterial and venous EAVs was determined separately. Iliff noted that leakage from one segment did not influence leakage from the other[22] such that the relative contributions from the arterial and venous EAVs could be added together. This suggests that approximately one-half of the total transvascular fluid flux could come from

EAVs. In the human lung, arterial and venous EAVs do seem to be located in different interstitial spaces. The pulmonary arteries and arterioles are in the center of the pulmonary lobule, running adjacent to the bronchial tree. The veins are located at the periphery of the lobules in the interlobular septae.[52] However, edema is known to increase the EAV Pxf[24,30,50] and, if the interstitial spaces around the arterial and venous EAVs are not anatomically separate, leakage from either segment would decrease the EAV transmural pressures and retard leakage from the other.

Because all of the studies reporting the relative contribution of EAVs were done with methods that were insensitive to edema-induced changes in the EA Pxf, we recently reported preliminary data on the relative contribution using techniques that would account for differences in the initial level of interstitial edema and for the progressive accumulation of edema during the course of the experiment.[53] By estimating filtration coefficients (Kf's), we found that EAV permeability was similar to, or even greater than, the AV permeability depending on what the relative surface area of these two types of vessels is per unit of lung tissue. Using data from Horsfield et al.[54,55] and from Weibel,[56] it would seem that the surface area of EAVs is only a small fraction of the AV surface area. If so, the permeability of EAVs must be many times higher than that of the AVs to account for the Kf's we observed.

Clinical Settings in Which EAV Leakage May Be Seen

EAVs may leak when vascular permeability is normal and P_A is high, even if Pvas is very low. Such a condition could exist with mechanical ventilation at high inspiratory and zero end-expiratory pressures, as well as with positive end-expiratory pressure breathing.[57,58] An EAV Ptm sufficient to cause leakage may also be produced by high Pvas regardless of P_A. The increased lung water seen with cor pulmonale,[59] high-altitude pulmonary edema[21] (when wedge pressures are low[60] and increasing flow has recently been shown not to alter vascular permeability[61]) or pulmonary emboli may result from an elevated Ppa causing arterial EAV leakage. Any condition that increases Ppv (LVF, mitral stenosis) will raise the vascular pressure in both the venous EAVs and the AVs. When P_A is high and EAV Pxf is more negative, increases in Ppv may exceed the Ptm needed to produce venous EAV leakage without doing so in AVs. There is morphologic evidence suggesting that certain models of increased permeability edema (ANTU,[19] air emboli[62,63]) damage the EAVs and result in EAV leakage.

The site of fluid and protein leakage may have some important therapeutic implications. Positive end-expiratory pressure with its resultant increase in lung volume and decrease in EAV Pxf could markedly increase lung edema if the primary site of leakage is the EAVs. Agents that alter the distribution of pulmonary vascular resistance could also have an effect on the formation or clearance of edema, depending on the specific site of leakage. Pmv could increase in the AVs or in the arterial EAVs, depending on whether these agents dilated or constricted the precapillary vessels.

Bronchial Circulation

There are several lines of evidence suggesting that leakage from the bronchial circulation may contribute to the increased extravascular lung water seen in various types of pulmonary edema. Borgstrom investigated why patients with uremia typically had a perihilar distribution of edema on chest roentgenograms. He tried to reproduce this pattern by intravascular infusion of bile salts. When the bile salts were injected into the bronchial arteries, the central pattern of edema resulted. Infusion into the pulmonary circulation caused edema, but of a much more diffuse pattern.[64] Pietra et al.[65-67] used colloidal carbon to trace the pathway of fluid leakage into the interstitium after histamine, bradykinin, serotonin, or endotoxin were administered either systemically or subpleurally. Carbon deposits were observed in endothelial gaps of bronchial venules and in the surrounding interstitium. No pathologic changes or carbon particles were observed in the pulmonary circulation. The lack of morphologic change in the pulmonary circulation after histamine infusion has been confirmed by other groups.[68,69] When Goetzman et al.[68] and Grega et al.[69] infused histamine into an isolated lung (no bronchial circulation), no edema resulted.

However, histamine has been shown to increase the permeability of bovine pulmonary artery explants.[70] Brigham and Owen demonstrated that histamine infusion into sheep caused a dose-dependent, reversible increase in lung lymph flow (Q_L) without a fall in the lymph-to-plasma protein ratio (L/P), and without an increase in the Ppa.[71] They concluded that histamine increased pulmonary vascular permeability. In an attempt to determine whether histamine increased bronchial or pulmonary vascular permeability, Nakahara, Ohkuda, and Staub measured Q_L and the L/P protein ratio in sheep while infusing histamine into either the bronchial or pulmonary circulations.[72] Similar dose-dependent effects were observed with infusions into either circulation. Using assumptions they made regarding the local concentration of histamine, the authors concluded that the pulmonary circulation was the likely site of the histamine effect.

Studies infusing histamine into the pulmonary or bronchial circulation are difficult to interpret because of extensive anastomoses between the two[73-75] and because of the high solubility of histamine. As summarized by Hyde at the annual meeting of the Federation of American Societies for Experimental Biology in April 1984, if histamine increased permeability of the bronchial vessels, and if edema from bronchial vessels were only a minor contribution to the lung lymph, then an increase in left atrial pressures should decrease the L/P ratio even after histamine administration, as has been observed.[76-78] When administered intravenously, histamine has also been found to cause pulmonary edema in lungs when the pulmonary circulation is occluded.[79] However, this does not exclude the pulmonary circulation as a site of leakage as these vessels could have been perfused and exposed to histamine via the bronchopulmonary anastomoses, particularly in that these anastomoses markedly increase within minutes of pulmonary vascular occlusion.[80] Preliminary data from Charan et al.[81] suggest that increasing azygous venous pressure (which will increase bronchial venous pressure and impede venous drainage from the caudal mediastinal lymph node) causes lung weight and Q_L to increase without decreasing the L/P ratio.

Site of Leakage as a Safety Factor

Previously described safety factors in pulmonary edema include the increase in Ppmv and πmv together with the fall in πpmv that would occur with edema of low protein content when epithelial permeability is intact. An additional factor that could work to keep the gas exchange areas of the lung functioning normally until later in the course of the edema-producing problem is the distribution of the transmural hydrostatic gradients that would result from an increased intravascular pressure.

Using the estimates for Pxf around EA arteries and veins (Fig. 4), together with estimates of the intravascular hydrostatic pressure in the various segments (based upon studies of the segmental distribution of pulmonary vascular resistance[82,83]), it is possible to estimate the transmural hydrostatic gradient for the various vascular segments. The largest gradient would be across the arterial EAVs as the intravascular pressure would be the greatest and the perivascular pressure would be the most negative relative to P_A. The alveolar septal vessels would have the smallest transmural gradient, assuming that the septal interstitial pressure approximated P_A.[41] The alveolar corner vessels would have an intravascular pressure that was similar or slightly higher than that of the septal vessels, but the perivascular pressure of the corner vessels would be lower than P_A, increasing their Ptm. The EA veins would have the lowest intravascular pressure but a more negative perivascular pressure than the corner vessels. Given comparable Kf's, this distribution of transmural gradients suggests the AVs would be least likely to leak in response to the hydrostatic stress.

Site of Epithelial Leakage

The site of fluid movement from the interstitium into the alveoli (particularly in normal permeability edema) is also unknown. Just as the estimates of comparative surface area suggest that AVs are the primary site of endothelial leakage, these estimates would also suggest that leakage occurs through the alveolar epithelium. However, this epithelium has repeatedly been found to be relatively impermeable,[11,84-86] as would be suggested by the structure of the alveolar epithelial intercellular junctions.[87]

Leakage might occur at the level of the bronchiolar epithelium. This concept can be traced to Drinker in 1945,[86] who suggested that alveolar edema might result from fluid flowing from peribronchial cuffs across the airways and down to the alveoli. A similar hypothesis was suggested by Macklin in 1955,[87] and was supported by studies of Gee and Staub.[88] Yoneda induced normal permeability pulmonary edema in mice and studied the pathway of fluid leakage across the epithelial surface using horseradish peroxidase as an ultrastructural marker.[89] Tracer was observed in the intercellular junctions within arterial endothelial cells. It was found to track into the media and adventitia of small arteries and then to outline each bronchial epithelial cell up to the luminal surface. No tracer was seen in the junctions between alveolar epithelial cells. Yoneda suggested this intraepithelial cell junction at the terminal bronchial level was the site of leakage into the airspace.

Mason and Effros filled airways with a solution containing tracers, perfused the lungs with other markers for 30 minutes, and then removed the airway fluid.[90] The highest concentrations of vascular markers were found in the initial samples pumped from airways. These data also suggest a proximal airway site of leakage.

Summary and Conclusions

The arterial and venous EAVs may be as important as the AVs are relative to transvascular fluid and protein exchange in the lung. In addition, the bronchial circulation may also contribute to pulmonary edema formation or clearance. Because of these observations, the differences in intravascular and interstitial hydrostatic pressures around the various vascular segments or beds,[91] and the differences in vascular morphology, it becomes apparent that fluid and protein exchange in the lung cannot be described by single values for the variables described in equation [1]. Anatomical and physiological relationships in the lung suggest that the vessels exposed to the smallest transmural hydrostatic gradient resulting from a hydrostatic stress will be those located in the alveolar septum. In addition, recent studies suggest that fluid leaks from the interstitium into the alveolar space at a site in the airway while alveolar epithelial permeabililty remains intact.

REFERENCES

1. Staub, N.C.: Pulmonary edema. *Physiol. Rev.* 54:678–811, 1974.
2. Staub, N.C.: Proposed pulmonary space nomenclature. In *Central Hemodynamics and Gas Exchange, Appendix III.* Giutini, C., ed. Turin, Italy, Minerva Med., 1971, pp. 465–467.
3. Macklin, C.C.: Evidences of increase in the capacity of the pulmonary arteries and veins of dogs, cats, and rabbits during inflation of freshly excised lung. *Revue Canadienne Biologie* 5:199–232, 1946.
4. Howell, J.B.L., Permutt, S., Proctor, D.F., et al.: Effect of inflation of the lung on different parts of pulmonary vascular bed. *J. Appl. Physiol.* 16:71–76, 1961.
5. Staub, N.C., Hitoshi, N., and Pearce, M.L.: Pulmonary edema in dogs, especially the sequence of fluid accumulation in lungs. *J. Appl. Physiol.* 22:227–246, 1967.
6. Rous, P., Gilding, H.P., and Smith, F.: The gradient of vascular permeability. *J. Exp. Med.* 51:807–830, 1930.
7. Landis, E.M.: Heteroporosity of the capillary wall as indicated by cinematographic analysis of the passage of dyes. *Ann. N.Y. Acad. Sci.* 116:765–773, 1964.
8. Majno, G., Palade, G.E., and Schoefl, G.I.: Studies on inflammation. II. The site of action of histamine and serotonin along the vascular tree: A topographic study. *J. Biophys. Biochem. Cytol.* 11:607–626, 1961.
9. Pietra, G.G., Szidon, J.P., Leventhal, M.M., et al.: Hemoglobin as a tracer in hemodynamic pulmonary edema. *Science* 166:1643–1646, 1969.
10. Shirley, H.H., Jr., Wolfram, L.G., Wasserman, K., et al.: Capillary permeability to macromolecules: Stretched pore phenomenon. *Am. J. Physiol.* 190:189–197, 1957.
11. Cottrell, T.S., Levine, O.R., Senior, R.M., et al.: Electron microscopic alterations at the alveolar level in pulmonary edema. *Circ. Res.* 21:783, 1967.
12. Ashbaugh, D.G., Bigelow, D.B., Petty, T.L.: Acute respiratory distress in adults. *Lancet* 2:319–323, 1967.
13. Bachofen, M. and Weibel, E.R.: Alterations of the gas exchange apparatus in adult respiratory insufficiency associated with septicemia. *Am. Rev. Respir. Dis.* 116:589–615, 1977.
14. Bachofen, M., Bachofen H., and Weibel, E.R.: Lung edema in the adult respiratory distress syndrome. In *Pulmonary Edema.* Fishman, A.P. and Renkin, E.M., eds. Bethesda, MD, American Physiological Society, 1979, pp. 241–252.

15. Bohm, G.M.G.: Vascular permeability changes during experimentally produced pulmonary edema in rats. *J. Pathol. Bacteriol.* 92:151–164, 1966.
16. Bohm, G.M., Machado, D.C., and Padovan, P.A.: Ultrastructural changes in rat lung arterioles in conditions of altered permeability. *J. Pathol.* 121:115–117, 1977.
17. Cunningham, A.L., and Hurley, J.V.: Alpha-naphthyl-thiourea-induced pulmonary edema in the rat: A topographical and electron microscope study. *J. Pathol.* 106:25–35, 1972.
18. Meyrick, B., Miller, J., and Reid, L.: Pulmonary oedema induced by ANTU, or by high or low oxygen concentrations in rat: An electron microscopic study. *Br. J. Exp. Pathol.* 53:347–358, 1972.
19. Michel, R.P.: Pulmonary microvascular permeability to dextran in alphanaphthyl-thiourea (ANTU)-edema: A light and electron microscopic study. *Fed. Proc.* 43:515(A1340), 1984.
20. Hovig, T., Nicolaysen, A., and Nicolaysen, G.: Ultrastructural studies of the alveolo-capillary barrier in isolated plasma-perfused rabbit lungs: Effects of EDTA and increased capillary pressure. *Acta Physiol. Scand.* 82:417–432, 1971.
21. Whayne, T.F., Jr. and Severinghaus, J.W.: Experimental hypoxic pulmonary edema in the rat. *J. Appl. Physiol.* 25:729–732, 1968.
22. Iliff, L.D.: Extra-alveolar vessels and edema development in excised dog lungs. *Circ. Res.* 28:524–532, 1971.
23. Smith, H.C., Gould, V.F., Cheney, F.W., et al.: Pathogenesis of hemodynamic pulmonary edema in excised dog lungs. *J. Appl. Physiol.* 37:904–911, 1974.
24. Mitzner, W. and Robotham, J.L.: Distribution of interstitial compliance and filtration coefficient in canine lung. *Lymphology* 12:140–148, 1979.
25. Morriss, A.W., Drake, R.E., and Gabel, J.C.: Comparison of microvascular filtration characteristics in isolated and intact lungs. *J. Appl. Physiol.: Respir. Environ. Exercise Physiol.* 48:438–443, 1980.
26. Albert, R.K., Lakshminarayan, S., Huang, T.W., et al.: Fluid leaks from extra-alveolar vessels in living dog lungs. *J. Appl. Physiol.: Respir. Environ. Exercise Physiol.* 44:759–762, 1978.
27. Hauge, A., Lande, P.K.M., and Waler, B.A.: Vasoconstriction in isolated blood-perfused rabbit lungs and its inhibition by cresols. *Acta Physiol. Scand.* 66:226–240, 1966.
28. Bo, G., Hauge, A., and Nicolaysen, G.: Alveolar pressure and lung volume as determinants of net transvascular fluid filtration. *J. Appl. Physiol.* 42:476–482, 1977.
29. Inoue, H., Inoue, C., and Hildebrandt, J.: Vascular and airway pressures, and interstitial edema affect peribronchial fluid pressure. *J. Appl. Physiol.: Respir. Environ. Exercise Physiol.* 48:177–184, 1980.
30. Lai-Fook, S.J.: A continuum mechanics analysis of pulmonary vascular interdependence in isolated dog lobes. *J. Appl. Physiol.* 46:419–429, 1979.
31. Smith, J.C. and Mitzner, W.: Analysis of pulmonary vascular interdependence in excised dog lobes. *J. Appl. Physiol.: Respir. Environ. Exercise Physiol.* 48:450–467, 1980.
32. Goshy, M., Lai-Fook, S.J., and Hyatt, R.E.: Perivascular pressure measurements by Wick-catheter technique in isolated dog lobes. *J. Appl. Physiol.: Respir. Environ. Exercise Physiol.* 46:950–955, 1979.
33. Albert, R.K., Lakshminarayan, S., Kirk, W., et al.: Lung inflation can cause pulmonary edema in zone I of in situ dog lungs. *J. Appl. Physiol.: Respir. Environ. Exercise Physiol.* 49:815–819, 1980.
34. Benjamin, J.J., Murtagh, P.S., Proctor, D.F., et al.: Pulmonary vascular interdependence in excised dog lobes. *J. Appl. Physiol.* 37:887–894, 1974.
35. Permutt, S., Howell, J.B.L., Proctor, D.F., et al.: Effect of lung inflation on static pressure-volume characteristics of pulmonary vessels. *J. Appl. Physiol.* 16:64–70, 1961.
36. Permutt, S.: Mechanical influences on water accumulation in the lungs. In *Pul-*

monary Edema. Fishman, A.P., and Renkin, E.M., eds. Bethesda, MD, American Physiological Society, 1979, pp. 175–194.

37. Goldberg, H.S., Mitzner, W., and Batra, G.: Effects of transpulmonary and vascular pressures on rate of pulmonary edema formation. *J. Appl. Physiol.* 43:14–19, 1977.

38. Mellins, R.B., Levine, O.R., Skalak, R., et al.: Interstitial pressure of the lung. *Circ. Res.* 24:197–212, 1969.

39. Woolverton, W.C., Brigham, K.L., and Staub, N.C.: Effect of positive pressure breathing on lung lymph flow and water content in sheep. *Circ. Res.* 42:550–557, 1978.

40. Glazier, J.B., Hughes, J.M.B., Maloney, J.E., et al.: Measurements of capillary dimensions and blood volume in rapidly frozen dogs. *J. Appl. Physiol.* 26:65–76, 1969.

41. Bruderman, I., Somers, K., Hamilton, W.K., et al.: Effect of surface tension on circulation in the excised lungs of dogs. *J. Appl. Physiol.* 19:707–712, 1964.

42. Lloyd, T.C., and Wright, G.W.: Pulmonary vascular resistance and vascular transmural gradient. *J. Appl. Physiol.* 15:241–245, 1960.

43. Rosenzweig, D.Y., Hughes, J.M.B., and Glazier, J.B.: Effects of transpulmonary and vascular pressures on pulmonary blood volume in isolated lung. *J. Appl. Physiol.* 28:553–560, 1970.

44. Weibel, E.R., and Bachofen, H.: Structural design of the alveolar septum and fluid exchange. In *Pulmonary Edema.* Fishman, A.P., and Renkin, E.M., eds. Bethesda, MD, American Physiological Society, 1979, pp. 1–20.

45. Mead, J., Takishima, T., and Leith, D.: Stress distribution in lungs: A model of pulmonary elasticity. *J. Appl. Physiol.* 28:596–608, 1970.

46. Gil, J., Bachofen, H., Gehr, P., et al..: Alveolar volume-surface area relation in air- and saline-filled lungs fixed by vascular perfusion. *J. Appl. Physiol.* 47:990–1001, 1979.

47. Nicolaysen, G., and Hauge, A.: Determinants of transvascular fluid shifts in zone I lungs. *J. Appl. Physiol.: Respir. Environ. Exercise Physiol.* 48:256–264, 1980.

48. Albert, R.K., Lakshminarayan, S., Charan, N.B., et al.: Extra-alveolar vessel contribution to hydrostatic pulmonary edema in in situ dog lungs. *J. Appl. Physiol.: Respir. Environ. Exercise Physiol.* 54:1010–1017, 1983.

49. Guyton, A.C., and Lindsey, A.W.: Effect of elevated left atrial pressure and decreased plasma protein concentration on the development of pulmonary edema. *Circ. Res.* 7:649–657, 1959.

50. Lai-Fook, S.J.: Perivascular interstitial fluid pressure measured by micropipettes in isolated dog lung. *J. Appl. Physiol.: Respir. Environ. Exercise Physiol.* 52:9–15, 1982.

51. Goldberg, H.S.: Pulmonary interstitial compliance and microvascular filtration coefficient. *Am. J. Physiol.* 239:H189–H198, 1980.

52. Kay, J.M.: Comparative morphologic features of the pulmonary vasculature in mammals. *Am. Rev. Respir. Dis.* 128:S53–56, 1983.

53. Albert, R.K., Kirk, W., Pitts, C., et al.: Pulmonary arterial and venous extra-alveolar vessels are leakier than alveolar vessels in excised dog lungs. *Fed. Proc.* 43:46A, 1984.

54. Horsfield, K.: Morphometry of the small pulmonary arteries in man. *Circ. Res.* 24:593–597, 1978.

55. Horsfield, K. and Gordon, W.I.: Morphometry of pulmonary veins in man. *Lung* 159:211–218, 1981.

56. Weibel, E.R.: *Morphometry of the Human Lung.* Berlin, FRG, Springer-Verlag, pp. 78–82, 1963.

57. Sladen, A., Laver, M.B., and Pontoppidan, H.: Pulmonary complications and water retention in prolonged mechanical ventilation. *N. Engl. J. Med.* 279:448–453, 1968.

58. Webb, H.H. and Tierney, D.F.: Experimental pulmonary edema due to intermittent positive pressure ventilation with high inflation pressures: Protection by positive end-expiratory pressure. *Am. Rev. Respir. Dis.* 110:556–565, 1974.

59. Turino, G.M., Edelman, N.H., Senior, R.M., et al.: Extravascular lung water in cor pulmonale. *Bull. Pathophysiol. Resp.* 4:47–64, 1968.
60. Hultgren, H.N., Lopez, C.E., Lundberg, E., et al.: Physiologic studies of pulmonary edema at high altitude. *Circulation* 29:393–408, 1964.
61. Landolt, C.C., Matthay, M., and Staub, N.C.: Lung resection, increased blood flow and pressure in sheep: Failure to detect pore stretching or high linear flow injury. *Microvasc. Res.* 20:117, 1980.
62. Moosavi, H., Utell, M.J., Hyde, R.W., et al.: Lung ultrastructure in non-cardiogenic pulmonary edema induced by air embolization in dogs. *Lab. Invest.* 45:456–464, 1981.
63. Albertine, K.H., Wiener-Kronish, J.P., Kolke, K., et al.: Quantification of ultrastructural damage to the microcirculation of the lung during air embolization in sheep. *Am. Rev. Respir. Dis.* 127:306(A), 1983.
64. Borgstrom, K.-E., Ising, U., Linder, E., et al.: Experimental pulmonary edema. *Acta Radiol.* 54:97–119, 1960.
65. Pietra, G.G., Szidon, J.P., Levanthal, M.M., et al.: Histamine and interstitial pulmonary edema in the dog. *Circ. Res.* 29:323–337, 1971.
66. Pietra, G.G., Szidon, J.P., Carpenter, H.A., et al.: Bronchial venular leakage during endotoxin shock. *Am. J. Pathol.* 77:387–406, 1974.
67. Pietra, G.G. and Magno, M.: Pharmacological factors influencing permeability of the bronchial microcirculation. *Fed. Proc.* 37:2466–2470, 1978.
68. Goetzman, B.N., and Visscher, M.B.: The effects of alloxan and histamine on the permeability of the pulmonary alveolocapillary barrier to albumin. *J. Physiol. Lond.* 204:51–61, 1969.
69. Grega, G.J., Daugherty, R.M., Scott, J.F., et al.: Effect of pressure, flow, and vasoactive agents on vascular resistance and capillary filtration in canine fetal, newborn, and adult lung. *Microvasc. Res.* 3:297–307, 1971.
70. Meyrick, B. and Brigham, K.L.: Increased permeability of bovine pulmonary artery intimal explants caused by histamine structure and function. *Fed. Proc.* 42:3650A, 1983.
71. Brigham, K.L. and Owen, P.J.: Increased sheep lung vascular permeability caused by histamine. *Circ. Res.* 37:647–657, 1975.
72. Nakahara, K., Ohkuda, K., and Staub, N.C.: Effect of infusing histamine into pulmonary or bronchial artery on sheep pulmonary fluid balance. *Am. Rev. Respir. Dis.* 20:875, 1979.
73. Krahl, V.E.: Anatomy of the mammalian lung. In *Handbook of Physiology and Respiration.* Washington, D.C., American Physiological Society, 1964, Section 3, Vol. 1, Chapter 6, pp. 213–284.
74. McLaughlin, R.F., Tyler, W.S., and Canada, R.O.: A study of the subgross pulmonary anatomy in various animals. *Am. J. Anat.* 108:149–166, 1961.
75. Magno, M.G. and Fishman, A.P.: Origin, distribution, and blood flow of bronchial circulation in anesthetized sheep. *J. Appl. Physiol.: Respir. Environ. Exercise Physiol.* 53:272–279, 1982.
76. Minnear, F.L., Mullins, R.J., Bell, D.R., et al.: Histamine-induced increase in pulmonary lymph flow: Hemodynamics versus permeability. *Physiology* 25:205A, 1982.
77. Bernard, G.R., Snapper, J.R., Hutchison, A.A., et al.: Effects of left atrial pressure elevation and histamine infusion on lung lymph in awake sheep. *J. Appl. Physiol.: Respir. Environ. Exercise Physiol.* 56:1083–1089, 1984.
78. Walkenstein, M.D., Peterson, B.T., Gerber, J.E., et al.: Histamine-induced pulmonary edema in sheep with unilateral occlusion of the pulmonary artery. *Fed. Proc.* 42:7197A, 1983.
79. Jindal, S.K., Lakshminarayan, S., Kirk, W., et al.: The acute increase in anastomotic bronchial blood flow after pulmonary artery obstruction. *J. Appl. Physiol.: Respir. Environ. Exercise Physiol.* 1984 (In press).

80. Charan, N.B., Turk, G.M., Jones, C.M., et al.: Leakage from the bronchial veins influences lung lymph flow. *Fed. Proc.* 42:5751A, 1983.
81. Charan, N.B., Turk, G.M., Bishop, D.T., et al.: Lung fluid balance is influenced by bronchial venous obstruction in anesthetized sheep. *Am. Rev. Respir. Dis.* 125:278A, 1982.
82. Schneeberger-Keeley, E.E. and Karnovsky, M.J.: The ultrastructural basis of alveolocapillary membrane permeability to peroxidase used as a tracer. *J. Cell Biol.* 37:781–793, 1968.
83. Schneeberger-Keeley, E.E.: The permeability of the alveolocapillary membrane to ultrastructural protein tracers. *Ann. N.Y. Acad. Sci.* 221:238–243, 1971.
84. Taylor, A.E. and Gaar, K.A., Jr.: Estimation of equivalent pore radii of pulmonary capillary and alveolar membranes. *Am. J. Physiol.* 218:1133–1140, 1970.
85. Schneeberger-Keeley, E.E. and Karnovsky, M.J.: Substructure of intercellular junctions in freeze-fractured alveolocapillary membranes of mouse lungs. *Circ. Res.* 38:404–411, 1976.
86. Drinker, C.R.: *Pulmonary Edema and Inflammation.* Cambridge, MA, Harvard University Press, 1945, p. 43.
87. Macklin, C.C.: Pulmonary sumps, dust accumulation, alveolar fluid and lymph vessels. *Acta Anat.* 23:1–33, 1955.
88. Gee, M.H. and Staub, N.C.: Role of bulk fluid in protein permeability of the dog lung alveolar membrane. *J. Appl. Physiol.* 42:144–149, 1977.
89. Yoneda, K.: Anatomic pathway of fluid leakage in fluid-overload pulmonary edema in mice. *Am. J. Pathol.* 101:7–13, 1980.
90. Mason, G.R. and Effros, R.M.: Flow of edema fluid into pulmonary airways. *J. Appl. Physiol. Respir. Environ. Exercise Physiol.* 55:1262–1268, 1983.
91. Bhattacharya, J. and Staub, N.C.: Direct measurement of microvascular pressures in the isolated, perfused dog lung. *Science* 210:327–328, 1980.

The Assessment of Pulmonary Microvascular Permeability and Edema

James C. Hogg

Introduction

The collection of edema fluid in the interstitium and airspace of the lungs interferes with the normal process of gas exchange. The purpose of this chapter is to review the techniques that are presently available for quantitating the edema and estimating the disruption of the air/blood barrier. These techniques can be divided into five general areas that include: (1) imaging of the lung; (2) the use of indicator dilution techniques; (3) the measurement of lung mechanics; (4) the clearance of material through the air/blood barrier; and (5) the measurement of markers of injury to the air/blood barriers in the circulating blood. Each of these broad areas is represented by a variety of individual methods that may be very old or very new. The majority of these techniques are of questionable value in most clinical situations. Some provide important investigative tools and others show promise as methods that might be usefully applied to the care of patients.

Imaging the Lung

The chest x-ray is a standard method of evaluating the severity of lung edema.[1-5] In skilled hands, this method has met with considerable success in diagnosing edema prior to the onset of signs and symptoms. The fact that edema collects in the interstitial space before it floods the airspace[6] has been used by radiologists to monitor the onset of edema. With heart failure these signs are preceded by signs of vascular congestion that can be used to help separate edema due to heart failure from edema due to microvascular injury.

Pistolesi and Guintini[7] provided a careful study comparing chest x-ray findings to measurements of extravascular lung water made with both a standard and modified indicator dilution curve. The chest x-rays were evaluated for

Supported by the Medical Research Council of Canada.

From Said, S.I. (ed.): *The Pulmonary Circulation and Acute Lung Injury*. Mount Kisco, N.Y., Futura Publishing Co., Inc., 1985.

the presence or absence of edema using standard criteria (Table I). They found significant relationships between a radiological score for the severity of edema and the extravascular water with both of these methods. When the standard method was used (Fig. 1), a linear relationship was found while the input-output method (Fig. 2) showed the x-ray score could double before there was any significant increase in extravascular water. The problems with this sort of analysis were thoroughly discussed by Staub[8] in an earlier review and were well recognized by Pistolesi and Guintini. However, the data in Figures 1 and 2 show the important point that the plain chest x-ray can provide evidence that edema is present before the most careful measurements of extravascular water increase. The importance of this work is that it correlated the chest x-ray findings with measurements of lung water and confirmed several previous studies that had shown that the chest x-ray becomes abnormal before signs and symptoms of edema develop.

Table I provides a list of the chest x-ray changes that occur with edema. The first is a distension of the vessels, particularly veins, in the upper lung zones with contraction of these vessels in the lower zones.[1] These changes reverse the normal vascular pattern but do not necessarily indicate a reversal of blood flow[9] even though they are often interpreted in that way. It seems more likely that the veins in the lower lobe become overdistended first and then constrict to produce this pattern. As the large veins do not normally contribute to vascular resistance, this contraction does not necessarily lead to a reduction in blood flow to the lower lobes. To this observer, it seems most likely that the reversed vascular pattern seen in pre-edema and the reversal of blood flow that is seen with alveolar flooding are separate events.

Hilar abnormalities are common and quite variable during the formation of

---

Table I
Criteria Used To Grade Pulmonary Edema
(Interstitial) By X-Ray Examinations*

Chest X-Ray Findings
    Reversed vascular pattern
    Hila enlarged
        increased density
        blurred
    Kerley's A lines
        B lines
        C lines
    Micronoduli
    Widening of fissures
    Peribronchial and perivascular cuffs
    Extensive perihilar haze
    Subpleural effusion
    Diffuse increase in density

Additional Findings of Rare Occurrence
    Perilobular lines and rosettes
    Unusual linear shadows

*Modified from ref. 7 with permission of the authors and publishers.

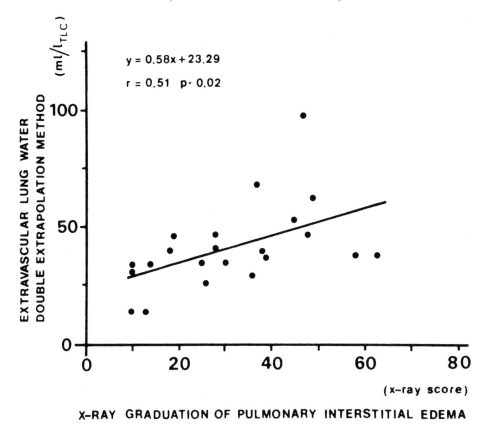

Figure 1: *This graph shows the relationship between the x-ray grading of pulmonary interstitial edema and extravascular water measured by the usual double indicator dilution method. The data show a linear increase in extravascular water in relation to increased interstitial edema with a relatively shallow slope. (Data from ref. 7 with permission of the authors and publisher.)*

edema in the lung (Fig. 3). Enlargement and increased density likely represent vascular distension alone, but when this is associated with a blurring or haze, it seems likely that extravascular fluid has accumulated in the interstitial space. This latter abnormality can occasionally be quite prominent and produce the so-called "bat's wing" or butterfly appearance on the radiograph. The peribronchial and perivascular cuffs of fluid that occur in early edema can be appreciated by the loss of a sharp outline between the bronchial and vascular walls[4] and can become prominent enough to form micronodules. The formation of septal lines are thought to represent engorgement of lymphatics and expansion of the surrounding connective tissue space.[1,10] These lines (Fig. 4) were first described by Kerley[1] who divided them into those that are several centimeters in length and radiate toward the hilum (type A), those that are short and sharp in outline and run in a horizontal direction (type B), and those that are fine and interlacing (type C). It is of interest that Kerley A and C lines are more commonly associated with acute edema and B lines with more chronic edema.

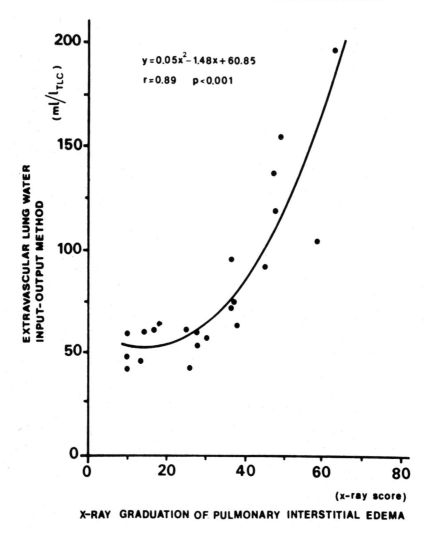

Figure 2: *This graph shows similar data with more careful measurements of extravascular lung water against the x-ray score of pulmonary edema. The data show that the x-ray score can increase substantially before there is any measurable increase in extravascular water. (Data from ref. 7 with permission of the authors and publisher.)*

Grainger[10] studied the appearance of septal lines in relation to pulmonary vascular pressures and showed that the lines were infrequent when the left atrial pressure was below 20 torr. As extravascular fluid continues to collect, the fluid can be seen in the fissures. This may be because of the distension of subpleural lymphatics at this site or because fluid is more easily visible when it is in the fissure adjacent to lung parenchyma.[11–13] Harrison et al.[12] drew attention to a diffuse haze that occurred just prior to alveolar flooding, which is associated with volume loss and the appearance of air bronchograms as the airspaces fill with fluid.

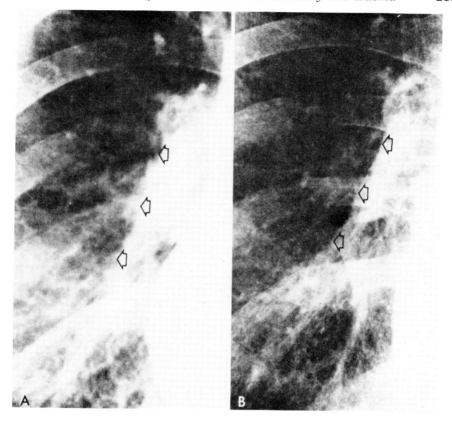

Figure 3: *The hilum from a patient with left ventricular failure.* **A:** *The hilum is enlarged and blurred.* **B:** *Shows the same patient following therapy where the hilar abnormalities have disappeared (large arrows). (Reproduced from ref. 7 with permission of the authors and publishers.)*

Taken together, these roentgenographic signs of pulmonary edema can provide qualitative information about the amount of water in the lung. They have been better studied in edema due to heart failure than in edema due to capillary injury. Milne[14] believes that it is possible to differentiate many forms of edema using the plain chest film, but his arguments are too extensive and controversial to be adequately discussed in this chapter.

Computed Tomography

The history of the development of mathematical methods of reconstructing images from projections has been very well reviewed by Gordon and his associates.[15] They state that the development of the mathematical reconstruction techniques occurred as early as 1917. These showed that a two- or three-dimensional object could be reconstructed uniquely from an infinite set of its projections. The introduction of x-ray tomography provided a method for obtaining these projected images of the body but it required modern computer-age techniques to produce useful three-dimensional reconstructions of these x-ray

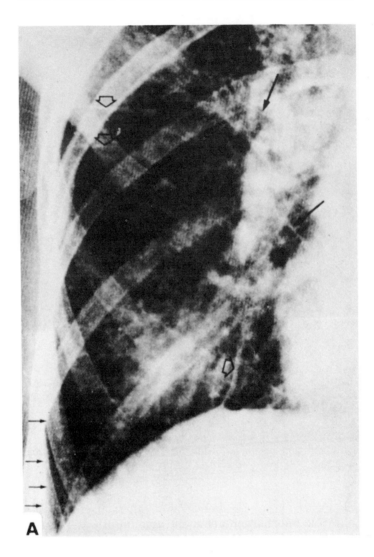

Figure 4: *The nature of the Kerley lines.* **A:** *Shows the A lines (long black arrows) and B lines (short black arrows) with the open arrows showing fluid in the fissure.* **B:** *At a higher magnification, the Kerley B lines (short arrows) can be better seen.* **C:** *The arrows indicate the C lines.*

images. It is of considerable interest that the same mathematical and computing procedures are now used to reconstruct two-dimensional images of celestial objects from their radio and x-ray signals into three-dimensional reconstructions of our galaxy. This technology has also provided the ability for the reconstruction of images obtained by nuclear magnetic resonance and positron emission tomography. Kreel[16] provided an interesting and early review of computed tomography of the thorax that outlines many of the problems facing the radiologist who uses this technique. The data that is accumulating indicates that this method may be of considerable interest in exploring chest disease. Its ability to

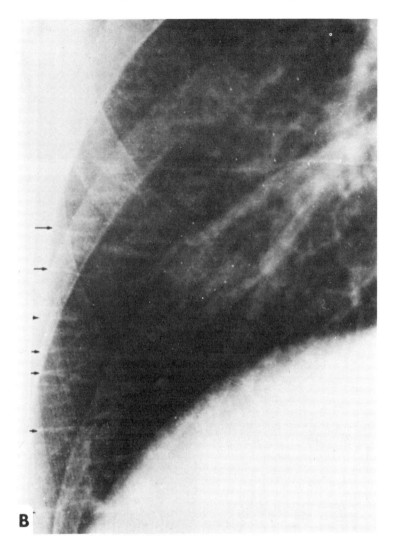

Figure 4B *(Continued)*

show regional changes in extravascular water has probably been incompletely explored at the present time. Indeed, it may be that its real value will be for lesions other than the edematous process.

Nuclear Magnetic Resonance

Purcell and Block were awarded the Nobel Prize in 1952 for laying the experimental foundation for nuclear magnetic resonance spectroscopy (NMR). However, the first NMR images were produced in the early 1960s by Lauterbur.[17] The later development of computerized tomography subsequently laid

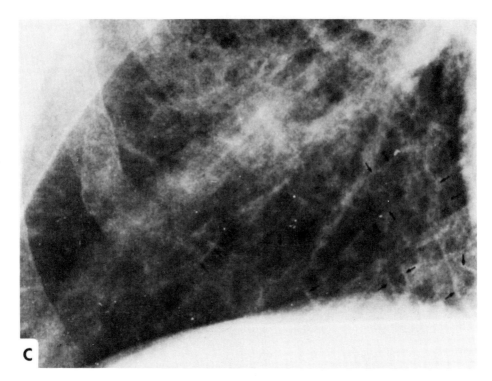

Figure 4C

the groundwork for the development of clinically useful NMR images. The technique involves placing the body in a homogeneous magnetic field so that the magnetic nuclei of the element of interest will align themselves in the direction of the magnetic field. A pulse of radio frequency energy is first superimposed on this field to alter the orientation of these nuclei relative to the static magnetic field and is then removed so that the nuclei return to the previous equilibrium state. The nucleus absorbs energy when the pulse frequency is applied and releases energy when the frequency is removed. The absorption and emission of this energy occurs at a specific resonant frequency that depends upon both the nature of the nucleus and the strength of the static magnetic field. The strength of the signal can then be related to the specific number of nuclei present so that quantitative information can be obtained. The time that the nucleus takes to return to its equilibrium alignment after the removal of the pulse is called T1, or the spin lattis relaxation time. If two or more nuclei follow a radio frequency pulse, they move out of phase with each other since each acts as a small magnet. This dephasing time can also be measured and is called T2, or the spin-spin relaxation time. The NMR signals are also sensitive to flow because the movement of magnetized nuclei through the region change the signal. NMR therefore provides information concerning the total number of specific nuclei present, the T1 and T2 relaxation times, and also gives information with respect to flow.

Hydrogen is the primary element that has been thus far imaged in vivo.[18] Body organs that have the same number of protons (water molecules) and would show little or no contrast differentiation on radiographic image can be differentiated easily by variations in their relaxation times. At the present time there is extensive experimental work going on with respect to measuring the elemental constitution of various body regions using NMR. The ease with which NMR measures hydrogen makes this an attractive method for imaging the thorax.[19] The major problem at the present moment is the time that it takes to create an image. This time is currently longer than the breath-holding time so that if one is to produce an image of the lung, a gaiting procedure must be used. There are also the problems of putting patients with lung edema in the confined apparatus required to make the measurements. This makes NMR of limited practical value in the measurement of pulmonary edema at the present state of the art but the method holds great promise for the future. The present state of development of NMR must be considered in relation to the development of x-ray diagnosis. Clearly, one cannot possibly compare the quality of x-rays available shortly after the discovery of the roentgen ray to those that are available today. Theoretically, NMR should be able to provide estimates of lung water, to differentiate intravascular from extravascular water, and provide information about blood flow. While a great deal of work will be required before these theoretical possibilities become a practical reality, the promise of the technique suggests a very bright future.

Digital Subtraction Angiography

The fundamental principle of digital subtraction angiography (DSA) is that the output of an image intensifier is coupled to a low noise video system.[20] A control image of the area is then generated and a small amount of contrast material is injected so that the image can be recorded as it passes through the area of interest. The digital array without contrast media is substracted from that with contrast media and the resultant signal converted to an analog format and displayed on an oscilloscope. Theoretically, this technique should allow a clear differentiation of the pulmonary circulation without the risk attended to the present methods of pulmonary bi-plane angiography. The technique should provide an advantage over the plain chest x-ray for relating the size of the vascular to the interstitial space, but only time will tell if it is useful in detecting the amount of fluid present in these regions of the lung in the early stages of edema.

Scanning Methods

Several investigators have used a dilution principle and external counting to measure the size of the lung water compartments. Isotope is injected IV and allowed to disperse throughout the compartment to which it is confined. Pritchard and Lee[21,22] used different ^{125}I-labeled compounds to mark the vascular (^{125}I-albumin), interstitial (^{125}I-iodine), and intracellular (^{125}I-iodoantipyrine) compartments successfully in open-chested dogs, but the method is not suitable for man because of the problems with the chest wall.

Gorin and his associates[23,24] have used the gamma camera to estimate the amount of a tracer protein in the vascular and extravascular space. In this method, they inject ^{113M}IN-transferrin and ^{99M}Tc-erythrocytes into the body and scan over the lung. They assume that the ratio of intravascular activity in the lung relative to that in the blood is directly proportional to a similar ratio for an intravascular reference usually counted over the heart. This proportionality constant is determined over the lung before the labeled transferrin escapes from the vascular space. In this way they can measure the extravascular accumulation of the tranferrin by subtracting the amount in the blood from the total amount of activity counted over the chest. They have shown that this procedure works in animals where permeability has been induced by injecting pseudomonas organisms.[24] The principal drawbacks of the method are the assumptions that there are no changes in distribution volumes of the indicators during the study, that the activity in the chest wall does not interfere, and that the intravascular label does not elute.

Sugerman and his associates[25] have recently used technetium-labeled human serum albumin to compare the ratio of counts over the lung to counts over the heart. They find that this ratio remains constant in normal lungs and rises when there is an albumin leak. This may provide a simple way of separating high pressure edema from situations where both high pressure and capillary injury are present.

Indicator Dilution Methods

This approach is based on a method of measuring cardiac output that was first introduced by Stewart in 1897[26] and modified by Henriques[27] for a single injection. Hamilton provided a systematic investigation of the method and a careful inquiry into the sources of error, which he summarized in the *Handbook of Physiology*.[28] The basis of the technique is the injection of a known amount of indicator in a flowing stream, the mixing of the indicator with the fluid, and measurement of the concentration of the indicator at a downstream site. The flow can then be calculated by dividing the amount of indicator injected (I) by the sum of the concentrations (C) over the time it passes the sampling site:

$$\text{flow} = I / \int C dt \qquad [1]$$

The mean transit time (MTT) for the indicator to pass from the injection to the sampling site can be calculated by dividing the sum of the concentrations by the sum of the concentration over time. It follows that the volume between the injection and sampling sites can be found by multiplying flow by the MTT.

This technique was modified by Chinard and Enns[29] to measure extravascular water space by comparing a reference indicator that stayed in the vascular space to tritiated water that diffused out of the vascular space. By measuring the mean transit time of the vascular (V) and diffusable (D) indicator, they calculated the extravascular lung water (EVLW) where $EVLW = CO \times (MTT_D - MTT_V)$. The problem with the technique seems to relate to the fact that normal values are extremely wide so that accuracy is difficult to achieve. Pistolesi and Guintini[7] thought that a major source of this error was in the uncertainty of forward extrapolation of the curve that is necessary because of recirculation of the indicator. They developed a method to avoid this that requires simultaneous sampling from the pulmonary artery and aorta allowing the dilution curve on the input side (pulmonary artery) to be compared to the dilution curve on the output side (aorta). They used a convolution integral to analyze the input and output to obtain the distribution of transit times between the two sampling sites. They showed that the previous forward extrapolation was subject to considerable error and compared both methods of measuring lung water to the chest x-ray (compare Figs. 1 and 2). The indicator dilution method for measuring extravascular water has also been modified by Lewis and his associates,[30] who used heat as the diffusable indicator. By injecting cold cardio-green dye, they were able to use cardiogreen as the vascular indicator and heat as the diffusable indicator. They also designed a small computer to allow rapid calculation of the data at the bedside. Although the error in the values obtained are open to question, the method provides a reasonable way of following edema in individual patients. The main problem with all of these techniques is that they are dependent on getting the indicator into the edematous region because the edema itself may reduce blood flow.

Crone[31] developed a method that allowed the indicator dilution technique to measure the product of permeability (P) and surface area (S). This product is calculated using the formula $PS = -F \times \ln(I - E)$ where F is the intravascular water flow and E is the fractional extraction calculated as the difference between the vascular and extravascular indicator to the peak of the vascular indicator curve. This method was designed to avoid the problem of diffusion of the extravascular indicator back into the vascular space. In calculating the intravascular water flow, Goresky and his associates[32] showed that a composite intravascular water flow curve must be constructed to take into account the hematocrit and water content of erythrocytes and plasma. Brigham and his associates[33] have recently reported data on measurements of the extravascular water and permeability surface area for urea in patients with adult respiratory distress syndrome (ARDS). They concluded that the amount of water measured in the lung by this technique did not relate to the severity of oxygenation defect nor did it correlate with survival. Interestingly, they found that the product of permeability and surface area was lower than normal in patients with ARDS that survived but very high in those that died. They interpreted this finding to mean that those who survived had the ability to reduce flow to the areas of the lung where the microvasculature was damaged. It seems doubtful if measurements of lung water or PS product will be very useful in the clinical setting because of the wide variability in the measurement. This is particularly true in ARDS where one would like to be able to detect early injury to the membrane and take steps to prevent it. As measurable edema in ARDS likely means severe injury to the membrane, lung water measurements are not likely to be that helpful.

Detection of Edema by Measuring Lung Mechanics

The effect of vascular distension and pulmonary edema on the mechanical properties of the lungs has been carefully studied.[34-38] Unfortunately, the usual measurements of elastic and flow resistance properties of the lungs have not been very helpful except when gross edema is present. Although total airways resistance is minimally changed by edema, the resistance of peripheral airways does incease as edema develops.[39] These studies also showed that the increase in peripheral airways resistance was readily reversible when LA pressure was below 15 torr but increased in an irreversible fashion at higher left atrial pressures. These authors also observed that the effect of rising LA on the peripheral airways was much greater at low lung volumes and they suggested that there might be a competition for space between vessel airway and edema fluid in the bronchovascular bundle. Since then several groups have attempted to use tests of peripheral airways function to detect interstitial lung edema. It has been shown that fluid accumulation leads to small airway closure,[40,41] raising the possibility that the closure might be detected by various tests.[42,43] Although the initial interest in this problem appears to have faded, the fact remains that a reduction in FEV_1 is one of the most common findings in patients with congestive heart failure.[44] This suggests that interstitial edema has an important effect on peripheral airway function but the nature of the peripheral airways tests make them difficult to perform or interpret at the bedside of severely ill patients.

Clearance Through the Blood/Air Barrier

Recently several groups of investigators have used radioactive aerosols of ^{99m}TC=dethytenetriaminepentaacetate (^{99m}TC=DTPA) to measure the permeability of the blood/air barrier.[45-48] Studies have been carried out in normal human subjects, smokers, and patients with interstitial and/or chronic obstructive pulmonary disease. Animal studies have also been carried out in situations of hydrostatic and acid-induced edema. Rizk and his associates[49] have examined the method carefully in dogs and have shown that it was reproducible, varied little with breathing frequency, but was affected by positive end-expiratory pressure. They also showed that the absorption was primarily from the portion of the lung supplied by the pulmonary circulation. The exact site and nature of the leaks that allow these molecules to pass through the air/blood barrier have not been determined, but it seems likely that the increased permeability is associated with a defect in the epithelial barrier. Early studies from our laboratory[50] suggested that the increased permeability was associated with disruption of the epithelial tight junctions, but this finding could not be confirmed when quantitative assessments of the junctions were made.[51] More recent studies by Walker and his associates[52] suggest that the site of increased permeability may be at the corners where three cells meet, and this possibility needs to be investigated more fully.

An interesting feature of airway epithelial permeability is that it can be greatly increased in the exudative phase of the acute inflammatory reaction, but it rapidly returns to normal at the later stages when the inflammatory cells have begun to migrate.[53] These observations might be rationalized by the histological observation that when normal epithelial cells slough from the airway, they are replaced by broad flat basal cells that eventually develop into a mature epithelium. The appearance of the basal cells may be responsible for returning the permeability to normal early in the repair phase of the inflammatory reaction by reducing the number of corners per unit surface area. This sort of argument would also fit with the observation that the permeability is increased in diffuse interstitial lung disease where the alveolar surface is covered with cuboidal epithelium that would have more corners per unit surface area than the alveolar surface covered with flat type II cells. Although much remains to be learned about the exact site and nature of epithelial permeability in both normal and diseased states, the aerosol tests of permeability could well provide a sensitive test of epithelial injury.

Circulating Markers of Endothelial Injury

It would be very useful if damaged endothelial cells released a marker that could be measured accurately in the blood. Although it seems likely that the converting enzyme, lipoproteinlipase, and factor 8 are released, it has not been possible to use them as markers of endothelial cell damage. Plasma fibronectin is a 44,000 molecular weight alpha-II globulin that is secreted primarily by the liver and possibly by endothelial cells and is involved in the nonimmunological opsonization process.[54] Fisher[55] has postulated that endothelial disruption may increase the levels of this protein in the plasma so that it would serve as a useful marker of endothelial injury. He has studied oxygen exposure in rats and shown that there is a steady increase in the serum fibronectin as the injury develops. Whether or not this turns out to be a useful measurement of pulmonary endothelial disruption remains to be seen but the idea is promising.

An alternative approach to measuring a product released by damaged cells is to try to obtain evidence of a response to the injured endothelium in the circulating blood. The studies of Craddock et al.,[56] showing that the polymorphonuclear leukocyte was activated by dialysis membranes has led to the suggestion that the measurement of complement proteins C_{5a} might be a useful prognostic sign of endothelial damage in ARDS. A study of Hammerschmidt et al.[57] provided data that were somewhat hopeful in this regard because it appeared that complement proteins did change in a way that would predict the onset of ARDS in high risk patients. More recent studies by Weinberg and his associates[58] failed to confirm these early findings. The fact that white blood cells are more easily measured than complement proteins caused Thommasen et al.[59] to undertake a prospective study of the WBC count in high risk patients. They measured the white count every 4 hours in ɹ attempt to predict the onset of ARDS and the data showed (Table II) that tلϵ white cells often fell dramatically just prior to the onset of ARDS. Although this finding could also be observed in some patients who did not develop the syndrome, a fall to below 4,000 cells was reasonably sensitive and specific with the predictive value of a negative test being 93% in this study (Table II). These preliminary data suggest that frequent measurements of the white blood cell count may turn out to be a useful and simple predictor of endothelial injury in this high risk group of patients.

Table II
Predictive Value of WBC Count*

	ARDS	No ARDS	Sensitivity	Specificity	Positive Predictive Value	Negative Predictive Value
Fall in WBC**	8	4				
			80%	87%	67%	93%
No fall in WBC	2	26				

*From ref. 59 with permission of authors and publisher.
**A fall in WBC was a decrease to less than 4,200 cells/mm^3. The relationship between a fall in WBC and ARDS was significant (p<.05).

Summary

In summary, there are a wide variety of methods available for measuring the disruption of the alveolar capillary barrier and the increase in fluid in the interstitial space. While many of these are intellectually stimulating and the source of great scientific debate, there appears to be no easy method of consistently measuring either of these important parameters. Clearly, accurate methods of measuring the disruption of the alveolar capillary barrier and the subsequent accumulation of fluid would be of great benefit to the management of the many patients who develop pulmonary edema. The methodology is advancing steadily, but a simple easy method of measuring either the injury to the membrane or the increased edema that results has not yet arrived.

REFERENCES

1. Kerley, P.: Cardiac failure. In *A Textbook of X-Ray Diagnosis,* 3rd Edition. Shank, S.C. and Kerley, P., eds. London, Lewis, 1962, Vol. 2, pp. 97–108.
2. Chait, A.: Interstitial pulmonary edema. *Circulation* 45:1323–1330, 1972.
3. Goodrich, W.A.: Pulmonary edema: Correlation of x-ray appearance and physiological changes. *Radiology* 51:58–65, 1948.
4. Gleason, D.C. and Steiner, R.E.: The lateral radial graph in pulmonary edema. *Am. J. Roentgenol.* 98:279–290, 1966.
5. Garnett, E.S., Webber, C.E., Coates, G., et al.: Lung density: Clinical method for quantitation of pulmonary congestion and edema. *Can. Med. Assoc. J.* 116:153–154, 1977.
6. Staub, N.C., Nagano, H., and Pierce, M.L.: Pulmonary edema in dogs, especially the sequence of fluid accumulation in the lungs. *J. Appl. Physiol.* 22:227–240, 1967.
7. Pistolesi, M. and Guintini, G.: Assessment of extravascular lung water. *Radiol. Clin. N. Am.* 16:551–574, 1978.
8. Staub, N.C.: Pulmonary edema. *Physiol. Rev.* 54:678, 1974.
9. Muir, A.L., Hall, D.L., Despas, P., et al.: The distribution of blood flow in acute pulmonary edema in dogs. *J. Appl. Physiol.* 33:763–769, 1972.
10. Grainger, R.G.: Interstitial pulmonary edema and the radiological diagnosis: A sign of pulmonary venous and capillary hypertension. *Br. J. Radiol.* 31:201–217, 1958.
11. Heitzman, E.R. and Ziter, F.M., Jr.: Acute interstitial pulmonary edema. *Am. J. Roentgenol.* 98:291–299, 1966.
12. Harrison, M.O., Conte, P.J., and Heitzman, E.R.: Radiological detection of clinically occult cardiac failure following myocardial infarction. *Br. J. Radiol.* 44:265–272, 1971.
13. Logue, R.B., Rodgers, J.V., Jr., Gay, B.B., Jr.: Subtle roentgenographic signs of left heart failure. *Am. Heart J.* 65:464–473, 1963.
14. Milne, E.N.C.: Advances in the physiologic interpretation of the chest radiograph. Fleischner Society, *14th Annual Symposium on Chest Disease,* Sante Fe, New Mexico, June 17–19, 1984, pp. 88–106.
15. Gordon, H.G.T., and Johnson, S.A.: Image reconstruction from projections. *Sci. Am.* 233:56–72, 1975.
16. Kreel, L.: Computed tomography of the Thorax. *Radiol. Clin. N. Am.* 16:575–584, 1978.
17. Lauterbur, P.C.: Image formation by induced local interactions: Examples employing nuclear magnetic resonance. *Nature* 242:190–191, 1973.
18. Crooks, L., Hoenninger, J., Arakawa, M., et al.: Tomography of hydrogen with nuclear magnetic resonance. *Radiology* 136:701–706, 1980.

19. Gamsu, G., Webb, W.R., Sheldon, P., et al.: Nuclear magnetic resonance imaging of the thorax. *Radiology* 147:473–480, 1983.
20. Pond, G.D., Ovitt, T.W., Capp, M.P.: Comparison of conventional pulmonary angiography with intravenous digital subtraction angiography for pulmonary embolic disease. *Radiology* 147:345–350, 1983.
21. Pritchard, J.S. and Lee, G.deJ.: Non-invasive measurement of regional interstitial spaces, capillary permeability and solute fluxes in the lungs using a radioisotope method. *Bull. Physiopathol. Respir.* 11:137, 1975.
22. Pritchard, J.S. and Lee, G.deJ.: Measurement of water distribution in transcapillary solute flux in dog lung by external radioactivity counting. *Clin. Sci.* 57:145, 1979.
23. Gorin, A.B., Kohler, J., and DeNardo, G.: Noninvasive measurement of pulmonary transvascular protein flux in normal man. *J. Clin. Invest.* 66:869, 1980.
24. Gorin, A.B., Weidner, W.J., Demling, R.M., et al.: Noninvasive measurement of pulmonary transvascular protein flux in sheep. *J. Appl. Physiol.* 45:225, 1978.
25. Sugerman, H.J., Tatum, J.L., Berg, T.S., et al.: Gamma scintographic analysis of albumin flux in patients with acute respiratory distress syndrome. *Surgery* 95:674–682, 1984.
26. Stewart, G.M.: Researches on the circulation time and on influences which effect it. IV: The output of the heart. *J. Physiol.* 22:159, 1897.
27. Henriques, V.: Uber die Verteilung des Blutes Vom linken Herzen Zwichen dem Hertzen und dem ubrigen organismus. *Biochem. Z.* 56:230, 1913.
28. Hamilton, W.F.: Measurements of the cardiac output. In *Handbook of Physiology,* Washington American Physiological Society, Section 2, Vol. 1, p. 551, 1962.
29. Chinard, F.P. and Enns, T.: Transcapillary pulmonary exchange of water in the dog. *Am. J. Physiol.* 178:197 -202, 1954.
30. Lewis, F.R., Elings, V.B., Hill, S.L., et al.: Measurement of extravascular lung water by thermal green dye indicator dilution method. *Ann. N.Y. Acad. Sci.* 384:394–410, 1982.
31. Crone, C.: Permeability of capillaries and various organs as determined by use of indicator diffusion methods. *Acta Physiol. Scand.* 48:292–305, 1963.
32. Goresky, C.A., Cronin, R.F.P., Wangel, B.E.: Indicatory dilution measurement of extravascular water in the lungs. *J. Clin. Invest.* 48:487–501, 1969.
33. Brigham, K.L., Kariman, K., Harris, T.R., et al.: Correlation of oxygenation with vascular permeability surface area but not with lung water in humans with acute respiratory failure and pulmonary edema. *J. Clin. Invest.* 72:339–349, 1983.
34. Borst, H.G., Berglund, E., Whittenberger, J.L., et al.: The effect of pulmonary vascular pressures on mechanical properties of the lungs of anesthetized dogs. *J. Clin. Invest.* 36:1708–1714, 1957.
35. Cook, C.D., Mead, J., Schreiner, G.L., et al.: Pulmonary mechanics during induced pulmonary edema in anesthetized dogs. *J. Appl. Physiol.* 14:177–186, 1959.
36. Levine, O.R., Mellens, R.B., and Fishman, A.P.: Quantitative assessment of pulmonary edema. *Circ. Res.* 17:414–426, 1965.
37. Sharp, J.T., Bunnel, I.L., Griffith, G.T., et al.: The effect of therapy on pulmonary mechanics and human pulmonary edema. *J. Clin. Invest.* 40:665–672, 1961.
38. Sharp, J.T., Griffith, G.T., Bunnell, I.L., et al.: Ventilatory mechanics in pulmonary edema in man. *J. Clin. Invest.* 37:111–117, 1958.
39. Hogg, J.C., Agarawal, J.B., Gardiner, A.J.S., et al.: Distribution of airway resistance with developing pulmonary edema in dogs. *J. Appl. Physiol.* 32:20–24, 1972.
40. Hughes, J.M.B. and Rosenzweig, D.Y.: Factors affecting trapped gas volume in perfused dog lung. *J. Appl. Physiol.* 29:332–339, 1970.
41. Hughes, J.M.B., Rosenzweig, D.Y., and Kivitz, P.W.: Site of airway closure in excised dog lung: Histologic demonstration. *J. Appl. Physiol.* 29:340–344, 1970.
42. Staub, N.: The effect of pulmonary edema on small airways in health and disease. In *Small Airways in Health and Disease.* Sadoul, P., Milic-Emili, J., Simonssen, B.G., et al., eds. Amsterdam, Excerpta Medica, 1979, pp. 53–60.

43. Fairley, H.B.: Airway closure. *Anesthesiology* 36:529–531, 1972.
44. Sloman, G. and Gandevia, B.: Ventilatory capacity and exercise, ventilation and congenitally acquired cardiac disease. *Br. Heart J.* 26:121–128, 1964.
45. Jones, J.G., Minty, B.D., Laller, P., et al.: Increased alveolar epithelial permeability in cigarette smokers. *Lancet* 1:66–68, 1980.
46. Jones, J.G., Minty, B.D., Bealey, J.M., et al.: Pulmonary epithelial permeability is immediately increased after embolization with oleic acid but not with neutral fat. *Thorax* 37:169–174, 1982.
47. Hugon, G.J., Little, J.W., and Murray, J.F.: Assessment of alveolar capillary membrane permeability of dogs by aerosolization. *J. Appl. Physiol.* 51:955–962, 1981.
48. Mason, G.R., Uszler, J.M., Effros, R.M., et al.: Rapidly reversible alterations in pulmonary epithelial permeability induced by smoking. *Chest* 83:6–11, 1983.
49. Rizk, N.W., Luce, J.M., Hoeffel, J.M., et al.: Site of deposition and factors affecting clearance of aerosolized solute from canine lung. *J. Appl. Physiol.* 56:723–729, 1984.
50. Simani, A.S., Inoue, S., and Hogg, J.C.: Penetrations of the respiratory epithelium of guinea pigs following the exposure to cigarette smoke. *Lab. Invest.* 31:75–81, 1974.
51. Walker, D.C., MacKenzie, A., Wiggs, B.R., et al.: Structure of tight junctions and the tracheal epithelium may not correlate with permeability. *Cell Tissue Res.* 235:607–613, 1984.
52. Walker, D.C., MacKenzie, A., Hulbert, W.C., et al.: A re-assessment of the tricellular region of epithelial cell tight junctions. *Acta Anatomica* (In press).
53. Hulbert, W.C., Walker, D.C., Jackson, A., et al.: Airway permeability to horseradish peroxidase in guinea pig: The repair phase after injury by cigarette smoke. *Am. Rev. Respir. Dis.* 123:320–326, 1981.
54. Czop, J.K., McGowan, S.E., and Centre, D.M.: Opsonan-independent sagocytosis by human alveolar macrophages augmented by human plasma fibronectin. *Am. Rev. Respir. Dis.* 125:607–609, 1982.
55. Fisher, A.B.: Circulating markers of lung microvascular injury, presented in A Symposium on New Approaches to the Clinical Assessment of Lung Microvascular Injury. *Am. Rev. Respir. Dis.* Annual Meeting 129:23, 1984.
56. Craddock, P.R., Fehr, R.J., Dalmasso, A.P., et al.: Hemodialysis leukopenia: Pulmonary vascular leukostasis resulting from complement activation by dialysis membranes. *J. Clin. Invest.* 59:879–888, 1977.
57. Hammerschmidt, D.E., Weaver, L.J., Hudson, L.D., et al.: Association of complement activation in elevated plasma C_{5a} with adult respiratory distress syndrome: Pathophysiological relevance and possible prognostic value. *Lancet* 947–949, 1980.
58. Weinberg, P.F., Mathay, M.A., Webster, R., et al.: Lack of relationship between complement activation and acute lung injury. *Am. Rev. Respir. Dis.* 127:95A, 1983.
59. Thommasen, H., Lee, S., Russell, J., et al.: Transient leukopenia associated with adult respiratory distress syndrome. *Lancet* 809–812, 1984.

CHAPTER 10

Neonatal Lung Edema

Richard D. Bland and
Thomas N. Hansen

Introduction

Infants with respiratory distress often have too much water and an abnormal distribution of protein in their lungs. In some cases, neonatal pulmonary edema is the result of hemodynamic abnormalities, but in many cases respiratory failure develops as a consequence of lung microvascular injury and epithelial protein leak. The purpose of this chapter is to present some of the mechanisms that are responsible for edema formation in the newborn lung and to provide rationale for appropriate treatment and prevention.

Table I lists several types of newborn lung disease in which pulmonary edema is a prominent feature. Persistent postnatal pulmonary edema is usually attributed to slow removal of fetal lung liquid after birth. It is frequently associated with operative delivery or severe birth asphyxia. Hyaline membrane disease is most common in babies who are born prematurely with stiff lungs secondary to a deficiency of surface active material in the airspaces. The pathology of this condition includes micro-atelectasis, interstitial fluid accumulation, plasma proteins in the airspaces that are patent, and dilated pulmonary lymphatics. Pneumonitis from group B, β-hemolytic Streptococcus is often difficult to distinguish clinically and radiographically from hyaline membrane disease. In this condition, granulocytes become trapped in the microcirculation of the lungs and there is abundant protein in the terminal air sacs. Aspiration of meconium at birth sometimes induces severe respiratory distress, in which pulmonary hypertension and edema are important components. Congestive heart failure frequently develops in babies with congenital cardiac malformations, especially those that are associated with left ventricular outflow obstruction, excessive pulmonary blood flow, or pulmonary venous obstruction. Lung edema sometimes occurs from impaired myocardial function, which may be the result of severe asphyxia, hypoglycemia, hypocalcemia, myocarditis, or an aberrant coronary artery. In babies who are born prematurely, persistent

From Said, S.I. (ed.): *The Pulmonary Circulation and Acute Lung Injury.* Mount Kisco, N.Y., Futura Publishing Co., Inc., 1985.

Table I
Newborn Lung Diseases Associated with Pulmonary Edema

Persistent postnatal pulmonary edema (slow removal of fetal lung liquid)
Hyaline membrane disease
Pneumonitis from group B, β-hemolytic *Streptococcus*
Meconium aspiration syndrome
Congestive heart failure
    Congenital cardiac malformation
    Impaired myocardial function
    Patent ductus arteriosus
Lung lymphatic obstruction
Chronic lung disease from hyperoxia and mechanical ventilation

---

patency of the ductus arteriosus often leads to pulmonary edema from too much blood flow, as lung vascular resistance decreases postnatally. Obstructed drainage of lung lymphatics also may cause pulmonary edema. Infants with respiratory distress from any of the above conditions often require a high concentration of inspired oxygen and mechanical ventilation with positive airway pressure to treat hypoxemia and respiratory failure. In some cases, these supportive measures aggravate the underlying lung injury and cause chronic lung disease, the pathology of which includes edema, overdistended airspaces, and fibrosis.

Much of our knowledge about the development of neonatal pulmonary edema derives from experiments done with fetal and newborn animals, to which we will refer frequently. As lung edema after birth often has a prenatal origin, we will include a brief discussion of the composition, secretion, and clearance of fetal lung liquid. We will also point out features of postnatal pulmonary development that may increase vulnerability of newborn lungs to edema formation.

Lung Fluid Dynamics Before and During Birth

Secretion of Fetal Lung Liquid

Before birth the lungs have no respiratory function. They are filled with liquid and receive less than 10% of total cardiac output.[85] Fetal lungs secrete into the trachea a liquid that is rich in chloride (>150 mEq/L) and almost free of protein (<0.3 mg/ml).[1,2,72] Active transport of chloride ion across the pulmonary epithelium generates an electrical potential difference that causes liquid to flow from the microcirculation through the interstitium into potential airspaces of the fetal lung[78] at an hourly rate of about 3 to 5 ml/kg body weight.[72] The volume of lung liquid within potential airspaces, including the trachea, is between 20 and 30 ml/kg body weight.[54,74,75]

Clearance of Fetal Lung Liquid Before and After Birth

Successful transition from placental to pulmonary gas exchange at birth requires rapid reversal of the direction of lung liquid flow. Several recent reports indicate that removal of liquid from the lungs of fetal animals may begin even before birth. Kitterman et al.[59] observed that secretion of liquid into the trachea of fetal lambs decreases before spontaneous vaginal delivery, and Bland et al.[11,15] demonstrated that events associated with labor reduce extravascular lung water content in fetal rabbits and lambs. The decrease in lung water that occurs during labor is the result of a decrease in the volume of fluid in potential airspaces relative to the volume of liquid in the interstitium of the lungs.[15,17] The mechanism responsible for this change remains unknown, but it may be the result of hormonal changes that occur in the fetus late in gestation.

Enhorning et al.[38] discovered that injection of β-adrenergic agonists into pregnant rabbits decreased the amount of water in the lungs of their pups. Walters and Olver[93] showed that intravenous infusion of epinephrine or iso-proterenol in fetal lambs late in gestation caused reabsorption of liquid from potential airspaces, an effect that β-adrenergic blockade prevented. Lawson et al.[64] confirmed the inhibitory effect of epinephrine on secretion of fetal lung liquid and also found that epinephrine increased the concentration of surface active material in that liquid. These observations suggest that β-adrenergic agonists, frequently used to inhibit premature labor, may benefit the fetus by reducing lung water content and by stimulating release of surfactant.

Perks and Cassin[81] reported that intravenous infusion of arginine vaso-pressin into fetal goats caused reabsorption of liquid from potential airspaces. Plasma concentrations of vasopressin increase several hours before birth in fetal lambs,[4,89] and concentrations of that hormone are very high in plasma from umbilical cord blood of human infants who experience labor.[27,82] Like-wise, plasma concentrations of epinephrine increase in fetal lambs late in labor[25,37] as lung liquid drains into the interstitium, with subsequent absorption into the pulmonary microcirculation.

The amount of fetal lung liquid decreases by more than 50% before vaginal birth,[15] after which the process of liquid clearance continues for several hours postnatally. In rabbits, there is a steady decrease in lung water content between 30 minutes and 24 hours after birth, and throughout this period rabbit pups delivered by cesarean section without prior labor have more water in their lungs than vaginally delivered pups have.[14]

Figure 1 shows the postnatal sequence of change in the distribution of fluid in the lungs of baby rabbits. Before breathing begins, potential airspaces are filled with liquid, and very little fluid surrounds large pulmonary blood vessels and airways. When breathing starts, transpulmonary pressure inflates the lungs and displaces residual liquid from terminal respiratory units into distensible perivascular spaces around large pulmonary blood vessels and airways. Puddling of fluid in these connective tissue spaces, which are distant from sites of respiratory gas exchange, allows time for smaller blood vessels and pulmonary lymphatics to expel the remaining water without serious impairment of lung function. By 6 hours after birth, the perivascular cuffs of fluid disappear.

What governs the rate of clearance of liquid from the lungs after birth? As noted previously, liquid in potential airspaces contains < 0.3 mg of protein/ml. When transpulmonary pressure drives that liquid into the interstitium, the concentration of protein in lung tissue decreases, thereby increasing the difference in protein osmotic pressure between plasma and interstitial fluid. Recent experiments performed with fetal[79] and adult[69] sheep indicate that active sodium transport in the pulmonary epithelium also may contribute to the flow of liquid from potential airspaces into the interstitium of the lung, where that liquid can be absorbed into the circulation. In vitro studies of ion transport in

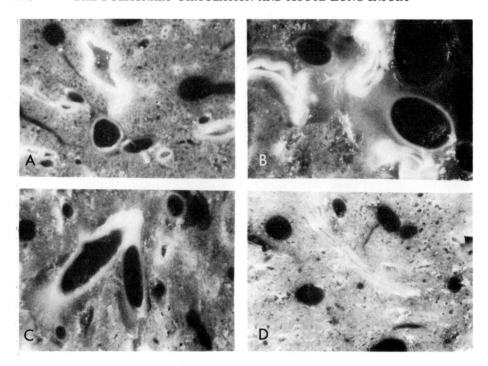

Figure 1: *Sections of lung obtained from vaginally delivered rabbit pups that were killed* **(A)** *without breathing (top left),* **(B)** *30 minutes after birth (top right),* **(C)** *1 hour after birth (bottom left), and* **(D)** *6 hours after birth (bottom right). Before birth airways are filled with fluid and there are small cuffs of fluid around pulmonary arteries. By 30 minutes of age, perivascular and peribronchial cuffs are large and airways are compressed in the absence of distending pressure. Fluid cuffs are smaller 1 hour after birth, and they are virtually absent several hours later. Original magnification, ×8.5. (From Bland, R.D., et al.,[14] with permission.)*

type II lung epithelial cells suggest that the same cells that secrete surface active material into the airspaces also may be responsible for pumping sodium in the opposite direction during labor and after birth.[18,67] Air entry into the lungs decreases hydraulic pressure in the pulmonary circulation and increases pulmonary blood flow,[31] which in turn increases lung blood volume and effective vascular surface area for fluid exchange.[15] These developments facilitate absorption of water into the pulmonary vascular bed. About 10% of the liquid leaves the lungs through lymphatics,[15] which drain into the systemic venous system. Postnatal reduction of intrathoracic pressure decreases systemic venous pressure, which may hasten lymphatic drainage, but the pulmonary microcirculation directly absorbs most of the liquid.

Fluid Balance in the Newborn Lung

Figure 2 shows the fluid compartments of the normal newborn lung. The epithelium, which separates airspaces from interstitium, is virtually impermeable to protein.[74,75] The endothelium, which divides the microcirculation from

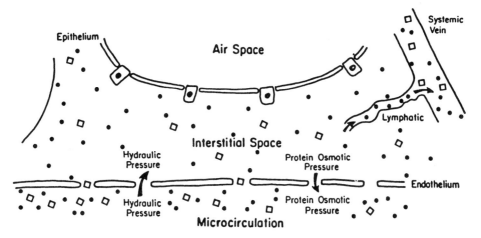

Figure 2: *Schematic drawing of the fluid compartments in the newborn lung and the variables that affect filtration in the pulmonary microcirculation. Dots represent albumin molecules, open squares indicate globulin molecules. (From Bland, R.D.: Edema formation in the newborn lung. Clin. Perinatol. 9:593–611, 1982, with permission.)*

the interstitium, allows macromolecules to pass through it, but it restricts passage of large molecules more than it restricts small ones.[20] Thus, the concentration of albumin in the interstitium of the newborn lung averages 75–80% of the concentration of albumin in plasma, whereas the concentration of globulins in interstitial fluid averages 50–55% of their concentration in plasma.[9] These tissue proteins generate an osmotic pressure of more than 10 cmH$_2$O,[7] which inhibits the flow of water into airspaces. As noted above, recent studies, both in vivo[69,79] and in vitro,[18,19,67] indicate that active ion transport by lung epithelial cells also may help to keep airspaces dry.

Flow of liquid across the microvascular membrane depends on differences between (a) intravascular and extravascular hydraulic pressure, and (b) intravascular and extravascular protein osmotic pressure (Fig. 2). Conditions that increase intravascular hydraulic pressure or decrease intravascular protein osmotic pressure hasten liquid flow into the interstitium; conditions that decrease filtration pressure or increase the concentration of protein in plasma tend to reduce fluid movement into the interstitium, thereby inhibiting edema formation. Other variables that contribute to lung water balance are microvascular surface area, endothelial permeability to protein, and the capacity of lymphatics to pump fluid out of the lungs.

Studies performed with adult and newborn sheep indicate that postnatal lung development has no significant influence on pulmonary microvascular permeability to protein; however, fluid filtration pressure and microvascular surface area per unit lung mass are greater in newborn lungs than in adult lungs.[9,16,90] These differences may reflect the fact that pulmonary blood flow per unit lung mass is considerably greater in newborn lungs than it is in adult lungs.[13] In addition, because the neonatal lung is one-quarter of the size of the mature lung,[9] it is likely that left atrial pressure exceeds alveolar pressure (West zone III) throughout a greater fraction of the pulmonary circulation in the newborn lung. Furthermore, plasma protein concentration of newborn animals is significantly less than it is in adult animals, so that the difference in protein osmotic pressure between plasma and lung interstitial fluid is less in the younger animals.[51] It is not surprising, therefore, that net lung fluid filtration is greater per unit lung mass in newborn lambs than it is in mature sheep.[9] It remains to be determined whether or not edema is more likely to develop in the newborn lung than it is in the adult lung when both lungs are subjected to comparable hemodynamic stress.

Mechanisms of Edema Formation

Increased Lung Microvascular Pressure

Pulmonary edema in newborn infants is often a consequence of increased pressure in the microcirculation of the lungs (Table II). This may occur when the heart fails and left atrial pressure increases, as it does in cases of obstruction to left ventricular outflow or mitral valve stenosis. Myocardial dysfunction from infection, metabolic abnormalities, or severe asphyxia also may cause an increase in lung microvascular pressure. Excessive intravascular infusions of fluid—either blood, protein-containing solutions, or crystalloid—may overload the pulmonary circulation and cause fluid to accumulate in the lungs. Increased blood flow to the lungs, associated with large left-to-right shunts, fever, hypoxia, noxious stimuli, or other stressful conditions, may increase lung microvascular pressure and thereby cause pulmonary edema. This probably is the source of respiratory distress in babies who are born prematurely and have large systemic-to-pulmonary shunts through a ductus arteriosus. When the lung vascular bed fails to develop normally before birth, as in cases of pulmonary hypoplasia, or when the lung vascular bed is reduced in size because of fibrosis or lung resection, increase in blood flow to the lungs is likely to elevate microvascular pressure and cause edema. Intravenous infusions of fat emulsion increase pulmonary microvascular pressure and transvascular filtration of fluid in the lungs of newborn lambs[91] and mature sheep,[70] and this may be responsible for the respiratory distress that sometimes occurs in human infants who receive intravenous infusion of lipid for nutritional support.[44] Recent studies indicate that both 5-hydroxytryptamine and cyclooxygenase products of arachidonic acid metabolism may be responsible for this lipid-induced increase in lung fluid filtration.[45,92]

When pulmonary microvascular pressure increases, net filtration of fluid

---

Table II
Conditions that Increase Pulmonary Microvascular Pressure and Thereby Facilitate Edema Formation in the Newborn Lung

Heart failure associated with congenital cardiac
   malformations or myocardial dysfunction
Excessive intravascular fluid infusions
Increased pulmonary blood flow
Hypoxia
Restricted lung vascular bed: pulmonary hypoplasia or fibrosis
Intravenous infusion of fat

into the lungs increases and the concentration of protein in interstitial fluid decreases (Fig. 3). Resultant increases in lymph flow and in the protein osmotic pressure difference between plasma and tissue fluid (lymph) protect the lungs from edema until the drainage capacity of lymphatics is overwhelmed by the increased rate of fluid filtration.

In the initial phase of pulmonary edema, liquid accumulates in the loose connective tissue of the lung interstitium, beneath the pleura, between lobes and surrounding large blood vessels and airways. In the early stage of edema, most of the extravascular fluid seeps to the dependent portions of the lung, where intravascular hydraulic pressure is greatest. When fluid accumulation exceeds the capacity of the interstitium, liquid flows abruptly into airspaces, pulling protein across the epithelium, which normally restricts the passage of large solutes. The lungs become boggy and congested, fluid distends the lymphatics, lung compliance and vital capacity decrease, and gas exchange is impaired.

Lung Fluid Filtration in the Newborn Lung During Hypoxia

In his classic monograph on pulmonary edema, published in 1945, Drinker wrote that "oxygen lack is the most potent and elusive cause of abnormal leakage from the lung capillaries."[34] To test that possibility, Bland et al. measured steady-state lung lymph flow, as an indicator of net transvascular filtration of fluid, in eight unanesthetized sheep[8] and in 14 lambs before and during alveolar hypoxia.[13,22] Figure 4 shows results of two such experiments,

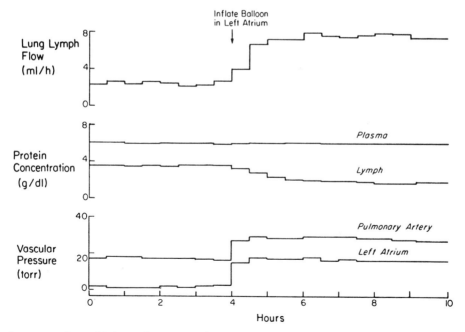

Figure 3: *Effect of left atrial pressure elevation on lung lymph flow and concentrations of protein in lymph and plasma of an unanesthetized lamb. (From Bland, et al.,[16] with permission.)*

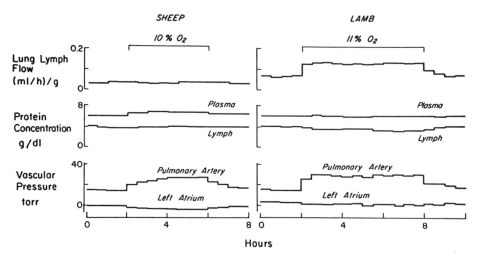

Figure 4: *Effects of sustained alveolar hypoxia on lung lymph flow (relative to dry lung tissue excluding blood), protein concentrations in lymph and plasma, and average vascular pressures in a sheep (left) and a lamb (right). (From Bland et al.,[13] with permission.)*

one in an adult sheep and the other in a 2-week-old lamb. The investigators measured lung lymph flow, concentrations of protein in lymph and plasma, and pressures in the pulmonary artery and left atrium during a 2-hour control period and then for 4 to 6 hours of hypoxia. In sheep, hypoxia caused pulmonary hypertension, but lymph flow and lymph protein concentration did not change significantly; that is, hypoxia had no apparent influence on net lung fluid filtration. In lambs, when pulmonary arterial pressure increased because of hypoxia, lymph flow also increased, and the concentration of protein in lymph decreased. Results were virtually identical in studies performed with anesthetized lambs and in lambs kept hypoxic for 12 hours.[49] These findings are similar to those observed when a balloon catheter in the left atrium is filled with saline to raise lung microvascular pressure in a lamb (Figs. 3 and 5). In newborn lambs, then, hypoxia either constricts lung vessels distal to sites of fluid exchange, or alternatively, intense vasoconstriction redirects the increased blood flow that occurs during hypoxia to fewer vessels and thereby transmits to fluid exchange sites a greater fraction of the pressure in the pulmonary artery. Recent angiographic studies by Hansen et al.[50] in newborn lambs before and during hypoxia indicate that the latter explanation most likely accounts for the increase in fluid filtration observed in lambs during hypoxia. It is noteworthy that Landolt et al.[63] also observed an increase in lung lymph flow and a decrease in lymph protein concentration during hypoxia in adult sheep following substantial lung resection. This finding also suggests that there is a threshold of pulmonary blood flow per unit lung mass above which lung fluid filtration begins to increase. We found no evidence that hypoxia alters lung vascular permeability to protein in either lambs or sheep. Even the most severe degree of sustained hypoxia and acidemia in lambs did not injure their pulmonary endothelium.[48]

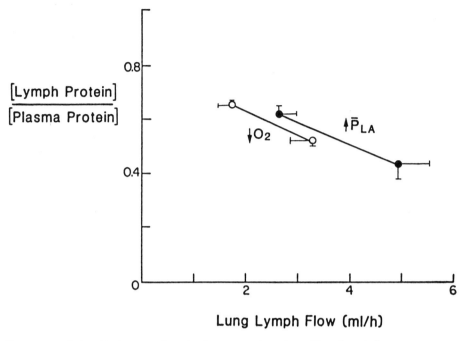

Figure 5: *Relationship between lymph:plasma protein ratio and lung lymph flow in two groups of unanesthetized lambs. One group (n=14) breathed 10−12% O_2 ($\downarrow O_2$) after a control period in air, and the second group (n=7) had left atrial hypertension from saline-filling of a balloon catheter in the left atrium. In both groups, the lymph:plasma protein ratio decreased as lymph flow increased, indicative of similar protein sieving in the pulmonary microcirculation during the two types of experiments. Points are mean ± SEM. (From Bland et al. Studies of lung fluid balance in newborn lambs. Ann. N.Y. Acad. Sci. 384:126−144, 1982, with permission.)*

Decreased Protein Osmotic Pressure

Another condition that may facilitate edema formation in the nowborn lung is decreased intravascular protein osmotic pressure. Hypoproteinemia may be the result of premature birth, fetal hydrops, excessive intravascular infusions of fluid, protein loss through the kidneys or intestinal tract, or inadequate nutrition (Table III).

Table III
Conditions that Decrease Intravascular Protein Osmotic Pressure and Thereby Facilitate Edema Formation in the Newborn Lung
Premature birth
Fetal hydrops
Excessive fluid and salt intake
Protein loss through the kidneys or intestinal tract
Poor nutrition

Several years ago Guyton and Lindsey[46] studied the importance of plasma protein concentration in the development of pulmonary edema. They reduced the plasma protein osmotic pressure of dogs by 50% and found that pulmonary edema occurred at a lower left atrial pressure than it did in dogs with normal concentrations of protein in plasma. They concluded that hypoproteinemia predisposes animals to pulmonary edema.

Zarins et al.[95] studied lung fluid balance in baboons and reported that hypoproteinemia, induced by plasmapheresis, increased lung lymph flow without changing the lymph:plasma protein ratio. They suggested that increased capillary permeability to protein may have been responsible for the increased filtration of fluid associated with hypoproteinemia. More recently, Kramer et al.[61,62] used plasmapheresis to reduce intravascular protein osmotic pressure of sheep, and they, too, observed an increase in lymph flow, but there was no evidence of a change in protein permeability. They attributed the increase in fluid filtration to an alteration in the hydraulic conductivity of the pulmonary microcirculation during protein depletion.

Hazinski et al.[51] measured steady-state lung lymph flow in lambs before and after gradual development of hypoproteinemia. In the first phase of each experiment (Fig. 6), they measured lung lymph flow, concentrations of protein in lymph and plasma, and pressures in the pulmonary artery and left atrium during a 2-hour baseline period, and then for 4 hours, during which pulmonary microvascular pressure was increased by saline-filling a balloon catheter in the left atrium. After the first phase of the experiment, the investigators inserted a catheter in the thoracic duct and drained protein-rich systemic lymph for 3 days. Fluid losses were replaced with feedings of a protein solution containing sugar and electrolytes, thereby keeping body weight, vascular pressures, and cardiac output constant. Following protein drainage, a repeat study showed that during the baseline period, lymph flow was greater than it was during the baseline portion of the first phase of the study. Vascular pressures were not appreciably different than they were during the control period 3 days earlier, but there was a small difference in the protein osmotic pressure difference between plasma and lymph during the second phase of the study. Elevation of lung microvascular pressure by balloon inflation of the left atrial catheter again increased lymph flow by the same fractional increment as it did when plasma protein concentration was normal. Reduction of plasma protein concentration did not influence the rate at which radioiodinated albumin, injected intravenously, reached equilibrium concentrations in lymph and plasma. These findings suggest that in newborn lambs hypoproteinemia increases transvascular filtration of fluid without changing endothelial permeability to protein in the lung. Despite the presence of hypoproteinemia and left atrial pressure elevation, pulmonary edema did not develop in these lambs because lung lymph flow kept pace with transvascular filtration of fluid.

Impaired Lymphatic Drainage

Impaired lymphatic drainage also may contribute to lung fluid accumulation (Table IV). Pulmonary edema often accompanies interstitial emphysema and fibrosis, in which air (Fig. 7) or scar tissue blocks lymphatic flow.[88] Recent studies indicate that elevated outflow obstruction reduces lymphatic drainage;[33] therefore, water may accumulate in the lungs if the lymphatics must

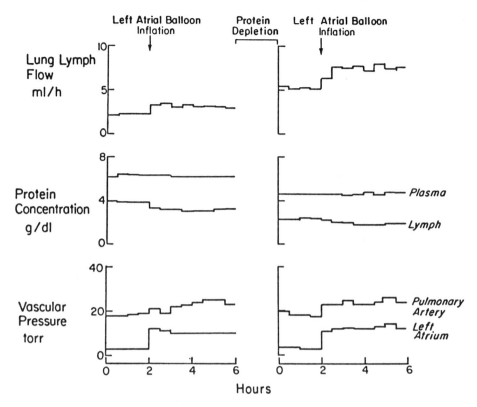

Figure 6: *Effects of hypoproteinemia and increased left atrial pressure on steady-state lung lymph flow and protein concentrations in lymph and plasma of a 2-week-old lamb. After the first phase of the study, plasma proteins drained through a thoracic duct fistula and fluid losses were replaced by crystalloid solution, followed by a repeat study during hypoproteinemia. (From Bland et al.,[16] with permission.)*

pump against an exceedingly high central venous pressure,[80] particularly if that pressure is sustained for a prolonged period. This may be the source of lung edema in some cases of right-sided heart failure, or blockage of the superior vena cava. Following lymphatic obstruction, edema persists until new channels form or until the damaged lymphatics heal.[29]

**Table IV
Conditions that May Interfere
with Lymphatic Drainage in the
Newborn Lung and Thereby
Facilitate Edema Formation**

Pulmonary interstitial emphysema
(air leak into the interstitium)
Pulmonary fibrosis
Superior vena cava obstruction
Systemic venous hypertension

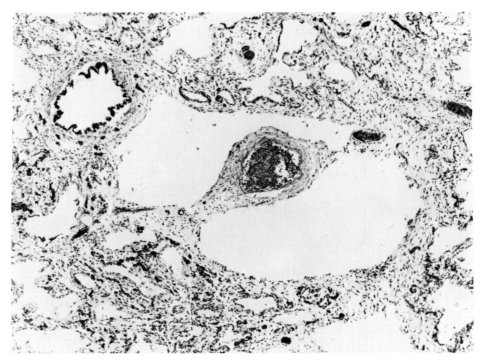

Figure 7: *Section of lung from an infant who died with severe pulmonary interstitial emphysema. The large space around the lung arteriole represents air that had dissected along a perivascular sheath of connective tissue, destroying lymphatics and causing considerable interstitial edema. Photograph provided by Dr. Martha Warnock, Professor of Pathology, University of California, San Francisco. (From Bland, R.D.: Edema formation in the newborn lung. Clin. Perinatol. 9:593−611, 1982, with permission.)*

Microvascular Endothelial Injury

Lung edema sometimes is the result of microvascular injury, in which disruption of the endothelial membrane allows protein-rich fluid to leak at an increased rate from the pulmonary microcirculation into the interstitium. If there is coexisting epithelial injury, proteinaceous fluid enters airspaces and interferes with respiratory gas exchange. Table V lists some of the conditions that have been shown to enhance microvascular permeability to protein in the lungs of experimental animals.

Table V
**Conditions that Increase Microvascular Permeability
to Protein in the Lungs**

Bacteremia: Pseudomonas[23]
Endotoxemia: *E. coli*,[24] group B β-hemolytic *Streptococcus*[84]
Pulmonary emboli[77]
Prolonged oxygen breathing[21]

An important source of lung injury in newborn infants is prolonged oxygen breathing. Bressack et al.[21] studied lung fluid balance in unanesthetized lambs that continuously breathed pure oxygen, and in every case, pulmonary microvascular permeability to protein increased within 3 to 4 days. Figure 8 is a summary of results from experiments in which six lambs breathed oxygen at a partial pressure of more than 700 torr for 5 days.[12] Lymph flow began to increase on the third day of sustained hyperoxia, and the concentration of protein in lymph increased progressively from the third to the fifth day, with no appreciable change in pulmonary vascular pressures. Radioactive tracer studies with intravenous injection of ^{125}I-albumin also demonstrated a substantial increase in permeability within 5 days, when all of the lambs were suffering respiratory distress associated with oxygen toxicity. Extravascular lung water content was increased and histology revealed severe pulmonary edema (Fig. 9). In a subsequent study, lambs pretreated with large doses of vitamin E, an antioxidant, acquired the same degree of oxygen-induced lung endothelial

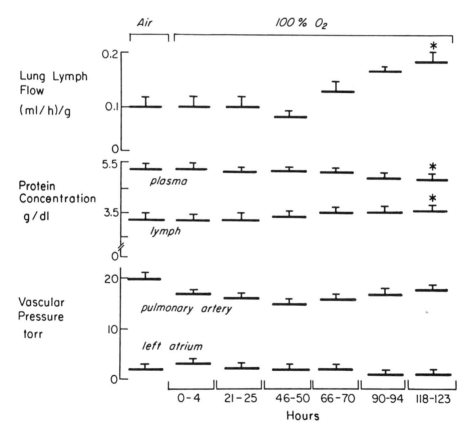

Figure 8: *Lung lymph flow (relative to dry lung tissue excluding blood), concentrations of protein in plasma and lymph, and average pressures in the pulmonary artery and left atrium of six unanesthetized lambs, 2−4 weeks old, during a 4-hour control period in air and then daily as the lambs spontaneously breathed 100% oxygen continuously for 5 days. Bars represent mean values and standard errors of the mean. Asterisks indicate significant changes relative to measurements made in the control period of air breathing. (From Bland, R.D.,[12] with permission.)*

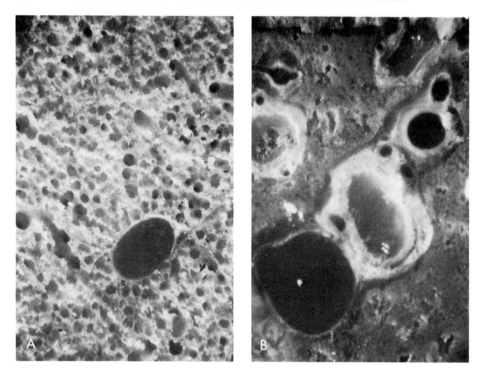

Figure 9: *Sections of lung, frozen in liquid nitrogen at an inflation pressure of 25 cmH$_2$O: normal lamb (left) and lamb killed after 5 days in 100% oxygen (right). The injured lung contains fluid in airspaces, as well as the perivascular tissue spaces around large blood vessels and airways. Original magnification, ×8.5. (From Bland, R.D.: Edema formation in the newborn lung. Clin. Perinatol. 9:593–611, 1982, with permission.)*

injury,[47] and subsequent clinical studies have confirmed the observation that vitamin E does not prevent or reduce the severity of chronic lung disease in human infants born prematurely.[36,86]

Several reports have indicated that granulocytes play an important role in the development of many types of pulmonary microvascular injury,[30,41,52,58] including endothelial damage and edema from prolonged oxygen breathing.[12,87] To study the importance of neutrophils as mediators in pulmonary oxygen toxicity, Raj et al.[83] produced neutropenia in rabbits and lambs by giving them nitrogen mustard or hydroxyurea; neutrophil depletion had no effect on survival time or on lung water content of either adult rabbits or newborn lambs that continuously breathed pure oxygen at 1 atmosphere pressure. These results indicate that polymorphonuclear leukocytes are not essential in the development of oxygen-induced lung endothelial injury. These findings are consistent with those of Martin et al.,[66] who demonstrated that prolonged hyperoxia, in the absence of inflammatory cells, directly damages lung parenchymal cells and causes them to release toxic oxygen radicals.

Epithelial Protein Leak

The pulmonary epithelium forms a tight barrier against protein movement between interstitium and airspaces.[69,74] Egan et al.[35] showed that epithelial leaks may develop, however, when transpulmonary pressure exceeds 35 to 40 cmH$_2$O, as it often does when surface tension at the air-liquid interface stiffens the lungs. Jobe et al.[57] found a direct relationship between peak airway pressure and epithelial protein leak in mechanically ventilated lambs born prematurely. These changes in epithelial permeability probably reflect overexpansion of some areas of the lung, with distortion of intercellular junctions and resultant transudation of interstitial protein into the airspaces.[73] Certainly the presence of plasma-derived fibrin in the airspaces of infants with hyaline membrane disease[43] is indicative of substantial epithelial injury.

Several studies have demonstrated that newborn infants with respiratory distress, especially those who are born prematurely, are deficient in protease inhibitors, both in their plasma[39,40,60,65,68] and in their lungs.[71] Merritt et al.[71] found an increase in the number of neutrophils, macrophages, and neutrophil-derived elastase activity in fluid suctioned from the airways of infants with respiratory distress. They also showed that elastase inhibitory capacity and α$_1$-proteinase inhibitor activity were reduced in infants with chronic lung disease following acute neonatal lung injury. These observations, confirmed recently by Ogden et al.,[76] suggest that degradative enzymes, released by inflammatory cells in the lungs, may play an important role in the development of lung epithelial injury in newborn infants. It is not surprising, therefore, that Jefferies et al.[56] recently observed rapid pulmonary clearance of radionuclides administered by aerosol into the lungs of infants with respiratory distress syndrome.

Clinical Implications

Pulmonary Edema in Premature Infants

Newborn babies who are born prematurely have an increased risk of respiratory distress from pulmonary edema. Filtration pressure in their pulmonary circulation is greater than normal, particularly if they experience hypoxia. Protein osmotic pressure in their plasma is low,[5] especially if they receive too much fluid. Because the airspaces of their lungs are often unstable from deficiency of surface active material, a large transpulmonary pressure often develops, with considerable heterogeneity in lung expansion. This may produce protein leaks in the epithelium and reduce interstitial pressure around extra-alveolar vessels,[55] which may contribute to edema formation.[3,28] Infants with respiratory distress frequently require mechanical ventilation and high concentrations of inspired oxygen, which may injure the lungs, cause release of proteolytic enzymes, and possibly interfere with lymphatic drainage. The result is fluid accumulation and an abnormal distribution of protein in the lungs (Fig. 9), with impaired respiratory gas exchange.

Prevention and Treatment of Neonatal Pulmonary Edema

Several measures may reduce the likelihood of edema formation or lessen its severity. These include fluid and salt restriction, especially in the first few days of life, cautious administration of blood transfusions, gentle ventilatory assistance designed to reduce the need for supplemental oxygen and excessive airway pressure, early closure of the ductus arteriosus if blood flow through it causes pulmonary overperfusion or heart failure, avoidance of conditions that increase blood flow to the lungs, such as hypoxia and painful or noxious stimuli, and adequate nutrition to promote protein synthesis and healing.

When edema occurs despite these measures, diuretic therapy is often helpful. Effective diuresis decreases pulmonary microvascular pressure and increases the concentration of protein in plasma. These two changes inhibit fluid filtration into the lungs and hasten the entry of water into the pulmonary microcirculation from the interstitium. Bland et al.[10] studied the influence of intravenous furosemide on lung fluid balance in lambs, with and without pulmonary edema. Diuresis caused an increase in plasma protein concentration and a decrease in pulmonary vascular pressures, with resultant reduction in lung lymph flow (Fig. 10). Furosemide also has an effect on lung fluid balance that is independent of the drug's diuretic action; in lambs without kidneys, intravenous infusion of furosemide consistently led to a small decrease in lymph

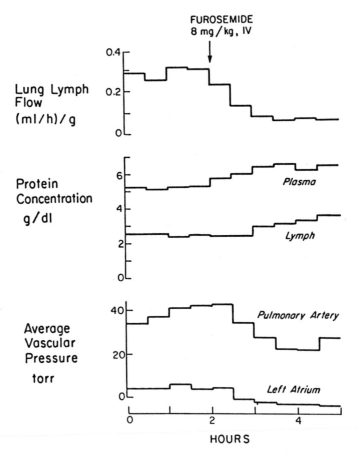

Figure 10: *Effect of intravenous furosemide on steady state lung lymph flow (relative to dry lung tissue excluding blood), protein concentrations in plasma and lymph, and pressures in the pulmonary artery and left atrium of an unanesthetized lamb with pulmonary edema, which had been induced by intravenous infusion of excess isotonic saline. (From Bland et al.,[10] with permission.)*

flow, without any change in pulmonary vascular pressure or plasma protein concentration. It is possible that this nondiuretic influence of furosemide is the result of increased capacitance of peripheral systemic veins,[32] with diminished pulmonary blood flow, causing a reduction in lung microvascular surface area for fluid exchange.

Although hypoproteinemia may predispose infants to pulmonary edema, infusions of albumin or plasma usually do not benefit infants with respiratory distress.[6] Such infusions tend to increase pulmonary microvascular pressure, and this offsets the effect of increased intravascular protein osmotic pressure. Furthermore, the infused protein leaks into the interstitium of the lungs within a short period of time, and this frequently aggravates the edema.

Ventilatory support with positive end-expiratory pressure is often beneficial in cases of severe pulmonary edema. Positive end-expiratory pressure does not reduce lung water content,[26,53,94] but it redistributes fluid in the airspaces and improves respiratory gas exchange. Ventilation also spares energy reserves by reducing the work of breathing. If ventilatory assistance becomes necessary, sedation may further decrease oxygen consumption and thereby facilitate recovery. In cases of longstanding pulmonary edema with associated fibrosis, it is especially important to avoid hypoxia and other conditions that increase blood flow, microvascular pressure, and filtration of fluid in the lungs.

Acknowledgments

Work presented in this paper was supported in part by National Heart, Lung and Blood Institute (NHLBI) Pulmonary Specialized Center of Research (SCOR) grant HL 19185, and by US Public Health Service Program Project grants HL/HD 24056 and HL 25816. R.D. Bland did part of this work during his tenure as an Established Investigator of the American Heart Association, and T.N. Hansen received support from NHLBI Pulmonary Faculty Training Grant HL 07159. The authors gratefully acknowledge the secretarial help of Mrs. Marilyn Biagini.

REFERENCES

1. Adams, F.H., Fujiwara, T., and Rowshan, G.: The nature and origin of the fluid in the fetal lamb lung. *J. Pediatr.* 63:881–888, 1963.
2. Adamson, T.M., Boyd, R.D.H., Platt, H.S., et al.: Composition of alveolar liquid in the foetal lamb. *J. Physiol. (London)* 204:159–168, 1969.
3. Albert, R.K., Lakshminarayan, S., Huang, T.W., et al.: Fluid leaks from extra-alveolar vessels in living dog lungs. *J. Appl. Physiol.* 44:759–762, 1978.
4. Alexander, D.P., Bashore, R.A., Britton, H.G., et al.: Maternal and fetal arginine vasopressin in the chronically catheterized sheep. *Biol. Neonate* 25:242–248, 1974.
5. Bland, R.D.: Cord-blood total protein level as a screening aid for the idiopathic respiratory-distress syndrome. *N. Engl. J. Med.* 287:9–13, 1972.
6. Bland, R.D., Clarke, T.L., Harden, L.B., et al.: Early albumin infusion to infants at risk for respiratory distress. *Arch. Dis. Child.* 48:800–805, 1973.
7. Bland, R.D., and Bressack, M.A.: Lung fluid balance in awake newborn lambs with pulmonary edema from rapid intravenous infusion of isotonic saline. *Pediatr. Res.* 13:1037–1042, 1979.

8. Bland, R.D., Demling, R.H., Selinger, S.L., et al.: Effects of alveolar hypoxia on lung fluid and protein transport in unanesthetized sheep. *Circ. Res.* 40:269–274, 1977.

9. Bland, R.D., and McMillan, D.D.: Lung fluid dynamics in awake newborn lambs. *J. Clin. Invest.* 60:1107–1115, 1977.

10. Bland, R.D., McMillan, D.D., and Bressack, M.A.: Decreased pulmonary transvascular fluid filtration in awake newborn lambs after intravenous furosemide. *J. Clin. Invest.* 62:601–609, 1978.

11. Bland, R.D., Bressack, M.A., and McMillan, D.D.: Labor decreases the lung water content of newborn rabbits. *Am. J. Obstet. Gynecol.* 135:364–367, 1979.

12. Bland, R.D.: Special considerations in oxygen therapy for infants and children. *Am. Rev. Resp. Dis.* (Suppl. 5, Part 2) 122:45–54, 1980.

13. Bland, R.D., Bressack, M.A., Haberkern, C.M., et al.: Lung fluid balance in hypoxic, awake newborn lambs and mature sheep. *Biol. Neonate* 38:221–228, 1980.

14. Bland, R.D., McMillan, D.D., Bressack, M.A., et al.: Clearance of liquid from lungs of newborn rabbits. *J. Appl. Physiol.: Respir. Environ. Exercise Physiol.* 49: 171–177, 1980.

15. Bland, R.D., Hansen, T.N., Haberkern, C.M., et al.: Lung fluid balance in lambs before and after birth. *J. Appl. Physiol.: Respir. Environ. Exercise Physiol.* 53: 992–1004, 1982.

16. Bland, R.D., Hansen, T.N., Hazinski, T.A., et al.: Studies of lung fluid balance in newborn lambs. *Ann. N.Y. Acad. Sci.* 384:124–144, 1982.

17. Bland, R.D.: Dynamics of pulmonary water before and after birth. *Acta Paediatr. Scand.* (Suppl.) 305:12–20, 1983.

18. Bland, R.D. and Boyd, C.A.R.: Birth activates cation exchange in rabbit lung epithelial cells. *Fed. Proc.* 43:1033, 1984.

19. Bland, R.D. and Boyd, C.A.R.: Ion transport in rabbit lung epithelial cells (Abstr.). *Clin. Res.* 32:60A, 1984.

20. Boyd, R.D.H., Hill, J.R., Humphreys, P.W., et al.: Permeability of lung capillaries to macromolecules in foetal and newborn lambs and sheep. *J. Physiol. (London)* 201: 567–588, 1969.

21. Bressack, M.A., McMillan, D.D., and Bland, R.D.: Pulmonary oxygen toxicity: Increased microvascular permeability to protein in unanesthetized lambs. *Lymphology* 12:133–139, 1979.

22. Bressack, M.A. and Bland, R.D.: Alveolar hypoxia increases lung fluid filtration in unanesthetized newborn lambs. *Circ. Res.* 46:111–116, 1980.

23. Brigham, K.L., Woolverton, W.C., Blake, L.H., et al.: Increased sheep lung vascular permeability caused by Pseudomonas bacteremia. *J. Clin. Invest.* 54:792–804, 1974.

24. Brigham, K.L., Bowers, R.E., and Haynes, J.: Increased sheep lung vascular permeability caused by Escherichia coli endotoxin. *Circ. Res.* 45:292–297, 1979.

25. Brown, M.J., Olver, R.E., Ramsden, C.A., et al.: Effects of adrenaline and of spontaneous labour on the secretion and absorption of lung liquid in the foetal lamb. *J. Physiol. (London)* 344:137–152, 1983.

26. Caldini, P., Leith, J.D., and Brennan, M.J.: Effect of continuous positive-pressure ventilation (CPPV) on edema formation in dog lung. *J. Appl. Physiol.* 39:672–679, 1975.

27. Chard, T., Boyd, N.R.H., Edwards, C.R.W., et al.: The release of oxytocin and vasopressin by the human fetus during labor. *Nature (London)* 234:352–354, 1971.

28. Clements, J.A.: Pulmonary edema and permeability of alveolar membranes. *Arch. Environ. Health* 2:280–283, 1961.

29. Cowan, G.S.M., Jr., Staub, N.C., and Edmunds, L.G., Jr.: Changes in the fluid compartments and dry weights of reimplanted dog lungs. *J. Appl. Physiol.* 40: 962–970, 1976.

30. Craddock, P.R., Fehr, J., Brigham, K.L., et al.: Complement and leukocyte-mediated pulmonary dysfunction in hemodiolysis. *N. Engl. J. Med.* 296:769–774, 1977.

31. Dawes, G.S., Mott, J.C., Widdicombe, J.G., et al.: Changes in the lungs of the newborn lamb. *J. Physiol. (London)* 121:141–162, 1953.

32. Dikshit, K., Vyden, J.K., Forrester, J.S., et al.: Renal and extrarenal hemodynamic effects of furosemide in congestive heart failure after acute myocardial infarction. *N. Engl. J. Med.* 288:1087–1090, 1978.

33. Drake, R., Giesler, M., Laine, G., et al.: Effect of outflow pressure on lung lymph flow in unanesthetized sheep. *J. Appl. Physiol.* 58:70–76, 1985.

34. Drinker, C.K.: *Pulmonary Edema and Inflammation.* Cambridge, MA, Harvard University Press, 1945, p. 72.

35. Egan, E.A., Olver, R.E., and Strang, L.B.: Changes in non-electrolyte permeability of alveoli and the absorption of lung liquid at the start of breathing in the lamb. *J. Physiol. (London)* 244:161–179, 1975.

36. Ehrenkrantz, R.A., Ablow, R.C., and Warshaw, J.B.: Prevention of bronchopulmonary dysplasia with vitamin E administration during the acute stages of respiratory distress syndrome. *J. Pediatr.* 95:873–877, 1979.

37. Eliot, R.J., Klein, A.H., Glatz, T.H., et al.: Plasma norepinephrine, epinephrine, and dopamine concentrations in maternal and fetal sheep during spontaneous parturition and in premature sheep during cortisol-induced parturition. *Endocrinolgoy* 108:1678–1682, 1981.

38. Enhorning, G., Chamberlain, D., Contreras, C., et al.: Isoxsuprine-induced release of pulmonary surfactant in the rabbit fetus. *Am. J. Obstet. Gynecol.* 129:197–202, 1977.

39. Evans, H.E., Levi, M., and Mandl, I.: Serum enzyme inhibitor concentrations in the respiratory distress syndrome. *Am. Rev. Respir. Dis.* 101:359–363, 1970.

40. Evans, H.E., Keller, S., and Mandl, I.: Serum trypsin inhibitory capacity and the idiopathic respiratory distress syndrome. *J. Pediatr.* 81:588–592, 1982.

41. Flick, M.R., Perel, A., and Staub, N.C.: Leukocytes are required for increased lung microvascular permeability after microembolization in sheep. *Circ. Res.* 48:344–351, 1981.

42. Fox, R.B., Hoidal, J.R., Brown, D.M., et al.: Pulmonary inflammation due to oxygen toxicity: Involvement of chemotactic factors and polymorphonuclear leukocytes. *Am. Rev. Respir. Dis.* 123:521–523, 1981.

43. Gitlin, D. and Craig, J.M.: The nature of the hyaline membrane in asphyxia of the newborn. *Pediatrics* 17:64–71, 1956.

44. Greene, H.L., Hazlett, D., and Demarec, R.: Relationship between intra-lipid induced hyperlipidemia and pulmonary function. *Am. J. Clin. Nutr.* 29:127–135, 1976.

45. Gurtner, G.H., Knoblauch, A., Smith, P.L., et al.: Oxidant- and lipid-induced pulmonary vasoconstriction mediated by arachidonic acid metabolites. *J. Appl. Physiol.: Respir. Environ. Exercise Physiol.* 55:949–954, 1983.

46. Guyton, A.C. and Lindsey, A.W.: Effect of elevated left atrial pressure and decreased plasma protein concentration on the development of pulmonary edema. *Circ. Res.* 7:649–657, 1959.

47. Hansen, T.N., Hazinski, T.A., and Bland, R.D.: Vitamin E does not prevent oxygen-induced lung injury in newborn lambs. *Pediatr. Res.* 16:583–587, 1982.

48. Hansen, T.H., Hazinski, T.A., and Bland, R.D.: Effects of asphyxia on lung fluid balance in baby lambs. *J. Clin. Invest.* 74:370–376, 1984.

49. Hansen, T.N., Hazinski, T.A., and Bland, R.D.: Effects of hypoxia on transvascular fluid filtration in newborn lambs. *Pediatr. Res.* 18:434–440, 1984.

50. Hansen, T.N., LeBlanc, A.L., and Gest, A.L.: Hypoxia and angiotensin II infusion redistribute lung blood flow in lambs. *J. Appl. Physiol.* (In press).

51. Hazinski, T.A., Bland, R.D., Hansen, T.N., et al.: Lung fluid filtration in unanesthetized newborn lambs. Effects of protein loss and left atrial hypertension. *J. Clin. Invest.* (Revision in review).

52. Heflin, A.C. and Brigham, K.L.: Prevention by granulocyte depletion of increased vascular permeability of sheep lung following endotoxemia. *J. Clin. Invest.* 68:1253–1260, 1981.

53. Hopewell, P.C. and Murray, J.F.: Effects of continuous positive-pressure ventilation and experimental pulmonary edema. *J. Appl. Physiol.* 40:568–574, 1976.

54. Humphreys, P.W., Normand, I.C.S., Reynolds, E.O.R., et al.: Pulmonary lymph flow and the uptake of liquid from the lungs of the lamb at the start of breathing. *J. Physiol. (London)* 193:1–29, 1967.

55. Inoue, H., Inoue, C., and Hildebrandt, J.: Vascular and airway pressures, and interstitial edema affect peribronchial fluid pressure. *J. Appl. Physiol.* 48:177–185, 1980.

56. Jefferies, A.L., Coates, G., and O'Brodovich, H.: Pulmonary epithelial permeability in hyaline-membrane disease. *N. Engl. J. Med.* 311:1075–1080, 1984.

57. Jobe, A., Ikegami, M., Jacobs, H. et al.: Permeability of premature lamb lungs to protein and the effect of surfactant on that permeability. *J. Appl. Physiol.: Respir. Environ. Exercise Physiol.* 55:169–176, 1983.

58. Johnson, A. and Malik, A.B.: Pulmonary edema after glass bead microembolization: Protective effect of granulocytopenia. *J. Appl. Physiol.: Respir. Environ. Exercise Physiol.* 52:155–161, 1982.

59. Kitterman, J.A., Ballard, P.A., Clements, J.A., et al.: Trachael fluid in fetal lambs: Spontaneous decrease prior to birth. *J. Appl. Physiol.: Respir. Environ. Exercise Physiol.* 47:985–989, 1979.

60. Kotas, R.V., Fazen, L.E., and Moore, T.E.: Umbilical cord serum trypsin inhibitor capacity and the idiopathic respiratory distress syndrome. *J. Pediatr.* 81:593–599, 1982.

61. Kramer, G.C., Harms, B.A., Gunther, R.A., et al.: The effects of hypoproteinemia on blood to lymph fluid transport in sheep lung. *Circ. Res.* 49:1173–1180, 1982.

62. Kramer, G.C., Harms, B.A., Bodai, B.I., et al.: Effects of hypoproteinemia and increased vascular pressure on lung fluid balance in sheep. *J. Appl. Physiol.: Respir. Environ. Exercise Physiol.* 55:1514–1522, 1983.

63. Landolt, C.C., Matthay, M.A., Albertine, K.H., et al.: Overperfusion, hypoxia, and increased pressure cause only hydrostatic pulmonary edema in anesthetized sheep. *Circ. Res.* 52:335–341, 1983.

64. Lawson, E.E., Brown, E.R., Torday, J.S., et al.: The effect of epinephrine on trachael fluid flow and surfactant efflux in fetal sheep. *Am. Rev. Resp. Dis.* 118:1023–1026, 1978.

65. Makram, W.E. and Johnson, A.M.: Serum proteinase inhibitors in infants with hyaline membrane disease. *J. Pediatr.* 81:579–587, 1972.

66. Martin, W.J., II, Gadek, J.E., Hunninghake, G.W., et al.: Oxidant injury of lung parenchymal cells. *J. Clin. Invest.* 68:1277–1288, 1981.

67. Mason, R.J., Williams, M.C., Widdicombe, J.H., et al.: Transepithelial transport by pulmonary alveolar type II cells in primary culture. *Proc. Natl. Acad. Sci.* 79: 6033–6037, 1982.

68. Mathis, R.K., Freier, E.F., Hunt, C.E., et al.: Alpha$_1$-antitrypsin in the respiratory distress syndrome. *N. Engl. J. Med.* 288:59–64, 1973.

69. Matthay, M.A., Landolt, C.C., and Staub, N.C.: Differential liquid and protein clearance from the alveoli of anesthetized sheep. *J. Appl. Physiol.: Respir. Environ. Exercise Physiol.* 53:96–104, 1982.

70. McKeen, C.R., Brigham, K.L., Bowers, R.E., et al.: Pulmonary vascular effects of fat emulsion in unanesthetized sheep. *J. Clin. Invest.* 61:1291–1297, 1978.

71. Merritt, T.A., Cochrane, C.G., Holcomb, K., et al.: Elastase and α_1-proteinase inhibitor activity in tracheal aspirates during respiratory distress syndrome. *J. Clin. Invest.* 72:656–666, 1983.

72. Mescher, E.J., Platzker, A.C.G., Ballard, P.L., et al.: Ontogeny of trachael fluid, pulmonary surfactant, and plasma corticoids in the fetal lamb. *J. Appl. Physiol.* 39:1017–1021, 1975.

73. Nilsson, R., Grossman, G., and Robertson, B.: Lung surfactant and the pathogenesis of neonatal bronchiolar lesions induced by artificial ventilation. *Pediatr. Res.* 12: 249–255, 1978.

74. Normand, I.C.S., Reynolds, E.O.R., and Strang, L.B.: Passage of macromolecules

between alveolar and interstitial spaces of foetal and newly ventilated lungs of the lamb. *J. Physiol. (London)* 210:151–164, 1970.

75. Normand, I.C.S., Olver, R.E., Reynolds, E.O.R., et al.: Permeability of lung capillaries and alveoli to non-electrolytes in the foetal lamb. *J. Physiol. (London)* 219:303–330, 1971.

76. Ogden, B.E., Murphy, S.A., Saunders, G.C., et al.: Neonatal lung neutrophils and elastase/proteinase inhibitor imbalance. *Am. Rev. Respir. Dis.* 130:817–821, 1984.

77. Ohkuda, K., Nakahara, K., Weidner, W.J., et al.: Lung fluid exchange after uneven pulmonary artery obstruction in sheep. *Circ. Res.* 43:152–161, 1978.

78. Olver, R.E. and Strang, L.B.: Ion fluxes across the pulmonary epithelium and the secretion of lung liquid in the foetal lamb. *J. Physiol. (London)* 241:327–357, 1974.

79. Olver, R.E., Ramsden, C.A., and Strang, L.B.: Adrenaline induced changes in net lung liquid volume flow across the pulmonary epithelium of the foetal lamb: evidence for active sodium transport (Abstr.). *J. Physiol. (London)* 316:55, 1981.

80. Paré, P.D., Brooks, L.A., and Baile, E.M.: Effect of systemic venous hypertension on pulmonary function and lung water. *J. Appl. Physiol.: Respir. Environ. Exercise Physiol.* 51:592–597, 1981.

81. Perks, A.M. and Cassin, S.: The effects of arginine vasopressin and other factors on the production of lung fluid in fetal goats. *Chest* 81(Suppl.):63–65, 1982.

82. Polin, R.A., Husain, M.K., James, L.S., et al.: High vasopressin concentrations in human umbilical cord blood—Lack of correlation with stress. *J. Perinat. Med.* 5:114–119, 1977.

83. Raj, J.U., Hazinski, T.A., and Bland, R.D.: Oxygen-induced lung microvascular injury in neutropenic rabbits and lambs. *J. Appl. Physiol.: Respir. Environ. Exercise Physiol.* Vol. 58 (In press) 1985.

84. Rojas, J., Green, R.S., Hellerquist, C.G., et al.: Studies on group B β-hemolytic Streptococcus. II. Effects on pulmonary hemodynamics and vascular permeability in unanesthetized sheep. *Pediatr. Res.* 15:899–904, 1981.

85. Rudolph, A.M. and Heymann, M.A.: Circulatory changes during growth in the fetal lamb. *Circ. Res.* 26:289–299, 1970.

86. Saldanha, R.I., Cepeda, E.E., and Poland, R.L.: The effect of vitamin E prophylaxis on the incidence and severity of bronchopulmonary dysplasia. *J. Pediatr.* 101:89–93, 1982.

87. Shasby, D.M., Fox, R.B., Harada, R.N., et al.: Reduction of the edema of acute hyperoxic lung injury by granulocyte depletion. *J. Appl. Physiol.: Respir. Environ. Exercise Physiol.* 52:1237–1244, 1982.

88. Stahlman, M.T., Cheatham, W., and Gray, M.E.: The role of air dissection in bronchopulmonary dysplasia. *J. Pediatr.* 85:878–882, 1979.

89. Stark, R.I., Daniel, S.S., Husain, K.M., et al.: Arginine vasopressin during gestation and parturition in the sheep fetus. *Biol. Neonate* 35:235–241, 1979.

90. Sundell, H.W., Brigham, K.L., Harris, T.R., et al.: Lung water and vascular permeability-surface area in newborn lambs delivered by cesarean section compared with the 3–5 day-old lamb and adult sheep. *J. Devel. Physiol.* 2:191–204, 1980.

91. Teague, W.G., Braun, D., Goldberg, R.B., et al.: Intravenous lipid infusion increases lung fluid filtration in lambs (Abstr.). *Pediatr. Res.* 18:313A, 1984.

92. Teague, W.G., Raj, J.U., Braun, D., et al.: Mechanism of increased lung fluid filtration during lipid infusion in lambs (Abstr.). *Clin. Res.* 33:144A, 1985.

93. Walters, D.W. and Olver, R.E.: The role of catecholamines in lung liquid absorption at birth. *Pediatr. Res.* 12:239–242, 1978.

94. Woolverton, W.C., Brigham, K.L., and Staub, N.C.: Effect of positive pressure breathing on lung lymph flow and water content in sheep. *Circ. Res.* 42:550–557, 1978.

95. Zarins, C.K., Rice, C.L., Peters, R.M., et al.: Lymph and pulmonary response to isobaric reduction in plasma oncotic pressure in baboons. *Circ. Res.* 43:925–930, 1978.

IV

Mechanisms of Lung Injury:
Role of Granulocytes, Free Oxygen
Radicals, Lipids, and Peptides
(Complement)

CHAPTER 11

Neutrophils, Oxygen Radicals, and the Adult Respiratory Distress Syndrome

John E. Repine

> Have we over-stimulated the phagocytes? Have they not only eaten up the bacilli, but attacked and destroyed the red corpuscles as well, a possibility suggested by the patient's pallor? Nay, have they finally begun to prey on the lungs themselves? Or on one another?
>
> G.B. Shaw,
> *The Doctor's Dilemma,* 1906

Introduction

The adult respiratory distress syndrome (ARDS) or acute noncardiogenic edematous lung injury is an important clinical problem. It has been estimated that 75,000 individuals die from ARDS each year. ARDS is associated with many inciting events including infection, embolism, hyperoxia, shock, trauma, aspiration, and burns. The association of ARDS with these diverse insults combined with the central alveolar-capillary membrane site of injury have prompted speculation that a wide variety of factors in vascular and/or alveolar spaces might contribute to ARDS (Fig. 1). Consequently, most reviews include long lists of potential mediators. These lists usually identify alveolar macrophages (AM), platelets, arachidonic acid metabolites, proteases, complement byproducts, fibrinogen degradation products, complement byproducts, fibrinogen degradation products, kallikrein, endotoxin, neutrophils, and/or highly reactive metabolites of activated oxygen (commonly called oxygen radicals) as potential participants. Many chapters in this volume dwell on the various contributions of these augmenting and/or protecting factors. This chapter will largely review our own work and ideas which are focused on the roles of neutrophils and oxygen radicals and their interactions with arachidonic acid metabolites and oxygen radical scavengers.

From Said, S.I. (ed.): *The Pulmonary Circulation and Acute Lung Injury.* Mount Kisco, N.Y., Futura Publishing Co., Inc., 1985.

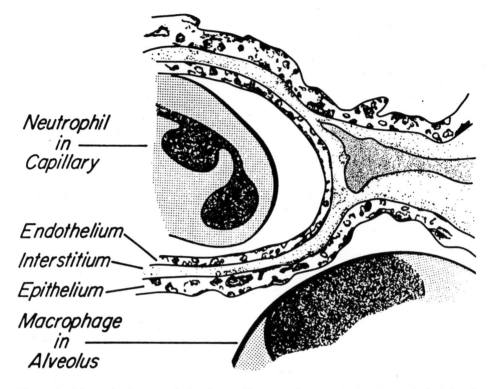

Neutrophil
in
Capillary

Endothelium
Interstitium
Epithelium

Macrophage
in
Alveolus

Figure 1: *Schematic diagram of alveolar capillary membrane unit showing endothelial cell, interstitial and epithelial layers. An alveolar macrophage is depicted in the alveolus; a neutrophil in the capillary.*

Do Neutrophils Contribute to the Development of ARDS?

Considerable evidence suggests that neutrophils contribute to the development of ARDS. Increased numbers of neutrophils are commonly found in lung lavages from patients with ARDS and often early during the course of their illness.[1] Moreover, neutrophil accumulation frequently occurs adjacent to damaged endothelial cells in lungs of ARDS patients. Indeed, electron microscopy shows neutrophils penetrating endothelial junctions and in close proximity to damaged endothelial cells in lungs of ARDS patients.[2] In addition, neutrophils possess multiple mechanisms that might alter alveolar capillary membrane structure and function. Stimulated neutrophils can make and release many substances that could directly or indirectly increase vascular permeability and/or cause pressor responses that potentiate vascular leak.[3] Substances released from neutrophils include arachidonic acid metabolites, proteases, and oxygen radicals (Fig. 2). Neutrophil-derived oxygen radicals include superoxide anion (O_2^-) and hydrogen peroxide (H_2O_2), which can react to form hydroxyl radical ($^{\cdot}OH$) as well as hypochlorous acid (HOCl), and perhaps singlet oxygen ($^1O_2$). We have also found stimulants of neutrophil oxygen radical production in lung lavages from some patients with ARDS. This latter finding suggests that mechanisms may also be available to activate neutrophils. Furthermore, neutro-

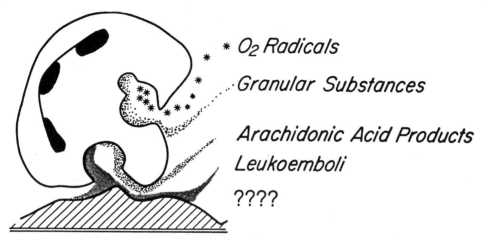

* O_2 *Radicals*

Granular Substances

Arachidonic Acid Products

Leukoemboli

????

Figure 2: *Schematic diagram of neutrophil releasing toxins that could potentially damage lung tissue.*

phils obtained from the blood of patients with ARDS are often activated, having an increased ability to produce oxygen metabolites in vitro.[4] These findings indicate that neutrophils may contribute to ARDS. First, neutrophils are present in crucial alveolar-capillary injury locations. Second, neutrophils can release potent toxins. Third, factors are present that can stimulate neutrophils to release potentially damaging oxygen radicals and/or other toxins. The possibility that these activating factors have also leaked into the periphery and "turned on" circulating neutrophils is intriguing. Likewise, the possibility needs to be explored that individual variations in the capabilities of neutrophils to adhere and/or release toxins account for individual variabilities in the severity of ARDS. Unfortunately, it is not obvious how the exact contribution of neutrophils will be more definitively established in patients with ARDS in the near future.

Do Neutrophils and Oxygen Radicals Contribute to Experimental Acute Edematous Lung Injury From Hyperoxia?

Exposure to hyperoxia can cause ARDS, but the nature of this process is not well understood. Characteristically, lung injury from hyperoxia is described as an acute noncardiogenic edematous lung damage that occurs in most species after exposure to high concentrations of normobaric oxygen ($>95\%$ O_2) for approximately 3 days. Oxygen toxicity is characterized by the development of endothelial and epithelial cell injury, inflammation, alveolar hemorrhage, and edema (Fig. 3). In most species that have been exposed to hyperoxia, death is well confined to a relatively narrow time period.[5] As shown in Figure 4, no deaths occur until rats have been breathing hyperoxia for about 66 hours. However, after exposure for 66 hours, a rapid increase in mortality begins and continues until most rats have died during the next 6–12 hours. The possibility that neutrophils might contribute to lung injury from hyperoxia was initially

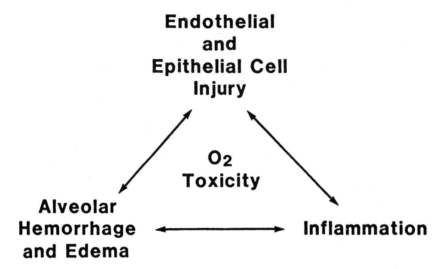

Figure 3: *Features of oxygen toxicity. Interactions between these three features may contribute to the development of acute injury from hyperoxia.*

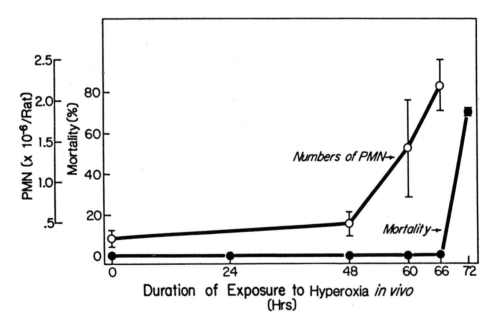

Figure 4: *Rats died precipitously (●) following continuous exposure to hyperoxia (>95% O_2) for more than 66 hours. Neutrophils (○) increased preterminally in lung lavages of rats exposed to hyperoxia.*

suggested when increased numbers of neutrophils were measured preterminally in lung lavages of rats or rabbits that had been exposed to hyperoxia for about 3 days (Fig. 4). In addition, the lung histology of these hyperoxia-exposed animals exhibited increased numbers of neutrophils in alveolar and interstitial spaces, and again, often near disrupted lung tissues (Fig. 5). However, while it was clear that neutrophils increased preterminally in lung lavages of rats or rabbits exposed to hyperoxia, a cause and effect relationship between these two events was not certain. Indeed, whether pulmonary neutrophil accumulation contributed to injury from hyperoxia or simply represented an unrelated response to injury was not known.

To address this issue, we examined the effect of neutropenia on the development of lung injury from hyperoxia.[6,7] Our results using nitrogen mustard pretreated neutropenic (<100 neutrophils/mm^3) rabbits suggested that neutrophils participated in lung injury from hyperoxia. Briefly, after exposure to hyperoxia for 66 hours, rabbits rendered neutropenic by nitrogen mustard pretreatment had decreased amounts of acute pulmonary edema, which was evidenced by decreased lung weight gains, lung lavage albumin concentrations, lung lavage angiotensin converting enzyme (ACE) activities, and mortalities when compared to control rabbits that were similarly exposed to hyperoxia.[6,7] In addition, the contribution of neutrophils to lung injury from hyperoxia was further evidenced when numbers of neutrophils initially circulating (or in lung lavages) correlated with degrees of lung injury (Fig. 6). The clinching experiment of transfusing normal neutrophils into neutropenic rabbits to help confirm their participation in the injury process was not done because of potential difficulties related to activation or subpopulation selection of neutrophils by their separation and problems related to the immediate transit of transfused

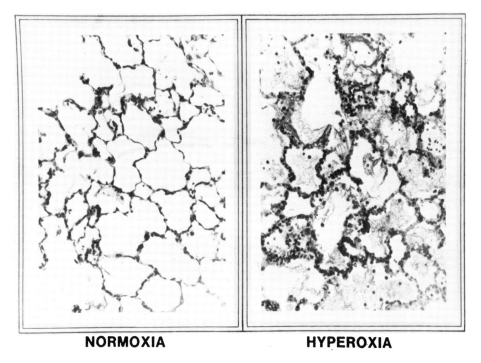

NORMOXIA   **HYPEROXIA**

Figure 5: *Histologic sections from lungs of rats exposed to hyperoxia for 48 hours (right panel) manifested increased cellularity and alveolar extravasation of fluid not seen in lungs from control rats that had been exposed to normoxia (left panel).*

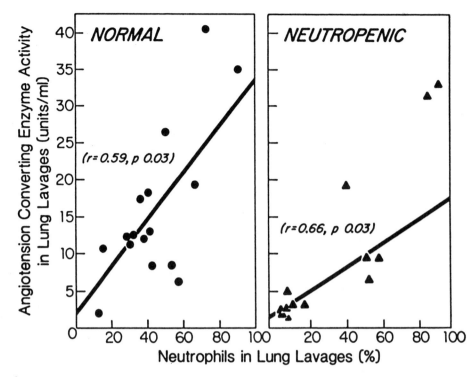

Figure 6: *Angiotensin converting enzyme (ACE) activities correlated with the numbers of neutrophils in lungs lavages from neutrophil-replete rabbits that had been exposed to hyperoxia for about 66 hours. Similarly, ACE activities also correlated with numbers of neutrophils in lung lavages from nitrogen mustard-treated rabbits given hyperoxia.*

neutrophils to lungs in the absence of any stimulus. However, in several neutropenic rabbits, neutrophils did spontaneously increase and were associated with increased lung injury (Fig. 6). Although these studies suggest that neutrophils can contribute to hyperoxia-induced lung injury, they do not imply that lung injury from hyperoxia will not occur in neutropenic rats or rabbits that are exposed to prolonged durations of hyperoxia. However, the contribution of neutrophils in the latter situation is difficult to exclude because of problems in determining and minimizing numbers of neutrophils circulating or sequestered in lung tissues.

The possibility that oxygen radicals participate in hyperoxic-induced injury rests primarily on indirect observations in which addition of scavengers of oxygen radicals prevents injury. Scavengers that decrease lung injury from hyperoxia include dimethylthiourea (DMTU),[8] liposomes containing superoxide dismutase (SOD) and catalase,[9] or polyethylene–attached SOD or catalase.[10] These results, combined with additional observations that exposure to hyperoxia can increase oxygen radical production by lung cells, suggest that oxygen radicals can contribute to lung injury from hyperoxia. However, until techniques are developed that provide direct measurement of oxygen radicals and better define the mechanism of action of purported oxygen radical scavengers, the contribution of oxygen radicals to lung injury in animals that have been exposed to hyperoxia will remain unproven.

How are Neutrophils Recruited and Activated in Lungs Exposed to Hyperoxia?

Our next studies were designed to examine mechanisms by which neutrophils were recruited into lungs of animals breathing high concentrations of oxygen. First, we explored the possibility that alveolar macrophages (AM) might mediate these events. Our initial presumption was that hyperoxic damage to AM might underly this process. Specifically, we hypothesized that hyperoxia damages AM, causing release of factors that (1) attract neutrophils to the lung, (2) stimulate neutrophils to adhere to lung endothelial cells, and (3) cause neutrophils to release toxic oxygen radicals (Fig. 7). The latter would injure endothelial cells, reduce the integrity of the alveolar capillary membrane, and lead to lung edema.

We then obtained evidence that supported these premises. First, AM recovered by lavage from lungs of rabbits breathing pure oxygen for about 66 hours had nuclear abnormalities, disorganized cytoplasms, and vacuolization not seen in AM recovered from rabbits breathing at normoxia (Fig. 8). In addition, these abnormalities in AM from rabbits exposed to hyperoxia resembled changes in cultured rabbit AM exposed to hyperoxia in vitro. Indeed, AM exposed to hyperoxia for 48 to 72 hours in vitro also developed nuclear abnormalities, vacuolization, and disorganized cytoplasms not seen in cultured AM exposed to normoxia for similar durations. Hyperoxic exposure also caused cultured AM to release increased amounts of cytoplasmic lactate dehydrogenase

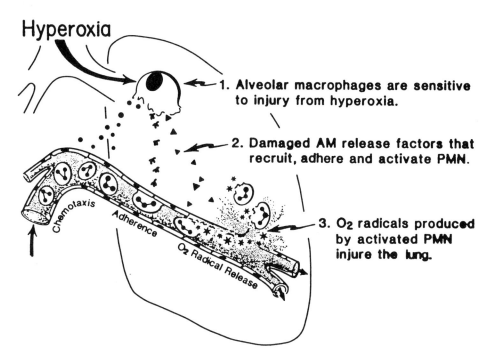

Figure 7: *Schematic diagram of our proposed mechanism for the development of acute edematous lung injury from hyperoxia.*

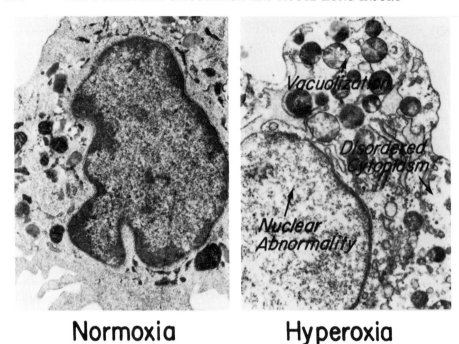

Normoxia   Hyperoxia

Figure 8: *Electron micrographs showed vacuolization, disordered cytoplasms, and nuclear abnormalities in alveolar macrophages recovered from lungs of rabbits that had been continuously exposed to hyperoxia for about 66 hours.*

(LDH). Hyperoxic damage to AM appeared to involve oxygen radicals since addition to the culture media of oxygen radical scavengers (catalase or DMTU) prevented injury.[11] Thus, hyperoxia was toxic to AM in lungs of animals or in cultures.

Next, we found increased chemotactic activity for neutrophils in lung lavages from rats or rabbits exposed to hyperoxia.[5] In addition, chemotactic activity for neutrophils increased in lung lavages just before death in animals exposed to hyperoxia (Fig. 9) and in close conjunction with increased concentrations of neutrophils in lung lavages (Fig. 4). In parallel studies, hyperoxia also stimulated cultured rabbit AM to produce chemotaxins for neutrophils.[12] To assess the possibility that AM were the source of neutrophil chemotaxins found in lung lavages of animals exposed to hyperoxia, we characterized the molecular weights of chemotaxins recovered from supernatants of lung lavages or media overlying cultured AM. Chemotaxins in supernatants from AM exposed to hyperoxia in vitro had molecular weights that were similar to chemotaxins from supernatants from lung lavages of rabbits exposed to hyperoxia.[12] By chromatographic analysis, two peaks were measured in both fractions. One peak was a small molecular weight fraction of less than 1,000 daltons; the other a larger molecular weight fraction of approximately 12,000 daltons. Supernatants from cultured AM exposed to hyperoxia (48 to 72 hours) also contained factors that increased the adherence of neutrophils to nylon fibers, a model simulating the increased adherence of neutrophils to endothelial cells.[13] Finally, supernatants

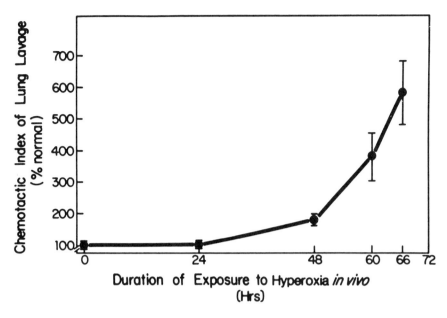

Figure 9: *Chemotactic activities for neutrophils (in vitro) increased just preterminally in lung lavages from rats that had been exposed to hyperoxia.*

from lung lavages from rats exposed to hyperoxia (Fig. 10) or cultured rabbit AM exposed to hyperoxia also contained factors that stimulate neutrophil production of oxygen radicals. Distinct differences in the molecular weights, chemical natures, and times of release of the various factors obtained from hyperoxia-exposed cultured rabbit AM that stimulate neutrophil chemotaxis, adherence, and/or oxygen radical production may allow further understanding of this mechanism of injury. In aggregate, these experiments support the proposed sequence that hyperoxia damages AM and that hyperoxic-damaged AM then release factors that attract neutrophils, augment neutrophil adherence to endothelium, and initiate release of toxic oxygen radicals from neutrophils (Fig. 7). The possibility that AM can recruit and activate neutrophils contrasts with other experiments that suggest that under normal conditions, AM may also release factors which decrease neutrophil-mediated attachment and activation within the lung. Accordingly, our hypothesis is that products from unstimulated AM can mediate both protective and destructive events in acute lung injury. Therefore, AM could contribute to lung injury not only by recruiting and activating neutrophils in the lung, but also by not releasing sufficient amounts of factors that decrease neutrophil recruitment and activation (Fig. 11).

While the aforementioned investigations suggested that AM might be intimately involved in recruitment and activation of neutrophils in lungs of animals exposed to hyperoxia, it was also apparent that another mechanism could participate in recruitment and activation of neutrophils in lungs exposed to hyperoxia. This mechanism involves direct endothelial cell injury by hyperoxia in conjunction with the ability of neutrophils to recognize and adhere in greater numbers to injured endothelial cells (Fig. 12). This impression is based on

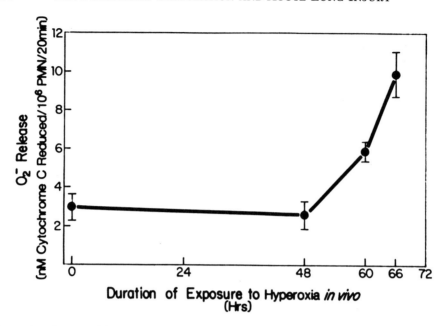

Figure 10: *Superoxide anion stimulating activities for neutrophils (in vitro) increased just preterminally in lung lavages from rats that had been exposed to hyperoxia.*

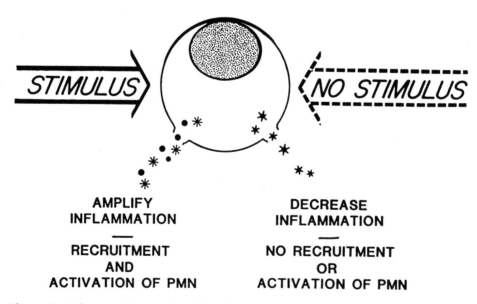

Figure 11: *Schematic diagram of our hypothesis regarding a central role for alveolar macrophages (AM) in modulating recruitment and activation of neutrophils in lungs. Stimulated AM release neutrophil activators; unstimulated AM release neutrophil inhibitors.*

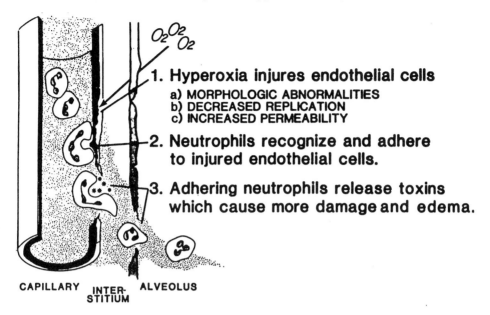

Figure 12: *Schematic diagram of a hypothetical mechanism for recruitment of neutrophils to lungs exposed to hyperoxia.*

observations made in an endothelial cell culture model in which more neutrophils adhered to endothelial cells that had been previously exposed to hyperoxia.[14] In these studies, hyperoxia caused endothelial injury which was manifested by cytoplasmic LDH release, decreased replication, and ultrastructural abnormalities. Once again, ultrastructural abnormalities in endothelial cells exposed to hyperoxia in vitro resembled morphological alterations seen in endothelial cells in lungs of animals breathing at hyperoxia. Moreover, more neutrophils adhered to cultured endothelial cells that had been damaged by prior exposure to hyperoxia than to similar cultures that had been exposed to normoxia.[14] In addition, close examination of these preparations suggested that neutrophils might be activated after adhering to hyperoxia-exposed endothelial cells. The precise mechanisms by which hyperoxia directly damages endothelial cells is unknown. However, one might speculate that it involves production of toxic oxygen radicals since addition of SOD or catalase decreases endothelial cell injury from hyperoxia.[9] In addition, preliminary evidence suggests that endothelial cells reduce nitroblue tetrazolium (NBT).[15] Moreover, since NBT reduction is inhibitable by SOD and diminished in endothelial cells that have been depleted of oxygen, it may reflect production of oxygen radicals (superoxide anion) by endothelial cells (Fig. 13). The association of these findings with the observation that SOD and catalase also prevented hyperoxia-induced decreases in the growth of endothelial cells suggests that hyperoxia may stimulate endothelial cells to injure themselves by making self-damaging oxygen radicals.

Thus, our investigations indicate there are at least two pathways by which neutrophils can be recruited and activated in lungs of animals exposed to hyperoxia. Undoubtedly, other mechanisms exist that can attract neutrophils to

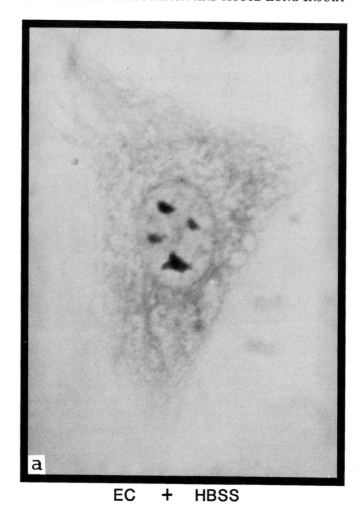

EC + HBSS

Figure 13: *Cultured bovine pulmonary artery endothelial cells (EC) treated with nitroblue tetrazolium (NBT) dye (***b***) have blue granules not seen in untreated endothelial cells (***a***). Addition of superoxide dismutase (SOD) decreased the number and blue intensity of granules in EC treated with NBT (***c***).*

lungs of animals exposed to hyperoxia. These may involve damage to other cell types and release of factors that are either similar or dissimilar to the factors identified. It does not appear that complement is directly involved in hyperoxic lung injury. Complement is not activated and prior complement depletion of rats with cobra venom factor does not alter neutrophil accumulation and/or the development of acute pulmonary edema following exposure to hyperoxia.[5]

What is the Mechanism of Acute Edematous Lung Injury Following Injection of Phorbol Myristate Acetate?

To further assess mechanisms by which neutrophils might participate in acute edematous lung injury, we examined another model of acute permeability

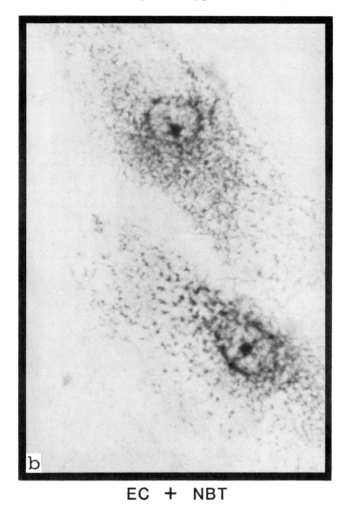

EC + NBT

Figure 13b *(Continued)*

pulmonary edema. In this model, phorbol myristate acetate (PMA), a potent neutrophil stimulant,[16] was injected intravenously into control (neutrophil replete) or nitrogen mustard–treated (neutropenic) rabbits. PMA was used because it resembled factors obtained from hyperoxia-treated AM. Both PMA- and AM-derived factors increase neutrophil adherence and neutrophil release of oxygen radicals in vitro. Following injection of PMA, circulating neutrophil concentrations rapidly decreased (<5 min) in control rabbits from approximately $2,000/mm^3$ to less than $100/mm^3$.[17] The number of circulating neutraphils remained very low in both control and neutropenic rabbits for the next 4 hours. In parallel, histologic examination revealed many neutrophils in lungs of control rabbits but not neutropenic rabbits given PMA. In addition, injection of PMA caused severe acute edematous lung injury in control rabbits but not in neutropenic rabbits.[17] Indeed, control rabbits given PMA had gross morphologic and histologic evidence of lung injury as well as lung weight and lavage albumin concentration increases which were not found in neutropenic rabbits

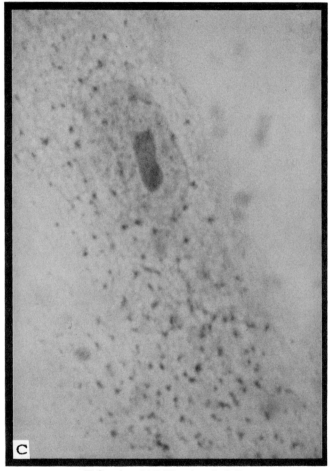

EC + NBT + SOD

Figure 13c

given PMA (Fig. 14). Moreover, protection from lung injury seen in neutropenic rabbits given PMA was so complete that no differences could be discerned between lungs from neutropenic rabbits given PMA and unpretreated control rabbits given intravenous saline. A role for neutrophils in the development of acute edematous lung injury in control rabbits given PMA was further indicated when individual increases in lung weights and lung lavage albumin concentrations correlated with concentrations of circulating and lavage neutrophils. Furthermore, pretreating rabbits with mepacrine (Fig. 15) or DMTU (Fig. 16), but not corticosteroids, prevented acute pulmonary lung edema following intravenous instillation of PMA. The latter supports the speculation that oxygen radicals may be important since mepacrine or DMTU, but not corticosteroids, also decreased oxygen radical generation by PMA-stimulated neutrophils in vitro.[18,19]

These studies demonstrated that injection of PMA caused acute pulmonary

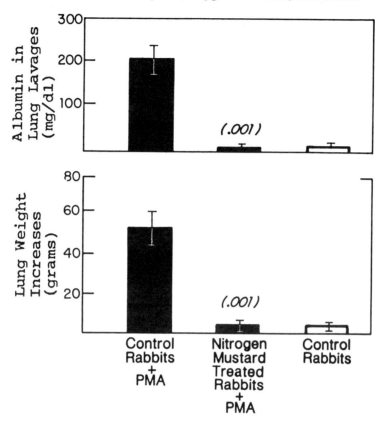

Figure 14: *Following intravenous injection of phorbol myristate acetate (PMA), lungs from control rabbits weighed more and had greater lung lavage albumin concentrations than nitrogen mustard-pretreated (neutropenic) rabbits given PMA or unpretreated control rabbits given saline.*

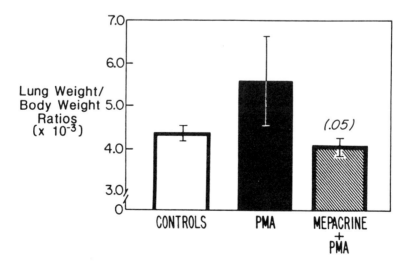

Figure 15: *Pretreatment with mepacrine prevented lung weight gains in rabbits given PMA.*

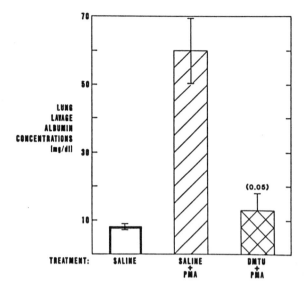

Figure 16: *Pretreatment with dimethylthiourea (DMTU) decreased lavage albumin concentrations in lungs of rabbits given PMA.*

edema and that neutrophils contributed to this process. However, because of the complexity of these intact animal studies in which many cells and mediators circulate in the blood, many questions remained. In particular, we wondered if stimulated neutrophils could cause edema in the absence of other circulating cells, and if so, by what mechanisms neutrophils mediated acute edematous lung injury. To address these questions, we studied isolated rabbit lungs whose vasculature had been washed out and perfused with only saline. This approach diminishes blood cells and other circulating factors that complicate interpretation. In addition, these surgically removed isolated lungs can be mechanically ventilated in a temperature-controlled humidified chamber, perfused through cannulas that enter through the pulmonary artery and exit through the left ventricle, and monitored using transducers to measure continuously changes in vascular pressures and lung weights (Fig. 17). Saline-perfused isolated rabbit lungs were acutely damaged by the addition of PMA and normal neutrophils.[17] Damage was manifested by increased lung weight gains and lung lavage albumin concentrations (Fig. 18). In contrast, adding PMA and oxygen radical-deficient neutrophils from patients with chronic granulomatous disease (CGD) did not cause lung injury (Fig. 18). The latter finding suggested that oxygen radicals might be central to neutrophil-mediated injury. To further address this possibility, we added DMTU, an oxygen radical scavenger, to isolated lungs perfused with neutrophils and PMA. The addition of DMTU prevented acute injury in isolated lungs perfused with neutrophils and PMA. Similarly, DMTU can (1) decrease lung injury in rats exposed to hyperoxia[8] or thiourea,[20] (2) scavenge toxic oxygen radicals and decrease bactericidal activities mediated by neutrophils or chemical reactions,[21] (3) decrease damage to alveolar macrophages exposed to hyperoxia,[12] and (4) decrease oxidant-induced pleural fibrosis[22] and decrease H_2O_2-mediated injury to endothelial cells and isolated lungs.[23] Another oxygen radical scavenger, mepacrine (but not corticosteroids), also prevented increases in lung weights and lavage albumin concentration seen in isolated lungs perfused with neutrophils and PMA. It should

Isolated Rabbit Lung Model

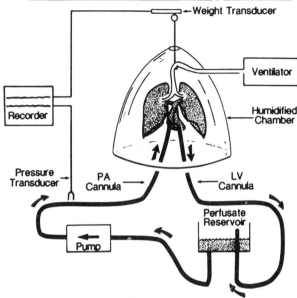

Figure 17: *Schematic diagram of isolated perfused lung apparatus.*

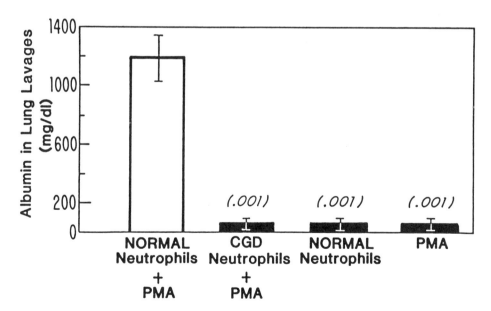

Figure 18: *Addition of normal human neutrophils and phorbol myristate acetate (PMA) increased lavage albumin concentrations in isolated perfused lungs. In contrast, addition of PMA and O_2 radical-deficient neutrophils from patients with chronic granulomatous disease (CGD) did not increase lavage albumin concentrations in isolated perfused lungs.*

be mentioned that how neutrophils are stimulated may be a very important determinant in the mechanism by which they cause injury. In vitro studies show that some stimuli are more effective at causing release of neutrophil oxygen radicals (PMA) while other stimuli are relatively better agonists for degranulation (FMLP). This concept is also emphasized by our recent studies that show that properly stimulated (high dose PMA) CGD neutrophils may be able to cause acute edematous injury in isolated lungs.[24] The mechanism of injury in the latter is unclear. It is possible that a combination type of injury might be occurring that results from interactions of small concentrations of oxygen radicals produced by arachidonic acid metabolism and other toxins from neutrophils.

We next added purine (P) and xanthine oxidase (XO) to chemically generate oxygen radicals in the cell-free isolated lung perfusate.[23] Purine and xanthine oxidase generate superoxide anion (O_2^-) and hydrogen peroxide (H_2O_2), which reacts with iron to form hydroxyl radical ($^{\cdot}OH$). Superoxide anion can then be converted by SOD to H_2O_2, which in turn can be converted by catalase to water and oxygen. Hydroxyl radical can be scavenged by DMTU or dimethyl sulfoxide (DMSO).[25-28] Concentrations of P and XO were used which made quantities of O_2^- that were comparable to those produced by neutrophils stimulated by PMA. Addition of P and XO to perfusates of isolated lungs caused increased lung weight gains and lung lavage albumin concentrations—changes that were not seen after addition of P or XO alone (Fig. 19). Moreover, addition of catalase or DMTU to perfusates prevented P- and XO-mediated increases in lung weights and lung lavage albumin concentrations while pretreatment with SOD or DMSO did not decrease acute edematous injury in isolated lungs perfused with P and XO (Fig. 19). These results indicated that oxygen radicals alone could cause acute edematous lung injury, and moreover, that H_2O_2 or an H_2O_2-derived product, such as $^{\cdot}OH$, mediated the damage.

During the previous studies, it became apparent that perfusion with chemically generated oxygen radicals also increased pulmonary artery perfusion pressures in isolated lungs.[23] This raised the pertinent question of whether oxygen radicals caused pulmonary edema by directly injuring the alveolar capillary membrane (permeability edema) and/or by increasing microvascular pressure (hydrostatic edema). This issue was addressed by injecting papaverine, a smooth muscle dilator, into isolated lungs perfused with P and XO. Papaverine prevented increases in mean perfusion pressures and lung weight increases that followed addition of P and XO. In addition, increases in perfusion pressures following injection of P and XO were inhibited by adding catalase or DMTU, confirming that oxygen radical production participated in pressor responses. To ascertain if oxygen radicals had a direct (pressure independent) effect on alveolar capillary membrane integrity, after the usual 55-minute perfusion period, left atrial pressures were increased mechanically in lungs given P, XO, and papaverine. This maneuver caused an immediate and permanent increase in the weights of rabbit lungs that were perfused with P, XO, and papaverine but not in lungs perfused with papaverine alone or papaverine, P, XO, and catalase (Fig. 20). This finding suggested that P and XO damaged the alveolar capillary membrane but that increases in perfusion pressures were needed to evidence edema. Thus, oxygen radicals may mediate their toxic effect on the isolated lung by both increasing perfusion pressures and causing pressure independent permeability damage to the alveolar capillary membrane (Fig. 20).

Increases in perfusion pressure involved oxygen radical-mediated increases

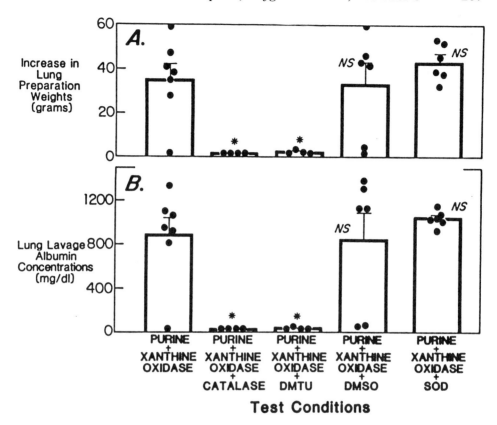

Figure 19: *Addition of purine and xanthine oxidase to perfusates of isolated lungs caused increases in lung weights lavage albumin concentrations that were inhibitable by co-addition of catalase and dimethylthiourea (DMTU) but not dimethylsulfoxide (DMSO) or superoxide dismutase (SOD).*

in thromboxane.[29] Following perfusion with hypoxanthine (HX) and XO (but not HX or XO) perfusate thromboxane activities increased more than 30 times in isolated lungs. In contrast, prostacyclin levels increased only about two times in isolated lungs perfused with HX and XO. Increases in thromboxane and perfusion pressures were similarly decreased by addition of catalase, ASA, indomethacin, or imidazole (Fig. 21). Since the latter three agents do not scavenge oxygen radicals (superoxide anion) well in vitro, it appeared that oxygen radical-induced increases in pulmonary artery perfusion pressures were related, at least in part, to thromboxane generation. Our findings in isolated lungs are summarized in Figure 22. They emphasize the combined importance of increases in perfusion pressures and alveolar capillary membrane permeability in the development of lung edema.

Do Interactions Occur Between Neutrophils and Other Cells?

Obviously, neutrophils may interact with other cells and humoral factors in the blood. Platelets are a prime example, especially since thrombocytopenia

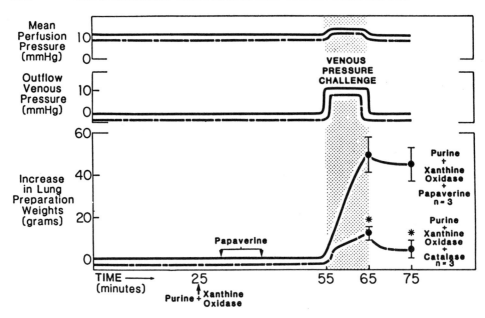

Figure 20: *In the presence of papaverine, no increases in pressures or lung weights were seen in isolated lungs perfused with purine and xanthine oxidase until a mechanical venous pressure challenge was applied. Co-addition of catalase prevented increases in lung weights following this mechanical venous pressure challenge in isolated lungs perfused with purine, xanthine oxidase, and papaverine. The results suggest that O_2 radicals can cause alveolar capillary membrane permeability defects that are independent of pressure. Perfusion pressure increases are required for the generation of edema.*

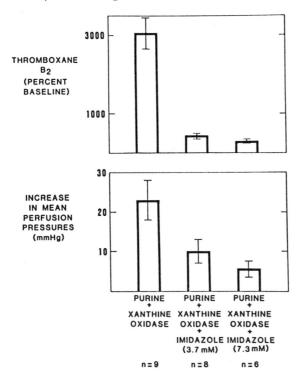

Figure 21: *Pretreatment with imidazole prevented purine- and xanthine oxidase-induced increases in perfusate thromboxane B_2 and pressure increases in isolated lungs.*

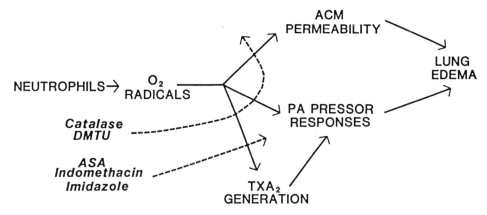

Figure 22: *Schematic diagram summarizing our findings in isolated perfused lungs. The dotted lines indicate inhibition by co-addition of O₂ radical scavengers, catalase and dimethylthiourea (DMTU) or arachidonic acid metabolism inhibitors, aspirin, indomethacin, and imidazole.*

with pulmonary platelet microthrombi and sequestration are often seen in patients with ARDS.[30,31] Our own studies suggest both direct and indirect roles for platelets in the pathogenesis of ARDS. First, addition of *Staphylococcus aureus* 502[30] or acetyl glyceryl ether phosphorylcholine (AGEPC) or platelet activating factor (PAF)[31] caused rapid decreases in the number of circulating platelets which were associated with increases in perfusate thromboxane concentrations, pulmonary artery hypertension, and hydrostatic edema in isolated lungs (Figs. 23, 24). In contrast, in the presence of aspirin, platelets did not disappear and hypertension (and edema) did not develop in isolated lungs perfused with *S. aureus* or PAF. The mechanism responsible for the pressor

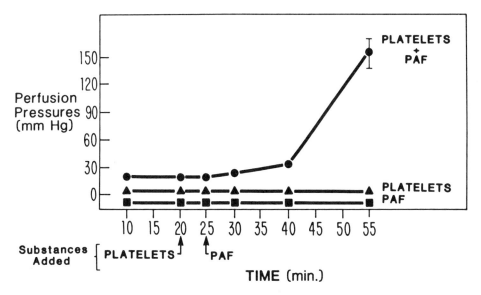

Figure 23: *Platelet activating factor (PAF) caused pulmonary hypertension in isolated lungs perfused with human platelets.*

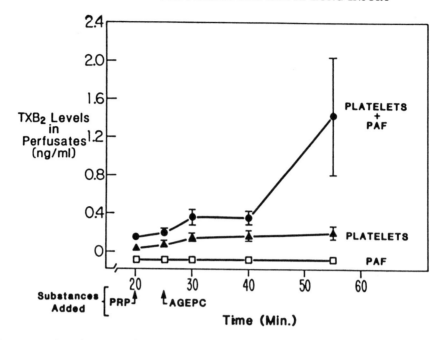

Figure 24: *Thromboxane B$_2$ levels increased in isolated lungs perfused with human platelets and platelet activating factor (PAF).*

responses appeared to involve elevations of thromboxane since they were in-hibited by addition of aspirin, indomethacin, imidazole, or 13 azoprostanoic acid—a thromboxane receptor site blocker. In contrast, addition of PAF and neutrophils did not cause pressor responses or edema in isolated lungs. These findings suggest that neutrophils can release O$_2$ radicals that cause alveolar capillary permeability and stimulate thromboxane and that platelets may con-tribute to this process, in part, by releasing more of the potent vasoconstricting thromboxane (Fig. 25). It also appears that platelets can augment the adherence of neutrophils to endothelial cells since they are able to increase neutrophil adherence to nylon fiber in vitro (Fig. 26).[32] These observations indicate the potentially complex interactions that may exist between neutrophils and plate-lets and underscore the diversity of responses possible in an intact organism.

How Can the Lung Be Protected Against Oxygen Radical-Mediated Injury?

As indicated, mechanisms are available that can recruit and activate neu-trophils in lungs of animals exposed to hyperoxia, stimulate oxygen radical production, and initiate complex mechanisms involving arachidonic acid meta-bolites and other cells, such as platelets. Accordingly, it was assumed that intrinsic or extrinsic increases in lung antioxidant enzymes might diminish neutrophil and/or oxygen radical-derived lung injury seen following exposure to hyperoxia or PMA. In addition, observations from other sources indicate that

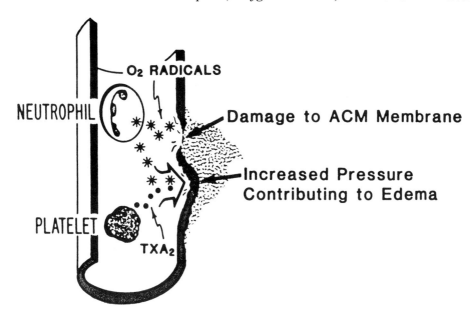

Figure 25: *Schematic diagram of possible platelet-neutrophil interactions contributing to the development of lung edema. O_2 radicals from neutrophils damage the alveolar capillary membrane and cause thromboxane (TXB_2)-mediated increases in perfusion pressure. Activated platelets also release thromboxane, which participates in pulmonary artery pressure increases.*

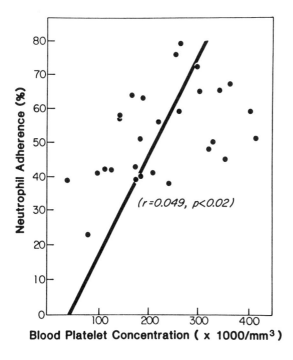

$(r = 0.049, p < 0.02)$

Figure 26: *Addition of increasing amounts of human platelets increased the adherence of human neutrophils to nylon fiber in vitro.*

preexposure to endotoxin (as well as sublethal hyperoxia or hypoxia) is associated with increases in lung antioxidant enzymes and protection against lung injury from hyperoxia in rats.[33,34] The latter may be relevant even though controversy exists regarding whether increased antioxidant mechanisms are themselves protective or only represent phenomena accompanying other changes that provide protection. To further ascertain if a cause and effect relationship existed between increases in lung antioxidant enzymes and protection against hyperoxia, we exposed rats to hypoxia, a maneuver used to increase lung antioxidant enzyme concentrations. We then removed lungs from hypoxia-preexposed rats and exposed them to chemically generated oxygen radicals. Lungs from rats that had been preexposed to hypoxia had slightly increased glutathione activities and were protected against injury following perfusion with oxygen radicals generated by hypoxanthine and XO.[35]

Another mechanism by which antioxidant enzymes might be increased in lungs of animals exposed to hyperoxia involves extrinsic amplification using liposomes (chemical agents or polyethylene glycol (PEG). In preliminary studies, lungs from rats injected with liposomes containing SOD and catalase did not develop acute pulmonary edema when injected with PMA. In addition, lungs from liposome-pretreated rats did not develop edema when subsequently isolated and perfused with neutrophils and PMA or hypoxanthine and xanthine oxidase. Liposomes may be able to deliver antioxidant enzymes to intracellular endothelial cell locations in the alveolar capillary membrane. This may be important since extracellular increases in concentrations of SOD and catalase do not protect well against lung injury, perhaps because these large proteins do not enter intracellular locations or tight interfaces joining neutrophils and endothelial cells. In addition, these large proteins may be cleared too rapidly from the circulation to provide appreciable protection. Addition of smaller, more permeable oxygen radical scavengers such as DMSO or DMTU is potentially another way to increase lung antioxidant defenses and protect against injury mediated by O_2 radicals.[20,21,23] Finally, attachment of antioxidants, such as SOD and catalase, to PEG can be used to protect against lung injury from hyperoxia.[36] Indeed, multiple daily doses of PEG attached SOD and catalase completely prevented lung injury from hyperoxia. All animals that received both PEG attached SOD and catalase survived while all untreated rats died, usually within 72 hours of exposure to hyperoxia. In addition, rats that received one preexposure dose of both PEG attached catalase and SOD had a decreased mortality rate in hyperoxia compared to untreated rats that had been exposed to hyperoxia. Specifically, rats given a single injection of PEG attached catalase and SOD lived 88 hours in hyperoxia comapred to about 52 hours for untreated controls. Administration of PEG attached catalase and SOD also decreased numbers of neutrophils, chemotaxins for neutrophils, and albumin concentrations in lung lavage of rats exposed to hyperoxia.[36] Pleural effusions were also decreased in lungs of PEG attached catalase and SOD treated rats that had been exposed to hyperoxia. The latter suggests that PEG attached antioxidants protect by decreasing lung injury but does not indicate whether PEG antioxidants protect by scavenging O_2 metabolites and/or whether neutrophils contributed to the process. Furthermore, since oxygen radicals also contribute to neutrophil bactericidal functions, it was reasoned that increases in antioxidants might also compromise oxygen radical-mediated bactericidal functions.[37] We found that this preparation of liposomes (with or without SOD) decreased neutrophil bactericidal activities in vitro and the clearance of intravenously injected *S. aureus* from the blood of rabbits. In contrast, pretreatment with PEG (with or without SOD) did not decrease neutrophil bactericidal activity in vitro or the clearance of intravenously injected *S. aureus*.

A novel defense mechanism is the recent observation that RBC (red blood cells) can decrease oxygen radical-mediated events.[38] Previous investigations had focused on the possibility that RBC might be injured by oxidants but none focused on the possibility that RBC could scavenge oxygen metabolites and protect other tissues. This is not so surprising since RBC contains large amounts of SOD, catalase, glutathione peroxidase, and hemoglobin which can scavenge O_2 radicals. The possibility that RBC can protect against oxygen radical-mediated injury was more clearly suggested when addition of increasing concentrations of RBC decreased hypoxanthine and xanthine oxidase mediated acute edematous injury in isolated perfused lungs[38] (Fig. 27). In addition, glutaraldehyde-treated RBC also decreased injury following perfusion with hypoxanthine and xanthine oxidase, suggesting that release of intracellular RBC contents was not needed for protection. The latter is consistent with observations that H_2O_2 can freely diffuse through RBC membranes and that glutaraldehyde-fixed RBC does not release intracellular contents when treated with H_2O_2. RBC also prevented H_2O_2-mediated injury to endothelial cells in suspension (Fig. 28) and H_2O_2-mediated oxidation of reduced cytochrome c.[38] The mechanism by which RBC scavenge H_2O_2 was not determined but very likely involves glutathione peroxidase at low concentrations of H_2O_2 and catalase at higher concentrations of H_2O_2 (Fig. 29). In parallel, insulflation of RBC also prevents lung injury from hyperoxia.[39] Furthermore, injury and inflammation occurs in areas that lack RBC while injury is relatively uncommon in areas that contain RBC. These observations raise many question. Do RBC routinely scavenge intravascularly generated oxygen radicals? Does influx of RBC into interstitial and alveolar spaces bring protective antioxidants to areas where they might not usually reside? Is it possible that RBC antioxidant defenses are different in different individuals, and accordingly, account for the different susceptibilities of certain individuals to injury? This latter issue of why certain individuals who undergo apparently the same insult develop severe or fatal ARDS while others do not must be intimately tied to alterations in heretofore undefined defense and/or repair mechanisms. Conditions that de-

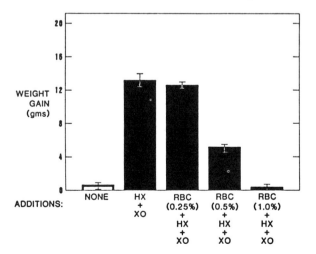

Figure 27: *Addition of increasing concentrations of human erythrocytes (RBC) progressively decreased lung weight gains in isolated lungs perfused with O_2 radicals generated by hypoxanthine (HX) and xanthine oxidase (XO). Addition of catalase, but not superoxide dismutase (SOD) also prevented HX- and XO-induced lung injury, suggesting that injury was mediated by H_2O_2 or H_2O_2 derived products, such as ·OH.*

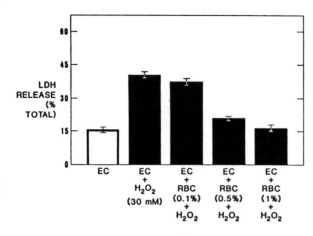

Figure 28: *Addition of increasing concentrations of human erythrocytes (RBC) progressively decreased lactate dehydrogenase (LDH) release from bovine pulmonary artery endothelial cells (EC) treated with hydrogen peroxide (H₂O₂).*

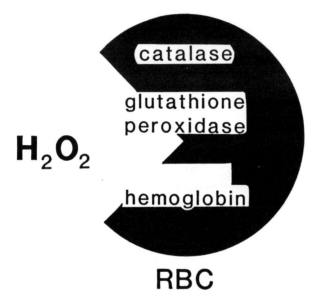

Figure 29: *Schematic diagram depicting potential intracelluar erythrocyte (RBC) scavengers of hydrogen peroxide (H₂O₂).*

crease RBC antioxidants may include oxidant stress (hyperoxia), transfusion, immaturity, and/or drugs. Our overall working hypothesis for the mechanism of lung injury from hyperoxia is shown in Figure 30. Antioxidants could be effective at a number of places in this proposed sequence.

What is Needed to Improve Our Understanding of the Pathogenesis of ARDS?

Very basic investigations are needed to improve our knowledge of the factors involved in the development of ARDS. As cited in this volume, many factors can be measured in lavages and vascular spaces following a massive lung

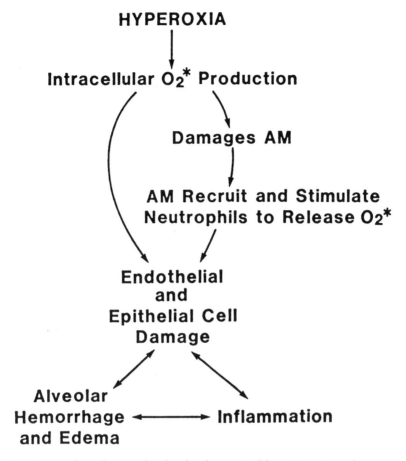

Figure 30: *Proposed mechanism for the development of lung injury in pulmonary oxygen toxicity.*

assault, such as that seen in ARDS. However, the significance of any of these factors remains largely unknown. Efforts must now be made to distinguish unrelated and secondary phenomena from primary inciting factors, remembering that since ARDS is associated with inciting events, key contributing factors may vary in different insults.

I propose the following as two immediate needs in ARDS research. First, a method is needed for measuring oxygen radicals in biological systems. In contrast to other substances that can be measured directly (or indirectly as their immediate by-product), oxygen radicals cannot be easily detected in biological systems. A way to measure oxygen radicals could be used to determine their presence and toxicity. It would also facilitate evaluation of the mechanism of purported scavengers of oxygen radicals. Ideally, the approach would be noninvasive so that frequent measurements of oxygen radical-mediated events could be undertaken. The approach should be relatively selective and facilitate measurement of oxygen radicals at intracellular sites. Our efforts in this regard have yielded the following approach involving measurement of the disappearance of DMTU. The approach was analogous to prior studies in which reaction of ·OH with DMSO led to the production of CH_4, which can be measured in expired air and theoretically used as an index of oxygen radical metabolite generation.[40] While background CH_4 production from contaminating gut bacteria has limited the effectiveness of this approach, we found that DMSO would disappear.[41] In parallel, we also found that DMTU disappeared in vitro following addition to H_2O_2 (but not oleic acid, histamine, leukotrienes, or elastase).[42] Furthermore, DMTU disappeared from perfusates of isolated lungs treated with H_2O_2 in proportion to both the amount of added H_2O_2 and the corresponding amount of injury (Fig. 31). The specificity of DMTU disappearance was suggested when addition of catalase (but not aminotriazole-inactivated catalase) prevented both H_2O_2-mediated acute edematous injury and corresponding DMTU disappearances. Furthermore, DMTU disappearance did not occur in isolated lungs perfused with oleic acid, elastase, or leukotrienes or in lungs given a perfusion pressure challenge even though these lungs developed comparable amounts of acute edematous injury. These findings suggest that measurement of DMTU disappearance might be a useful way of assessing the presence and/or toxicity of H_2O_2 in biological systems. Similarly, DMTU disappeared in proportion to the amount of added H_2O_2 and the corresponding degree of injury observed in suspensions containing cultured endothelial cells (Fig. 32).[43] Again, specificity was demonstrated when addition of trypsin caused endothelial cell injury but not DMTU disappearance and addition of catalase (but not SOD or urea) similarly prevented both injury and DMTU disappearance. Furthermore, DMTU disappearance helped establish that addition of RBC prevented endothelial cell (EC) damage by scavenging H_2O_2 since addition of RBC prevented both EC

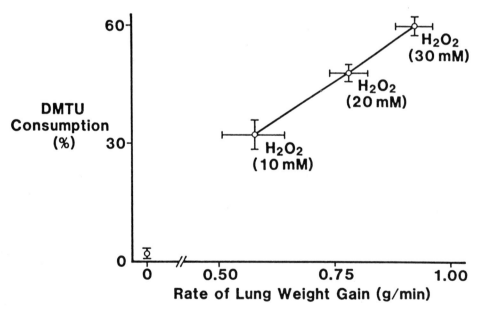

Figure 31: *Addition of increasing concentrations of H_2O_2 to perfusates of isolated lungs caused progressive increases in the consumption of dimethylthiourea (DMTU) and corresponding increases in acute edematous injury manifested by lung weight gain.*

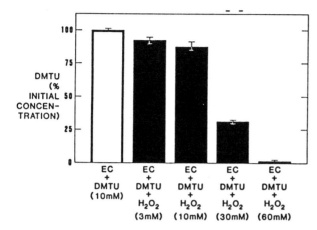

Figure 32: *Addition of increasing concentrations of H_2O_2 caused progressive increases in the concentrations of dimehtylthiourea (DMTU) present in suspensions of cultured bovine pulmonary artery endothelial cells (EC).*

injury (LDH release) and corresponding DMTU dissappearances (Fig. 33). We propose that use of DMTU disappearance, or this principle, should improve investigations of the contribution of oxygen radicals to lung injury. Hopefully, other techniques for measuring oxygen radicals in biological systems will be developed and used to test the validity of these hypotheses regarding the participation of oxygen radicals to lung injury.

A second immediate need for research in ARDS is the development of more sensitive and selective markers of lung injury. Our inability to detect subtle injury to cells early in the disease process remains a major limiting factor. The latter is especially crucial with respect to unraveling cause and effect relationships. Most of our injury markers are too insensitive. For example, by the time that measurable lung weight gains or appreciable increases in lung lavage albumin concentrations have occurred, many mechanisms have been activated. Better markers of lung injury might also serve eventually as diagnostic tools for determining which individuals are going to develop ARDS thereby facilitating a

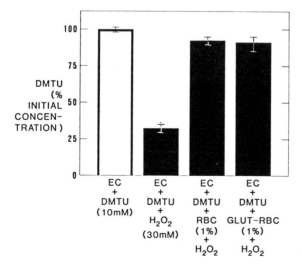

Figure 33: *Addition of intact (glutaraldehyde-treated) or untreated human erythrocytes (RBC) prevented dimethylthiourea (DMTU) disappearance in suspensions of bovine pulmonary artery endothelial cells (EC) treated with H_2O_2.*

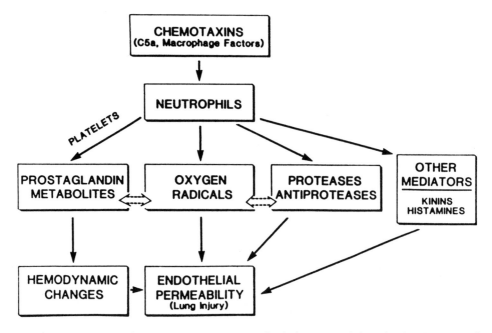

Figure 34: *Schematic diagram suggesting a central role for neutrophils in the development of acute edematous lung injury, such as that seen in the adult respiratory distress syndrome.*

more rapid initiation of appropriate therapy that could improve the presently dismal outcome in most cases of ARDS. With these specialized tools, an improved understanding of basic mechanisms underlying lung injury could be obtained. This would involve identification of factors that affect oxidant injury, such as metals and antioxidant enzymes, and the nature of oxygen radical-dependent reactions, such as the generation of thromboxanes or the inactivation of antiproteases or leukotrienes. Future investigation of ARDS will be very exciting and involve observations that extend from the bedside to very fundamental biochemical and biophysical levels, and hopefully, back to the bedside again.

Summary

The adult respiratory distress syndrome is an important clinical problem, the pathogenesis of which is largely unknown. Evidence from our own and other laboratories implicates neutrophils in the development of some forms of acute edematous lung injury.[44] Furthermore, it appears that oxygen radicals may also contribute directly and indirectly by interacting with arachidonic acid metabolites, antiproteases, platelets, and/or other factors (Fig.34).[45] Continued investigation of the contributions of neutrophils and oxygen radicals will improve our understanding of the pathogenesis of acute edematous lung injury and hopefully suggest more rational diagnostic and therapeutic approaches to this dreaded condition.

Acknowledgments

This work was supported in part by the National Institutes of Heath, Colorado and American Lung Associations, Colorado and American Heart Associations, the Council for Tobacco Research, the Kroc, Hill, Swan, and Kleberg Foundations. Dr. Repine was an Established Investigator of the American Heart Association during most of this work. The author acknowledges the invaluable contributions of his fellows, colleagues and assistants. Editors of *Chest* (Figs. 1, 12, 34), *American Review of Respiratory Diseases* (Figs. 9, 19,20), *Journal of Laboratory and Clinical Medicine* (Fig. 26), *Lung Biology in Health and Disease* (Figs. 1, 4, 5–7, 11, 12, 14, 18, 19, 34), and *The Journal of Clinical Investigation* (Fig. 21) gave permission to reprint figures.

REFERENCES

1. Lee, C.T., Fein, A.M., Lippman, M., et al.: Elastolytic activity in pulmonary lavage fluid from patients with adult respiratory distress syndrome. *N. Engl. J. Med.* 304:192–196, 1981.
2. Bachofen, M. and Weibel, E.R.: Alterations of the gas exchange apparatus in adult respiratory insufficiency associated with septicemia. *Am. Rev. Respir. Dis.* 116: 589–615, 1977.
3. Klebanoff, S.J.: Oxygen metabolism and the toxic properties of phagocytes. *Ann. Int. Med.* 93:380–389, 1980.
4. Zimmerman, G.A., Renzetti, A.D., and Hill, H.R.: Functional and metabolic activity of granulocytes from patients with adult respiratory distress syndrome. *Am. Rev. Respir. Dis.* 127:290–300, 1983.
5. Fox, R.B., Hoidal, J.R., Brown, D.M., et al.: Pulmonary inflammation due to oxygen toxicity: Involvement of chemotactic factors and polymorphonuclear leukocytes. *Am. Rev. Respir. Dis.* 123:521–523, 1981.
6. Shasby, D.M., Fox, R.B., Harada, R.N., et al.: Reduction of the edema of acute hyperoxic lung injury by granulocyte depletion. *J. Appl. Physiol.* 52:1237–1244, 1982.
7. Shasby, D.M., Shasby, S.S., Bowman, C.M., et al.: Angiotensin converting enzyme concentrations in the lung lavage of normal rabbits and rabbits treated with nitrogen mustard exposed to hyperoxia. *Am. Rev. Respir. Dis.* 124:202–203, 182.
8. Fox, R.B.: Prevention of granulocyte-mediated oxidant lung injury in rats by a hydroxyl radical scavenger, dimethylthiourea. *J. Clin. Invest.* 74:1456–1464, 1984.
9. Turrens, J.F., Crapo, J.D., Freeman, B.A.: Protection against oxygen toxicity by intravenous injection of liposome entrapped catalase and superoxide dismutase. *J. Clin. Invest.* 73:879–885, 1984.
10. White, C.W., Jackson, J.H., Freeman, B.A., et al.: Intravenous polyethylene glycol (PEG)-conjugated superoxide dismutase (SOD) and catalase (CAT) prolongs survival of rats exposed to hyperoxia. *Clin. Res.* 32:60A, 1984.
11. Harada, R.N., Vatter, A.E., and Repine, J.E.: Oxygen radical scavengers protect alveolar macrophages from hyperoxic injury in vitro. *Am. Rev. Respir. Dis.* 128: 761–762, 1983.
12. Harada, R.N., Vatter, A.E., and Repine, J.E.: Macrophage effector function in pulmonary oxygen toxicity: Hyperoxia damages and stimulates alveolar macrophages to make and release chemotaxins for polymorphonuclear leukocytes. *J. Leukocyte Biol.* 35:373–383, 1984.
13. Bowman, C.M., Harada, R.N., and Repine, J.E.: Hyperoxia stimulates alveolar macrophages to produce and release a factor which increases neutrophil adherence. *Inflammation* 7:331–338, 1983.

14. Bowman, C.M., Butler, E.N., and Repine, J.E.: Hyperoxia damages cultured endothelial cells causing increased neutrophil adherence. *Am. Rev. Respir. Dis.* 128: 469–472, 1983.

15. Bowman, C.M., Butler, E.M., Toth, K.M., et al.: Reduction of nitroblue tetrazolium (NBT) by cultured endothelial cells—a measure of superoxide anion (O_2^-) production. *Clin. Res.* 30:82A, 1982.

16. Repine, J.E., White, J.G., Clawson, C.C., et al.: Effects of phorbol myristate acetate on the metabolism and ultrastructure of neutrophils in chronic granulomatous disease. *J. Clin. Invest.* 54:83–90, 1974.

17. Shasby, D.M., Van Benthuysen, K.M., Tate, R.M., et al.: Granulocytes mediate acute edematous lung injury in rabbits and isolated rabbit lungs perfused with phorbol myristate acetate: Role of oxygen radicals. *Am. Rev. Respir. Dis.* 125: 443–447, 1982.

18. Canham, E.M., Shoemaker, S.A., Tate, R.M., et al.: Mepacrine but not methylprednisolone decreases acute edematous lung injury following injection of phorbol myristate acetate. *Am. Rev. Respir. Dis.* 127:594–598, 1983.

19. Jackson, J.H., White, C.W., Clifford, D.P., et al.: Dimethylthiourea (DMTU), an O_2 radical scavenger, prevents acute edematous lung injury (ARDS) following injection of phorbol myristate acetate (PMA). *Clin. Res.* 31:96A, 1983.

20. Fox, R.B., Tate, R.M., Harada, R.N., et al.: Prevention of thiourea-induced pulmonary edema by hydroxyl radical scavengers. *J. Appl. Physiol.* 55:1456–1459, 1983.

21. Jackson, J.H., Berger, E.M., and Repine, J.E.: Thiourea and dimethylthiourea inhibit neutrophil bactericidal activity in vitro. (Submitted for publication.)

22. Antony, V.B., Owen, C.L., and Sahn, S.A.: Dimethylthiourea prevents oxygen radical-mediated pleural fibrosis in experimental pleurisy. *Clin. Res.* 32:424A, 1984.

23. Tate, R.M., Van Benthuysen, K.M., Shasby, D.M., et al.: Oxygen radical-mediated permeability edema and vasoconstriction in isolated perfused rabbit lungs. *Am. Rev. Respir. Dis.* 126:802–806, 1982.

24. Jackson, J.H., White, C.W., Shroeder, W.R., et al.: High-dose phorbol myristate acetate (PMA) and oxygen metabolite (O_2^*) deficient chronic granulomatous disease (CGD) neutrophils cause acute edematous lung injury (ARDS) and leukotriene (LT) increases in isolated perfused rabbit lungs (IPRL). *Clin. Res.* 32:62A, 1984.

25. Repine, J.E., Johansen, K.S., and Berger, E.M.: Hydroxyl radical scavengers produce similar decreases in chemiluminescence responses and bactericidal activities of neutrophils. *Infect. Immunol.* 43:435–439, 1984.

26. Repine, J.E., Fox, R.B., and Berger, E.M.: Dimethyl sulfoxide inhibits killing of Staphylococcus aureus by polymorphonuclear leukocytes. *Infect. and Immunity.* 31: 510–513, 1981.

27. Repine, J.E., Fox, R.B. and Berger, E.M.: Hydrogen peroxide kills Staphylococcus aureus by reacting with staphylococcal iron to form hydroxyl radical. *J. Biol. Chem.* 256:7094-7097, 1981.

28. Repine, J.E., Pfenninger, O.W., Talmage, D.W., et al.: Dimethyl sulfoxide prevents DNA nicking mediated by ionizing radiation or iron/hydrogen peroxide-generated hydroxyl radical. *Proc. Natl. Acad. Sci.* 78:1001–1003, 1981.

29. Tate, R.M., Morris, H.G., Schroeder, W.R., et al.: Oxygen metabolites stimulate thromboxane generation and cause vasoconstriction in isolated saline-perfused rabbit lungs. *J. Clin. Invest.* 74:608–613, 1984.

30. Shoemaker, S.A., Heffner, J.E., Canham, E.M. et al.: Staphylococcus aureus and human platelets cause pulmonary hypertension and thromboxane generation in isolated saline-perfused rabbit lungs. *Am. Rev. Respir. Dis.* 129:92–95, 1984.

31. Heffner, J.E., Shoemaker, S.A., Canham, E.M., et al.: Acetyl glyceryl ether phosphorylcholine (AGEPC)-stimulated human platelets cause pulmonary hypertension and edema in isolated rabbit lungs: Role of thromboxane A_2. *J. Clin. Invest.* 71:351–358, 1983.

32. Rasp, F.L., Clawson, C.C., and Repine, J.E.: Platelets increase neutrophil adherence in vitro to nylon fiber. *J. Lab. Clin. Med.* 97:812–816, 1981.

33. Frank, L., Summerville, J., and Massaro, D.: Protection from oxygen toxicity with endotoxin: Role of the endogenous antioxidant enzymes of the lung. *J. Clin. Invest.* 65:1104–1111, 1980.

34. Crapo, J.D., Marsh-Salin, J., Ingram, P., et al.: Tolerance and cross-tolerance using NO_2 and O_2. II. Pulmonary morphology and morphometry. *J. Appl. Physiol.* 44: 370–379, 1978.

35. White, C.W., Bowman, C.M., Berger, E.M., et al.: Preexposure to hypoxia increases lung catalase activity and decreases hydrogen peroxide dependent permeability pulmonary edema in isolated perfused rat lungs. *Clin. Res.* 31:423A, 1983.

36. White, C.M., Jackson, J.H., Freeman, B.A., et al.: Pretreatment with polyethylene glycol conjugated superoxide dismutase and catalase (PEG-SOD + CAT) decreases lung inflammation (lavage neutrophils and chemotaxins for neutrophils) and acute edematous injury (lavage albumin and mortality) in rats exposed to hyperoxia. *Clin. Res.* 32:530A, 1984.

37. McDonald, R.J., Berger, E.M., White, C.W., et al.: Pretreatment with liposome (LIP) encapsulated, but not polyethylene glycol (PEG) conjugated superoxide dismutase (SOD) or catalase (CAT) decrease clearance of bacteria in vitro and killing of bacteria by neutrophils in vitro. *Clin. Res.* 32:252A, 1984.

38. Toth, K.M., Clifford, D.P., White, C.W., et al.: Intact human erythrocytes prevent hydrogen peroxide-mediated damage to isolated perfused rat lungs and cultured bovine pulmonary artery endothelial cells. *J. Clin. Invest.* 74:292–295, 1984.

39. vanAsbeck, S., Hoidal, J., Schwartz, B., et al.: Insufflated red cells protect lungs from hyperoxic damage: Role of RBC glutathione in scavenging toxic O_2 radicals. *Clin. Res.* 32:563A, 1984.

40. Repine, J.E., Eaton, J.W., Anders, M.W., et al.: Generation of hydroxyl radical by enzymes, chemicals and human phagocytes in vitro: Detection using the anti-inflammatory agent—dimethyl sulfoxide. *J. Clin. Invest.* 64:1642–1651, 1979.

41. Parker, N.B., Berger, E.M., and Repine, J.E.: Reaction with hydroxyl radical (˙OH) causes disappearance of dimethyl sulfoxide (DMSO). *Clin. Res.* 32:15A, 1984.

42. Jackson, J.H., White, C.W., Schroeder, W.B., et al.: Dimethylthiourea (DMTU) consumption reflects hydrogen peroxide (H_2O_2) concentrations and severity of acute edematous injury (ARDS) in isolated rat lungs perfused with H_2O_2. *Clin. Res.* 32:528A, 1984.

43. Toth, K.M., Parker, N.B., Clifford, D.P., et al.: Intact human erythrocytes (RBC) prevent hydrogen peroxide (H_2O_2)-mediated damage to cultured bovine pulmonary artery endothelial cells (EC) and corresponding disappearance of dimethylthiourea (DMTU). *Clin. Res.* 32:88A, 1984.

44. Tate, R.M. and Repine, J.E.: Neutrophils and the Adult Respiratory Distress Syndrome. *Am. Rev. Respir. Dis.* 128:552–559, 1983.

45. Repine, J.E. and Tate, R.M.: Oxygen radicals and lung edema. *The Physiologist* 26:177–181, 1983.

CHAPTER 12

Oxidant Injury to Pulmonary Endothelium

Lee Frank

Introduction

> Before I built a wall I'd ask to know what I was walling in or
> walling out. . .
>
> Robert Frost
> *Mending Wall*

The complex barrier function of the lung endothelium has been discussed at length in earlier chapters. Likening the pulmonary endothelium to a wall is, of course, a gross oversimplification that obviates the very *active* role the endothelium plays in determining what is "walled in or walled out." In addition, the "nonrespiratory" functions of the endothelium—its metabolism (degradation, activation, synthesis) of potent vasoactive blood-borne substances, its coagulant-anticoagulant role, etc.—attest to the pulmonary endothelium being much more than a passive physical barrier between blood and air in the lung. And, it's because the pulmonary endothelium does, as we now know, have such interesting activities to contribute to overall homeostasis in the lung that toxic agents may have such serious sequelae when the lung endothelium is a target organ of toxicity.

In this chapter we will try to look specifically at the mechanism of toxicity posed by hyperoxidant stresses and their effect on endothelial integrity, plus the responses of the endothelium to these not uncommon toxic challenges. While we will concentrate on hyperoxia as the toxic agent, we will look also at the toxicity produced by a variety of other seemingly diverse agents that may share a mechanism of toxicity which is actually quite similar to that of hyperoxia (see Table I). All these agents that threaten disruption of pulmonary endothelial integrity (and function) constitute the

> Something there is that doesn't love a wall, That sends the frozen-
> ground-swell under it, And spills the upper boulders in the sun;
> And makes gaps even two can pass abreast.
>
> (Ibid)

From Said, S.I. (ed.): *The Pulmonary Circulation and Acute Lung Injury.* Mount Kisco, N.Y., Futura Publishing Co., Inc., 1985.

Table I
Agents That Can Cause Oxidant Lung Damage

Inhalants	Chemotherapeutic Agents
Hyperoxia	Bleomycin (anticancer)
Photochemical smog	Adriamycin (anticancer)
Ozone	Nitrofurantoin (antibacterial)
Nitrogen dioxide	
Phosgene	**Other drugs**
	Phenylhydrazine
X-irradiation	6-OH-dopamine
	Alloxan
Herbicide	Streptozotocin
Paraquat	Nitrofurans
	Thiourea?
	α-Methyldopa?

Mechanism of Oxygen Toxicity

Although the toxic consequences of prolonged exposure to high concentrations of O_2 are well appreciated now, there are still many clinical situations in which vigorous hyperoxic therapy is a necessity for the care of respiratory distressed patients. Unfortunately, there are still no pharmacological agents available to help the clinician circumvent the lung damage associated with prolonged high O_2 treatment. However, in the past two decades or so, our understanding of why life-giving O_2 is also a universal cell toxin in higher than normal ambient concentrations has been extended considerably. Since understanding of the mechanism of a toxic process usually precedes the development of effective means to prevent or interfere with the toxic process, there is reason (as discussed below) to be optimistic that the wisdom to develop pharmacological agents to protect against hyperoxidant toxicity may be forthcoming.

The mechanism of O_2 toxicity is now believed to be related to the intracellular production of partially reduced species of O_2—O_2 free radicals—highly reactive and cytotoxic by-products of a variety of normal processes in aerobic metabolism (Table II). The "free radical theory of O_2 toxicity" maintains that these toxic O_2 metabolites are not biological curiosities or anomalies but are generated by specific enzymes, by autoxidiation, and by energy transfer reactions in all O_2-using life forms (Table III). All aerobic life forms have also evolved sophisticated antioxidant defense systems to prevent these reactive O_2

Table II
Cytotoxic O_2 Species

$O_2\cdot$	Superoxide radical
H_2O_2	Hydrogen peroxide
$OH\cdot$	Hydroxyl radical
$^1O_2$	Singlet oxygen
$ROO\cdot$	Peroxide radical
	(R = Lipid)

Table III
Intracellular Sources of Superoxide Radical (O$_2^-$) and Other Cytotoxic Species

Enzymes
  Xanthine oxidase
  Aldehyde oxidase
  Tryptophan dioxygenase
  Indoleamine dioxygenase
  Flavoprotein dehydrogenase, etc.
Autoxidation
  Reduced $\rightarrow$ oxidized Ferrodoxin
  Adrenaline $\rightarrow$ Adrenochrome
  Hemoglobin $\rightarrow$ Methemoglobin
  Certain Flavins, Thiols, Hydroquinones, etc.
Mitochondria
  Ubiquinone - cytochrome b portion of respiratory chain
Microsomes
  "Uncoupled" cytochrome P$_{450}$ reactions

Evidence for these sources discussed in refs. 27, 37, 50, 53, 54.

metabolites from potential injurious interaction with critical cell components (Tables IV and V). Under usual normoxic conditions, cytotoxicity is adequately held in rein; however, under conditions of hyperoxidant stress, the O$_2$ radical-antioxidant defense equilibrium is upset, as the rate of generation of toxic O$_2$ species overwhelms the detoxifying capacity of the defensive systems. Unless intracellular balance is restored either by removal of the hyperoxidant stress or by augmentation of the antioxidant defenses of the cell, serious cell damage and

Table IV
Antioxidant Defenses

Enzymatic
  Superoxide dismutase (SOD)
    ($O_2^- + O_2^- + 2 H^+ \rightarrow O_2 + H_2O_2$)
  Catalase
    ($2 H_2O_2 \rightarrow O_2 + 2 H_2O$)
  Glutathione peroxidase
    (+ Glutathione reductase and G-6-PD)
    ($2 H_2O_2 \rightarrow O_2 + 2 H_2O$)
    ($2 ROO^- + 2 H^+ \rightarrow 2 ROH + O_2$)
                    ("nontoxic" lipid alcohol)
Nonenzymatic
  Vitamin E
    (reduces peroxide radicals to terminate chain reaction membrane lipid peroxidation)
  β-carotene
  Ascorbate
                    (free radical scavenging effects)
  Glutathione
  also Cysteamine, cysteine, nonessential PUFA
    (polyunsaturated fatty acids), other thiols

Table V
Cell Components Damaged by Reactive O_2 Species

Lipids—peroxidation of unsaturated fatty acids in organelle, plasma
    membranes
Proteins—oxidation of sulfhydryl-containing enzymes → enzyme inacti-
    vation
Carbohydrates—polysaccharide depolymerization
Nucleic Acids—base hydroxylations, "nicking," cross-linkage, scission of
    DNA strands (mutations)
Also inhibitory effects on protein, nucleotide, fatty acid biosynthesis

---

Discussion of components damaged and consequences in refs. 15, 27, 50, 53, 54,
62, 82.

---

cell death can ensue.[28,37,47,50,53] Figure 1 summarizes these current concepts that are encompassed by the "free radical theory of O_2 toxicity."

The formulation and establishment of these concepts about O_2 toxicity over the past two decades is an exciting affair to review, representing a paradigm for "the scientific process." In addition to providing a testable mechanism for the biochemical/molecular basis of O_2 toxicity, additional dividends have resulted from this theory, including: (1) the realization that a variety of seemingly diverse toxic agents may damage the lung by a rather similar biochemical mechanism; (2) a better understanding of how pulmonary tolerance or resistance to these toxins may develop; (3) the knowledge about how excess O_2 free radical production may be exploited for the offensive purpose of bacterial killing by normal inflammatory cells; and (4) how this offensive weapon may be inappropriately turned against the host organism in a variety of inflammatory conditions (see Chapters 11 and 13), and also how it may perhaps be used as a biological argument for gun control.[87,119,125] Additionally, this theory has provided a rational basis for the design of pharmacological interventions to help prevent or reduce the serious toxicity associated with exposure to hyperoxidant agents such as O_2 (and those listed in Table I).

Pathology of Oxygen Toxicity

The normally thin ($\sim$0.2 μ) alveolar septae or respiratory membranes of the lung—the structures that impart to the lung its fine lace-like architecture—are markedly altered during exposure of animals or man to high concentrations of O_2. Figure 2 diagrams the basic morphological changes in the O_2-toxic lung, separating them into (1) an acute or exudative phase, and (2) a chronic or proliferative phase of toxicity. This separation is useful as an aid to understanding the pathophysiology of O_2 toxicity and also in providing insight into the differing sensitivities to O_2-induced injury and cell death of the predominant cell types that make up the respiratory exchange membrane of the lung. In experimental animals of many species and ages, this sequence of lung alterations has been well characterized,[5,67,75,77] and by combining the findings from a variety of reports on O_2 toxicity in man,[6,58,73,100] it is possible to conclude that a rather similar pattern of pathological changes occurs in man also when long-term exposure to elevated levels of O_2 becomes a clinical

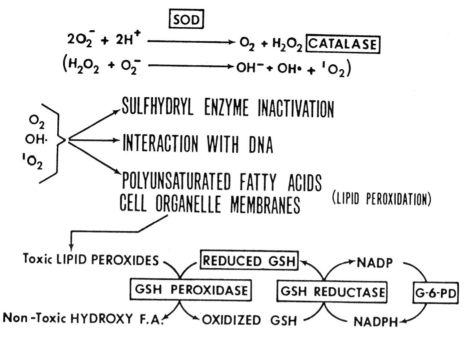

Figure 1: Oxygen free radicals and antioxidant defense systems. *Illustrated are the highly reactive O_2 metabolites: O_2^- = superoxide anion; OH· = hydroxyl radical; H_2O_2 = hydrogen peroxide; and $^1O_2$ = singlet oxygen. Also shown are the antioxidant enzyme defense systems: SOD = superoxide dismutase; catalase; and glutathione (GSH) peroxidase, glutathione (GSH) reductase, and glucose-6-phosphate dehydrogenase (G-6-PD). These enzymes function to protect the cell from the types of damaging biochemical interactions with O_2 radicals listed: critical sulfhydryl oxidations; DNA scism, alteration; membrane lipid peroxidations. The reaction between H_2O_2 and O_2^- to form other toxic O_2 metabolites is the so-called Haber-Weiss reaction (in parentheses). This reaction requires trace amounts of metals such as iron. (From Frank and Massaro,[47] with permission of* The American Journal of Medicine.)

necessity. The early prospective studies of Barber in irreversibly brain-damaged patients ventilated with 21% or 100% O_2[6] and the sequential human pathological studies of Gould and others have been particularly supportive of this conclusion.[58]

A key to understanding the progression of lung damage due to hyperoxia (or any other toxin for that matter) is recognition of the difference in susceptibility of the different cell types of the alveolar wall to O_2 poisoning: in terms of comparative sensitivity to O_2-induced cytotoxicity, endothelial cell >type I cell (membranous pneumocyte) >>type II cell (granular pneumocyte) and interstitial cells. Thus, detectable O_2 toxicity changes occur first in the endothelial cells lining the capillaries of the lung.[5,6,67,75,77] Microscopically, one sees swelling of organelles, increased vacuolarization, separation of thinned portions of the cells from their capillary basement membrane, eventual nuclear pyknosis, and cell sloughing (Fig. 3). Even before these morphological changes are manifested (after approximately 48 hours in >95% O_2), functional endothelial cell alterations are detectable. For example, after <24 hours of hyperoxic exposure, the pulmonary clearance of 5-hydroxytryptamine (serotonin) and epinephrine from

Pulmonary O₂ Toxicity

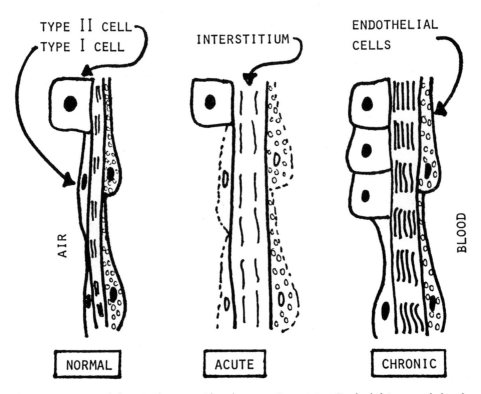

Figure 2: Acute and chronic changes with pulmonary O_2 toxicity. *On the left is normal alveolar wall or "respiratory membrane" of lung with capillary endothelial cells, thin interstitium, and airspace lined predominantly by type I cells. Acute changes (center) include damage/death of O_2-sensitive capillary endothelial cells and type I epithelial cells with widened interstitium due to capillary leakage and edema. Chronic phase changes (right) include regeneration of intact endothelium, proliferation of relatively O_2-resistant type II epithelial cells, and often permanent widening of interstitium with increased collagen/elastin fiber deposition. End result is much thickened respiratory or gas exchange membrane.*

lung perfusate, which is an active process localized in the pulmonary endothelium, is already significantly reduced.[8,9] Similarly, early O_2-induced reduction in endothelial cell angiotensin converting enzyme activity has recently been reported.[123]

With progressive damage to the pulmonary endothelium by O_2, progressive permeability changes ensue and leakage of watery and then more protein-rich plasma fluid occurs. This fluid leakage will be confined in its early stages to the interstitial space, with drainage centrally so that the larger lymphatic spaces in the perivascular-peribronchiolar region become increasingly dilated. As the capacity for lymphatic system drainage is exceeded by the progressive destruction and leakiness of the endothelial barrier, and as the type I cell epithelial barrier shows progressive O_2-induced toxic changes, this barrier too is breached and the alveolar spaces themselves begin to fill with proteinaceous edema fluid.

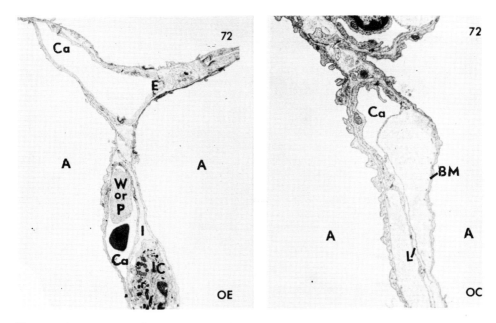

Figure 3: Transmission electron micrographs of adult rat lungs exposed to >95% O_2 for 72 hours. *(OC) on right is O_2-control (untreated) lung, which shows endothelial damage with elevation of thin portion of endothelium from its basement membrane (BM) with resulting appearance of occlusion of capillary lumen (L). (OE) on left is endotoxin-treated O_2-exposed lung showing intact endothelium (E) with patent capillaries (Ca). (A = alveolus; R = red blood cells; W or P = white blood cell or platelet; I = interstitium, with IC = interstitial cell). Original magnification ×11,000. (From Frank and Roberts,[48] with permission of* Toxicology and Applied Pharmacology.*)*

The initial manifestations of O_2 toxicity therefore reflect the sensitivity of the endothelial cell barrier to hyperoxidant stress. After 60–72 hours of exposure to >95% O_2, there is near total destruction of 50% of the capillary endothelial cells of the rat lung![21,24] And, in a morphometric study of prolonged O_2 exposure in man, the volume of the endothelial cells per cubic centimeter of alveolar tissue was reduced from 0.22 to 0.08 after 3 days in hyperoxia and to < 0.05 after 13 days in 60–100% O_2![74] Why the endothelium is so O_2 sensitive has been one of the key enigmas in O_2 toxicity research. In Table VI, some of the hypotheses proposed to explain this consistent observation in all species studied have been summarized. While the inflammatory cell theory (see Fig. 4) has received a great deal of recent attention, there is no convincing evidence that inflammatory cells *initiate the endothelial cell injury.* To the contrary, there has been ample demonstration that altered integrity and function of the capillary endothelial cells is the consequence of intracellular O_2 toxicity events.[22,104,117] The endothelial cell appears to be somehow more prone to develop O_2 radical-antioxidant defense system imbalance, and/or to be less able to respond to this toxic imbalance with adaptive increases in its detoxifying capacity. The recent findings that endothelial cells have comparatively very high rates of cyanide-resistant O_2 consumption (a relative index of the rate of production of partially reduced O_2 species) in 21% O_2 (approximately 20% vs.

Table VI
Endothelial Cell Sensitivity to O$_2$ Toxicity: Possible Explanations

(1) *Morphological*—related to squamoid cytoplasmic extensions that have large lipid membrane surface area with little cytoplasmic matrix and relatively few organelles → increased vulnerability to lipid peroxidation damage with reduced capacity for repair.

(2) *Morphological*—endothelial cells (and type I cells) have relatively reduced complement of organelles compared to O$_2$-resistant type II cells → smaller reserves of mitochondria (energy-production) and endoplasic reticulum (biosynthesis) to continue vital functions of cell as damage to some organelles occur.

(3) *Biochemical*—increased susceptibility to O$_2$-induced inhibition of nucleotide/protein synthesis [may be related to (2)].

(4) *Biochemical*—increased proportion of normal O$_2$ use via CN-resistant respiration → increased O$_2$ free radical production under normoxic and under hyperoxic conditions.

(5) *Biochemical*—possible decreased antioxidant defense system reserves.

(6) *Extraneous*—susceptibility to blood-borne factors (Fe^{++}?) that serve to promote toxic O$_2$ radical-mediated reactions such as lipid peroxidation.

(7) *Extraneous*—juxtaposition to blood stream makes endothelium more prone to inflammatory cell and platelet interactions that produce extracellular O$_2$ toxic species.

Some of these ideas are discussed in refs. 22, 75, 77, 125.

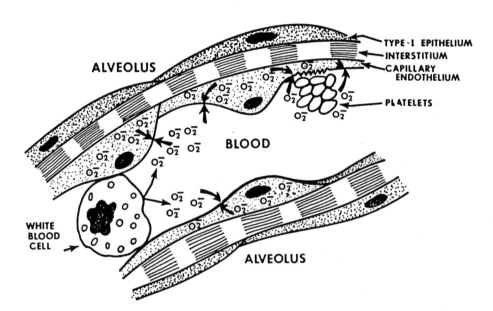

Figure 4: Vulnerability of pulmonary endothelium to oxygen toxicity. *Plasma membrane of endothelial cells are subjected to two-pronged attack by oxygen free radicals (O$_2^-$): (1) increased intracellular production of O$_2^-$ due to increased O$_2$ tension, and (2) extracellular O$_2^-$ released by circulating blood cells. At right, platelets have attached to O$_2^-$-damaged site on endothelial plasma membrane, aggregated, and released additional toxic O$_2^-$ radicals. Type I (and type II) epithelial cells are removed from intimate contact with blood-borne O$_2^-$ radicals. This proposed schema may help to explain why pulmonary endothelial cells are the cells of the lung most extensively damaged by hyperoxic exposure. (From Frank and Massaro,[47] with permission of* The American Journal of Medicine.).

only 4% for whole lung slices) and that CN-resistant O_2 consumption increases markedly in endothelial cells on exposure to hyperoxia (to 43% of total O_2 consumption) certainly suggest that the imbalance hypothesis may be a valid explanation for the marked sensitivity of the lung endothelium to O_2 toxicity.[22] Further support for this hypothesis is provided by the very recent demonstration that manipulations that increase the intracellular antioxidant capacity of endothelial cells in culture (exogenous SOD and catalase supplied in liposomal carriers) will largely prevent the manifestations of O_2-induced injury to the endothelial cells in this in vitro system.[51]

One of the biochemical alterations known to be associated with exposure to elevated concentrations of O_2 is the inhibition of DNA and protein synthesis.[84,88,91,92] The heightened sensitivity of the endothelial cells to hyperoxia may in fact be related to a comparatively increased susceptibility of these cells to inhibition of biosynthetic processes by hyperoxia. Evans and Hackney were able to demonstrate that in contrast to alveolar macrophages and type II cells, DNA synthesis was significantly impaired in endothelial cells early during exposure to 60% O_2 or even to 40% O_2.[32,33] Additionally, while ~72 hours of in vivo 100% O_2 exposure was required to produce substantial inhibition of DNA synthesis in alveolar macrophages, and ~48 hours of continuous 100% O_2 exposure would significantly inhibit DNA synthesis in type II cells, endothelial cells evidenced DNA inhibition (by ^{3}H-thymidine assay) after ≤24 hours of similar hyperoxic challenge[32,33] (Table VII). Early inhibition of biosynthetic processes in the pulmonary capillary endothelium may help account for the already discussed inability of these cells to reinforce their antioxidant defenses by new antioxidant enzyme production during high O_2 exposure. The comparatively increased susceptibility of the biosynthetic machinery in the endothelial cell to inhibition by O_2 can perhaps be related to the comparative key functional alterations produced in the various alveolar cells by hyperoxia, i.e., impairment of alveolar macrophage bactericidal capability and type II cell surfactant production requires comparatively more prolonged >95% O_2 exposure time (≥48 hours) than is required to demonstrate significant reductions in important endothelial cell functions (amine uptake depressed in <24 hours in >95% O_2).[8,9,56,60,68,103]

Table VII
Effect of 100% O_2 Exposure on Lung Cell Renewal*

Time in O_2	Labeling Index (number of actively-dividing cells/1,000 alveolar cells)		
	Alveolar Macrophages	Type II Cells	Endothelial Cells
0	1.0−1.5	0.9−1.7	5.0−7.0
8 hrs	1.1−1.4	0.8−1.2	3.5−4.1
24 hrs	0.1−1.5	0.5−1.3	<u>0−1.1</u>
48 hrs	0.1−1.1	<u>0</u>	0−1.2
72 hrs	<u>0−0.4</u>	0	0−1.0
96 hrs	0−0.4	0	0−0.9

‡Uptake of ^{3}H-thymidine and autoradiography. Data abstracted from Evans, Hackney, and Bills.[33] Underlined values denote earliest significant inhibition of lung cell renewal.

edema and its physiological sequelae (including atelectasis and pronounced pulmonary shunting) become so diffuse that respiratory exchange function is severely compromised and hypoxemia develops, then recovery from the acute exudative changes caused by hyperoxia can be a rapid process. The principal features of the chronic phase of experimental O_2 toxicity are: (1) absorption of exudates; (2) proliferation of type II pneumocytes and restoration of an intact epithelial lining cell layer; (3) proliferation of interstitial cells/fibroblasts with deposition of new collagen and elastin; and (4) restoration of an intact capillary endothelial lining. While the pattern of acute phase changes of O_2 toxicity are quite predictable in animal models, the extent of these chronic phase changes and the degree of restoration of the lung to relative structural normalcy are quite variable. Severe permanent alterations (diffuse pulmonary fibrosis and/or emphysematoid changes) are the eventual outcome in some experimental models.[5,16,19,64] Factors such as species, age, duration of exposure and O_2 level used, and undefined individual variations in reparative responses all seem to play a role in determining the final structural and pulmonary functional outcome of the chronic (or reparative-proliferative) phase of O_2 poisoning.

The endothelial cell response during the chronic phase of O_2 toxicity must intuitively be a critical factor in determining the end-stage picture of the O_2-damaged lung. Unless a relatively impermeable capillary barrier is restored and the blood conduit of the respiratory exchange membrane reasonably normalized, then cessation of fluid exudation into the lung can't occur, the proliferative response of the epithelial cells will be compromised, and gas exchange function may not be adequate enough to allow successful return of the patient/animal to room air O_2 tension. In actuality though, during the regenerative-proliferative phase of O_2 toxicity, the endothelial cells usually respond quite rapidly and vigorously post-O_2 exposure. Typical responses have been demonstrated autoradiographically (^{3}H-thymidine incorporation) by Bowden and Adamson,[14] who concluded from their studies that the endothelium of the pulmonary capillaries was the target site of hyperoxic damage, not the endothelium lining either larger hilar vessels or systemic vessels. During the second and third day after exposure of mice to 90% O_2 (6 days), ~50% of the regenerating cells in the alveolar wall were identified as endothelial cells.[14]

The unique problem of O_2 toxicity in the newborn merits special consideration because of the large number of newborn (premature) infants who require prolonged hyperoxic therapy, and also in light of some newly reported aspects about the sequelae of experimental O_2 toxicity in the neonatal animal. Prematurely born human infants very often require vigorous and prolonged respiratory support with elevated FI_{O_2} levels, and the progressive development of acute and chronic pulmonary O_2 toxicity (bronchopulmonary dysplasia or BPD) is unfortunately a not unusual complication of the necessary hyperoxic therapy.[4,13,29,86,93] Only recently have long-term follow-up studies of premature infants surviving respiratory distress syndrome/hyaline membrane disease and lung injury due to BPD been carried out, and several of these studies report what may be permanent pulmonary functional abnormalities and impaired respiratory reserve capacity due to O_2-induced lung injury incurred during the early days and weeks of life.[20,38,55]

While hyperoxic depression of cell nucleotide and protein biosynthesis during O_2 exposure will seriously interfere with ongoing repair capabilities in the adult lung, the problem is compounded when inhibition of cell proliferation by O_2 occurs during a normally active growth phase of the lung. Several studies in neonatal animals have now looked specifically at this effect and considered its implications for the clinical situation.[45,105,109] These studies have shown that an unappreciated consequence of prolonged O_2 exposure during the neonatal period is marked inhibition of the normal developmental process of alveolarization. When the newborn rat is exposed to hyperoxia during the early postnatal period when new alveoli formation should be occurring, with resultant expansion of the surface area of the lung involved in respiratory exchange, the process is very definitely blocked by the toxic effect of O_2 (Fig. 5). All of the predominant cell types of the lung are likely to be involved in the normal process of new alveolar wall formation. That the normal participation of the endothelium of the lung in this process is specifically inhibited by hyperoxia is suggested by the recent elegant demonstration of the blunting of normal lung vascular development by early postnatal O_2 exposure[105] (Fig. 6). These types of studies can be related to the fascinating biological concept of "critical periods" of maturation/development, i.e., if important maturational changes in an organ are interfered with when they are normally supposed to be occurring, will the

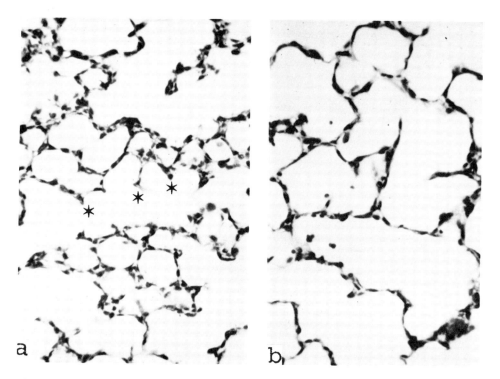

Figure 5: Inhibition of lung alveolarization by hyperoxia. *Lungs from 7-day-old rat pups maintained in room air (***a***) or exposed to 96–98% O_2 (***b***) from time of birth. Lungs fixed by inflation with 10% buffered formalin at 20 cm H_2O constant pressure. Hematoxylin and eosin stain. Original magnification ×100. Note presence of newly formed small air sacs (alveoli) adjacent to alveolar ducts in normal air-control lung at 7 days (***a***), and the virtual absence of small air sacs of similar size in O_2-exposed lungs (***b***). Developing alveolar septae or buds (∗) are also more prominent in air-control (***a***) than O_2-exposed lung (***b***). (From Frank and Groseclose,[45] courtesy of* The Journal of Applied Physiology.)

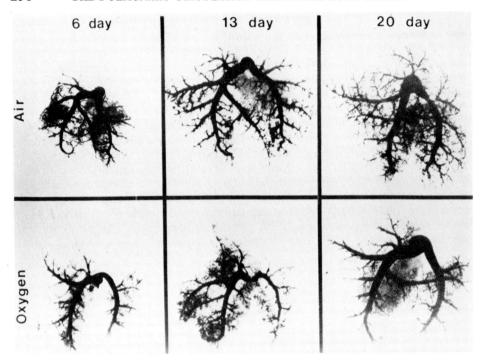

Figure 6: Inhibition of lung vascularization by hyperoxia. *Barium pulmonary artery angiograms performed in rat pups exposed to 21% O_2 (top panel) or >95% O_2 (bottom panel) for 6 days (left) and after recovery in room air for 1 week (center, 13 days), and 2 weeks (right, 20 days). Stunting of normal growth of finer distal vessels in O_2-exposed pup lungs is apparent. (From Roberts, et al (109), with permission of Pediatric Research/International Pediatric Research Foundation, Inc.)*

specific maturational changes merely be delayed, or will such changes be permanently bypassed once the normal "critical period" for their timed occurrence has passed? The hyperoxia studies in neonatal rats and other recent studies with hormonal interruption of the normal process of postnatal lung maturation (alveolarization) all suggest that permanent inhibition of alveolar formation and associated pulmonary vascular development may result.[85,109]

A morphological study by Sobonya et al.[122] on late survivors of BPD (died at age 3 years) in effect seems to confirm what the newborn animal studies suggested—that a consequence of prolonged hyperoxic therapy during the "critical period" of postnatal lung maturation can permanently impair normal lung development. The lungs of the BPD infants in this study had only 10×10^6 alveoli compared to a total of $125-175 \times 10^6$ alveoli in the lungs of age-matched control infants (accidental deaths), and a calculated surface area for respiratory exchange that was only one-third to one-half normal.[122]

Finally, to conclude this section on O_2 toxicity, we should reiterate that the effect of hyperoxic exposure on the nonrespiratory functions of the lung has been specifically examined in a variety of in vivo and in vitro systems.[8,9,11,123,124,128] Alterations of lung processing of a variety of vasoactive substances are a rather direct reflection of oxidant-induced injury to the endothelium. The studies, in effect, have uniformly shown that after 24 hours or less of exposure to >95% O_2, at a time when no endothelial cell morphological alterations are yet detectable, marked functional impairment is already manifested. This has now been shown to be the case with many of the substances normally processed by the endothelium, including serotonin and epinephrine,[8,9,124] angiotensin I,[123,124] and various prostanoids.[123,124] What has not been well investigated to date, surprisingly, are the possible systemic consequences of O_2-induced inhibition of these endothelial uptake and metabolic functions.[11,114] Intuitively, it would seem that passage of many of these potent vasoactive substances into the systemic circulation could produce serious perturbations of normal circulatory flow to various organ systems and perhaps contribute to some of the toxic effects in other organ systems (also poorly investigated to date) reported to occur in association with pulmonary O_2 toxicity.[5,19,44]

The Toxic Effects of Other Important Toxic Oxidants on the Pulmonary Endothelium

The various lung toxins listed in Table I are now believed to produce serious lung injury by means of a biochemical/molecular mechanism very similar to hyperoxia (O_2 free radical-induced cytotoxicity). Our appreciation of the similarity of the mechanism of toxic insult caused by hyperoxia and these other lung poisons has come about only gradually and through the interdisciplinary research work of many toxicologists, biochemists, chemists, radiation physicists, etc., too numerous to cite. Figure 7 presents examples of three clinically important oxidants whose toxic action on the cells of the lung are related to production of excess reactive O_2 species which presumably overwhelm the lung's antioxidant detoxifying capacity. As might be expected, each of these agents shows very accelerated or exacerbated lung-damaging effects when combined with hyperoxic exposure[40,61,76,102] and, conversely, a lessened toxicity under hypoxic conditions.[59,78,108]

Although these agents share a biochemical basis with hyperoxia for toxic interactions in the lung, there are some key differences in the overall pathological pattern of lung injury they produce which, in turn, can be related to the specific lung cells that they primarily injure. For example, the topically important herbicide, paraquat,[83,106] can be associated with damage to and necrosis of all the major cell types of the alveolus, yet its most extensive toxic action appears to be targeted for the type II cell, which has an avid uptake system for paraquat and related (poly)amines.[110,121,130] Initial edematous changes in the lung due to paraquat ingestion are primarily a reflection of increased permeability of the epithelial lining of the alveolus, which is different from the pathophysiology of early edema due to O_2 toxicity (endothelial cell permeability changes). Endothelial cell destruction in paraquat poisoning has been shown to be a more delayed toxic action of paraquat, and results in further edematous change and the appearance of characteristic pulmonary hemorrhages in experimental animals.[26,90,113] This delayed toxic effect may simply reflect the lessened uptake of paraquat in the endothelial cell compared to the more concentrated paraquat action in the epithelial cells. That higher concentrations of paraquat can definitely rapidly damage the lung endothelium has been demonstrated in a variety of in vitro and isolated lung studies, with monitoring

O$_2$ FREE RADICAL PRODUCTION BY LUNG TOXINS

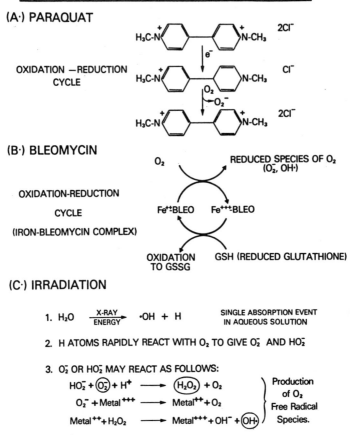

Figure 7: Free-radical production by lung toxins: (**A**) Paraquat; (**B**) Bleomycin; and (**C**) Irradiation. *Repeat oxidation-reduction cycles of paraquat and iron-bleomycin complex in the lung results in production of excess amounts of O_2^- (and, by subsequent interactions, other reactive O_2 species). Lung irradiation produces bursts of reactive O_2 species in target tissues, which are the same toxic O_2 metabolites involved in hyperoxic lung toxicity (O_2^-, H_2O_2, OH·). (From Frank,[43] courtesy of Trends in Pharmacological Sciences (TIPS) and Elsevier Science Publishers.)*

of toxicity by a combination of functional impairment and cell viability.[17,18,94] These and other studies have also provided important confirmatory evidence that protection from paraquat-induced endothelial cell injury is associated with the antioxidant defensive capacities of the lung cells.[17,18,41]

This last statement is also true of the findings of a variety of experimental studies of irradiation-induced lung damage. As Figure 7 indicates, irradiation produces the same cytotoxic O_2 species that are associated with hyperoxic exposure, and as might be predicted, the degree of lung damage that results has been related experimentally to the antioxidant complement of the lung (or the specific lung cells) tested. Augmentation of normal antioxidant enzyme levels has been demonstrated to reduce the expected degree of lung pathology post-irradiation,[46,81,96] while antioxidant enzyme inhibition or vitamin E depletion markedly increases the toxic effects of similar irradiation dosages.[79,80] There is conflicting information in the literature about the comparative sensitivity-resistance of the lung endothelial cell to the damaging effects of irradiation, but at least several well-wrought studies have demonstrated very early and progressive endothelial cell alterations after thoracic irradiation[2,99,132] and, in addition, imply that loss of capillary surface area and microvascular occlusion is a principal pathologic determinant of the chronic fibroemphysematous lung changes that are produced months after the provocative irradiation event.[2,99,132]

Capillary endothelial cell injury in the ozone or NO_2-exposed lung is not considered to be a prominent or consistently reproducible finding. The chemical reactivity of these two oxidant inhalants is such that only relatively small concentrations of the gases reach beyond the terminal conducting airways of the lung and into the distal alveoli. Most of the cellular injury is thus localized to the small airways and only the proximal alveolar ducts and acini.[23,34,118] Recent cross-tolerance experiments have shown that preexposure to O_3 results in increased lung antioxidant enzyme activities and, in turn, an increased protection of the O_3-preexposed animals from subsequent hyperoxia-induced lung injury and lethality (survival of non-preexposed rats in >95% $O_2 \times 7$ days = 2/18 (11%) vs. 28/32 (88%) for the O_3-preexposed groups).[71] The decreased edematous response to subsequent O_2 exposure that was observed in this study suggests that there was some influence of the 7-day exposure to 0.8 ppm O_3 on the lung endothelial cells which increased their subsequent tolerance to hyperoxic challenge.

Various in vivo and/or in vitro systems have been used to demonstrate a deleterious effect of some of the other clinically important hyperoxidant toxins such as bleomycin, nitrofurantoin, etc., on the integrity and/or function of the pulmonary endothelial cell population.[1,66]

Protection of the Lung (Endothelium) From Oxidant-Induced Toxicity

It's very often true that an understanding of the mechanism of a toxic process precedes the development of effective means to circumvent the toxic effects of that agent or process. The "free radical theory of O_2 toxicity" has helped us conceptualize why hyperoxia is associated with toxic lung damage and what normal defenses have evolved to control the potential toxicity of O_2, and has also provided us with some rational avenues of approach to therapeutic prevention of O_2 free radical-induced lung injury.

One clinically tested means to try to augment the lung's antioxidant defenses has been the administration of exogenous vitamin E and superoxide dismutase (SOD). Although initial success was reported from an early clinical trial of parenteral vitamin E as a prophylactic agent to prevent serious lung injury (BPD) in O_2-requiring premature infants,[31] several subsequent studies have unfortunately failed to show any positive effect of supplemental vitamin E on the incidence or severity of acute and chronic O_2 toxicity (BPD) in respiratory distressed premature infants.[30,101,115,133] Parenteral SOD therapy in O_2-requiring premature infants is just now being tested clinically.[111,112] The experimental effectiveness of parenteral SOD to prevent hyperoxidant-induced lung injury has been far from convincing, despite some reports of its successful use in animals versus hyperoxia, paraquat, and lung irradiation.[3,96-98,116,131] Many other studies have reported an inability to reproduce the positive protective effects of SOD claimed by earlier reports.[35,57,63,95,107] The inability of the 32,000 MW SOD protein to penetrate into the intracellular compartments of the lung cells where the excess O_2^- (superoxide radical) it detoxifies is being produced [69,70] makes it unlikely that standard preparations of SOD will be able to exert a significant beneficial effect against lung injury caused by the hyperoxidant toxins. However, the very recent use of liposomally encapsulated preparations of SOD and catalase to improve substantially the intracellular penetration of these antioxidant enzymes has been associated with exciting evidence for partial protection against O_2 toxicity and its edematous manifestations.[129] In addition, in vitro uptake of SOD and catalase in liposomes by cultured endothelial cells has been associated with significant protection of endothelial cell structural and functional integrity during high O_2 exposure.[51,52,89] The large surface area of the pulmonary microvascular lining with its apparent huge capacity for endocytosis and caveolae intracellulares formation and transport make the lung endothelium appear to be a prime site for effective augmentation of antioxidant enzyme levels by means of liposomally encapsulated enzyme treatment.

The stimulation of *endogenous* antioxidant enzyme activity represents another experimental approach to a similar end. For example, the preexposure of adult rats to sublethal levels of O_2 (80–85% O_2) for 5–7 days is associated with both the stimulation of increased lung antioxidant enzyme levels (SOD, CAT, GP, and G-6-PD) and a protective effect against the expected lethality from subsequent exposure to 100% O_2.[25,127] The morphological basis for the protective effect achieved in this experimental model has been recently related specifically to the endothelial cell changes found after the O_2-preexposure regimen, i.e., hypertrophied endothelial cells with a denser than normal distribution of intracellular organelles.[21,24] These morphologically altered endothelial cells are considered to be tolerant to further injury by 100% O_2 challenge. The authors also suggest that the tolerant endothelial cell population may be the site of augmented antioxidant enzyme activity as well. In another series of experimental studies, the use of small doses of bacterial endotoxin during hyperoxic exposure has been shown to markedly protect adult rats from pulmonary O_2 toxicity (survival in >95% O_2 increased from ~25% in untreated rats to >95% in endotoxin-treated groups).[42,43,48,49] Interestingly, associated with the protective action of endotoxin is the consistent finding in the treated animals of significant elevations of all the lung antioxidant enzymes during O_2 exposure, a response to >95% O_2 not found in O_2-susceptible untreated adult rats during similar exposure periods.[41-44,48,49,65]

Specific protection of the lung endothelium by endotoxin treatment has been hypothesized since marked reduction of the usual edematous manifestations of hyperoxia in the treated rats would suggest a preservation of capillary endothelial cell integrity. Morphological studies have provided evidence of decreased endothelial damage in endotoxin-treated O_2-exposed rats[48] (Fig. 3), and very recent in vitro studies have confirmed that endothelial cell function (amine uptake and normal membrane fluidity) after 24 hours in hyperoxia is significantly protected by endotoxin.[7,10] Even after 7 days of exposure to 100% O_2, in fact, the lung uptake of serotonin and norepinephrine in endotoxin-treated rats has been reported to be no different than in air control rats.[7]

While at present there are no specific agents available clinically to help circumvent the severe acute and chronic lung damage that may result from prolonged treatment with elevated concentrations of O_2, there is reason to be optimistic that a little more experimental study will result in clinical trials of some of the experimentally quite successful modes of prophylaxis against hyperoxidant toxicity. In addition to the possible use of liposomally encapsulated antioxidant enzymes and perhaps the use of chemical antioxidants such as the "nontoxic" O_2 radical scavenger dimethylthiourea (DMTU),[39,126] endotoxinlike agents that stimulate the endogenous antioxidant defense system activity in the lung all represent promising approaches to prophylaxis against clinical O_2 toxicity.

Summary

Under normoxic conditions, the pulmonary endothelium seems ideally suited for its complex barrier-metabolic role in maintaining lung fluid balance. Under hyperoxic conditions, the failure of the endothelial cell barrier function due to its apparent hypersensitivity to elevated levels of alveolar O_2 initiates the cascade of exudative changes that can progress to the full-fledged pathology of pulmonary O_2 toxicity. If, indeed, "Nature never says one thing and wisdom another" (Juvenal, *Satire XIV*), then we simply must learn more than we now know in order to understand why the endothelial cell is the lung cell most sensitive to altered O_2 tension and, perhaps, why this should be a part of the overall design of the lung. At the same time, continued study of methods to augment the antioxidant defense capacity of the lung may provide us with a means of augmenting the ability of the endothelium to act as an effective barrier even under unnatural hyperoxidant stress conditions.

Addendum

Retrolental fibroplasia (RLF) is a clinically important problem in premature newborn infants. The damaging effect of hyperoxia on the endothelium of the developing microvasculature of the peripheral retina may lead to various degrees of permanent visual impairment, even complete blindness. The reader interested in this O_2-endothelial cell interaction is referred to several fine recent reviews on RLF.[36,72,120]

REFERENCES

1. Adamson, I.Y.R.: Pulmonary toxicity of bleomycin. *Environ. Health Perspect.* 16:119–126, 1976.
2. Adamson, I.Y.R., Bowden, D.M., and Wyatt, J.P.: A pathway to pulmonary fibrosis: An ultrastructural study of mouse and rat following radiation to the whole body and hemithorax. *Am. J. Pathol.* 58:481–498, 1970.
3. Autor, A.P.: Reduction of paraquat toxicity by superoxide dismutase. *Life Sci.* 14:1309–1319, 1974.
4. Avery, M.E., Fletcher, B.D., and Williams, R.G. eds.: *The Lung and Its Disorders in the Newborn Infant*. Philadelphia, W.B. Saunders, 1981, pp. 222–262.

5. Balentine, J.D.: Experimental pathology of oxygen toxicity. In *Oxygen and Physiologic Function*, Jobsis, J.J., eds. Dallas, Professional Information Library, 1977, pp. 311–378.

6. Barber, R.E., Lee, J., and Hamilton, W.K.: Oxygen toxicity in man: A prospective study in patients with irreversible brain damage. *N. Engl. J. Med.* 273:1478–1484, 1970.

7. Block, E.R.: Endotoxin protects against hyperoxic alterations in lung endothelial cell metabolism. *J. Appl. Physiol.* 54:24–30, 1983.

8. Block, E.R. and Cannon, J.K.: Effect of oxygen exposure on lung clearance of amines. *Lung* 155:287–295, 1978.

9. Block, E.R. and Fisher, A.B.: Depression of serotonin clearance by rat lungs during oxygen exposure. *J. Appl. Physiol.* 43:33–38, 1977.

10. Block, E.R. and Patel, J.M.: Endotoxin protects against hyperoxic decrease in membrane fluidity in endothelial cells but not in fibroblasts. *Am. Rev. Respir. Dis.* (In press).

11. Block, E.R. and Stalcup, S.A.: Metabolic functions of the lung. Of what clinical relevance? *Chest* 2:215–223, 1981.

12. Block, E.R. and Stalcup, S.A.: Depression of serotonin uptake by cultured endothelial cells exposed to high O_2 tension. *J. Appl. Physiol.* 50:1212–1219, 1981.

13. Bonikos, D.S., Bensch, K.G., Northway, W.H., Jr., et al.: Bronchopulmonary dysplasia: The pulmonary pathologic sequelae of necrotizing bronchiolitis and pulmonary fibrosis. *Human Pathol.* 7:643–666, 1976.

14. Bowden, D.H. and Adamson, I.Y.R.: Endothelial regeneration as a marker of the differential vascular responses in oxygen-induced pulmonary edema. *Lab. Invest.* 30:350–357, 1974.

15. Brawn, K. and Fridovich, I.: Superoxide radical and superoxide dismutases: threat and defense. *Acta Physiol. Scand. Suppl.* 492:9–18, 1980.

16. Brooksby, G.A.: Experimental emphysema: Histologic changes and alterations in pulmonary circulation. *California Med.* 107:391–395, 1967.

17. Bus, J. S., Aust, S.D., and Gibson, J.E.: Lipid peroxidation as a proposed mechanism for paraquat toxicity. In *Biochemical Mechanisms of Paraquat Toxicity*. Autor, A. P., ed. New York, Academic Press, 1977, pp. 152–172.

18. Bus, J.S., Cagen, S.Z., Olgaard, R., et al.: A mechanism of paraquat toxicity in mice and rats. *Toxicol. Appl. Pharmacol.* 35:501–513, 1976.

19. Clark, J.M. and Lamberston, C.J.: Pulmonary oxygen toxicity: A review. *Pharmacol. Rev.* 23:37–133, 1971.

20. Coates, A.L., Desmond, K., Willis, D., et al.: Oxygen therapy and long-term pulmonary outcome of respiratory distress syndrome in newborns. *Am. J. Dis. Child* 136:892–895, 1982.

21. Crapo, J.D., Barry B.E., Foscue, H.A., et al.: Structural and biochemical changes in rat lungs occurring during oxygen exposures to lethal and adaptive doses of oxygen. *Am. Rev. Respir. Dis.* 122:123–143, 1980.

22. Crapo, J. D., Freeman, B.A., Barry, B. E., et al.: Mechanisms of hyperoxic injury to the pulmonary microcirculation. *The Physiologist* 26:170–176, 1983.

23. Crapo, J.D., Marsh-Salin, J., Ingram, P., et al.: Tolerance and cross-tolerance using NO_2 and O_2. II. Pulmonary morphology and morphometry. *J. Appl. Physiol.* 44:370–379, 1978.

24. Crapo, J.D., Peters-Golden, M., Marsh-Salin, J., et al.: Pathologic changes in the lungs of oxygen-adapted rats: A morphometric analysis. *Lab Invest.* 39:640–653, 1978.

25. Crapo, J.D. and Tierney, D.F.: Superoxide dismutase and pulmonary oxygen toxicity. *Am. J. Physiol.* 226:1401–1407, 1974.

26. Dearden, L.C., Fairshter, R.D., Morrison, J.T., et al.: Ultrastructural evidence of pulmonary capillary endothelial damage from paraquat. *Toxicol.* 24:211–222, 1982.

27. DelMaestro, R.F.: An approach to free radicals in medicine and biology. *Acta Physiol. Scand. Suppl.* 492:153–168, 1980.

28. Deneke, S.M. and Fanburg, B.L.: Normobaric oxygen toxicity. *N. Engl. J. Med.* 303:76–86, 1980.

29. Edwards, D.K., Dyer, W.M., and Northway, W.H., Jr.: Twelve years experience with bronchopulmonary dysplasia. *Pediatrics* 59:839–846, 1977.

30. Ehrenkrantz, R.A., Ablow, R.C., and Warshaw, J.B.: Prevention of bronchopulmonary dysplasia with vitamin E administration during the acute stages of respiratory distress syndrome. *J. Pediatr.* 95:373–378, 1979.

31. Ehrenkrantz, R.A., Bonta, B.W., Ablow, R.C., et al.: Amelioration of bronchopulmonary dysplasia after vitamin E administration: A preliminary report. *N. Engl. J. Med.* 299:564–569, 1978.

32. Evans, M.J. and Hackney, J.D.: Cell proliferation in lungs of mice exposed to elevated concentrations of oxygen. *Aerospace Med.* 43:620–622, 1972.

33. Evans, M.J., Hackney, J.D., and Bils, R.F.: Effects of a high concentration of oxygen on cell renewal in the pulmonary alveoli. *Aerospace Med.* 40:1365–1368, 1969.

34. Evans, M.J., Johnson, L.V., Stephens, R.J., et al.: Cell renewal in the lungs of rats exposed to low levels of ozone. *Exp. Mol. Pathol.* 24:70–73, 1976.

35. Fairshter, R.D., Rosen, S.M., Smith, W.E., et al.: Paraquat poisoning: New aspects of therapy. *Quart. J. Med.* 45:551–565, 1976.

36. Flower, R.W. and Patz, A.: Retinopathy of prematurity and the role of oxygen. In *Oxygen and Living Processes. An Interdisciplinary Approach.* Gilbert, D. L., ed. New York, Springer-Verlag, 1981, pp. 368–375.

37. Forman, H.J. and Fisher, A.B.: Antioxidant defenses. In *Oxygen and Living Processes. An Interdisciplinary Approach.* Gilbert, D.L., ed. New York, Springer-Verlag, 1981, pp. 235–249.

38. Fox, W.N.: Bronchopulmonary dysplasia: Clinical course and outpatient therapy. *Pediatr. Annals* 7:75–85, 1978.

39. Fox, R.B. and Murphy, K.A.: Scavenging oxygen radicals in vivo: Prevention of pulmonary oxygen toxicity by the hydroxyl radical scavenger, dimethylthiourea. *Am. Rev. Respir. Dis.* 125:149, 1982 (Abstr.).

40. Fisher, H.K., Clements, J.A., and Wright, R.R.: Enhancement of oxygen toxicity by the herbicide paraquat. *Am. Rev. Respir. Dis.* 107:246–252, 1973.

41. Frank, L.: Prolonged survival after paraquat: Role of the lung antioxidant enzyme systems. *Biochem. Pharmacol.* 30:2319–2324, 1981.

42. Frank, L.: Endotoxin reverses the decreased tolerance of rats to >95% O_2 after preexposure to lower O_2. *J. Appl. Physiol.* 51:577–583, 1981.

43. Frank, L.: Superoxide dismutase and lung toxicity. *Trends Pharmacol. Sci.* 4:124–128, 1983.

44. Frank, L.: Oxygen toxicity in eukaryotes. In *Superoxide Dismutase, Vol. III, Pathological States.* Oberley, L.W., ed. Boca Raton, Florida, CRC Press (In press).

45. Frank, L. and Groseclose, E.E.: Oxygen toxicity in newborns: The adverse effects of undernutrition. *J. Appl. Physiol.* 53:1248–1255, 1982.

46. Frank, L., Lapidus, R., and Ahmad, K.: Protection against radiation pneumonitis in rats: Role of the lung antioxidant enzymes. *Fed. Proc.* 40:425, 1981 (Abstr.).

47. Frank, L. and Massaro, D.: Oxygen toxicity. *Am. J. Med.* 69:117–126, 1980.

48. Frank, L. and Roberts, R.J.: Oxygen toxicity: Protection of the lung by bacterial lipopolysaccharide (endotoxin). *Toxicol. Appl. Pharmacol.* 50:371–380, 1979.

49. Frank, L., Summerville, J., and Massaro, D.: Protection from oxygen toxicity with endotoxin: Role of the endogenous antioxidant enzymes of the lung. *J. Clin. Invest.* 65:1104–1110, 1980.

50. Freeman, B.A. and Crapo, J.D.: Biology of disease. Free radicals and tissue injury. *Lab. Invest.* 47:412–426, 1982.

51. Freeman, B.A., Turrens, J.F., Crapo, J.D., et al.: Protection against oxygen toxicity in rats and in cultured endothelial cells following treatment with liposome-

entrapped superoxide dismutase and catalase. *Am. Rev. Respir. Dis.* 127:273, 1983 (Abstr.).

52. Freeman, B.A., Young, S.L., and Crapo, J.D.: Liposome-mediated augmentation of superoxide dismutase in endothelial cells prevents oxygen injury. *J. Biol. Chem.* 258:12534–12542, 1983.

53. Fridovich, I.: Oxygen radicals, hydrogen peroxide, and oxygen toxicity. In *Free Radicals in Biology*, Vol. I. Pryor, W.A., ed. New York, Academic Press, 1976, pp. 239–277.

54. Fridovich, I.: The biology of oxygen radicals. *Science* 201:875–880, 1978.

55. Gerhardt, T., Tapia, J.L., Goldman, S.L., et al.: Serial lung function measurements in infants with chronic lung disease. *Pediatr. Res.* 17:376, 1983 (Abstr.).

56. Gilder, H. and McSherry, C.K.: Phosphatidylcholine synthesis and pulmonary oxygen toxicity. *Biochim. Biophys. Acta* 441:48–56, 1976.

57. Giri, S.N., Hollinger, M.A., and Schiedt, M.J.: The effects of paraquat and superoxide dismutase on pulmonary vascular permeability and edema in mice. *Arch. Environ. Health* 36:149–154, 1981.

58. Gould, V.E., Tosco, R., Wheelis, R.F., et al.: Oxygen pneumonitis in man. Ultrastructural observations on the development of alveolar lesions. *Lab. Invest.* 26: 499–508, 1972.

59. Gray, L.H.: Oxygenation in radiotherapy. I. Radiobiological considerations. *Br. J. Radiol.* 30:403–406, 1957.

60. Gross, N.J., and Smith, D.M.: Impaired surfactant phospholipid metabolism in hyperoxic mouse lungs. *J. Appl. Physiol.* 51:1198–1203, 1981.

61. Hakkinen, P.J., Whiteley, J.W., and Witschi, H.P.: Hyperoxia, but not thoracic X-irradiation, potentiates bleomycin- and cyclophosphamide-induced lung damage in mice. *Am. Rev. Respir. Dis.* 126:281–285, 1982.

62. Halliwell, B.: Biochemical mechanisms accounting for the toxic action of oxygen on living organisms: The key role of superoxide dismutase. *Cell Biol. Intern. Rep.* 2:113–128, 1978.

63. Harley, J.B., Grinspan, S., and Root, R.K.: Paraquat suicide in a young woman: Results of therapy directed against the superoxide radical. *Yale J. Biol. Med.* 50:481–488, 1977.

64. Harrison, G.A.: Ultrastructural changes in rat lung during long-term exposure to oxygen. *Exp. Med. Surg.* 29:96–107, 1971.

65. Hass, M.A., Frank, L., and Massaro, D.: The effect of bacterial endotoxin on synthesis of (Cu, Zn) superoxide dismutase in lung of oxygen-exposed rats. *J. Biol. Chem.* 257:9379–9383, 1982.

66. Hijiya, K.: Ultrastructural study of lung injury induced by bleomycin sulfate in rats. *J. Clin. Electron Microscopy* 11:245–292, 1978.

67. Huber, G.L. and Drath, D.B.: Pulmonary oxygen toxicity. In *Oxygen and Living Processes. An Interdisciplinary Approach.* Gilbert, D.L., ed. New York, Springer-Verlag, 1981, pp. 273–342.

68. Huber, G.L., LaForce, F.M., and Mason, R.J.: Impairment and recovery of pulmonary antibacterial defense mechanisms after oxygen administration. *J. Clin. Invest.* 49:47–58, 1970.

69. Huber, W. and Saifer, M.G.P.: Orgotein, the drug version of bovine Cu-Zn superoxide dismutase. I. A summary account of safety and pharmacology in laboratory animals. In *Superoxide and Superoxide Dismutases*. Michelson, A.M., Cord, J.M., and Fridovich, I., eds. New York, Academic Press, 1977, pp. 517–536.

70. Huber, W., Saifer, M.G.P., and Williams, L.D.: Superoxide dismutase pharmacology and orgotein efficacy: New perspectives. In *Biological and Clinical Aspects of Superoxide and Superoxide Dismutase.* Bannister, W.H. and Bannister, J.V., eds. New York, Elsevier/North Holland, 1980, pp. 395–407.

71. Jackson, R.M. and Frank, L.: Ozone and oxygen cross-tolerance: Demonstration and common biochemical adaptations. *Am. Rev. Respir. Dis.* 129:425–429, 1984.

72. James, L.S. and Lanman, J.T.: History of oxygen therapy and retrolental fibroplasia. *Pediatrics* (Suppl.)57:591–642, 1976.

73. Kafer, E.R.: Pulmonary oxygen toxicity: A review of the evidence for acute and chronic oxygen toxicity in man. *Br. J. Anesthesiol* 43:687–695, 1971.

74. Kapanci, Y., Tosco, R., Eggermann, J., et al.: Oxygen pneumonitis in man: Light and electron-microscopic morphometric studies. *Chest* 62:162–169, 1972.

75. Kapanci, Y., Weibel, E.R., Kaplan, H.P., et al.: Pathogenesis and reversibility of the pulmonary lesions of oxygen toxicity in monkeys. II. Ultrastructural and morphometric studies. *Lab. Invest.* 20:101–118, 1969.

76. Kehrer, J.P., Haschek, W.M., and Witschi, H.: The influence of hyperoxia on the acute toxicity of paraquat and diquat. *Drug Chem. Toxicol.* 2:397–408, 1979.

77. Kistler, D.C., Caldwell, P.R.B., and Weibel, E.R.: Development of fine structural damage to alveolar and capillary lining cells in oxygen-poisoned rat lung. *J. Cell Biol.* 32:605–628, 1967.

78. Koch, C.J., Kruuv, J., and Frey, H.E.: Variation in radiation response of mammalian cells as a function of oxygen tenson. *Radiat. Res.* 53:33–42, 1973.

79. Konings, A.W.T., Damen, J., and Trieling, W.B.: Protection of liposomal lipids against irradiation-induced oxidative damage. *Int. J. Radiat. Biol.* 35:343–350, 1979.

80. Konings, A.W.T. and Drijver, E.B.: Radiation effects on membranes. I. Vitamin E deficiency and lipid peroxidation. *Radiat. Res.* 80:494–501, 1979.

81. Krizala, J., Kovarova, M., Kratochvilova, V., et al.: Importance of superoxide dismutase for the acute radiation syndrome. In *Biological and Clinical Aspects of Superoxide and Superoxide Dismutase*. Bannister, W.H. and Bannister, J.V., eds. New York, Elsevier/North Holland, 1980, pp. 327–334.

82. Lavelle, F., Michelson, A.M., and Dimitrijevic, L.: Biological protection by superoxide dismutase. *Biochem. Biophys. Res. Commun.* 55:350–357, 1973.

83. Marshall, E.: Pot-spraying plan raises some smoke. *Science* 217:429, 1982.

84. Massaro, G.D. and Massaro, D.: Adaption to hyperoxia. Influence on protein synthesis by lung and on granular pneumocyte ultrastructure. *J. Clin. Invest.* 53:705–709, 1974.

85. Maxwell, S., Whitney, P., Ryan, U., et al.: Lung lectin: Cell source and potential role in alveolarization. *Clin. Res.* 31:916A, 1983 (Abstr.).

86. Mayes, L., Perkett, E., and Stahlman, M.T.: Severe bronchopulmonary dysplasia: A retrospective review. *Acta Paediatr. Scand.* 72:225–229, 1983.

87. McCord, J.M. and Wong, K.: Phagocyte-produced free radicals: Roles in cytotoxicity and inflammation. In *Oxygen Free Radicals and Tissue Damage*. CIBA Foundation Symposium No. 65, Amsterdam, Excerpta Medica, 1979, pp. 343–360.

88. Michelson, A.M.: Toxicity of superoxide radical ions. In *Superoxide and Superoxide Dismutases*. Michelson, A.M., McCord, J.M., and Fridovich, I., eds. New York, Academic Press, 1977, pp. 245–255.

89. Michelson, A.M., Puget, K., Perdereau, B., et al.: Scintigraph studies on the localization of liposomal superoxide dismutase injected into rabbits. *Mol. Physiol.* 1: 71–84, 1981.

90. Modée, J., Ivemark, B.I., and Robertson, B.: Ultrastructure of the alveolar wall in experimental paraquat poisoning. *Acta Pathol. Microbiol. Scand.* 80:54–60, 1972.

91. Mustafa, M.G. and Tierney, D.F.: Biochemical and metabolic changes in the lung with oxygen, ozone, and nitrogen dioxide. *Am. Rev. Respir. Dis.* 118:1061–1090, 1978.

92. Northway, W.H., Jr., Rezcan, L., Petriceks, R., et al.: Oxygen toxicity in the newborn lung: Reversal of inhibition of DNA synthesis in the mouse. *Pediatrics* 57:41–46, 1976.

93. Northway, W.H., Jr., Rosan, R.C., and Porter, D.Y.: Pulmonary disease following respiratory therapy of hyaline-membrane disease: Bronchopulmonary dysplasia. *N. Engl. J. Med.* 276:357–368, 1967.

94. Ody, C. and Junod, A.F.: Paraquat induced cytotoxicty in cultured endothelial cells. *Am. Rev. Respir. Dis.* 127:285, 1983 (Abstr.).

95. Patterson, C.E. and Rhodes, M.L.: The effect of superoxide dismutase on paraquat mortality in mice and rats. *Toxicol. Appl. Pharmacol.* 62:65–72, 1982.

96. Petkau, A.: Radiation protection by superoxide dismutase. *Photochem. Photobiol.* 28:765–774, 1978.

97. Petkau, A., Kelly, K., Chelack, W.S., et al.: Protective effect of superoxide dismutase on erythrocytes of X-irradiated mice. *Biochem. Biophys. Res. Commun.* 70:452–458, 1976.

98. Petkau, A., Kelly, K., Chelack, W.S., et al.: Radioprotection of mice by superoxide dismutase. *Biochem. Biophys. Res. Commun.* 65:886–893, 1975.

99. Phillips, T.L.: An ultrastructural study of the development of radiation injury in the lung. *Radiology* 87:49–54, 1966.

100. Pratt, P.C.: Pathology of pulmonary oxygen toxicity. *Am. Rev. Respir. Dis.* 110:51–57, 1974.

101. Puklin, J.E., Simon, R.M., and Ehrenkranz, R.A.: Influence on retrolental fibroplasia of intramuscular vitamin E administration during respiratory distress syndrome. *Ophthalmology* 89:96–102, 1982.

102. Quintiliana, M.: Modification of radiation sensitivity: The oxygen effect. *Int. J. Radiat. Oncol. Biol. Phys.* 5:1069–1076, 1979.

103. Raffin, T.A., Simon, L.M., Braun, D., et al.: Impairment of phagocytosis by moderate hyperoxia (40–60% oxygen) in lung macrophages. *Lab. Invest.* 42:622–626, 1980.

104. Raj, J.U. and Bland, R.D.: Neutrophil depletion does not prevent oxygen-induced lung injury in rabbits. *Am. Rev. Respir. Dis.* 125:274, 1982 (Abstr.).

105. Raub, J.A., Mercer, R.R., O'Neil, J.J., et al.: Alterations in lung function of rat pups following postnatal alveolarization in 60% O_2. *Am. Rev. Respir. Dis.* 125:169, 1982 (Abstr.).

106. Revkin, A.C.: Paraquat: A potent weed killer is killing people. *Science Digest*, June 1983, pp. 36–42, 100–104.

107. Rhodes, M.L. and Patterson, C.E.: Effect of exogenous superoxide dismutase on paraquat toxicity. *Am. Rev. Respir. Dis.* 117:255, 1978 (Abstr.).

108. Rhodes, M.L., Zavala, D.C., and Brown, D.: Hypoxic protection in paraquat poisoning. *Lab. Invest.* 35:496–500, 1976.

109. Roberts, R.J., Weesner, K.M., and Bucher, J.R.: Oxygen-induced alterations in lung vascular development in the newborn rat. *Pediatr. Res.* 17:368–375, 1983.

110. Rose, M.S. and Smith, L.L.: The relevance of paraquat accumulation by tissues. In *Biochemical Mechanisms of Paraquat Toxicity.* Autor, A.P., ed. New York, Academic Press, 1977, pp. 71–91.

111. Rosenfeld, W., Evans, H., Concepcion, L., et al.: Prevention of bronchopulmonary dysplasia by administration of bovine superoxide dismutase in preterm infants with respiratory distress syndrome. *J. Pediatr.* 105:781–784, 1984.

112. Rosenfeld, W., Evans, H., Jhaveri, R., et al.: Safety and plasma concentrations of bovine superoxide dismutase administered to human premature infants. *Dev. Pharmacol. Ther.* 5:151–161, 1982.

113. Roth, R.A., Wallace, K.B., Alper, R.H., et al.: Effect of paraquat treatment of rats on dispositon of 5-hydroxy-tryptamine and angiotensin I by perfused lung. *Biochem. Pharmacol.* 28:2349–2355, 1979.

114. Ryan, J.W. and Ryan, U.S.: Humoral control of arterial blood pressure: A role for the lung? *Cardiovasc. Med.* 3:531–552, 1978.

115. Saldana, R.K., Cepeda, E.E., and Poland, R.L.: The effect of vitamin E prophylaxis on the incidence and severity of bronchopulmonary dysplasia. *J. Pediatr.* 101:89–93, 1982.

116. Schwartz, D.J., Ballis, J.U., and Jensen, R.: Parenteral superoxide dismutase (SOD) prophylaxis for thoracic irradiation. *Am. Rev. Respir. Dis.* 125:228, 1982 (Abstr.).

117. Schwartz, F.A., Niewoehner, D.E., and Hoidal, J.R.: Neutrophil depletion does not protect rats from hyperoxic lung injury. *Clin. Res.* 31:746A, 1983 (Abstr.).

118. Schwartz, L.W., Dungsworth, D.L., Mustafa, M.G., et al.: Pulmonary responses of rats to ambient levels of ozone. Effects of 7-day intermittent or continuous exposure. *Lab. Invest.* 34:565–578, 1976.

119. Shasby, D.M., Fox, R.B., Harada, R.N., et al.: Reduction of edema of acute hyperoxic lung injury by granulocyte depletion. *J. Appl. Physiol.* 52:1237–1244, 1982.

120. Silverman, W.A.: The lesson of retrolental fibroplasia. *Sci. Am.* 236:100–107, 1977.

121. Smith, L.L., Rose, M.S., and Wyatt, I.: The pathology and biochemistry of paraquat. In *Oxygen Free Radical and Tissue Damage.* CIBA Foundation Symposium No. 65, Amsterdam, Excerpta Medica, 1979, pp. 321–341.

122. Sobonya, R.E., Logvinoff, M.M., Taussig, L.M., et al.: Morphometric analysis of the lung in prolonged bronchopulmonary dysplasia. *Pediatr. Res.* 16:969–972, 1983.

123. Stalcup, S.A. and Mellins, R.B.: Endothelial cells injured by 20 hours of hyperoxia have augmented bradykinin-stimulated prostacyclin release, a higher thromboxane A_2: Prostacyclin ratio and decreased angiotensin converting enzyme activity. *Am. Rev. Respir. Dis.* 125:275, 1982 (Abstr.).

124. Stalcup, S.A., Turino, G.M., and Mellins, R.B.: Endothelial cell function in altered oxygen environments. In *Pathobiology of the Endothelial Cell.* Nossel, H.L. and Vogel, H.J., ed. New York, Academic Press, 1982, pp. 455–469.

125. Tate, I.M. and Repine, J.E.: Neutrophils and the adult respiratory distress syndrome. *Am. Rev. Respir. Dis.* 128:552–559, 1983.

126. Tate, R.M., Van Benthuysen, K.M., Shasby, D.M., et al.: Dimethylthiourea, a hydroxyl radical scavenger, blocks oxygen radical-induced acute edematous lung injury in an isolated perfused lung. *Am. Rev. Respir. Dis.* 123:243, 1981 (Abstr.).

127. Tierney, D.F., Ayers, L., and Kasuyama, R.S.: Altered sensitivity to oxygen toxicity. *Am. Rev. Respir. Dis.* 115:59–65, 1977.

128. Toivonon, H., Hartiala, J., and Bakhle, Y.S.: Effects of high oxygen tension on the metabolism of vasoactive hormones in isolated perfused rat lungs. *Acta Physiol. Scand.* 111:185–192, 1981.

129. Turrens, J.F., Crapo, J.D., and Freeman, B.A.: Protection against oxygen toxicity by intravenous injection of liposome-entrapped catalase and superoxide dismutase. *J. Clin. Invest.* 73:87–95, 1984.

130. Waddell, W.J. and Marlowe, C.: Tissue and cellular distribution of paraquat in mice. *Toxicol. Appl. Pharmacol.* 56:127–140, 1980.

131. Wasserman, B. and Block, E.R.: Prevention of acute paraquat toxicity in rats by superoxide dismutase. *Aviat. Space Environ. Med.* 49:805–809, 1978.

132. Watanabe, S., Watanabe, K., Ohishi, T., et al.: Mast cells in the rat alveolar septa undergoing fibrosis after ionizing irradiation: Ultrastructural and histochemical studies. *Lab. Invest.* 31:555–567, 1974.

133. Watts, J.L., Pocs, B.A., Milner, R.A., et al.: Randomized control trial of vitamin E and bronchopulmonary dysplasia. *Pediatr. Res.* 15:686, 1981 (Abstr.).

CHAPTER 13

Oxygen Radicals and Pulmonary Edema

Aubrey E. Taylor,
Denis J. Martin,* and
Mary I. Townsley*

Introduction

During the past 10 years, a great deal of experimental information has accumulated indicating that the reduction of molecular oxygen to superoxide (O_2^-), hydrogen peroxide (H_2O_2), and hydroxyl radicals $(OH^{\cdot})$ results in damage to biological membranes and extracellular constituents. These primary oxygen radicals can be generated by damaged pulmonary epithelium and endothelium and by activated tissue macrophages. In addition, neutrophils that enter the pulmonary tissues because of some chemical signal produced by the damaged tissues release these toxic compounds. The result is lipid peroxidation, nucleic acid damage, and protein denaturation. The purpose of this chapter is not to discuss each form and type of free radical production, but to acquaint the reader with the basic chemistry thought to be involved in producing oxygen radicals and to indicate how these compounds are involved with several seemingly unrelated forms of pulmonary pathology.[6,9,10,13,21,23,39,52–54,56,65]

In order to present the available information concerning the effects of free radicals in producing lung pathology, this chapter is divided into three major subdivisions. The first section presents the basic chemical pathways in which free radicals can be produced by either pulmonary tissues or the macrophage-leukocyte systems. The concepts of how the various superoxides can be eliminated or removed from lung tissue either by altering their removal enzymatically or by preventing their formation will also be presented. The second section of this chapter discusses how different oxygen radical generating systems are thought to be involved in producing the lung pathology associated with hyperoxia, thiourea, α-napthylthiourea (ANTU), *E. coli* endotoxin, microemboli challenge, or complement activation. The third and final section of this chapter presents the many other types of lung damage that could be related to free radical production and have not yet been studied in detail.

*D. Martin and M. Townsley were both Parker B. Francis - Puritan-Bennet Foundation Pulmonary Research Fellows.

From Said, S.I. (ed.): *The Pulmonary Circulation and Acute Lung Injury.* Mount Kisco, N.Y., Futura Publishing Co., Inc., 1985.

The overall aim of this chapter is to acquaint the reader with a basic understanding of the free radical system as it relates to the inflammatory response and related pathology in lung tissue. However, the reference material will direct the reader to sources that present more in-depth analyses of this important biological system in both plants and animals. This is a most timely research topic and we hope that the reader will enjoy the content of this chapter as much as the authors have enjoyed producing it.

Superoxide Production

$$O_2 \xrightarrow{e^-} O_2^- \xrightarrow{e^- + 2H^+} H_2O_2 \xrightarrow[\searrow H_2O]{e^- + H^+} OH^{\cdot} \xrightarrow{e^- + H^+} H_2O$$

The complete reduction of O_2 results in the formation of the superoxide anion radical (O_2^-), hydrogen peroxide (H_2O_2), and the hydroxyl radical ($OH^{\cdot}$) as the intermediates of the process. These compounds are highly reactive in tissues and must be removed (scavenged) and/or their formation must be controlled or the tissues will ultimately be destroyed.

A variety of enzymatic processes act as defense mechanisms to bypass or prevent the formation of these radicals as O_2 is reduced.

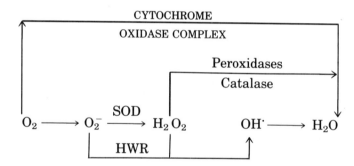

The majority of the O_2 reduction by aerobic cells is carried out tetravalently by cytochrome oxidase,[1] which totally bypasses the production of any toxic oxygen radicals. However, O_2^- can be normally produced within cells by a variety of means. For example, autoxidation of hemoglobin or myoglobin, enzymatic oxidations catalyzed by xanthine oxidase (hypoxanthine $\longrightarrow$ xanthine) and NADPH-oxidase (neutrophils and macrophages), and mitochondrial autoxidation of reduced electron transport systems all result in the production of O_2^-.[22,23] In fact, the O_2^- production by neutrophils is actually an important biochemical defense mechanism, since those cells kill invading bacteria by forming $OH^{\cdot}$ by the Haber-Weiss reaction (HWR) as H_2O_2 and O_2^- combine.[27] In addition, hydrogen peroxide can combine with chloride in the presence of myeloperoxidase to form hypochlorus acid (HOCL), a very potent bactericide (it is actually laundry bleach) that can cause severe structural damage to both cellular membranes and extracellular constituents.[57]

Hydrogen peroxide is produced when O_2^- is dismutated to H_2O_2[43] and by divalent reduction of O_2^- by enzymes such as glycolate-oxidase.[9,42] H_2O_2 is not present in any significant quantities in most cells, indicating that H_2O_2 is probably decomposed as reduced glutathione is oxidized by H_2O_2 in the presence of glutathione peroxidase.[44] H_2O_2 or O_2 generation alone are usually not thought to be too damaging to the cell since the amount of scavengers present can efficiently detoxify these species, but when HOCl or hydroxyl radicals are found, severe tissue damage will always result.

When the superoxide radical is formed, the enzyme superoxide dismutase (SOD)[41] rapidly converts this compound to hydrogen peroxide (H_2O_2), which is subsequently reduced by peroxidases to H_2O. Since these enzymes exist in all tissues, it is obvious that the tissues have been geared to detoxify or scavenge this compound and its products. In addition to SOD and the peroxidases, other compounds such as vitamin E (α-tocopherol), β-carotene, and glutathione peroxidase can reduce the degree of lipid peroxidation of membranes in the presence of oxygen radicals.[53,54] Other compounds that may also control radical formation, detoxify them, or reduce the amount of lipid peroxidation once formed in cellular membranes or extracellular fluid compartments are ascorbic acid, cysteine, reduced glutathione, ceruloplasmin, and transferrin.[4,11,26,39,45,53,54]

If radical intermediates are not rapidly scavenged by the cell, however, a variety of deleterious effects can result, including lipid peroxidation, nucleic acid damage, and protein denaturation.[9,21] Lipid peroxidation is directly related to loss of membrane viability and cell death. In additon, H_2O_2 may lead to cell death directly by some as yet unknown chemical mechanism independent of its involvement in lipid peroxidation.[59,71] Thus, cell membranes are very susceptible to free radical damage. In addition,the various structural components of the interstitial matrix such as hyaluronic acid are also damaged by free radicals.[8,41] The cell normally has an adequate supply of oxygen radical scavengers, so almost no damage occurs under usual circumstances. However, the extracellular fluids contain only very low levels of catalase and SOD, so the interstitial matrix may be easily damaged by only small concentrations of oxygen radicals.[60]

Figure 1 is a schematic diagram indicating how the processes discussed above are involved in generating products that will be toxic to biological tissues. In addition to the pathways discussed above, production of superoxides will also activate the arachidonic acid cascade system (block 19) possibly due to the destruction of biological membranes.[47] When this occurs, lipoxygenase products of arachidonic acid are formed that will act as signals for neutrophils to infiltrate into the tissues and ultimately liberate their bactericidal oxygen radicals.[13,16,60,71] Also, when the cyclooxygenase system is activated and the endoperoxide PGG_2 is converted to PGH_2, an O_2^- is generated (blocks 5 and 6). Therefore, when biological membranes are damaged by any process, oxygen radicals will also be produced through stimulation of the arachidonic acid cascade system. Neutrophils will be attracted to tissues by the lipoxygenase products or oxygen radicals (blocks 8 and 9) and they will subsequently produce additional toxic oxygen radicals.[49,61] The oxygen radicals will then form H_2O_2 (block 10) or O_2^- and H_2O_2 will combine to form $OH^\cdot$ (Haber-Weiss reaction). The compounds can both destroy more tissue and signal more neutrophil infiltration and macrophage activation. Thus, a vicious cycle is set up that will result in massive tissue destruction if not checked.

Also shown in Figure 1 (blocks 11, 12, 13) is the very interesting finding that minor tissue damage results in a greater production of SOD. This finding has been demonstrated in rat lung tissue[2,16,19,20,63] and indicates that small,

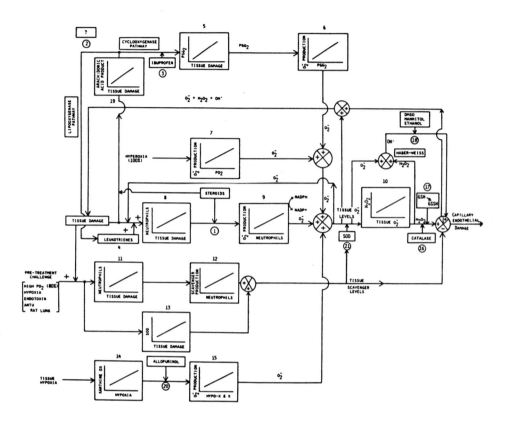

Figure 1: *Schematic model of how oxygen radicals (O_2^-), hydroxyl radicals (OH·), and hydrogen peroxide (H_2O_2) are produced in damaged lung tissue. Starting at the far left, tissue damage causes neutrophil infiltration into tissues with the subsequent release of O_2^- formed by NADPH $\longrightarrow$ $NADP^+$ reaction. These oxygen radicals combine with those produced by the formation of O_2^- by the arachidonic acid system (blocks 19, 5, and 6). In addition, the effects of hyperoxia on the generation of O_2^- is also shown (block 7). The effects of small challenge on the production of SOD and other free radical scavengers is shown in blocks 11, 12, and 13. At block 10, the formation of H_2O_2 is shown and above this block the formation of OH· by the Haber-Weiss reaction of O_2^- and H_2O_2 is shown. The free radicals, leukotrienes, and O_2^- feedback to cause further damage and neutrophil and/or macrophage activity. Finally, all radicals will cause vascular endothelial and alveolar epithelial damage. At several portions of the schematic (shown as circled numbers) different blockers or scavengers of the oxygen radicals are shown, e.g., ① effect of steroids on membrane stabilizaton and neutrophil activities; ③ effect of ibuprofen on blocking the cyclooxygenase pathway; ㉑ effect of allopurinol on blocking xanthine oxidase activity; ㉑ the effect of SOD either from exogenous or endogenous sources on dismutating O_2^- to H_2O_2; ⑯ the effects of catalase on converting H_2O_2 to H_2O; ⑪ the effects of the glutathione reductase system on detoxifying H_2O_2; and finally ⑱ which represents the scavenging of OH· radicals by DMSO, mannitol, etc. In order to simplify the schema, tissue macrophage activation can replace neutrophil activation to explain experimental findings at the appropriate point in the model. (Modified from Taylor and Parker.[67])*

supposedly nontoxic challenges of endotoxin, hyperoxia, ANTU, etc. can cause the cell machinery to generate more radical scavengers, especially SOD. Whether or not this process occurs in all species is not presently known, but it indicates that animals may have the innate ability to regulate their levels of oxygen radical scavenging compounds when challenged by several different types of damaging systems. This would certainly constitute a valuable survival mechanism, and its relationship to lung pathology is evident as it is the only schema in Figure 1 that intrinsically decreases the amount of free radical formation (summation at far right of figure).

Also designated in Figure 1 are portions of the proposed schematic at which specific compounds can prevent the production of different oxygen radicals or detoxify (scavenge) them once formed. First, consider the schemes that produce superoxides: in order to prevent the formation of O_2^- associated with the xanthine oxidase system, allopurinol (block 20) can be used, which inhibits the formation of xanthine oxidase from xanthine dehydrogenase.[24] Secondly, the formation of cyclooxygenase products from arachidonic acid can be inhibited by indomethacin, ibuprofen, or other cyclooxygenase blockers (block 3).[36,37] Also, if the lipoxygenase pathway can be blocked (block 2),[61] then these chemotaxic substances will not be released and neutrophils may not enter the tissue or macrophages may not be activated. Also, the effects of cortisol type compounds (block 1) seem to be related to the inhibition of neutrophil infiltration into the tissues, which is possibly related to the inhibition by cortisol of phopholipase and the subsequent blockade of arachidonic acid release from membranes. In addition, the number of circulating leukocytes (including neutrophils) can be reduced by nitrogen mustard and other types of leukocyte-depleting compounds to lessen their effect on lung damage.[15,28]

Pretreatment with small challenges may also cause a greater production of SOD and, of course, pretreatment of tissues with SOD (block 21) will scavenge the O_2^- produced when lungs are subjected to damaging agents.[46] In fact, it is now known that SOD can cross cell membranes and catalyze the reduction of O_2^- to H_2O_2 within the cell environment.[40]

Once O_2^- has been converted to H_2O_2, three things can occur: (1) catalase or glutathione peroxidase will convert H_2O_2 to water; or (2) H_2O_2 will form $HOCl$;[57] or, (3) H_2O_2 will combine with O_2^- to form $OH^.$. Either catalase (block 16) or glutathione peroxidase (block 17) can eliminate this potentially toxic compound and cysteine can increase the production of reduced glutathione which is oxidized by H_2O_2.[9]

Once $OH^.$ radicals are formed, they can be scavenged by several compounds such as ethyl alcohol, dimethylsulfoxide (DMSO), methylthiourea, and mannitol (block 18), provided that these scavengers can obtain access to the site at which $OH^.$ radicals are produced and detoxify them before damage occurs.[17]

Oxygen Radical Production in Lung Tissue

Several different indices of tissue damage have been used to evaluate free radical formation after various types of lung pathology. For the most part, vascular endothelial, epithelial, or interstitial disruption have been assessed by using lymph protein fluxes to assess vascular permeability damage, and either edema fluid formation or transepithelial albumin fluxes to assess airway epithelial membrane damage. Ultrastructural studies have been used to assess damage of these membranes and alterations in the interstitial compartment following the production of oxygen radicals. It is of interest to note that many of the oxygen radical generating systems appear first to alter the microcirculatory endothelial integrity, so estimates of vascular permeability can be extremely sensitive indices of oxygen radical formation.

Several compounds known to induce oxygen radical formation in lung tissues are shown in Table I. The first studies to demonstrate the involvement of superoxide production in lung pathology were those of oxygen toxicity. It appears that high levels of O_2 overrides the mitochondrial cytochrome oxidase machinery for bypassing O_2^- production, and after 50–70 hours of breathing

Table I
Conditions for Which Scavengers Have Been Effective in Preventing Tissue Damage

Compound or condition	Scavengers, Detoxifying Enzymes	Mechanism(s)
Thiourea[17]	DMSO, ethanol, mannitol catalase	OH˙ formation (no neutrophil requirement)
α-napthlythiourea[66]	DMSO, SOD, catalase ibuprofen	OH˙ formation arachidonic acid products (no neutrophil requirement)
Microemboli-Air Bubbles[14]	SOD	OH˙ formation? O_2^-? (neutrophil requirement)
Microemboli-Glass Beads[29]	—	—? (neutrophil requirement)
Hyperoxia[7]	SOD (intercellular)	OH˙? O_2^- (no neutrophil requirement)
Irradiation[17]	Dimethylthiourea	OH˙ (no neutrophil requirement)
Endotoxin (Traber et al. Fed. Proc. 42:1105, 1984)	(SOD caused more damage)	H_2O_2 or HOCl (neutrophil requirement)
Complement[48] Activation	Ibuprofen, SOD (capillary endothelial study)	OH˙ arachidonic acid products (neutrophil requirement)?
Complement[68] Activation	Catalase (capillary endothelial study)	H_2O_2, HOCl (neutrophil requirement)
Glucose-glucose oxidase	SOD (early)	O_2^-? OH˙ (early)
Myeloperoxidase or Lactoperoxidase[43]	Catalase (late) (Alveolar epithelial study)	H_2O_2, HOCl (late) (neutrophil requirement)
Phorbal Myristate[32] Acetate	Catalase (alveolar epithelial study)	H_2O_2, HOCl, *macrophage involvement* (no neutrophil requirement)
ARDS[35]	DMSO	OH˙? (neutrophils?)

100% O_2, severe lung tissue damage results. Crapo et al.[7] were able to reduce the damage by pretreating the lungs with a superoxide dismutase, which was attached to phospholipid vesicles that allowed SOD to enter the pulmonary cells. Extracellular SOD was not effective in preventing the damage. The neutrophils, although augmenting the hyperoxic damage, did not appear to be the primary mediators of the massive lung damage associated with breathing high levels of oxygen.[7,16,56]

Another series of studies[64,66] (including the authors' unpublished observations) in which a thiourea compound (ANTU) was used to produce damage indicates that SOD, DMSO, and catalase are all equally effective in preventing the lung damage. Further, these studies are particularly striking because ANTU always causes severe intraalveolar edema, but when the scavengers are present there is no apparent lung damage. The results of the ANTU studies strongly indicate that OH· radicals are responsible for the damage since all enzymes and scavengers block the damaging effects of oxygen radicals. A recent study by Fox et al. indicates that thiourea causes OH· generation in lung tissue, but the damage is the result of a reaction involving cyanide production when the OH· reacts with thiourea. In this study, dimethylthiourea, ethanol, and mannitol scavenge the OH· radicals, but they differ in their ability to scavenge OH· radicals, yielding 91%, 63%, and 53% protection, respectively.[17]

Radiation also causes the formation of OH· radicals, and Fox et al.[17] have also shown that dimethylthiourea is a potent scavenger of OH· in this model and prevents the radiation damage.

Recently Flick et al. partially reversed the endothelial damage associated with air microemboli by using SOD.[14] Other scavengers were not tested, but other studies from the same laboratory indicate that leukocyte depletion also partially prevented the damage associated with embolic challenge.[15] Also, glass bead emboli appear to cause a neutrophil-dependent type of capillary wall damage.[29] To gain more insight into the mechanisms involved in microemboli damage, OH· scavengers and catalase should be evaluated relative to protective effects.

Endotoxin appears also to require neutrophil activation to produce vascular lesions in sheep,[28] but the response is either absent or very weak in dog lungs.[34] A very recent study indicates that SOD may actually accentuate the lung damage, indicating that perhaps HOCl is formed by H_2O_2 more rapidly when excess SOD is present.[68a] This hypothesis could easily be tested by the addition of catalase to the system.

Complement activation has also been studied in sheep models and it is interesting to note that both ibuprofen and SOD partially reversed the damage associated with the challenge.[48] ANTU may also activate the complement system since both SOD and ibuprofen can block the damaging effects in 50% of the animals studied.[40a] These studies indicate that the oxygen radical generation with complement activation may be a result of the breakdown of arachidonic acid to its products in which O_2^- is generated with the conversion of PGG_2 to PGH_2 as shown clearly by Kontos' group in the cerebral circulation.[36,37,58]

Peter Ward's group, in an elegant study, has demonstrated that H_2O_2 production within the airways is the most damaging of the generated free radicals, most likely because of the subsequent hypochlorus production.[30] Furthermore, SOD administered after the instillation of immune complexes protects for a few hours, but later catalase is required to protect the epithelial membrane from disruption.[31] C_3 activator from cobra venom infused directly into the pulmonary artery causes neutrophil aggregation and H_2O_2 production, which most likely represents a C_{5a}-mediated reaction.[68] And finally, when phorbal myristate acetate (PMA) was instilled into rat lungs, SOD is ineffective in inhibiting the damage, but catalase is fully protective. A most important finding from this study is that neutrophils *are not* required. It appears that phorbal myristate acetate activates the tissue macrophages.[32] This finding has led these authors to postulate that PMA activates phagocytic cells within the pulmonary interstitial matrix and that the scavengers administered will primarily effect the phagocytic cell release of oxygen radicals, not those generated within pulmonary tissue cells.[55]

Klein et al.[35] have recently treated patients with ARDS using DMSO and found that both PaO_2 and $PaCO_2$ markedly improved in these patients. However, no other studies have been conducted in the human model. Whether or not this represents a nonspecific effect of DMSO or specific scavenging of OH· requires much further study. It is of interest to note that SOD is now added to solutions used to perfuse patients during cardiac surgery and for transplant organ perfusates. The SOD-containing solutions appear to protect the organs better than previously used perfusates.

The studies outlined in this section do not present a detailed discussion of the experimental protocols used to assess superoxide production or the possible problems associated with interpreting lung damage in each experimental design. But it is clear from these studies that oxygen radicals are involved in many forms of lung pathology. It appears that many forms of lung pathology require the presence of neutrophils and that the production of O_2^-, OH·, and H_2O_2 are responsible for much of the lung damage. However, it should be pointed out that neutrophil depletion produces different results when produced by different compounds such as hydroxyurea or nitrogen mustard (unpublished data, authors' laboratory), which may be related to the compound's direct effects on macrophage or leukocyte action. Also, it is safe to say that the production of O_2^- is related to the membrane damage. The subsequent formation of cyclooxygenase products from arachidonic acid which causes further O_2^- production and a greater neutrophil infiltration constitutes a positive feedback system with a final result of severely damaged lung tissue.

Other Forms of Lung Pathology That May Involve Oxygen Radical Formation

From the previous section, it is quite obvious that lung damage can result from the production of oxygen radicals. Either O_2^-, OH·, or H_2O_2 are responsible for the lung pathology associated with several different types of experimental models of ARDS. And, in addition, lipid peroxidation caused by oxygen radicals may occur by two different mechanisms. The radicals or H_2O_2 may directly result in lipid peroxidation, a toxic effect that can be prevented by antioxidants such as vitamin E or promethazine. While *this* damage cannot be blocked with catalase, lipid peroxidation may also result from H_2O_2 secondary to some chemical alteration that is inhibitable by catalase.[59] These responses are similar to those seen with complement activation, where SOD protected initially (preventing the lipid peroxidation by O_2^-) but catalase was required for long-term protection.[31] The differences in effects of the various radicals appear to be related to whether or not the oxygen radical damage is produced by tissue cells or by the more phagocytic tissue macrophages and infiltrated neutrophils. The cell damage caused by challenges such as hyperoxia, thiourea, and ANTU appears to be primarily mediated by OH· radicals since SOD, DMSO, and catalase protect while the damage due to activation of complement macrophage-neutrophil system appears to be related to the generation of H_2O_2 and the formation of HOCl. It should be pointed out that some compounds such as paraquat (similar to the carbon tetracholoride radical formation in liver damage) forms a free radical (in the presence of O_2^-), which can in itself cause lipid peroxidation and cell damage independent of H_2O_2 and OH· production.

Table II presents several compounds that are known occasionally to cause fulminating pulmonary edema. Pulmonary edema can result from either high vascular pressures (hydrostatic edema) or alterations in vascular permeability to plasma proteins, which cause edema at low vascular pressures (permeability edema). The table shows possible mechanisms of injury, with the most likely mechanisms noted by asterisks. In some instances, the mechanism of edema formation has been evaluated experimentally and these are indicated in the table.

A very careful assessment of these experimental models for producing edema reveals that the endothelial cells were damaged by the challenge and

Table II
Factors That Cause Pulmonary Edema

Factor/Compound	Mechanism	
Acid aspiration	Permeability*	Hydrostatic*
Alloxan	Permeability*	Hydrostatic
Alveolar hypoxia	Permeability	Hydrostatic*
Ammonium chloride	Permeability*	Hydrostatic
Ca^{++} removal	Permeability*	--
Coronary occlusion	--	Hydrostatic*
Ethchlorvynol	Permeability*	Hydrostatic
Fibrin degradation products	--	Hydrostatic*
Hemorrhagic shock	--	Hydrostatic*
Heroin	Permeability*	Hydrostatic*
Histamine	--	Hydrostatic*
High altitude pulmonary edema	Permeability	Hydrostatic*
Iprindole	Permeability*	Hydrostatic
Ketoacidosis	Permeability*	--
Lung reexpansion	Permeability	Hydrostatic*
Neurogenic pulmonary edema	--	Hydrostatic*
Oleic acid	Permeability*	--
Pancreatitis	Permeability*	Hydrostatic*
Paraquat	Permeability*	Hydrostatic
Salicylates	Permeability*	Hydrostatic*
Septic shock	Permeability*	Hydrostatic*
Serotonin	--	Hydrostatic*
Slow-reacting substances	Permeability	Hydrostatic*
Thermal burns	Permeability*	Hydrostatic*
War gases	Permeability*	Hydrostatic*

*indicates mechanism most likely responsible for edema formation;
--indicates mechanism eliminated by proper experimental validaton.
(Modified from Taylor and Parker.[67])

that large tissue infiltration of neutrophils had occurred.[67] This is especially true for acid aspiration,[25] alloxan,[70] ethchlorvynol,[12] high altitude pulmonary edema,[69] ketoacidosis,[51] lung re-expansion,[5] pancreatitis,[33] septic shock,[28] and iprindole.[3] Certainly the activation of neutrophils and the tissue macrophages could result in additional tissue damage, but they may be present because of the initial tissue damage with subsequent liberation of oxygen radicals which then serve as chemotactic agents.[49] Previous studies indicate that these activated cells could result in additional tissue damage mediated by oxygen metabolites. The inflammatory response is an important mechanism for ridding the body of foreign invaders, but we must begin to ask the question of whether or not certain types of tissue damage cause neutrophils and tissue macrophages to turn on their own tissues, as in an autoimmune response. Are there good and bad neutrophils?

Clearly, the etiology of lung injury is complex, though oxygen and other free radicals seem to be involved. Table III indicates just how complex the oxygen radical system really is when we attempt to study how the different scavengers protect against lung injury. In the first condition, SOD blocked the damaging effect while DMSO and catalase, which scavenge $OH^.$ and H_2O_2, respectively, have no effect. But O_2^- produces lipid peroxides that may be blocked in the presence of antioxidants such as vitamin E. This is a rather clear-cut case. The second condition indicates that all scavengers are beneficial, which implicates the $OH^.$ as the primary mediator of the tissue damage, again another clear experimental conclusion.

The third condition is one in which SOD and DMSO fail to protect, but catalase and the antioxidants partially protect when given alone. However, in a recent study in which H_2O_2 was generated in a hepatocyte culture, when calatase and promethazine (an antioxidant) were combined, total protection resulted. This indicates that H_2O_2 caused an initial lipid preoxidation followed by some secondary effect that was inhibited by catalase.[59]

The final condition indicates how confusing results can be when different scavengers are used at different time frames in intact animal experiments. For example, SOD blocked the initial damage associated with complement activation, but the effect lasted only 1 hour. Most likely an antioxidant would also

Table III
Schema for Determining Which Oxygen Metabolites are Responsible for Tissue Damage Based on the Pattern of Effective Scavengers

Pathological Challenge Type	SOD	DMSO	Catalase	Antioxidants (i.e., vitamin E)	Responsible Metabolite(s)
1	+	−	−	±	O_2^-
2	+	+	+	+	$OH^.$
3	−	−	±	±	lipid peroxidation and/or other effect of H_2O_2
4	+ (early) − (late)		+ (late)	+ (early)	lipid peroxidation (early) H_2O_2 (late)

+ = protective effect; ± = partial protective effect; − = no protective effect.

have protected at this time. The important finding is that catalase was later protective, implicating H_2O_2 as well. It was also shown in these studies that neutrophils were necessary for the H_2O_2 effect. Thus when lungs are challenged by any substance, the protective effects of any scavenger may be time-dependent and possibly related to either neutrophil or macrophage involvement.[43]

The major point to be made concerning Table III is that very unexpected results may occur when attempts are made to logically scavenge oxygen radicals or metabolites. A single scavenger experiment would probably not be useful in defining the oxygen metabolite responsible for the lung injury. And, in fact, a combination of two scavengers may be required to block totally the damage (condition 3). Table III, although complex, presents ideal cases. When the oxygen radical system is studied in intact animals, many more side effects may be present that severely limit the interpretation of the data collected from whole animal studies.

While there is little doubt that oxygen radicals are involved in most types of lung pathology, much more research is required before we can accurately assess the questions raised here: (1) how are the various oxygen radicals generated in these forms of pulmonary edema? (2) which is the specific oxygen metabolite responsible for the damage? (3) what are the specific contributions of neutrophils and tissue or alveolar macrophages in producing lung injury? and (4) what is the best approach to prevent their generation before irreversible tissue damage results? The field is certainly an intriguing one that is expanding at a rapid rate, and we refer the interested reader to several authoritative texts that now exit.[52]

REFERENCES

1. Antonini, E., Brunori, M., Greenwood, C., et al.: Catalytic mechanism of cytochrome oxidase. *Nature* 228:936–937, 1970.
2. Autor, A.P.: Reduction of paraquat toxicity by superoxide dismutase. *Life Sci.* 14:1309–1319, 1974.
3. Bean, J.W., Zee, D., and Thom, B.: Pulmonary changes with convulsions induced by drugs and oxygen at high pressure. *J. Appl. Physiol.* 21:865–872, 1966.
4. Borg, D.C. and Schaich, K.M.: Cytotoxicity from coupled redox cycling of autoxidizing xenobiotics and metals. *Israel J. Chem.* 24:38–53, 1984.
5. Brennan, N.J. and Fitzgerald, M.X.: Anatomically localized re-expansion pulmonary edema following pneumothorax drainage: Case report and literature review. *Respiration* 38:233–237, 1979.
6. Buckley, G.B. (ed.): The role of oxygen free radicals in human disease process. *Surgery* 94:407–438, 1983.
7. Crapo, J.D., Freeman, B.A., Barry, B.E., et al.: Mechanisms of hyperoxic injury to the pulmonary microcirculation. *The Physiologist* 26:170–176, 1983.
8. Del Maestro, R.F., Arfors, K.E., and Lindblom, R.: Free radical depolymerization of hyaluronic acid: Influence of scavenger substances. *Bibl. Ana.* (Suppl.) 18:132–135, 1979.
9. Del Maestro, R.F.: An approach to free radicals in medicine and biology. *Acta Physiol. Scand.* (Suppl) 492:153–168, 1980.
10. Del Maestro, R., Bjork, J., and Arfors, K.E.: Free radicals and microvascular permeability. In *Pathology of Oxygen.* New York, Academic Press, pp. 157–173, 1982.

11. Dormandy, T.L.: Free radical oxidations and anti-oxidants. *Lancet I:* 647–650, 1978.
12. Fairman, R.P., Glauser, F.L., and Falls, R.: Increases in lung lymph and albumin clearance with ethchlorvynol. *J. Appl. Physiol.* 50:1151–1155, 1981.
13. Fantone, J.C. and Ward, P.A.: A review: Role of oxygen-derived free radicals and metabolites in leukocyte-dependent inflammatory reactions. *Am. J. Pathol.* 107: 395–418, 1982.
14. Flick, M.R., Hoeffel, J., and Staub, N.C.: Superoxide dismutase prevents increased lung vascular permeability after microemboli. *Fed. Proc.* 40:405, 1981.
15. Flick, M.R., Perel, A., and Staub, N.C.: Leukocytes are required for increased lung microvascular permeability after microembolization in sheep. *Circ. Res.* 48: 344–351, 1981.
16. Fox, R.B., Hoidal, J.R., Grown, D.M., et al.: Pulmonary inflammation duc to oxygen toxicity: Involvement of the chemotactic factors and polymorphonuclear leukocytes. *Am. Rev. Respir. Dis.* 123:521–523, 1981.
17. Fox, R.B., Harada, R.N., Tate, R.M., et al.: Prevention of thiourea-induced pulmonary edema by hydroxyl-radical scavengers. *J. Appl. Physiol.* 55:1456–1459, 1983.
18. Frank, L. and Roberts, R.L.: Endotoxin protection against oxygen-induced acute and chronic lung injury. *J. Appl. Physiol.* 47:577–581, 1979.
19. Frank, L. and Summerville, L.F.: A mechanism of protection from pulmonary oxygen toxicity by endotoxin treatment. *Am. Rev. Respir. Dis.* 121:340, 1980.
20. Frank, L., Summerville, L.F., and Massaro, D.: Protection from oxygen toxicity with endotoxin: Role of the endogenous antioxidant enzymes of the lung. *J. Clin. Invest.* 65:1104–1110, 1980.
21. Freeman, B.A. and Crapo, J.D.: Biology of disease: Free radical and tissue injury. 47:412–426, 1982.
22. Fridovich, I.: Quantitative aspects of the production of superoxide anion radical by milk xanthine oxidase. *J. Biol. Chem.* 215:4053–4057, 1970.
23. Fridovich, I.: The biology of oxygen radicals. *Science* 201:875–880, 1978.
24. Granger, D.N., Rutili, G., and McCord, J.M.: Superoxide radicals in feline intestinal ischemia. *Gastroenterology* 81:22–29, 1981.
25. Grimbert, F.A., Parker, J.C., and Taylor, A.E.: Increased pulmonary vascular permeability following acid aspiration. *J. Appl. Physiol.* 51:335–345, 1981.
26. Gutteridge, J.M.C.: The protective action of superoxide dismutase on metal-ion catalysed peroxidation of phospholipids. *Biochem. Biophysiol. Res. Comm.* 77: 379–386, 1977.
27. Haber, F. and Weiss, J.: The catalytic decomposition of hydrogen peroxide by iron salts. *Proc. Royal Soc. Ser. A.* 147:332–351, 1934.
28. Heflin, A.C. and Brigham, K.L.: Prevention by granulocyte depletion of increased vascular permeability of sheep lung following endotoxemia. *J. Clin. Invest.* 68: 1253–1260, 1981.
29. Johnson, A. and Malik, A.B.: Pulmonary edema after glass bead microembolization: Protective effective of granulocytopenia. *J. Appl. Physiol.* 52:155–161, 1982.
30. Johnson, K.J., Fantone, J.C., III, Kaplan, J., et al.: In vivo damage of rat lungs by oxygen metabolites. *J. Clin. Invest.* 67:983–993, 1981.
31. Johnson, K.J. and Ward, P.A.: Role of oxygen metabolites in immune complex injury of lung. *J. Immunol.* 126:2365–2369, 1981.
32. Johnson, K.J. and Ward, P.A.: Acute and progressive lung injury after contact with phorbol myristate acetate. *Am. J. Pathol.* 107:29–35, 1982.
33. Kimura, T., Toung, J.K., Margolis, S., et al.: Respiratory failure in acute pancreatitis: A possible role for triglycerides. *Ann. Surg.* 189:509–514, 1979.
34. Kinnebrew, D.S., Parker, J.C., Falgout, H.J., et al.: Pulmonary microvascular permeability following *E. Coli* endotoxin and hemorrhage. *J. Appl. Physiol.* 52: 403–409, 1982.
35. Klein, H.A., Samant, S., Herz, B.L., et al.: Dimethyl sulfoxide in adult respiratory

distress syndrome. Abstract of preliminary report. *Ann. NY Acad. Sci..* 411: 389–390, 1983.

36. Kontos, H.A., Wei, E.P., Ellis, E.F., et al.: Prostaglandins in physiological and in certain pathological responses of the cerebral circulation. *Fed. Proc.* 40:2326–2330, 1981.

37. Kontos, H.A., Wei, E.P., Christman, C.W., et al.: Free oxygen radicals in cerebral vascular responses. *The Physiologist* 26:165–169, 1983.

38. Kosower, N.S. and Kosower, E.M.: The glutathione-glutathione disulfide system. In *Free Radicals in Biology*, Vol. 2. Pryor, W.A., ed. London, Academic Press, pp. 55–84, 1976.

39. Lewis, D.H., Del Maestro, R., and Arfors, K.E. (eds.): Free radicals in medicine and biology. *Acta. Physiol. Scand.* (Suppl) 492:1–168, 1980.

40. Lynch, R.E. and Fridovich, I.: Permeation of the erythrocyte stroma by superoxide radical. *J. Biol. Chem.* 253:4697–4699, 1978.

40a. Martin, D., Korthuis, R.J., Perry, M., et al.: Oxygen radical-mediated lung damage associated with alpha/napthylthiourea. *Acta Physiol. Scand.* (In press) 1985.

41. McCord, J.M.: Free radicals and inflammation, protection of synovial fluid by superoxide dismutase. *Science* 185:529–531, 1974.

42. McCord, J.M. and Fridovich, I.: Superoxide dismutase: An enzymatic function for erythrocuprien (hemocuprien). *J. Biol. Chem.* 244:6049–6055, 1969.

43. McCormich, J.R., Harkin, M.M., Johnson, K.J., et al.: Suppression by superoxide dismutase of immune complex-induced pulmonary alveolitis and dermal inflammation. *Am. J. Physiol.* 102:55–61, 1981.

44. Meister, A.: Selective modification of glutathione metabolism. *Science* 220: 472–478, 1983.

45. Nishikimi, M. and Yagi, K.: Oxidations of ascorbic acid and α-tocopherol by superoxide. In *Biochemical and Medical Aspects of Active Oxygen*. Hayaishi, O. and Asada, K., eds. Baltimore, MD, University Park Press, pp. 79–87, 1977.

46. Parker, J.C., Martin, D.J., Rutili, G., et al.: Prevention of free radical-mediated vascular permeability increase in lung using superoxide dismutase. *Chest* 83: 525–528, 1983.

47. Perez, H.D. and Goldstein, J.M.: Generation of a chemotactic lipid from arachidonic acid by exposure to a superoxide generating system. *Fed. Proc.* 38:1170, 1979.

48. Perkowski, S.Z., Havill, A.W., Flynn, J.T., et al.: Role of intrapulmonary release of eicosanoids and superoxide anion as mediators of pulmonary dysfunction and endothelial injury in sheep with intermittent complement activation. *Circ. Res.* 53:574–583, 1983.

49. Petrone, W.F., English, D.K., Wong, K., et al.: Free radicals and inflammation: The superoxide dependent activation of a neutrophil chemotactic factor in plasma. *Proc. Natl. Acad. Sci. USA* 77:1159–1163, 1980.

50. Pingleton, W.W., Coalson, J.J., and Guenter, C.A.: Significance of leukocytes in endotoxin shock. *Exp. Mol. Pathol.* 22:183–194, 1975.

51. Powner, D., Snyder, J.V., and Grenvile, A.: Altered pulmonary capillary permeability complicating recovery from diabetic ketoacidosis. *Chest* 68:253–255, 1975.

52. Pryor, W.A (ed.): *Free Radicals in Biology*. New York, Academic Press, Volumes IV (1980) and V (1982).

53. Pryor, W.A.: The function of free radicals and the consequences of their reactions in vivo. *Photochem. Photobiol.* 28:787–801, 1978.

54. Pryor, W.A.: The role of free radical reactions in biological systems. In *Free Radicals in Biology*, Vol. 1. Pryor, W., ed. New York, Academic Press, pp. 1–49, 1976.

55. Reiko, T., and Web, Z.: Secretory products of macrophages and their physiological functions. *Am. J. Physiol.* 246:C1–C9, 1984.

56. Repine, J.E. and Tate, R.M.: Oxygen radicals and lung edema. *The Physiologist* 26:177–181, 1983.

57. Rosen, H. and Klebanoff, S.J.: Bactericidal activity of a superoxide anion generating system: A model for the polymorphonuclear leukocyte. *J. Exp. Med.* 149: 27–39, 1979.

58. Rosenblum, W.I.: Effects of free radical generation on mouse pial arterioles: Probable role of hydroxyl radicals. *Am. J. Physiol.* 245:H139–H142, 1983.

59. Rubin, R. and Farber, J.L.: Mechanisms of the killing of cultured hepatocytes by hydrogen peroxide. *Arch. Biochem. Biophysiol.* 228:450–459, 1984.

60. Salin, M.L. and McCord, J.M.: Free radicals in leukocyte metabolism and inflammation. In *Superoxide and Superoxide Dismutases.* Michelson, A.M., McCord, J. M., and Fridovich, I., eds. New York, Academic Press, pp. 257–270, 1977.

61. Samuelsson, B.: Leukotrienes: Mediators of immediate hypersensitivity reactions and inflammation. *Science* 220:568–575, 1983.

62. Shasby, D.M., Van Bethuysen, K.M., Tate, R.M., et al.: Granulocytes mediate acute edematous lung injury in rabbits and in isolated lungs perfused with phorbol myristate acetate: Role of oxygen free radicals. *Am. Rev. Respir. Dis.* 125:443–447, 1981.

63. Stevens, J.B. and Autor, A.P.: Induction of superoxide dismutase by oxygen in neonatal rat lung. *J. Biol. Chem.* 252:3509–3513, 1977.

64. Taylor, A.E. and Martin, D.: Oxygen radicals and the microcirculation. *The Physiologist* 26:152–155, 1983.

65. Taylor, A.E. (ed.): Oxygen radicals and the microcirculation. *The Physiologist* 26: 151–181, 1983.

66. Taylor, A.E., Martin, D., and Parker, J.C.: The effects of oxygen radicals on pulmonary edema formation. *Surgery* 94:433–438, 1983.

67. Taylor, A.E. and Parker, J.C.: The pulmonary interstitial spaces and lymphatics. In *Handbook of Physiology Vol. 4, Pulmonary Circulation and Non-Respiratory Functions of the Lung.* Fishman, A.P., Fisher, A.B., eds. Baltimore, MD, Williams & Wilkins (In press).

68. Till, G.O., Johnson, K.J., Kunkel, R., et al.: Intravascular activation of complement and acute lung injury. *J. Clin. Invest.* 69:1126–1135, 1982.

68a. Traber, D.L., Adams, T., Ziebert, L., et al.: Potentiation of the lung vascular response to endotoxin by superoxide dismutase. *J. Appl. Physiol.* (In press) 1985.

69. Viswanathan, R., Jain, E.K., and Subramanian, S.: Pulmonary edema of high altitude. *Am. Rev. Respir. Dis.* 100:342–349, 1969.

70. Vreim, C.E. and Staub, N.C.: Protein composition and lung fluids in acute alloxan edema in dogs. *Am. J. Physiol.* 230:376–379, 1976.

71. Ward, P.A.: Role of toxic oxygen products from phagocytic cells in tissue injury. *Adv. Shock Res.* 10:27–34, 1983.

CHAPTER 14

Arachidonate Products as Mediators of Diffuse Lung Injury

James R. Snapper* and
Kenneth L. Brigham

Introduction

Arachidonic acid is a long chain unsaturated fatty acid strategically poised as a phospholipid in extracellular and intracellular membranes.[1-4] Phospholipase stimulation results in the release of free arachidonate and its subsequent metabolism into a wide variety of potential mediators.[1-4] These eicosanoids, including the bisenoic prostaglandins and leukotrienes, may be important in maintaining homeostasis as well as in the pathogenesis of injury. They are ubiquitous in their distribution throughout the body and appear to function mainly locally. These agents are probably not stored and are synthesized immediately before release, and most active arachidonate products have very short half-lives in the circulation. Arachidonate products can be thought of as "local hormones."[1-4] Figure 1 contains a simplified schema of the arachidonate metabolic pathway.

This chapter examines the possible role of products of arachidonic acid metabolism in diffuse lung injury. The lungs are a rich source of arachidonate products as well as enzymes, such as the 15-hydroxy prostaglandin dehydrogenase system, which initiate the breakdown of prostaglandins.[5,6] The lungs are exposed to the entire cardiac output, plasma-containing eicosanoids and other possible mediators, and cells such as leukocytes and platelets, which are themselves capable of generating arachidonate products.[7] The lung can be perceived as a metabolic organ as well as a respiratory organ which, under normal conditions, maintains homeostasis partially through the release and local metabolism of arachidonate products. These same mediators, under pathologic conditions, such as those observed in the diffuse lung injury associated with the adult respiratory distress syndrome (ARDS), may directly contribute to lung injury.

Supported by the grants no. HL 19153 (SCOR in Pulmonary Vascular Diseases) and no. HL 27274 from the National Heart, Lung and Blood Institute. *This work was done during the tenure of an Established Investigatorship from the American Heart Association and with funds contributed in part by the Middle Tennessee Chapter of the American Heart Association.

From Said, S.I. (ed.): *The Pulmonary Circulation and Acute Lung Injury*. Mount Kisco, N.Y., Futura Publishing Co., Inc., 1985.

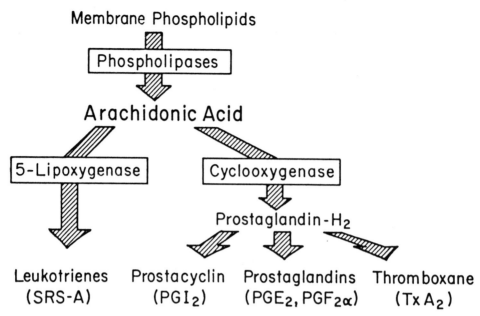

Figure 1: *Abbreviated schema of arachidonate metabolism.*

The pathogenesis of alterations in lung mechanics as well as in the pulmonary vasculature and lung fluid and solute exchange will be discussed since airway and vascular changes are not readily separated in severe diffuse lung injury and changes in the airways may contribute greatly to lung dysfunction.[8,9] Leukotrienes C_4 and D_4 have now been identified as major constituents of slow reacting substances of anaphylaxis (SRS-A),[10-13] long considered important mediators of bronchospasm in asthma but only recently proposed as mediators of pulmonary vascular injury and increased microvascular permeability.[14-16] This review will focus on animal models of ARDS since it is from these models that the most direct evidence has accumulated for a role of arachidonate products in diffuse lung injury.

Evidence for a possible role of arachidonate products in diffuse lung injury comes in three different forms: (1) studies of the effect of infused and aerosolized arachidonate products on the lungs;[14-23] (2) measurements of arachidonate products in blood and lung lymph after the infusion of agents, such as endotoxin, which cause diffuse lung injury;[9,16,17,23-26] and (3) studies of the effects of pharmacologic agents that inhibit different parts of the arachidonate metabolic pathway in the response to injurious stimuli.[8,9,28-30] These types of experiments have clear limitations. Exogenously delivered arachidonate products, for example, may not accurately reproduce the effects of these same agents when released and metabolized locally. Similarly, measurement of stable arachidonate products in blood and lung lymph may not accurately reflect concentrations of their short-lived active parent compounds at their reactive sites. The so called "specific" pharmacologic inhibitors of different parts of the arachidonate metabolic pathway may have other pharmacologic actions that are, in fact, responsible for observed effects of these agents in models of diffuse lung injury.

Still, these types of studies, in toto, form strong evidence of a role for products of arachidonate metabolism in diffuse lung injury.

The effects of exogenously delivered arachidonate products have been widely studied in many different animal preparations and in man.[17-21] The same agent may have different effects, depending on the species and the age of the animals studied.[21] Fetal and neonatal preparations may, for example, have different responses from those observed in adult animals of the same species.[21] The predominant pulmonary vascular effect of infused arachidonate is vasoconstriction.[22] Figure 2 is an example of the effects of infused arachidonate in the awake adult sheep. Thromboxane-A_2, prostaglandins-H_2,-$F_{2\alpha}$,-D_2, and -E_2 as well as leukotriene-D_4 are all pulmonary vasoconstrictors.[17-21] Most of these agents also cause constriction of airway smooth muscle. Prostacyclin (PGI_2) and the nonendogenously produced linolenic acid metabolite prostaglandin-E_1 are pulmonary vasodilators.[17-21] Leukotriene-D_4 can increase capillary permeability in the skin[13-15] and may have a similar effect in the lungs.[23] Arachidonate products can also activate the complement system and

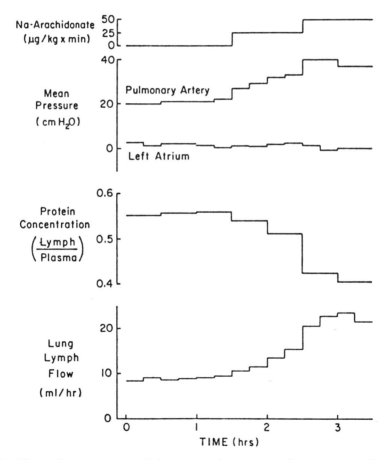

Figure 2: *Effects of intravenous arachidonate on pulmonary vascular pressures and lung lymph in a sheep. (From ref. 22, with permission.)*

stimulate various cell lines. They can function as chemotaxins, platelet aggregators and disaggregators, or cause or oppose leukostasis.[13-21] Arachidonate products may thus act directly or indirectly by affecting other systems involved in the maintenance of homeostasis or the pathogenesis of disease. The specific effects of a given arachidonate product depend on the age and the species studied.

Hypoxic Pulmonary Vasoconstriction

The regulation of perfusion in the lungs has been proposed as a process that may, in part, be controlled by arachidonate products.[5,6,8,9,22,28-34] Much attention has been given to the role of these agents as modulators of hypoxic pulmonary vasoconstriction.[22,31-34] When arachidonic acid is infused into the pulmonary circulation during hypoxic pulmonary vasoconstriction, it causes dilation,[31] in contrast to its normal potent constrictor effects.[22] This vasodilatory effect appears to result from the increased production, during hypoxia, of prostacyclin, a potent pulmonary vasodilator, in excess of constrictor cyclooxygenase arachidonate products.[31] Sublethal doses of endotoxin cause, in dogs, a loss of hypoxic pulmonary vasoconstriction.[32] When dogs are pretreated with the cyclooxygenase inhibitor, meclofenamate, hypoxic pulmonary vasoconstriction is not lost.[32] Newman et al. observed that isolated lungs from rats that had been exposed to high concentrations of inspired oxygen for several days did not constrict normally to hypoxia.[33] Normal hypoxic pulmonary vasoconstriction was restored, in this preparation, when meclofenamate was added to the perfusate.[33] These results are far from conclusive and conflicting data exist,[34] but the studies do illustrate the three types of experimentation that yield evidence for a role of arachidonate products in diffuse lung injury:(1) studies of infused agents, (2) measurements of arachidonate products, and (3) studies with pharmacologic inhibitors.

Endotoxemia

ARDS is characterized by severe hypoxemia, a chest radiograph compatible with pulmonary edema, stiff noncompliant lungs, and normal pulmonary capillary wedge or left atrial pressure.[8] Gram negative sepsis is a common precipitating factor for ARDS.[8,25] Endotoxemia causes diffuse lung

Table I	
Effects of Endotoxemia in Sheep	
Early (0–1 HR)	• Pulmonary hypertension • Altered lung mechanics • High flow of protein-poor lung lymph
Late (2–5 HR)	• High flow of protein-rich lung lymph
Early & Late (0–5 HR)	• Hypoxemia • Leukopenia

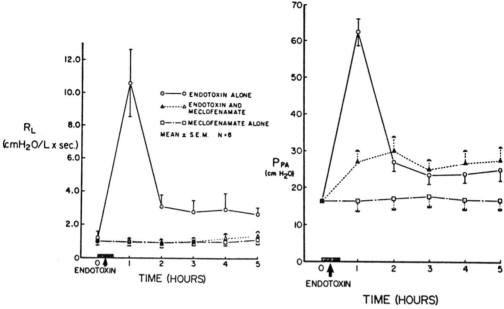

Figure 3: *Effect of meclofenamate on endotoxin-induced changes in resistance to airflow across the lungs, R_L (left) and pulmonary artery pressure, P_{PA} (right). The data from the endotoxin alone experiments are shown as (⊙——⊙); the data from the meclofenamate and endotoxin experiments are shown as (△ --- △); the data from the meclofenamate alone experiments are drawn as (⊡ ---⊡). (From ref. 9, with permission.)*

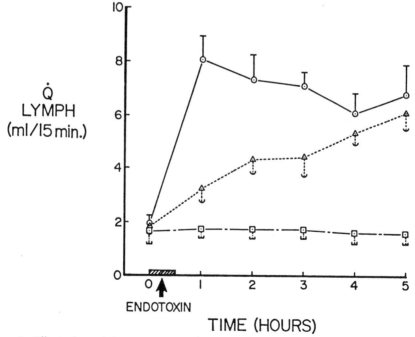

Figure 4: *Effect of meclofenamate on endotoxin-induced changes in lung lymph flow, $\dot{Q}$ lymph. The data from the endotoxin alone experiments are shown as (⊙——⊙); the data from the meclofenamate and endotoxin experiments are shown as (△ --- △); the data from the meclofenamate alone experiments are shown as (⊡ ---⊡). (From ref. 9, with permission.)*

injury in the unanesthetized sheep and is employed as an animal model of ARDS.[8,9,16,17,24,−30,34−44] Endotoxemia causes, in this preparation, a well-characterized sequence of pathophysiologic changes (Table I), including early (occurring within the first hour of endotoxemia) marked pulmonary hypertension (Figs. 2, 3) and altered lung mechanics (Fig. 3). From 2 to 5 hours after endotoxemia, pulmonary vascular pressures have returned toward normal but there is the high flow of protein-rich lung lymph (Fig. 4). It is this phase of the sheep's response to endotoxemia that has been interpreted as representing increased pulmonary microvascular permeability and as being analogous to ARDS.[35,36] Endotoxemia can cause radiographic changes in sheep analogous to those seen in ARDS as well as respiratory failure.[36] Endotoxemia causes early profound leukopenia (Fig. 5) and hypoxemia (Fig. 6).[9,39] The pathologic changes caused by endotoxemia have been well characterized and include pulmonary leukocyte sequestration and migration into the pulmonary interstitium, endothelial damage, and edema formation (Table II).[45] Endotoxemia causes production and release from the lungs of both constrictor and dilator cyclooxygenase products of arachidonate as well as lipoxygenase products

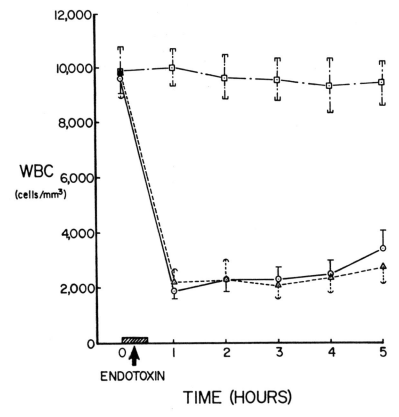

Figure 5: *Effect of meclofenamate on endotoxin-induced changes in WBC. The data from the endotoxin alone experiments are shown as (⊙——⊙); the data from the meclofenamate and endotoxin experiments are shown as (△ --- △); the data from the meclofenamate alone experiments are drawn as (☐ ⋯☐). (From ref. 9, with permission.)*

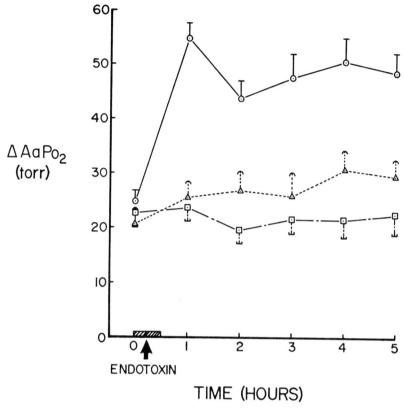

Figure 6: *Effect of meclofenamate on endotoxin-induced changes in room air ΔAaPO₂. The data from the endotoxin alone experiments are shown as (⊙——⊙); the data from the meclofenamate and endotoxin experiments are shown as (△ --- △); the data from the meclofenamate alone experiments are shown as (▫ -··-▫). (From ref. 9, with permission.)*

Table II
Structural Changes Caused By Endotoxin Infusion in the Sheep

Time following Endotoxemia	Structural Changes
15 minutes	Accumulation, margination, degranulation, and fragmentation of granulocytes and accumulation of activated lymphocytes in pulmonary micro-circulation
30 minutes	More severe; migration of granulocytes and lymphocytes into interstitium; some interstitial edema
60 minutes	Interstitial leukocytes; endothelial and vessel wall damage; damaged type I and interstitial cells; perivascular edema
2 hours and onward	Endothelial layers disruption

(Fig. 7).[9,16,26–30] Compelling evidence that these products may actually modulate the lung injury caused by endotoxemia comes from studies with inhibitors of different aspects of the arachidonate metabolic pathways.[8,9,28–30]

Cyclooxygenase inhibitors markedly attenuate the early alterations in pulmonary hemodynamics (Fig. 3), lung mechanics (Fig. 3), and hypoxemia (Fig. 6) caused by endotoxemia.[9] Meclofenamate, a cyclooxygenase inhibitor, does not inhibit the later increases in lung fluid and solute exchange (Fig. 4) or the marked leukopenia (Fig. 5).[9,39] These data argue strongly for a role of cyclooxygenase products of arachidonate in the early changes in pulmonary hemodynamics and lung mechanics caused by endotoxemia. The thromboxane synthetase inhibitor, imidazole, attenuates both the early pulmonary hypertension and the late increases in lung fluid and solute exchange caused by endotoxemia in the awake sheep.[30] Preliminary results with the competitive SRS-A antagonist FPL 55712 demonstrate no effects on the sheep's response to endotoxemia. More specific lipoxygenase and thromboxane synthetase inhibitors are the subject of ongoing research attempting to further define the exact arachidonate products that may contribute to the lung injury caused by endotoxemia. Pretreatment of sheep with steroidal antiinflammatory agents attenuate all as-

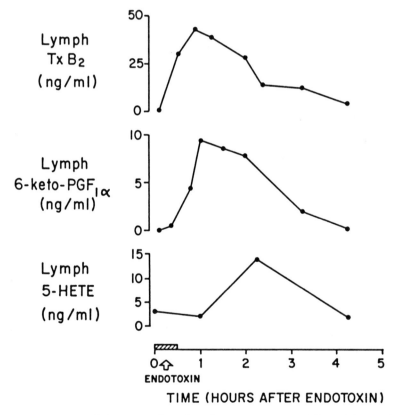

Figure 7: *Time course of changes in lung lymph concentrations of the stable metabolite of thromboxane-A₂, thromboxane-B₂ (TxB₂), and prostacyclin (6-keto-PGF₁α), and the lipoxygenase product 5-HETE following endotoxin infusion in a sheep.*

pects of the sheep's response to endotoxemia.[28,42] If steroids are given 45 minutes after endotoxin during the period of severe pulmonary hypertension and altered lung mechanics, they attenuate the later changes in lung fluid and solute exchange.[42] The mechanisms through which steroids act are not known but may involve inhibition of arachidonate metabolism.

Arachidonate products may modulate the injury caused by endotoxemia indirectly through interactions with the complement system or platelet and leukocyte function.[13-21] Granulocytes appear to play a significant role in the lung injury caused by endotoxemia.[26,39-41] Hydroxyurea granulocyte depletion attenuates the early alterations in lung mechanics (Fig. 8) and late increased lung fluid and solute exchange (Fig. 9) caused by endotoxemia but not

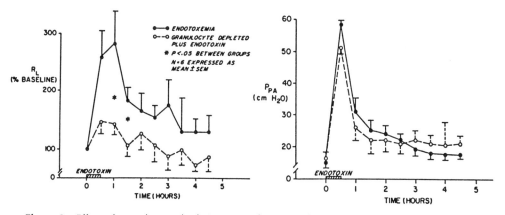

Figure 8: *Effect of granulocyte depletion on endotoxin induced changes in resistance to airflow across the lungs; R_L (left) and pulmonary artery pressure, P_{PA} (right). (From ref. 26, with permission.)*

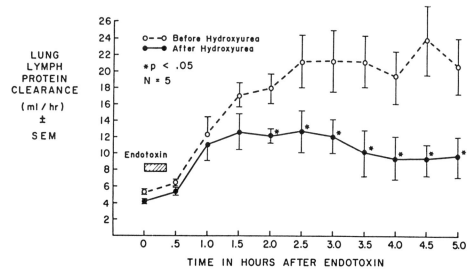

Figure 9: *Effect of granulocyte depletion on endotoxin-induced changes in lung lymph protein clearance (lung lymph flow X lymph to plasma protein concentration ratio). (From ref. 41, with permission.)*

the early pulmonary hypertension (Fig. 8).[4,26] Thus, if cyclooxygenase arachidonate products are responsible for both the early alterations in lung mechanics and pulmonary hemodynamics, the origin of the mediators may differ. Normal circulatory granulocyte counts are not necessary for the pulmonary hypertension but appear necessary for the alterations in lung mechanics. Hydroxyurea, used for granulocyte depletion, may in these studies affect more than circulating granulocytes. Hydroxyurea does decrease lymphocyte counts but does not affect platelet counts or the distribution or number of lung mast cells.[26] It is therefore possible that cells other than granulocytes are the source of arachidonate products that modulate the lung injury caused by endotoxemia. Table III summarizes the experimental results from studies using the endotoxemia model in sheep as a model of ARDS.

Arachidonate products of leukocyte origin may affect airway functions in diffuse lung injury by modulating airway reactivity.[43,44] Viral infections,[46] as well as recovery from ARDS,[47] have been associated with airway hyperreactivity in man. Endotoxemia (Fig. 10) in sheep,[43] ozone in dogs,[48] activated complement in rabbits,[49,50] and cigarette smoke[51] in guinea pigs are all associated with pulmonary inflammation and increased airway reactivity. Hydroxyurea granulocyte depletion decreases airway reactivity to aerosol histamine (Fig. 11) in sheep,[44] and there is a positive correlation between airway reactivity and circulating granulocyte counts in this model (Fig. 12).[44] Leukocyte production of arachidonate products thus may directly cause the early alterations in lung mechanics observed following endotoxemia.[26] Later, when inflammatory cells have sequestered and infiltrated into the lungs,[45] they may be a rich source for these potential mediators of bronchospasm. Nonspecific stimuli then cause the local release of large quantities of constrictor eicosanoids, resulting in increased airway reactivity.

Experimental evidence suggests that arachidonate products of platelet origin are not important in the pathogenesis of the lung injury caused by glass bead microembolization,[52] complement activation,[53] or endotoxemia.[27] Platelet depletion with antiplatelet antibodies does not attentuate the sheep's response to endotoxemia (Figs. 13, 14) or the usual increases observed in plasma and lung lymph concentrations of arachidonate metabolites, including thromboxane-B_2.[27] Lymphocytes, pulmonary macrophages, and many other of the some 40 cell types found in the lungs are capable of producing arachidonate products, and presumably different cells may produce arachidonate products depending on the experimental conditions. Further research is required to fully delineate the source and local action of released eicosanoids.

This chapter has briefly outlined some of the research, indicating a possible role for arachidonate products in diffuse lung injury. There is considerable evidence that arachidonate products are involved in diffuse lung injury as well as in the maintenance of homeostasis in the lungs. Arachidonate products may modulate lung injury through direct actions causing vaso- or bronchoconstriction or dilation, endothelial damage and increased microvascular permeability, or they may act indirectly by stimulating complement, leukocytes, or platelets. The eicosanoids appear to form part of a complex system of checks and balances involving the eicosanoids themselves as well as other systems and cells which they stimulate or inhibit. It is unlikely that diffuse lung injury such as observed in ARDS will be explained by the actions of a single arachidonate product. It is likely, on the other hand, that these agents

Table III
Mechanisms of Lung Injury Following
Endotoxemia in Sheep

Early (0−1 HR)

Pulmonary Hypertension	Altered Lung Mechanics
cyclooxygenase products	cyclooxygenase products
nongranulocyte	granulocytes
nonplatelet	nonplatelet

Late (2−5 HR)
"Increased Permeability"
granulocytes
Noncyclooxygenase product
nonplatelet
probably non-SRS-A

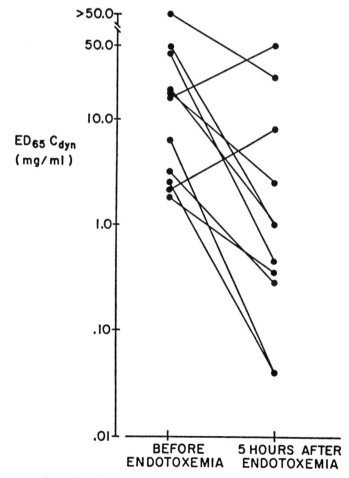

Figure 10: *Acute effects of endotoxemia on aerosol histamine responsiveness. $ED_{65}C_{dyn}$ is the concentration of aerosol histamine that causes a decrease in dynamic compliance of the lungs to 65% of control. The higher the $ED_{65}C_{dyn}$, the less responsive the sheep to aerosol histamine. (From ref. 43, with permission.)*

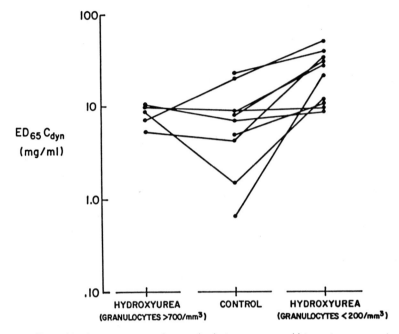

Figure 11: *Effect of hydroxyurea granulocyte depletion on aerosol histamine responsiveness in sheep. $ED_{65}C_{dyn}$ is the concentration of aerosol histamine that causes a decrease in dynamic compliance of the lungs to 65% of control. The higher the $ED_{65}C_{dyn}$, the less responsive the sheep to aerosol histamine. (From ref. 44, with permission.)*

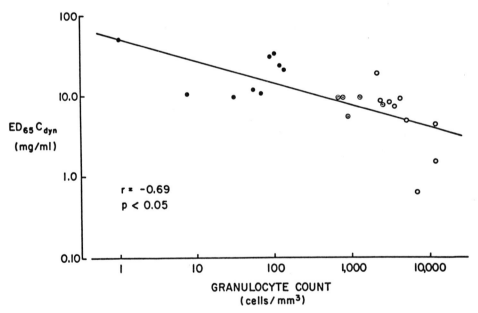

Figure 12: *Relationship of aerosol histamine responsiveness to peripheral blood granulocyte count. Data from nondepleted sheep are shown as (○), from partially depleted sheep as (◉), and from granulocyte depleted sheep as (●). $ED_{65}C_{dyn}$ is the concentration of aerosol histamine that causes a decrease in dynamic compliance of the lungs to 65% of control. The higher the $ED_{65}C_{dyn}$, the less responsive the sheep to aerosol histamine. (From ref. 44, with permission.)*

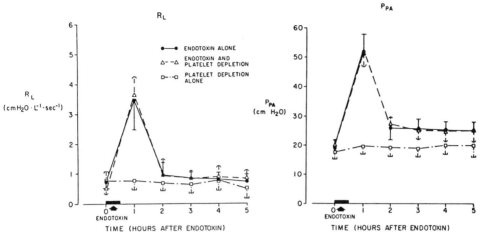

Figure 13: *Effect of platelet depletion on the endotoxin-induced changes in resistance to airflow across the lungs; R_L (left) and pulmonary artery pressure, P_{PA} (right).*

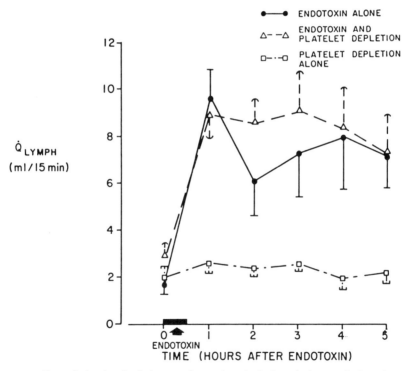

Figure 14: *Effect of platelet depletion on the endotoxin-induced changes in lung lymph flow $(\dot{Q}_{LYMPH})$.*

are important modulators of lung injury and that future research will help to delineate a complex system through which arachidonate products modulate diffuse lung injury.

References

1. Marcus, A.J.: The role of lipids in platelet function, with particular reference to the arachidonic acid pathway. *J. Lipid Res.* 19:793, 1978.
2. Flower, R.J. and Blackwell, G.J.: The importance of phospholipase-A_2 in prostaglandin biosynthesis. *Biochem. Pharmacol.* 25:285, 1976.
3. Samuelsson, B., Goldyne M., Granstrom E., et al.: Prostaglandins and thromboxanes. *Ann. Rev. Biochem.* 47:997, 1978.
4. Ramwell, P.W., Leovey, E.M.K., and Sintetos, A.L.: Regulation of the arachidonic acid cascade. *Biol. Reprod.* 16:70, 1977.
5. Bahlke, Y.S. and Vane, J..R.: Pharmacokinetic function of the pulmonary circulation. *Physiol. Rev.* 54:1007, 1974.
6. Vane, J.R.: The role of the lungs in metabolism of vasoactive substances. In *Pharmacology and Pharmacokinetics*. Teorell, T., Dedrick, R.L. and Condliffe, P.G., eds. New York, Plenum Press, 1979, p. 195.
7. Borgeat, P. and Samuelsson, B.: Transformation of arachidonic acid by polymorphonuclear leukocytes. *J. Biol. Chem.* 254:2643, 1979.
8. Snapper, J.R.: Septic pulmonary edema. *Semin. Respir. Med.* 3(2):92, 1981.
9. Snapper, J.R., Hutchison, A.A., Ogletree, M.L., et al.: Effects of cyclooxygenase inhibitors on the alterations in lung mechanics caused by endotoxemia in the unanesthetized sheep. *J. Clin. Invest.* 72(1):63, 1983.
10. Bach, M.K., Brashler, J.R., Hammarstrom, S., et al.: Identification of leukotriene C as a major component of slow reacting substances from rat mononuclear cells. *J. Immunol.* 125:115, 1980.
11. Bach, M.K., Brashler, J.R., Hammarstrom, S., et al.: Identification of a component of rat mononuclear cell SRS as leukotriene D. *Biochem. Biophys. Res. Commun.* 93:1121, 1980.
12. Lewis, R.A., Austen, K.F., Drazen, J.M., et al.: Slow reacting substances of anaphylaxis: Identification of leukotrienes C-1 and D from human and rat sources. *Proc. Natl. Acad. Sci. USA* 77:3710, 1980.
13. Samuelsson, B., Hammerstrom, S., Murphy, R. C., et al.: Leukotrienes and slow reacting substance of anaphylaxis (SRS-A). *Allergy* 35:375, 1980.
14. Hedqvist, P., Dahlen, S.-E., Gustafsson, L., et al.: Biological profile of leukotriene C_4 and D_4. *Acta Physiol. Scand.* 110:331, 1980.
15. Williams, T. and Piper, P. The action of chemically pure SRS-A on the microcirculation in vivo. *Prostaglandins* 19:779, 1980.
16. Ogletree, M., Oates, J., Brigham, K., et al.: Evidence for pulmonary release of 5-hydroxyeicosatetraenoic acid (5-HETE) during endotoxemia in unanesthetized sheep. *Prostaglandins* 23:459, 1982.
17. Brigham, K. and Ogletree, M.: Effects of prostaglandins and related compounds on lung vascular permeability. *Bull. Eur. Physiopathol. Respir.* 17:703, 1981.
18. Hyman, A., Spannhake, E., and Kadowitz, P.: Prostaglandins and the lung. In *Lung Disease: State of the Art, 1977–78*. New York, American Lung Association, 1978, pp. 229–254.
19. Ogletree, M.L., Snapper, J.R., and Brigham, K.L.: Immediate pulmonary vascular and airways responses after intravenous leukotriene (LT) D_4 injections in awake sheep. *The Physiologist* 25(4):275, 1982.
20. Snapper, J.R., Drazen, J.M., Loring, S.H., et al.: Vagal effects on histamine, carbachol and prostaglandin $F_{2\alpha}$ responsiveness in the dog. *J. Appl. Physiol: Respir. Environ. Exercise Physiol.* 47(1):13, 1979.
21. Kadowitz, P.J., Lippton, H.L., McNamara, D.B., et al.: Actions and metabolism of prostaglandins in the pulmonary circulation. In *Prostaglandins and the Cardiovascular System*. Oates, J.A., ed. New York, Raven Press, 1982, pp. 333–356.
22. Ogletree, M. and Brigham, K.: Arachidonate increases pulmonary vascular resis-

tance without changing lung vascular permeability in unanesthetized sheep. *J. Appl. Physiol.: Respir. Environ. Exercise Physiol.* 48:581, 1980.

23. Greenberg, G.M., Henderson, W.R., and Albert, R.K.: Vascular resistance and permeability are increased and lipoxygenase products are produced in excised rabbit lungs perfused with arachidonic acid. *Am. Rev. Respir. Dis.* 127(4):304, 1983.

24. Bernard, G.R., Lucht, W.D., Niedermeyer, M.L., et al.: Effect of N-acetylcysteine on the pulmonary response to endotoxin in the awake sheep and upon in vitro granulocyte function. *J. Clin. Invest.* (In press.)

25. Brigham, K.L., Begley, C.J., Bernard, G.R., et al.: Septicemia and lung injury. *Clin. Lab. Med.* 3(4):719, 1983.

26. Hinson, J.M., Jr., Hutchison, A.A., Ogletree, M.L., et al.: Effect of granulocyte depletion on altered lung mechanics after endotoxemia in sheep. *J. Appl. Physiol.: Respir. Environ. Exercise Physiol.* 55(1):92, 1983.

27. Snapper, J.R., Hinson, J.M., Jr., Lefferts, P.L., et al.: Effect of anti-platelet antibody (APA) on the awake sheep and platelet depletion on the sheep's response to endotoxemia. *Fed. Proc.* 42(2):1107, 1983.

28. Ogletree, M., Begley, C., and Brigham, K.: Combination of steroidal and non-steroidal anti-inflammatory agents inhibits early and late effects of endotoxin in awake sheep. *Am. Rev. Respir. Dis.* 4:303, 1983.

29. Ogletree, M. and Brigham, K.: Effect of cyclooxygenase inhibitors on pulmonary vascular responses to endotoxin in unanesthetized sheep. *Prostaglandins Leukotrienes Med.* 8:489, 1982.

30. Ogletree, M.L. and Brigham, K.L.: Imidazole, a selective inhibitor of thromboxane synthesis, inhibits pulmonary vascular responses to endotoxin in awake sheep. *Am. Rev. Respir. Dis.* 123:247, 1981.

31. Gerber, J., Voelkel, N., Nies, A., et al.: Moderations of hypoxic vasoconstriction by infused arachidonate acid: Role of PGI_2. *J. Appl. Physiol.* 49:107, 1980.

32. Weir, K., Mlczoch, J., Reeves, J., et al.: Endotoxemia and the prevention of hypoxic pulmonary vasoconstriction. *J. Lab. Clin. Med.* 88:975, 1976.

33. Newman, J., McMurtry, I., and Reeves, J.: Vascular responses of the lungs from rats exposed to high oxygen tensions. *Prostaglandins* 22:11, 1981.

34. Ogletree, M.L., Hutchinson, A.A., Snapper, J.R., et al.: Effects of alveolar hypoxia and endotoxin on lung prostacyclin and thromboxane metabolites in unanesthetized sheep. *Fed. Proc.* 41(5):1686, 1982.

35. Brigham, K., Bowers, R., and Haynes, J.: Increased sheep lung vascular permeability caused by E. coli endotoxin. *Circ. Res.* 45:292, 1979.

36. Esbenshade, A., Newman, J., Lams, P., et al.: Respiratory failure after endotoxin in sheep: Lung mechanics and lung fluid balance. *J. Appl. Physiol.* 53:967, 1982.

37. Snapper, J.R., Brigham, K.L., Heflin, A.C., et al.: Effects of endotoxemia on cyclic nucleotides in the unanesthetized sheep. *J. Lab. Clin. Med.* 102:240, 1983.

38. Brigham, K., Bowers, R., and Owen, P.: Effects of antihistamines on the lung vascular response to histamine in unanesthetized sheep: Diphenhydramine prevention of pulmonary edema and increased permeability. *J. Clin. Invest.* 58:391, 1976.

39. Snapper, J.R., Bernard, G.R., Hinson, J.M., Jr., et al.: Endotoxemia-induced leukopenia in sheep: Correlation with lung vascular permeability and hypoxemia but not with pulmonary hypertension. *Am. Rev. Resp. Dis.* 127:306, 1983.

40. Brigham, K.L., Loyd, J.E., Newman, J.H., et al.: Granulocytes in acute lung vascular injury in unanesthetized sheep. *Chest* 81S:56S, 1982.

41. Heflin, C. and Brigham, K.: Prevention by granulocyte depletion of increased vascular permeability of sheep lung following endotoxemia. *J. Clin. Invest.* 68:1253, 1981.

42. Brigham, K., Bowers, R., and McKeen, C.: Methylprednisolone prevention of increased lung vascular permeability following endotoxemia in sheep. *J. Clin. Invest.* 67:1103, 1981.

43. Hutchison, A.A., Hinson, J.M., Jr., Brigham, K.L., et al.: Effect of endotoxin on

airway responsiveness to aerosol histamine in sheep. *J. Appl. Physiol.: Respir. Environ. Exercise Physiol.* 54(6):1463, 1983.

44. Hinson, J.M., Jr., Hutchison, A.A., Brigham, K.L., et al.: Effects of granulocyte depletion on pulmonary responsiveness to aerosol histamine. *J. Appl. Physiol.: Respir. Environ. Exercise Physiol.* 56(2): 411, 1984.

45. Meyrick, B. and Brigham, K.: Acute effects of E. coli endotoxin on the pulmonary microcirculation of anesthetized sheep: Structure–function relationships. *Lab. Invest.* 48:548, 1983.

46. Empey, D.W., Laitinen, L.A., Jacobs, L., et al.: Mechanisms of bronchial hyperreactivity in normal subjects after upper respiratory tract infection. *Am. Rev. Respir. Dis.* 113:131, 1976.

47. Simpson, D.L., Goodman, M., Spector, S.L., et al.: Long-term follow-up and bronchial reactivity testing in survivors of the adult respiratory distress syndrome. *Am. Rev. Respir. Dis.* 117:449, 1978.

48. Holtzman, J.M., Fabbri, L.M., O'Byrne, P.M., et al.: Importance of airway inflammation for hyperreactivity induced by ozone in dogs. *Fed. Proc.* 42:1377, 1983 (Abstr.).

49. Irwin, C.G., Henson, P.M., and Bevens, N.: Acute effects of airways inflammation on airway function and reactivity. *Fed. Proc.* 41:1358, 1982.

50. Henson, P.M., Larsen, G.L., Webster, R.O., et al.: Pulmonary microvascular alterations and injury induced by complement fragments: Synergistic effect of complement activation, neutrophil sequestration, and prostaglandins. *Ann. NY Acad. Sci.* 284:287, 1982.

51. Hulbert, W. C., Walker, D. C., Jackson, A., et al.: Airway permeability to horseradish peroxidase in guinea pigs: The repair phase after injury by cigarette smoke. *Am. Rev. Respir. Dis.* 123:320, 1981.

52. Binder, A. S., Kageler, W., Perel, A., et al.: Effect of platelet depletion on lung vascular permeability after microemboli in sheep. *J. Appl. Physiol.: Respir. Environ. Exercise Physiol.* 48(3):414, 1980.

53. McDonald, J. W. D., Ali, M., Morgan, E., et al.: Thromboxane synthesis by causes other than platelets in association with complement-induced pulmonary leukostasis and pulmonary hypertension in sheep. *Circ. Res.* 52:1, 1983.

CHAPTER 15

Possible Role of Leukotrienes in the Pathogenesis of Pulmonary Hypertensive Disorders

John T. Reeves,
Kurt R. Stenmark, and
Norbert F. Voelkel

Introduction

Pulmonary hypertension is a serious clinical problem that arises from a variety of disease states. Unfortunately, we have little understanding of the pathological mechanisms leading to the pulmonary hypertension. For example, in chronic bronchitis, interstitial pneumonitis, cystic fibrosis, and pulmonary arteritis, it is not clear how the interstitial injury and/or inflammation affect the lung vasculature. With left-to-right shunts and pulmonary embolism, there is chronic or recurring injury to the vascular endothelium, which accompanies the thickening of the medial smooth muscle. Chronic endothelial injury and chronic elevation of left atrial pressure set the stage for chronic vascular leak into lung interstitium which could, by evoking release of chemotaxins, vasoactive substances, and mitogens, affect the pulmonary microcirculation (Fig. 1) although such mechanisms have not been established. Because the various forms of chronic pulmonary hypertension are often associated with chronic lung injury, inflammation, and vascular damage, we wondered whether substances known to mediate such events might be involved in the pathogenesis of pulmonary hypertension. Metabolites of arachidonic acid have recently received attention in this regard. The present discussion concerns the leukotrienes because they have potent effects on the lung and its vessels. It is the purpose of this review to examine the evidence that they may or may not be involved in pulmonary hypertensive states. Because the substances have been relatively recently characterized, most of the evidence derives from experimental work in animals, from perfused lungs, and even from cell cultures. As yet we have little evidence in human diseases, but we believe that the evidence to date is sufficient to warrant the following discussion.

From Said, S.I. (ed.): *The Pulmonary Circulation and Acute Lung Injury.* Mount Kisco, N.Y., Futura Publishing Co., Inc., 1985.

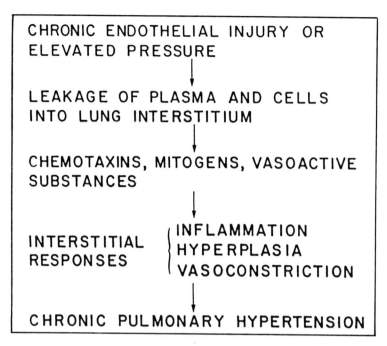

Figure 1: *Hypothetical schema for development of some forms of chronic pulmonary hypertension.*

Leukotrienes

The chemistry and pharmacology of leukotrienes has been expertly reviewed.[5] Briefly, leukotrienes are products of arachidonic acid metabolism (Fig. 2). Arachidonic acid is an essential fatty acid found, esterified, in the membrane of most mammalian cells. Once released in a free form, it appears to be rapidly metabolized along two pathways. One metabolic pathway is catalysed by cyclooxygenase, giving rise to substances such as prostacyclin (PGI_2, a vasodilator and an inhibitor of platelet aggregation) and thromboxane A_2 which causes platelet aggregation, vasoconstriction, and bronchoconstriction. Another pathway is catalysed by lipoxygenases, and gives rise to a variety of substances including leukotrienes. The leukotrienes arise from a metabolic cascade involving 5-HPETE and leukotriene A_4 as precursors. Leukotriene B_4 is known to be chemotactic for leukocytes. Leukotrienes C_4, D_4, and E_4 (Fig. 3) are known to cause edema and to constrict smooth muscle including that in airways and pulmonary arteries. 5-HETE does not appear to cause vascular smooth muscle contraction or edema in the lung.[99]

It was the capacity for smooth muscle contraction that led to the discovery of the class of substances now known as leukotrienes. Harkavy in 1930 found that the sputum of asthmatics contained a smooth muscle constrictor only when the patient was having an asthmatic attack.[38] The term *slow reacting substance of anaphylaxis* (SRS-A) was given to the active principle(s)[10,53] because it caused a slow, persistent smooth muscle constriction and it originated from immuno-

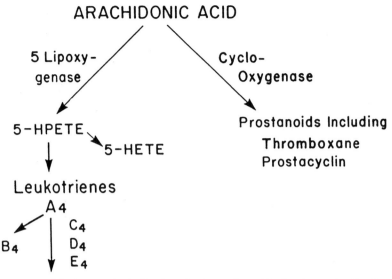

Figure 2: *A simplified cascade, indicating the formation of leukotrienes A_4, B_4, C_4, and D_4 from arachidonic acid. 5-HPETE = 5-hydroperoxyeicosatetraenoic acid; 5-HETE = 5-hydroxy-eicosatetraenoic acid.*

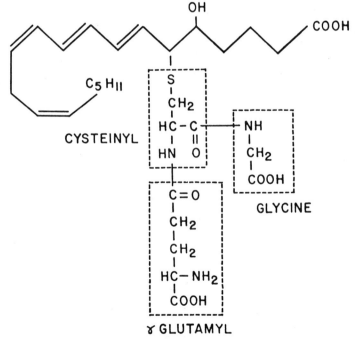

Figure 3: *Structure of leukotriene C_4. Progress in the study of SRS stemmed from Muryphy's[67] key discovery that the peculiar tripeptide glutathione (γ-glutamyl-cysteinyl-glycine) was attached to a lipid backbone derived from arachidonic acid. The "leuko" portion of the name refers to the origin from leukocytes. The "triene" refers to those conjugated double bonds that give the characteristic three absorption peaks by ultraviolet spectroscopy. The subscript "$_4$" refers to the total of four double bonds. The transformation from LTC_4 to LTD_4 is rapid and associated with the loss of the γ-glutamyl moiety. The transformation to the more stable compound LTE_4 is associated with further loss of the glycine moiety.*

logical disorders. In fact, the characteristic constriction caused by SRS when applied to the guinea pig ileum is the basis of the bioassay often currently used to screen for the presence of leukotrienes. The identity of SRS (now called leukotrienes) and its chemical structure have only recently been established.[67] The origin of the term *leukotrienes* has been presented.[85]

Possible Relation of Leukotrienes to Human Pulmonary Vascular Disease

A possible link between the presence of leukotrienes and one form of pulmonary hypertensive disease was recently suggested by findings in infants with persistent pulmonary hypertension of the newborn.[90] This is a disorder of unknown cause, with a significant morbidity and mortality, which is characterized by pulmonary hypertension in the newborn infant.[42] It is as though the high vascular resistance of the fetal lung does not regress with the onset of air breathing. A chest roentgenogram of an afflicted infant compared to a normal infant is shown in Figure 4.

The main features of the illness in the newborn are: pulmonary hypertension, bronchoconstriction, pulmonary edema, and hypoxemia. These features seem to match known or suspected actions of the leukotrienes as illustrated below:

Features of the pulmonary hypertensive illness in the newborn:	*Known or suspected lung actions of leukotrienes:*
1. Pulmonary hypertension	Vasoconstriction[37,99,104]
2. High airway resistance	Bronchoconstriction[37,102]
3. Pulmonary edema	Edema[3,13,18]
4. Hypoxemia secondary to items 1–3 above	

Thus it seemed reasonable to seek the presence of leukotrienes in newborns with pulmonary hypertension. However, because leukotriene measurements in blood are beset with difficulties, they were sought in pulmonary lavage fluid for the following reasons:

1. Lavage fluid was readily available. Infants with the disorder require for their clinical management an endotracheal tube. For care of the infants' airway, saline was flushed into and removed via the tube, thus providing lavage for analysis.

2. Sputum from another class of patients with pulmonary hypertension, i.e., cystic fibrosis, had been shown to contain leukotrienes.[17]

3. Leukotriene administered via the airways causes an increase in pulmonary arterial pressure and edema, suggesting that it can traverse the lung from the airway to the vascular compartment.[98]

The authors found that the lung lavage fluid from all five infants with the clinical diagnosis of persistent pulmonary hypertension, but fluid from none of the 14 control infants, had evidence of the presence of leukotrienes. Thus leukotrienes could be important in the pathogenesis of the disease process.

However, merely seeking and finding a particular substance in a body fluid

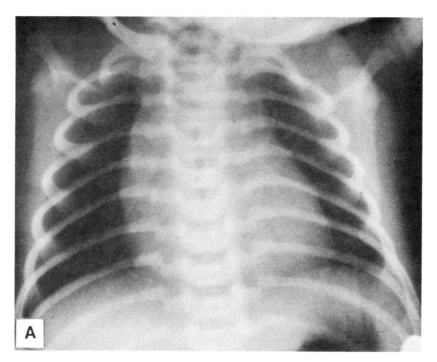

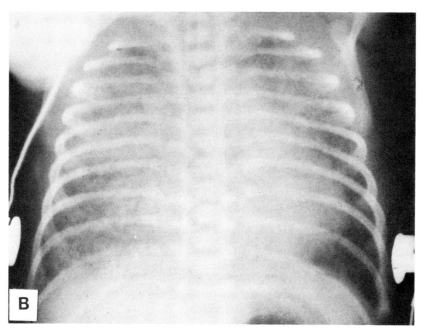

Figure 4: *Chest roentgenograms of newborn infants.* **A**: *The x-ray of an infant with no evidence of heart or lung disease.* **B**: *An x-ray of an infant, 60 hours old, with persistent pulmonary hypertension of the newborn. There is cardiomegaly and diffuse opacity compatible with pulmonary edema.*

in a complex disease process does not establish cause and effect between the substance and the disease. There are a number of criteria that need to be established before leukotrienes can be implicated in pulmonary hypertensive injury:

1. Leukotriene must be produced by the lung itself.
2. Leukotriene must have pulmonary vascular effects similar to those of the disease (i.e., edema, pulmonary hypertension, bronchoconstriction, inflammation, etc.).
3. Specific blockade of leukotriene production should prevent or reduce the abnormalities in animal models of edema and pulmonary hypertension.
4. It must be shown that leukotriene is the offending substance rather than being a response to other substances that might be causing the disease process.

Because the mechanism of possible leukotriene involvement in pulmonary hypertension cannot be evaluated in humans, investigators have turned to experimental animals. The four points listed above are considered in order.

Experimental Studies With Leukotriene

Leukotriene Production by the Lung

Given the early direction, much of the subsequent work centered around lung production of SRS-A under abnormal immunological states.[24,26,78] It is now clear that many cells including those in lung, joint, kidney, spleen, as well as leukocytes, monocytes, and basophils in blood and macrophages and mast cells in various tissues produce leukotrienes.[5] Within the lung, leukotriene may be produced by several cell types.[65,86] Also, mechanisms other than immunological stimuli may evoke lung leukotriene formation and release, for example, as may be seen when platelet activating factor (PAF) is given to isolated rat lungs (Fig. 5). If so, one wonders whether production proceeds with minimal pathologic stimulation or even occurs normally as a physiological event as might be implied by the work of Turnbull et al.[95]

The problem of "physiological release" in the isolated rat lung perfused with a salt solution was studied in our laboratory.[99] We found no leukotriene-like substances of bioassay in the effluent of unstimulated but perfused rat lungs. However, when we gave exogenous arachidonic acid to act as a substrate for leukotriene production, a small amount of SRS-like material could be detected in lung effluent. The experiment was repeated with indomethacin present in the perfusate. We expected an increase of lipoxygenase products because cyclo-oxygenase blockade might force metabolism down the lipoxygenase pathway.[11,23] We found that with indomethacin added, more SRS-A-like bioactivity was present in the effluent and LTC_4 could be identified by high pressure liquid chromatography (HPLC). These results raised the possibility that the lung might produce leukotrienes in response to minor manipulations. Although one could hardly conclude that removing the lung from the body, pump perfusing it with a salt solution, and administering arachidonate was a "minor manipulation," it is certainly less traumatic than the induction of pulmonary anaphy-

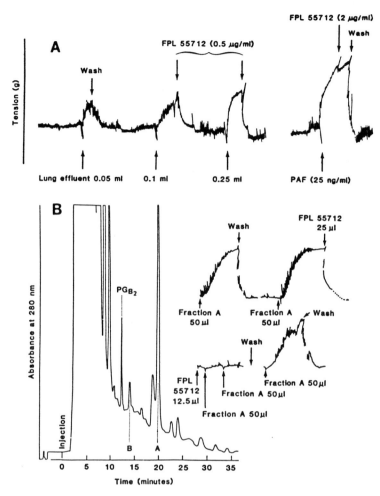

Figure 5: A: *Contractions of the isolated guinea pig ileum suspended in Tyrode solution, pH 7.3, containing $10^{-6}M$ atropine and $10^{-6}M$ pyrilamine, and bubbled with air. Effluent from lungs that received a 1 μg bolus injection of PAF contracted the guinea pig ileum; the contractions were immediately terminated upon addition of FPL 55712 (0.5 μg/ml) to the bath fluid. The direct application of PAF to the guinea pig ileum caused a contraction that was not terminated by FPL 55712.* **B:** *Reverse phase HPLC of partially purified extract of perfusate of rat lungs stimulated with PAF. The column was Sphereosorb C-18, 5 μm, 25 by 200 mm. The mobile phase used was methanol, water, and acetic acid (65:35:0.02 by volume), pH 5.1. The flow rate was 1 ml/min; the ultraviolet monitor was set at 280 nm. Prostaglandin B_2 was added as the elution reference.* **Inset:** *Guinea pig ileum bioassay of portions of fraction A illustrating inhibition of SRS-A-like response by FPL 55712 added to the assay cuvette as indicated by arrows. FPL 55712 inhibits ongoing contraction and in a lower dose prevents contraction if it is added to the ileum before application of fraction A. (Used with permission.[96])*

laxis in the perfused or chopped lung.[24] The work to date indicates that lung production of leukotrienes is not limited to immunological reactions and may in fact extend to a variety of pathological or even physiological responses.

Effects of Exogenously Administered Leukotrienes on the Lung

While there is agreement that the lung produces leukotrienes, there is less agreement on how the leukotrienes affect the lung, particularly in different species. When leukotriene is given intravenously to sheep,[50] cats,[28] or rats,[99] there is a rise in pulmonary arterial pressure and airway resistance that is transient and is blocked in some preparations by inhibitors of cyclooxygenase, such as indomethacin or meclofenamate. There appears to be interaction between the lipoxygenase and the cyclooxygenase pathways such that leukotrienes apparently can stimulate the synthesis of cyclooxygenase products. The responses to leukotrienes in vivo differ from the sustained contraction, not inhibited by cyclooxygenase blockade, seen with the addition of leukotrienes to the guinea pig lung strips[55a] or to the ileum. When leukotriene D_4 was given intravenously to guinea pigs, it caused a transient bronchoconstriction apparently mediated by thromboxane. However, when administered by aerosol to the airways, it caused a sustained bronchoconstriction that could be blocked by a lipoxygenase inhibitor and was increased by a cyclooxygenase inhibitor.[36] It is possible that the presence of blood cells or the binding of leukotriene to protein when given intravenously might cause the response to exogenous leukotrienes to differ from the response observed when they are given to the airways or administered to the perfusate of a more isolated system.

Indeed, in the rat lung LTC_4[99] and LTE_4[25] caused a sustained pulmonary pressor response when the lung was perfused with a physiological salt solution (but not when albumin or blood was present) and the responses were not abolished by indomethacin. Sustained bronchoconstriction and lung edema has been found in primates[88] and rats[97] following administration of leukotriene by the airways. In the rat, exogenous leukotrienes may act directly on the lung vessels rather than acting exclusively via the cyclooxygenase pathway, but leukotrienes have effects of their own. Further work needs to be done to establish for other species whether or not leukotriene has pulmonary vascular effects independent of cyclooxygenase metabolites. The concept is important because if leukotrienes contribute to the pathogenesis of pulmonary hypertension independent of cyclooxygenase metabolites, then cyclooxygenase inhibitors alone would not constitute effective treatment against leukotriene actions.

Lung Effects of Endogenously Generated Leukotrienes

Leukotrienes are locally produced within the lung. If they are effectively bound to proteins, then even if found in circulating blood,[79] they may not be active. If so, they might function primarily as local hormones to attract leukocytes, constrict smooth muscle, and cause edema. In such cases it is important to know the effects of endogenously produced leukotrienes. The two general approaches to the problem have been either to stimulate leukotriene production or to block leukotriene synthesis or action.

Stimulation of leukotriene synthesis, as indicated above, has been attempted by administration of arachidonate to provide additional substrate and the simultaneous blockade of the cyclooxygenase pathway in an attempt to force metabolism via the lipoxygenase pathway. In the rat lung, this has resulted in a sustained increase in pulmonary perfusion pressure and edema formation.[99]

Both pressure rise and edema formation were blocked by administration of diethylcarbamazine (DEC), an inhibitor of leukotriene synthesis.[60]

However, interpreting the results after the administration of exogenous arachidonic acid to an intact organism or to an isolated lung or even a cell culture is beset with difficulties. There may be more than one pool of esterified membrane arachidonate, and the fate of exogenous arachidonate is not known. Arachidonate and leukotrienes have different effects depending on the species, tissue, or cells studied and the conditions under which the studies are conducted.[4,16,32,50,70,83] For example, in the anesthetized dog during hypoxia[32] and during normoxia,[66] the net effect of arachidonate was vasodilation probably via production of prostacyclin. Yet other workers have found pulmonary pressor effects of arachidonic acid[49,72,103] and these were blocked with an inhibitor of cyclooxygenase. From the above, it seems that arachidonate given intravenously to an intact animal has lung vascular effects (either vasoconstriction or vasodilation), which are mediated, largely or exclusively, via the cyclooxygenase pathway. These findings differ from those in which arachidonate is given to the isolated rat lung perfused with a physiological salt solution. These discrepancies have not been fully resolved.

Because platelet activating factor (PAF) appears to stimulate lung leukotriene production,[96] this is also one way to observe the effects of endogenously produced leukotrienes, which could be characterized as leukotriene C_4 and D_4 (Fig. 5). The administration of PAF to the rat lung also caused a sustained pressor response followed by weight gain (Fig. 6). Neither the pressor response nor the weight gain was affected by indomethacin but both were blocked by DEC, which was considered to be consistent with the inhibition of leukotriene synthesis (Fig. 6). These initial findings in the rat lung have been confirmed following administration of PAF to the guinea pig lung in that PAF caused pulmonary edema and pulmonary vasconstriction.[35] These authors also made the additional observation that PAF stimulated bronchoconstriction. In fact, in the guinea pig lung the bronchoconstriction was of greater magnitude than the pulmonary vasoconstriction and appeared largely but not completely to be the result of thromboxane release.

At the present time our view is that leukotrienes C_4, D_4, and presumably also E_4 are produced by the mammalian lung (with the important differences between species as indicated above) and can cause pulmonary vasoconstriction, bronchoconstriction, and pulmonary edema. However, the factors regulating lung leukotriene synthesis, release, and action are still unknown.

Animal Models of Edema and Pulmonary Hypertension

Acute Lung Injury

Brigham,[9] in reviewing the experience with sheep in his laboratory, noted an increase in 5-HETE after endotoxin[73] and the failure of cyclooxygenase inhibitors to prevent the edema development. He postulated that lipoxygenase products could be mediators of the edema in this lung injury. Also, thiourea has long been known to cause pulmonary edema.[57] Recently, a hydroxyl radical scavenger, dimethyl sulfoxide, and also ethanol, mannitol, and dimethylthiourea were all shown to block the pulmonary edema from thiourea.[27] This suggested

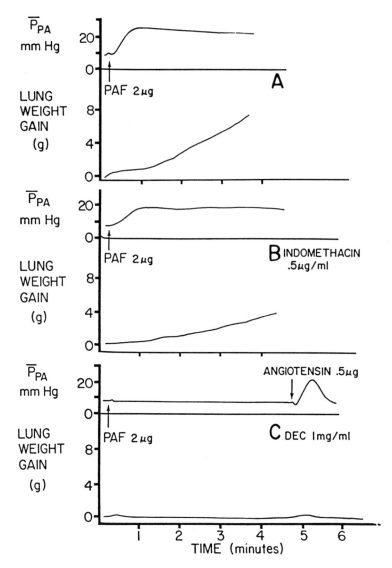

Figure 6: *Representative examples of three different experiments showing pulmonary artery pressure (PPA) tracing and lung weight gain. **A:** Physiological salt solution was used as the perfusate. **B:** The rats received an intraperitoneal injection of indomethacin (5 mg/kg) before they were killed and the lungs were perfused with a physiological salt solution containing indomethacin (0.5 μg/ml). **C:** The perfusate contained diethylcarbamazine (DEC, 1 mg/ml); angiotensin II was injected into the pulmonary artery 5 minutes after PAF. (Used with permission.[99])*

that the thiourea edema might be an oxidant-mediated injury, involving a reactive oxygen species, possibly different from H_2O_2. Preliminary evidence[19] suggests that luekotrienes are produced in thiourea-induced lung edema and that they may in fact mediate the edema. In Dauber's study, the leak was demonstrated both by a sensitive noninvasive method[82] as well as by the traditional wet/dry weight ratios following thiourea administration. The lung lavage was positive for SRS by bioassay using the guinea pig ileum and by radioimmunoassay in the dogs that received thiourea but not in the controls. Diethylcarbamazine reduced both the noninvasive estimate of leak and the lung wet/dry weight ratio following thiourea administration. Thus, it seemes likely that leukotrienes may contribute to the acute pulmonary edema in these dog and sheep models.

In vitro. One convenient form of lung injury for experimental study is that caused when reactive oxygen species such as H_2O_2 are produced in the fluid perfusing the lung. H_2O_2 may be produced by adding an oxidative enzyme such as glucose oxidase or xanthine oxidase to a fluid containing, respectively, either glucose or xanthine.[10a,47,48,76,94] The reaction consumes molecular oxygen with the result that the reaction is dependent on the presence of oxygen, but as it proceeds the PO_2 in the system falls[10a] and reactive oxygen species such as H_2O_2 are produced.[47,76,94] Reactive oxygen species activate circulating leukocytes that may be found in the lung[87] and contribute to the lung damage itself.[101] Oxygen radicals also have damaging effects on the lung itself,[47,59] in that in lungs perfused with a salt solution, the damage is independent of circulating cells and is prevented by oxygen radical scanvengers.[27,94]

Because active oxygen species can stimulate lipid peroxidation[15] and activate phospholipase[20] with the liberation of arachidonic acid,[20,29] one might expect oxidant lung injury to be associated with increased arachidonate metabolism. Indeed, evidence of activation of arachidonate metabolism has been presented for a wide variety of lung injuries including those from complement activation,[80] pulmonary thrombin embolism,[6,46] administration of phorbol myristate acetate,[68] and endotoxemia.[22,89] The activation of the arachidonate pathway in lung injury has recently been reviewed.[9]

With either phorbol myristate acetate in the awake sheep[69] or with H_2O_2 in the rat lung,[10a] the injury is not prevented by cyclooxygenase inhibition even though the cyclooxygenase pathway was activated by these interventions. In the rat lung, three different inhibitors of leukotriene synthesis or action did inhibit the edematous injury. At the same time the blockers inhibited the activation of the lipoxygenase pathway, because they blocked the H_2O_2-induced rise of 5-HETE. Leukotrienes themselves were not demonstrated in this injury, either because they were not the mediators of the injury or because they were rapidly destroyed by the oxygen radicals present.[33,41]

From these studies, in the intact sheep and in the isolated rat lung preparation, we conclude that lipoxygenase metabolites may be important in edematous lung injury. In other species, such as the rabbit, arachidonate activation may entail primarily the production of cyclooxygenase metabolites. In all of the animal models studied, the extent to which the leukotrienes mediate the increased vascular permeability needs to be established.

Possible Role of Leukotrienes in Animal Models of Chronic Pulmonary Hypertension

We wondered whether leukotrienes were invloved in chronic pulmonary hypertension. One form of pulmonary hypertension is that produced in rats by the pyrrolizidine alkaloid monocrotaline.[40] Monocrotaline induces lung injury not confined to the pulmonary vessels, but also involving a wide variety of lung cell types.[51,52,55,100] After the administration of a single 40 mg/kg dose of monocrotaline subcutaneously to young rats, there is development not only of a progressive pulmonary hypertension along a predictable time course, but also an increase in lung dry weight.[93] The increase in lung dry weight apparently indicates a lung hyperplastic response to the monocrotaline-induced injury because there is an increase in protein synthesis[56] along with the microscopic evidence of increased numbers of the various lung cell types.

Monocrotaline may have as one of its very early actions the damage of endothelial cells since large doses cause early pulmonary edema development[45] and smaller doses lead to a lung vessel leak without frank lung edema.[93] The leak is of interest because: (1) it appears early, preceding the development of right ventricular hypertrophy, pulmonary hypertension, and lung cell hyperplasia; (2) it is a permeability defect that persists at least for several days; (3) it may be causally related to the subsequent burst in lung protein synthesis (even brief pulmonary edema is followed by a burst of protein synthesis lasting for several days[30]); and (4) the sequence of lung vessel leak followed by lung cell hyperplasia and pulmonary hypertension is not unique to monocrotaline but also occurs in altitude-exposed rats.[93] One wonders if the leak might be more than a simple marker of the monocrotaline effect. For example, one could propose that endothelial cell injury would be followed by events such as the release of chemotaxins[71] and mitogens that would stimulate a vascular and/or interstitial cellular response that in turn would minimize the vascular leak. The cellular response in turn could be a factor in the pulmonary hypertension because the time course of the right ventricular hypertrophy coincides with the increase in dry lung weight and is closely related to it (Fig. 7).

A finding related to the cellularity of the lung was that young rats had a much greater pulmonary hypertensive response to monocrotaline than did older rats. The growth rate and the pulmonary hypertensive effect of monocrotaline were closely correlated. The possibility that there might be a causal link between the potential for lung growth and monocrotaline-induced pulmonary hypertension was supported by the finding of no monocrotaline effect when food intake of the rat was limited to prevent body growth.[31] If so, then the hyperplastic cellular response may be a requirement for the development of the pulmonary hypertensive disease. In the rat, for whatever reason, early in life when the lung is rapidly growing appears to be a time of particular susceptibility to monocrotaline.

Leukotrienes could have a role in monocrotaline-induced pulmonary hypertension. As indicated above, leukotrienes have pulmonary pressor activity and promote lung vessel leak, both of which are components of the monocrotaline injury model. Also leukotriene B_4 is chemotactic for leukocytes, which could elaborate mitogens and lead to pulmonary cell hyperplasia.[8] Macrophages that are prominent in monocrotaline lung injury[92] are known to generate leukotrienes B_4[44] and C_4[86] and thus they could be part of the pathogenesis of the lung injury. If leukotrienes were important in the genesis of the pulmonary hypertensive lung injury, then by inhibiting leukotriene synthesis, one might inhibit the injury. Stenmark[91] administered diethylcarbamazine because it has been shown to inhibit leukotriene synthesis in isolated cells stimulated by calcium ionophore.[60] In addition, it inhibited SRS production following anaphylactic challenge in rats[77] and it inhibited the edema associated with SRS-A appearance in lung lavage fluid in dogs given thiourea.[19] In monocrotaline-treated rats given diethylcarbamazine, the development of pulmonary hypertension was prevented as was the inflammatory cell response. Taken together,

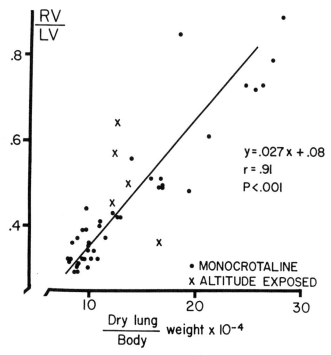

Figure 7: *Relationship of degree of right ventricular hypertrophy (RV/LV) to dry weight of lung, related to body weight. ● = values in rats killed at varying intervals after monocrotaline. Regression line indicates significant relationship; 5 altitude-exposed rats (X) fell around regression line. (Used with permission.[92])*

these data suggest that in rats given monocrotaline, as measured by leukocyte and macrophage number and activity, leukotrienes may be playing a role in the pulmonary hypertensive lung injury. The role could include the leukotriene actions of chemotaxis, increased permeability, and pulmonary vasoconstriction. If so, it is a curious anomaly that in this form of injury there has been no bronchoconstriction described. Perhaps this relates to the vascular route by which the injury is delivered.

Hypoxia

Alveolar hypoxia is known to increase pulmonary arterial pressure, particularly in the young, and thus one wonders if leukotrienes might be involved in hypoxic pulmonary vasoconstriction. A recent study by Ahmed[2] in the adult sheep suggested that disodium chromoglycate will inhibit hypoxic pulmonary vasoconstriction. Disodium chromoglycate (or Cromylin ®) is a putative inhibitor of mast cell release. It also is structurally related to FPL 55712, an end organ blocker of leukotriene action. Thus disodium chromoglycate could inhibit leukotrienes by one or more mechanisms.

In the newborn lamb, as in other mammals, pulmonary arterial pressure and vascular resistance fall rapidly with the first breaths after birth. While a part of the fall in resistance is due to mechanical factors, such as replacing the fetal alveolar fluid with air and expanding the lung, there is also a major contribution from the increased alveolar oxygenation. Hypoxic pulmonary vasoconstriction is thereby relieved. This fall in resistance is attenuated and may even be reversed by the administration of cyclooxygenase inhibitors.[14] Presumably such inhibition blocks the production of vasodilator prostaglandins. Also, the blockade of the cyclooxygenase pathway could shunt arachidonate metabolites to the lipoxygenase pathway.

Thus, a role for leukotrienes in hypoxic pulmonary vasoconstriction was sought and Morganroth[62-64] observed that DEC, U60,257, and FPL-55712 (agents that inhibit leukotriene synthesis or action) blocked hypoxic pulmonary vasoconstriction. Less affected was the angiotensin II-induced constriction in isolated perfused rat lungs. The inhibition of hypoxic pulmonary vasoconstriction did not appear to depend upon the generation of cyclooxygenase vasodilators, or on calcium inhibitory properties of the inhibitors used. Subsequently, it was demonstrated that DEC inhibits also the development of chronic hypoxic pulmonary hypertension in rats at high altitude.[63,64] Thus relatively selective inhibition of hypoxic pulmonary vasoconstriction by three dissimilar inhibitors of leukotriene synthesis or action suggested that leukotrienes were somehow involved in the mechanism of hypoxic constriction.

Problems

Leukotrienes have been found in infants who have evidence of lung edema, pulmonary hypertension, and hypoxemia. In animal models, lung production of leukotrienes and leukotriene action have been found where there was also edema, pulmonary hypertension, and hypoxia. However, there are a number of problems that remain to be solved:

1. The specificity of the inhibitors used is open to question. Even if each has been shown to inhibit leukotriene synthesis release or action, we do not know what other effects they might have. For example, BW 755C prevents synthesis of prostaglandins and other lung and platelet enzymes.[43] ETYA may block the 12-HETE but not the 5-HETE pathway.[7] Although FPL 55712 inhibits lipoxygenase but not cyclooxygenase in rat basophil leukemia cells, in other systems it inhibits histamine release, cyclic AMP and GMP, phosphodiesterase, and thromboxane synthetase.[12] DEC is a piperazine derivative that has been used for decades in the treatment of human parasites and a wide variety of effects have been described.[39] Among these are myocardial depression,[75] platelet inhibition,[54] sympathetic stimulation,[1] histamine release,[21] and depolarization of smooth muscle.[58]

2. With regard to a role of leukotrienes in hypoxic pulmonary vasoconstriction, a dilemma exists in that leukotrienes are potent inducers of lung edema, and lung edema is not apparent during hypoxic pulmonary vasoconstriction.

3. Leukotrienes are ephemeral substances that are difficult to identify with certainty and are even harder to measure. There may be in some pathologic states inhibitors of leukotriene action.[91] Thus the investigations are beset with technical and biological difficulties.

4. Leukotrienes are probably locally produced and locally active within a

given tissue, increasing further the difficulties of identifying and studying them.

5. Leukotrienes may not be the active substances in the above responses or they may not be the only active substances. There are complex interactions between leukotrienes and other pathways.[5,81] Further, the release of arachidonate from esterified membrane lipids is not an isolated event, but is accompanied by release of other potent substances including platelet activating factor. Surely many of these substances are unknown. Assays of those that are known are still in the development stages.

Summary

Leukotrienes are present in the lung lavage fluid in human pulmonary hypertension. The important question is, are they cause or effect of the disease state? Because the question cannot be effectively addressed in human beings, animal models have been employed. Because a single animal model of pulmonary hypertension does not closely mimic the human condition, several such animal models have been used. In animal models of edema, chronic pulmonary hypertension, and acute hypoxic pulmonary hypertension, lipoxygenase products have been implicated. Although we cannot draw conclusions regarding cause and effect relating leukotrienes to hypertensive lung injury, we can say that the problem deserves further investigation.

REFERENCES

1. Abaitey, A.K. and Parratt, J.R.: Cardiovascular effects of diethylcarbamazine citrate. *Br. J. Pharmacol.* 55:219–227, 1975.
2. Ahmed, T. and Oliver, W.: Does slow-reacting substance of anaphylaxis mediate hypoxic pulmonary vasoconstriction? *Am. Rev. Respir. Dis.* 127:566–571, 1983.
3. Albert, R.L. and Henderson, W.R.: Leukotriene C_4 increases pulmonary vascular permeability in excised rabbit lungs. *Fed. Proc.* 41:1503, 1982.
4. Armstead, W.H., Lippton, H.L., Hyman, A.L., et al.: Vasoconstrictor activity of leukotrienes in the feline mesenteric vascular bed. *Fed. Proc.* 42:500, 1983.
5. Bach, M.K.: The leukotrienes: Their structure, action, and role in diseases. *Current Concepts*, Kalamazoo, Michigan, UpJohn, 1983.
6. Bizios, R., Minnear, F.L., Hoyle, V.Z., et al.: Effects of cyclooxygenase and lipooxygenase inhibition on lung fluid balance after thrombin. *J. Appl. Physiol.* 55: 462–471, 1983.
7. Borgeat, P., Fruteau de Laclas, B., and Maclouf, J.: New concepts in the modulation of leukotriene synthesis. *Biochem. Pharmacol.* 32:381–387, 1983.
8. Bray, M.A., Hutchinson, A.W., and Smith, M.J.H.: Leukotriene B_4: Biosynthesis and biological activities. In *SRS-A and Leukotrienes*. Piper, P.J., ed. Chichester, Research Studies Press, Inc., 1981.
9. Brigham, K.L.: Mechanisms of lung injury. *Clin. Chest Med.* 3:9–24, 1982.
10. Brocklehurst, W.E.: The release of histamine and formation of slow reacting substance (SRS-A) during anaphylactic shock. *J. Physiol.* (London) 151:416–435, 1960.
10a. Burghuber, O., Methias, M.M., McMurtry, I.F., et al.: Lung edema due to hydro-

gen peroxide is independent of cyclooxygenase products. *J. Appl. Physiol.* 56: 900–905, 1984.

11. Burka, J.F. and Eyre, P.: Effects of bovine SRs-A (SRS-A bov) on bovine respiratory tract and lung vasculature in vivo. *Eur. J. Pharmacol.* 44:169–177, 1977.

12. Casey, F.B., Appleby, B.J., and Buck, D.C.: Selective inhibition of lipoxygenase metabolic pathway of arachidonic acid by the SRS-A antagonist FPL 55712. *Prostaglandins* 25:1–9, 1983.

13. Casey, L., Clarke, J., Fletcher, J., et al.: Cardiovascular, respiratory, and hematologic effects of leukotriene D_4 in primates. In *Leukotrienes and Other Lipoxygenase Products.* Samuelsson, B., Paoletti, R., eds. New York, Raven Press, 1982, pp. 201–210.

14. Cassin, S.: Humoral factors affecting pulmonary blood flow in the fetus and newborn infants. In *Report of 83rd Ross Conference on Pediatric Research.* Columbus, Ohio, Ross Laboratories, 1982, pp. 1–26.

15. Chan, P.M., Yurko, M., Fishman, R.A.: Phospholipid degradation in cellular edema induced by free radicals in brain cortical slices. *Neurochemistry* 38:525–531, 1982.

16. Chapnick, B.M. and Smart, K.J.: Differential effect of leukotriene D_4 on canine mesenteric and renal flow. *Fed. Proc.* 42:639, 1983.

17. Cromwell, O., Walport, M.J., Morris, H.R., et al.: Identification of leukotrienes D and B in sputum from cystic fibrosis patients. *Lancet* 2:164–165, 1981.

18. Dahlen, S.E., Bork, J., Hedquist, P., et al.: Leukotrienes promote plasma leakage and leukocyte adherence in postcapillary venules: In vivo effects of relevance to acute inflammatory response. *Proc. Natl. Acad. Sci. USA* 78:3887–3891, 1981.

19. Dauber, I., Pluss, W., Stenmark, K., et al.: Leukotriene in thiourea-induced lung injury. *Am. Rev. Resp. Dis.* 127:304, 1983 (Abstr.).

20. Del Maestro, R.F., Bjork, J., and Arfors, K.E.: Increase in microvascular permeability induced by enzymatically generated free radicals. II: Role of superoxide anion radical, hydrogen peroxide, and hydroxyl radical. *Microvasc. Res.* 22: 255–270, 1981.

21. Deline, T.R., Eyre, P., and Wells, P.W.: Histamine releasing properties of the anhelminthic 1-diethylcarbamyl-4-methylpiperazine citrate (Diethylcarbamazine). *Arch. Int. Pharmacol. Ther.* 205:192–198, 1973.

22. Demling, R.H., Smith, M., Gunther, R., et al.: Pulmonary injury and prostaglandin production during endotoxemia in conscious sheep. *Am. J. Physiol.* 240:H348–H353, 1981.

23. Engineer, D.M., Niederhausen, V., Piper, P.J., et al.: Release of mediators of anaphylaxis. Inhibition of prostaglandin synthesis and the modification of release of slow reacting substance of anaphylaxis and histamine. *Br. J. Pharmacol.* 62:61–66, 1978.

24. Farmer, J.B., Richards, I.M., Sheard, P., et al.: Mediators of passive lung anaphylaxis in the rat. *Br. J. Pharmacol.* 55:57–64, 1975.

25. Fedderson, O.C., Mathias, M.M., Murphy, R.C., et al.: Leukotriene E_4 causes pulmonary vasoconstriction not inhibited by meclofenamate. *Prostaglandins* 26: 869–883, 1983.

26. Fleisch, J.H., Haisch, K.D., and Paethe, S.M.: Slow reacting substance of anaphylaxis (SRS-A) release from guinea pig lung parenchyma during antigen- or ionophore-induced contraction. *J. Pharmacol. Exp. Ther.* 221:146–151, 1982.

27. Fox, R.B., Harada, R.N., Tate, R.M., et al.: Prevention of thiourea-induced pulmonary edema by hydroxyl-radical scavengers. *J. Appl. Physiol.* 55:1456–1459, 1983.

28. Fox, R.B. and Murphy, K.A.: Scavenger oxygen radicals in vivo: prevention of pulmonary oxygen toxicity by the hydroxyl radical scavenger, dimethylthiourea. *Am. Rev. Resp. Dis.* 125:149A, 1982.

29. Freeman, B.A. and Crapo, J.D.: Biology of disease: free radicals and tissue injury. *Lab. Invest.* 67:412–426, 1982.

30. Fricke, R.F. and Secker-Walker, R.H.: Recovery from ethchloruynal-induced pulmonary edema in the rat. *Clin. Res.* 28:425A, 1980.

31. Ganey, P. and Roth, R.A.: Dietary restriction and cardiopulmonary toxicity of monocrotaline pyrrole. *Fed. Proc.* 42:353, 1983 (Abstr.).

32. Gerber, J.G., Voelkel, N.V., Nies, A.S., et al.: Arachidonic acid induced pulmonary vasodilation during hypoxia: The role of PGI_2. *J. Appl. Physiol.* 49:107–112, 1980.

33. Goetz, E.J.: The conversion of leukotriene C_4 of isomers of leukotriene B_4 by human eosinophil peroxidase. *Biochem. Biophys. Res. Comm.* 106:270–275, 1982.

34. Greybar, G.B., Cowen, K.H., Spannake, E.W., et al.: Cyclooxygenase-mediated airway response to leukotriene D_4 in the cat. *Circulation* 68 (Suppl. III): 406, 1983.

35. Hamasaki, Y., Mojarad, M., Saga, T., et al.: Platelet activating factor raises airway pressure and vascular pressures and induces edema in lungs perfused with platelet free solution. *Am. Rev. Resp. Dis.* 129:742–746, 1984.

36. Hamel, R., Masson, P., Ford-Hutchinson, A.W., et al.: Differing mechanisms for leukotriene D_4-induced bronchoconstriction in guinea pigs following intravenous and aerosol administration. *Prostaglandins* 24:419–430, 1982.

37. Hanna, C.J., Bach, M.K., Pane, P.D., et al.: Slow-reacting substances (leukotrienes) contract human airway and pulmonary vascular smooth muscle in vitro. *Nature* 290:343–344, 1981.

38. Harkavy, J.: Spasm producing substance in the sputum of patients with bronchial asthma. *Arch. Int. Med.* 45:641–646, 1930.

39. Hawking, F. and Ross, W.F.: Miracil D, its toxicity, absorption, and excretion in animals and human volunteers. *Br. J. Pharmacol.* 3:167–173, 1948.

40. Hayaski, J., Hussa, J.F., and Lalich, J.J.: Cor pulmonale in rats. *Lab. Invest.* 16:875–881, 1967.

41. Henderson, W.R., Jorg, A., and Klebanoff, S.D.: Eosinophil peroxidase-mediated in activation of leukotrienes B_4, C_4, and D_4. *J. Immunol.* 128:2609–2613, 1983.

42. Heymann, M.A. and Hoffman, J.I.E.: Persistent pulmonary hypertension syndromes in the newborn. In *Pulmonary Hypertension*. Weir, E.K. and Reeves, J.T., eds. Mount Kisco, NY, Futura Publishing Co., 1984, pp. 45–72.

43. Higgs, G.A. and Vane, J.R.: Inhibition of cyclooxygenase and lipoxygenase. *Br. Med. Bull.* 39:265–270, 1983.

44. Hseuh, W. and Sun, F.F.: Leukotriene B_4 biosynthesis by alveolar macrophages. *Biochem. Biophys. Res. Comm.* 106:1085, 1982.

45. Hurley, J.V. and Jago, M.V.: Pulmonary edema in rats given monocrotaline: A topographic and electron micrographic. *J. Pathol.* 117:23–32, 1975.

46. Johnson, A., Bizios, R., Kern, D.F., et al.: Comparison of the effects of indomethacin (INDO) and ibuprofen (IBU) on thrombin-induced increase in lung vascular permeability. *Am. Rev. Respir. Dis.* 127:309, 1983 (Abstr.).

47. Johnson, K.J. and Ward, P.A.: Role of oxygen metabolites in immune complex injury of lung. *J. Immunol.* 126:2365–2369, 1981.

48. Johnson, K.J., Fantone, J.C., Kaplan, J., et al.: In vivo damage of rat lungs by oxygen metabolites. *J. Clin. Invest.* 67:983–993, 1981.

49. Kadowitz, P.J., Spannhake, E.W., Greenberg, S., et al.: Comparative effects of arachidonic acid, bisensic prostaglandins, and an endoperoxide analog on the canine pulmonary vascular bed. *Can. J. Physiol. Pharmacol.* 55:1369–1377, 1977.

50. Kadowitz, P.J. and Hyman, A.L.: Analysis of responses to leukotriene D_4 in the sheep pulmonary vascular bed. *Circulation* 63 (Suppl. III):35, 1983.

51. Kay, J.M., Smith, P., and Heath, D.: Electron microscopy of crotalaria pulmonary hypertension. *Thorax* 24:511–526, 1969.

52. Kay, J.M. and Heath, D.: *Crotalaria Spectabilis, the Pulmonary Hypertension Plant*. Charles C. Thomas, Springfield, Ill, 1969.

53. Kellaway, C.H. and Threthewic, E.R.: Liberation of a slow reacting smooth muscle stimulating substance in anaphylaxis. *Q. J. Exp. Physiol.* 30:121–145, 1940.

54. Kowalski, K.A., McConnell, L.A., Sadoff, D.A., et al.: Modulation of equine platelet function of diethylcarbamazine (DEC). *Am. J. Pathol.* 113:1–7, 1983.

55. Kuriyama, T., Sugita, T., Takisawa, H., et al.: Experimental study of pulmonary hypertension: Correlation between histopathological changes of pulmonary vas-

culature and elevation of pulmonary arterial pressure. *J. Jap. Thorac. Soc.* 14: 496–505, 1976.

55a. Leitch, A.G., Austen, K.F., Coney, E.J., et al.: Effects of indomethacin on the contractile response of guinea pig parenchymal strips to leukotrienes B_4, C_4, D_4 and E_4. *Fed. Proc.* 41:1047, 1982.

56. Lafranconi, M. and Huxtable, R.J.: The time course of lung hyperplasia and right heart hypertrophy produced by the pyrrolizide alkaloid, monocrotaline. *Fed. Proc.* 40:629, 1981 (Abstr.).

57. MacKensie, J.B. and Maclausie, C.G.: Production of pulmonary edema by thiourea in the rat and its relation to age. *Proc. Soc. Biol. Med.* 54:34–37, 1943.

58. Martin, R.J.: Electrophysiological effects of piperazine and diethylcarbamazine on Ascarissuum somatic muscle. *Br. J. Pharmacol.* 77:255–265, 1982.

59. Martin, W.J., Gadek, J.E., Hunninghake, G.W., et al.: Oxidant injury of lung parenchymal cells. *J. Clin. Invest.* 68:1277–1288, 1981.

60. Mathews, W.R. and Murphy, R.C.: Inhibition of leukotriene biosynthesis in mastocytoma cells by diethylcarbamazine. *Biochem. Pharmacol.* 31:2129–2132, 1982.

61. Meyrick, B., Gamble, W., and Reid, L.: Development of crotaline pulmonary hypertension: Hemodynamic and structural study. *Am. J. Physiol.* 239:H692–H702, 1980.

62. Morganroth, M.L., Murphy, R.C., and Voelkel, N.F.: Diethylcarbamazine, DEC, a leukotriene synthesis blocker, blocks hypoxic pulmonary vasoconstriction. *Fed. Proc.* 42:303, 1983 (Abstr.).

63. Morganroth, M.L., Reeves, J.T., Murphy, R.C., et al.: Leukotriene synthesis and receptor blockers block hypoxic pulmonary vasoconstriction. *J. Appl. Physiol.* 56:1340–1346, 1984.

64. Morganroth, M.L., Stenmark, K., Reeves, J.T., et al.: Diethylcarbamazine (DEC), a leukotriene synthesis blocker, blocks pulmonary hypertension in intact rats exposed to chronic hypobaric hypoxia. *Am. Rev. Resp. Dis.* 129:A344, 1984.

65. Morris, H.R., Piper, P.J., Taylor, G.W., et al.: The role of arachidonate lipoxygenase in the release of SRS-A from guinea pig chopped lung. *Prostaglandins* 19: 371–379, 1980.

66. Mullane, K.M., Dusting, G.J., Salmon, J.A., et al.: Biotransformation and cardiovascular effects of arachidonic acid in the dog. *Eur. J. Pharmacol.* 54:217–228, 1979.

67. Murphy, R.C., Hammarstrom, S., and Samuelsson, B.: Leukotriene C: A slow reacting substance from murine mastocytoma cells. *Proc. Natl. Acad. Sci. USA* 76:4275–4279, 1979.

68. Newman, J.H., Lloyd, J.E., Ogletree, M.L., et al.: Effects of melcofenamate on the pulmonary vascular response to PMA. *Am. Rev. Respir. Dis.* 124:282, 1982 (Abstr.).

69. Newman, J.H., Lloyd, J.E., Meyrick, B.O., et al.: Cyclooxygenase inhibition during phorbol-induced granulocyte stimulation in awake sheep. *J. Appl. Physiol.* 56: 999–1007, 1984.

70. Noonan, T.C., Garcia-Szabo, R.R., and Malik, A.B.: Pulmonary microcirculatory effects of leukotriene D_4 (LTD_4) and D_4 (LTD_4). *Fed. Proc.* 42:731, 1983.

71. O'Brien, R., Seton, M., Markarski, J., et al.: Endothelial cells (EC) treated with thiourea (TU) release a chemoattractant for neutrophils (PMN). *Am. Rev. Respir. Dis.* 1256:229, 1982 (Abstr.).

72. Ogletree, M.L. and Brigham, K.L.: Arachidonate raised vascular resistance but not permeability in the lungs of awake sheep. *J. Appl. Physiol.* 48:581–586, 1980.

73. Ogletree, M., Brigham, K.L., and Oates, J.: Increased flux of 5-HETE in sheep lung lymph during pulmonary leukostasis after endotoxin. *Fed. Proc.* 40:767, 1981.

74. Ogletree, M.L., Snapper, J.R., and Brigham, K.L.: Immediate pulmonary vascular and airways responses after intravenous leukotriene injections in awake sheep. *The Physiologist* 25:41, 1982.

75. Ojewole, J.A.O. and Vonejeme, I.: Myocardial depressant effects of diethylcarbamazine citrate in vivo. *Eur. J. Pharmacol.* 87:242–252.

76. Olson, J.S., Ballouk, D.P., Palmer, G., et al.: The reaction of xanthine oxidase with molecular oxygen. *J. Biol. Chem.* 249:4350–4362, 1974.

77. Orange, R.P., Valentine, M.D., and Austen, K.F.: Inhibition of the release of slow-reacting-substance of anaphylaxis in the rat with diethylcarbamazine. *Proc. Soc. Exp. Biol. Med.* 127:127–132, 1968.

78. Orange, R.P. and Austin, K.F.: Slow reacting substance of anaphylaxis in the rat. In *Cellular and Humoral Mechanisms in Anaphylaxis and Allergy.* Movat, H.Z., ed. Karger, Basel, 1969, 196–206.

79. Parker, C.W., Koch, D., Huber, M.M., et al.: Formation of the cysteinyl form of slow reacting substance (leukotriene E_4) in human plasma. *Biochem. Biophys. Res. Comm.* 97:1038–1046, 1980.

80. Perkowski, S.Z., Havill, A.M., Flynn, J.T., et al.: Role of intrapulmonary release of eicosanoids and superoxide anion as mediators of pulmonary dysfunction and endothelial injury in sheep with intermittent complement activation. *Circ. Res.* 53: 574–583, 1983.

81. Piper, P.J., Samhoun, M.N., Tippins, J.R., et al: Pharmacological studies on pure SRS-A and synthetic leukotrienes C_4 and D_4. In *SRS-A and Leukotrienes.* Piper, P.J., ed. New York, John Wiley and Sons, 1981, pp. 81–99.

82. Pluss, W., Dauber, I., van Grondelle, A., et al.: Specificity and sensitivity of non-invasive measurement of pulmonary vascular protein leak. *Am. Rev. Respir. Dis.* 127:306, 1983 (Abstr.).

83. Pozenbeck, M.J., Baez, A., and Kaley, G.: Effects of intracoronary leukotriene D_4 and a prostaglandin endoperoxide analogue in the chloralase anesthetized dog. *Fed. Proc.* 42:639, 1983.

84. Said, S. and Mutt, V.: Relationship of spasmogenic and smooth muscle relaxant peptides from normal lung to other vasoactive compounds. *Nature* 265:84–86, 1977.

85. Samuelsson, B., Borgeat, P., Hammarstram, S., et al.: Introduction of a nomenclature: Leukotrienes. *Prostaglandins* 17:785–787, 1979.

86. Scott, W.A., Rougen, C.A., and Cohn, Z.A.: Leukotriene C release by macrophages. *Fed. Proc.* 42:129–133, 1983.

87. Shasby, D.M., VanBenthuysen, K.M., Tate, R.M., et al.: Granulocytes mediate acute edematous lung injury in rabbits and isolated rabbit lungs perfused with phorbol myristate acetate: Role of oxygen radicals. *Am. Rev. Resp. Dis.* 125: 443–447, 1982.

88. Smedegard, G., Hedquist, R., Dahlen, S.E., et al.: Leukotriene C_4 affects pulmonary and cardiovascular dynamics in monkey. *Nature* 295:327–329, 1982.

89. Snapper, J.R., Ogletree, M.L., Hutchinson, A.A., et al.: Meclofenamate prevents increased resistance of the lung (R_L) following endotoxemia in unanesthetized sheep. *Am. Rev. Respir. Dis.* 123:200, 1981 (Abstr.).

90. Stenmark, K.R., James, S.L., Voelkel, N.F., et al.: Leukotriene C_4 and D_4 in neonates with hypoxemia and pulmonary hypertension. *N. Engl. J. Med.* 309: 77–80, 1983.

91. Stenmark, K.R., Morganroth, M.L., Voelkel, N.F., et al.: Time course and possible role of eicosonoids in monocrotaline induced pulmonary hypertension. *Am. Rev. Resp. Dis.* 129:A330, 1984.

92. Sugita, T., Hyers, T.M., Dauber, I.M., et al.: Lung vessel leak precedes right ventricular hypertrophy in monocrotaline-treated rats. *J. Appl. Physiol.* 54:371–374, 1983.

93. Sugita, T., Stenmark, K.R., Wagner Jr., W.W., et al.: Abnormal alveolar cells in monocrotaline induced pulmonary hypertension. *Exp. Lung Res.* 5:201–215, 1983.

94. Tate, R.M., VanBenthuysen, K.M., Shasby, D.M., et al.: Oxygen radical mediated permeability edema and vasoconstriction in isolated perfused rabbit lungs. *Am. Rev. Resp. Dis.* 126:802–806, 1982.

95. Turnbull, L.S., Jones, D.G., and Kay, A.B.: Slow reacting substance as a preformed mediator from human lung. *Immunology* 31:813–829, 1976.
96. Voelkel, N.F., Worthen, S., Reeves, J.T., et al.: Non-immunological production of leukotrienes induced by platelet activating factor. *Science* 218:286–289, 1982.
97. Voelkel, N.F., Morganroth, M., Stenmark, K., et al.: Leukotrienes in the lung circulation: Actions and interactions. In *Hypoxia, Exercise and Altitude*, Proceedings of the third Banff International Symposium. New York, Alan R. Liss, Inc., 1983, pp. 141–152.
98. Voelkel, N.F., Simpson, J., Worthen, S., et al.: Platelet-activating factor causes pulmonary vasoconstriction and edema due to platelet independent leukotriene formation. In *Advances in Prostaglandin and Thromboxane Research*. Samuelsson, B., Ramwell, P., Paoletti, R., eds. New York, Raven Press, 1983, Vol. 12, pp. 179–183.
99. Voelkel, N.F., Stenmark, K., Reeves, J.T., et al.: Actions of lipoxygenase metabolites in isolated rat lungs. *J. Appl. Physiol.* 57:860–867, 1984.
100. Wagenvoort, C.A. and Wagenvoort, N.: Pathology of pulmonary hypertension. In *Dietary Pulmonary Hypertension*. New York, John Wiley and Sons, 1977, pp. 103–118.
101. Weis, S.J., Young, J., LoBuglio, A.F., et al.: Role of hydrogen peroxide in neutrophil-mediated destruction of cultured endothelial cells. *J. Clin. Invest.* 68:714–721, 1981.
102. Weiss, J.W., Draxen, J.M., Coles, N., et al.: Bronchoconstrictor effects of leukotriene C in humans. *Science* 216:196–198, 1982.
103. Wicks, T.C., Rose, J.C., Johnson, M., et al.: Vascular responses to arachidonic acid in the perfused canine lung. *Circ. Res.* 38:167, 1976.
104. Yokochi, K., Olley, P.M., Sideris, E., et al.: Leukotriene D_4: A potent vasoconstriction of the pulmonary and systemic circulations in the newborn lamb. In *Leukotrienes and Other Lipoxygenase Products*. Samuelsson, B., Paoletti, R., eds. New York, Raven Press, 1982, pp. 211–214.

CHAPTER 16

Role of PAF-Acether (Platelet-Activating Factor) in Neutrophil Activation

Bernard Poitevin,
Jean Michel Mencia-Huerta,
Régine Roubin, and
Jacques Benveniste

Introduction

The role of PAF-acether (platelet-activating factor), a potent platelet-activating agent, was initially thought to be restricted to immediate hypersensitivity reactions because it originates from basophils. Basophil degranulation and release of PAF-acether have been suspected in the pathogenesis of glomerulonephritis and during acute serum sickness, exemplifying the relationship between allergic reactions and inflammatory processes. PAF-acether is now recognized as a mediator of inflammation since it is released from a variety of inflammatory cell types such as platelets, monocytes, macrophages, and polymorphonuclear neutrophils (PMN). PAF-atheter is also produced by alveolar macrophages and could be a component of the cellular and molecular pathways leading to asthma.

PAF-acether is the first example of a powerful mediator of inflammation belonging to the phospholipid class. Besides acting on platelets it acts in vitro on various cell types, including PMN, and organs. In vivo PAF-acether induces several pathobiological effects such as bronchoconstriction associated with pulmonary and cardiac vascular injuries in guinea pigs, baboons, and humans. PAF-acether also causes an increase in vascular permeability in the skin and exhibits an antihypertensive property identical to that of the hormone from the rat renal medulla described by Muirhead's group.[16] Recently, PAF-acether has been shown to cause the release of secondary mediators, leukotrienes (LT), and prostaglandins (PG) from various cell types and organs. In this respect, PAF-acether represents a good example of a mediator released from and acting on inflammatory cells and organs, by thus enhancing and/or perpetuating the inflammatory process.

From Said, S.I. (ed.): *The Pulmonary Circulation and Acute Lung Injury.* Mount Kisco, N.Y., Futura Publishing Co., Inc., 1985.

Historical Background, Definition, and Assay

A leukocyte-dependent histamine-releasing mechanism was described by Barbaro and Zvaifler[4] and a soluble intermediate was detected in 1971.[67] It was considered as lytic for platelets and remained uncharacterized. The methodology for its routine preparation was described by Benveniste et al.,[6] who started its characterization, named it platelet-activating factor (PAF), and demonstrated its release from immunoglobulin E-sensitized rabbit basophils. Its human origin,[7] its effect on human platelets,[8] and most of its known physicochemical characteristics including its phospholipid nature[9] were unveiled thereafter. The structure initially proposed was that of a glycerophospholipid with a choline polar head group, an ester-linked acyl chain at the carbon 2 of the glycerol, and no ester link at the carbon 1 position,[9] thereby proposing a new class of phospholipid mediator. Finally, the procedure for its purification was described,[70] its structure was elucidated as being a 1-O-alkyl-2-acetyl-*sn*-glycero-3-phosphocholine (hence named PAF-acether),[10,27] and its chemical synthesis was achieved[32] (Fig. 1). Given the numerous substances present in biological fluids and cell supernatants that can activate platelets, it is necessary to strictly define PAF-acether. The criteria used to distinguish it precisely from, for example, arachidonic acid, thrombin, adenosine diphosphate (ADP), and PG are: (1) platelet aggregation (or release of labeled serotonin) in the presence of aspirin or indomethacin and of ADP scavengers, (2) an elution pattern identical to that of synthetic PAF-acether during high pressure liquid chromatography, and (3) inactivation by phospholipases A_2, C, and D, and resistance to lipase from *Rhizopus arrhizus*.[9]

Release of PAF-Acether from PMN

Rabbit and human PMN synthesize PAF-acether when stimulated with the ionophore A 23187, immune complexes, C_{5a}, or phagocytosable particles such as serum-treated zymosan (STZ).[11,13,17,44,45,64,75] Only 50% of the PAF-acether synthesized is released in the extracellular medium.[11] Human neutrophils depleted of granule constituents as well as those from patients with chronic granulomatous disease—which is associated with a defect in the oxydative burst—release normal levels of PAF-acether when stimulated with STZ, demonstrating a dissociation of the PAF-acether release with degranulation and superoxide anion production.[13] The release of PAF-acether is Ca^{2+}-

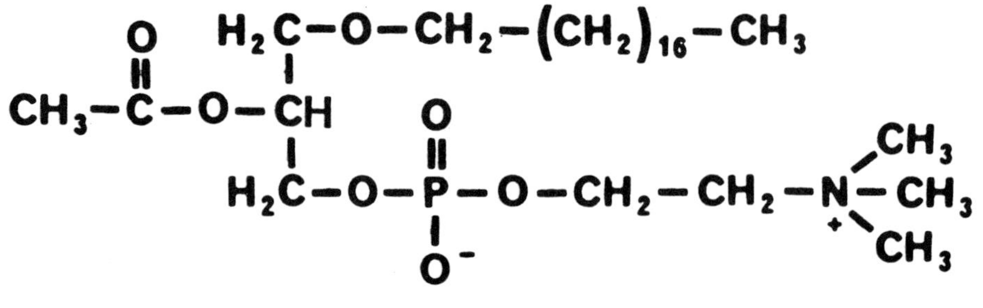

Figure 1: *Structure of PAF-acether.*

dependent,[13] and Jouvin-Marche et al. observed a dose-dependent inhibition of PAF-acether release and its reversal with Ca^{2+} when neutrophils are incubated with the Ca^{2+} antagonist nifedipine.[40] Nifedipine inhibited not only the secretion of PAF-acether but also that of slow-reacting substances much more efficiently than that of β-glucuronidase. This can be explained by the Ca^{2+} dependency of phospholipase A_2 (PLA_2) activity, which plays a critical role in the synthesis of these lipid mediators.[48]

Besides neutrophils, in blood, basophils, eosinophils, platelets and monocytes and, in tissues, alveolar and peritoneal macrophages, endothelial cells, renal and cardiac cells are capable of synthesizing PAF-acether upon stimulation with the specific secretagogue and/or through an IgE-dependent mechanism (reviewed in references 12 and 62).

In many cell types, biosynthesis of PAF-acether involves two steps: (1) deacylation of membrane ether-lipids by a PLA_2 yielding 2-lyso PAF-acether,[1,49,61] and (2) acetylation of 2-lyso PAF-acether into PAF-acether by an acetyltransferase.[1,2,52,78] In PMN, the amount of 1-O-alkyl-2-acyl-*sn*-glycero-3-phosphocholine (the substrate for PLA_2) is sufficient to insure the formation of 2-lyso PAF-acether. However, the amount of 2-lyso PAF-acether generated appears to be a limiting factor because the synthesis of PAF-acether is increased when exogenous synthetic 2-lyso PAF-acether is added during cell stimulation.[41] In addition, kinetic experiments indicate that PMN form transiently 2-lyso PAF-acether, which appears to be rapidly transformed into PAF-acether.[11,41] The latter data fit well with the high level of acetyltransferase activity detected in PMN.[41] Upon stimulation of PMN by the ionophore A 23187, the acetyltransferase activity is doubled,[41] suggesting that in addition to 2-lyso PAF-acether availability, the acetyltransferase also regulates the biosynthesis of the mediator.

Effect of PAF-Acether on PMN

PAF-acether stimulates most of the neutrophil functions since it induces aggregation, adherence, degranulation, chemotaxis and chemokinesis, release of superoxide anions and of LTB_4, and an increase in C_3 receptor expression (Table I).

Aggregation and Adherence

Consequence of Intravenous Injection of PAF-Acether

The effect of PAF-acether on neutrophils was initially suggested by experiments showing that intravenous injection of this phospholipid (1 μg/kg) into rabbits induces not only a thrombocytopenia, a reflect of the platelet-aggregating activity of the mediator, but also a neutropenia.[18,36] The latter effect is related to a massive sequestration of PMN aggregates in the capillary network, and primarily in the lung.[18,34,46] This neutropenia, as well as the thrombocytopenia induced by PAF-acether, is inhibited by prostacyclin.[20] Intravenous injection of PAF-acether (28 μg/kg) to baboons also induces an acute neutropenia and thrombocytopenia associated with an intravascular release of platelet factor 4 and thromboxane A_2.[47] The maximal decrease in the circulat-

Table I
In Vitro Effect of PAF-Acether and Analogs on PMN Functions

Phospholipid	PMN Function	Activation	No Effect
PAF-acether	Aggregation	18,30,53,57 66	
	Adherence	33,73	
	Degranulation	24,25,33,39 53,54,56,66 69,79,80	
	Chemotaxis and/or chemokinesis	25,26,33,66	
	Superoxide anion production	39,60,63,66	33
	LTB$_4$ production	23,43,50	
	C$_3$ receptor expression	72	
PAF-acether enatiomer	Degranulation		79
	Superoxide anion production		60
2-lyso PAF-acether	Aggregation		57,66
	Degranulation		39,57,66,79
	Chemotaxis and/or chemokinesis	25,26	33,66
	Superoxide anion production		39,60
2-ethyl analog	Aggregation	53	
	Degranulation	53,79	
2-methyl analog	Degranulation	79	
2-maleyl analog	Adherence	33	
	Degranulation		33
	Chemotaxis and/or chemokinesis		33
2-succinyl analog	Adherence	33	
	Degranulation		33
	Chemotaxis and/or chemokinesis		33
1-ester analog	Superoxide anion production		60
Lyso-phosphatidyl-choline	Degranulation		39
	Superoxide anion production		39,60

ing neutrophil and platelet counts occurs within 30 seconds after PAF-acether injection. Although thrombocytopenia is reversed within 2 to 3 minutes, neutrophils do not return into the circulation until 30 minutes after PAF-acether injection.

Effect of Intratracheal Administration of PAF-Acether

The initial observation on the platelet-dependent cyclooxygenase-independent bronchomotor effect of PAF-acether was obtained in the guinea pig.[74] Intratracheal administration of PAF-acether (60 µg/kg) to premedicated baboons provokes a bronchomotor effect determined as an increase in the peak inspiratory pressure (5.7 ± 1.5 and 9.6 ± 3.3cm H_2O, respectively, before and after instillation), and a decrease of oxygen blood tension (78.8 ± 10.0 *vs.* 43.0 ± 7.5 mmHg) 10 minutes after. As for intravenous injection, a decrease in circulating platelets (227 ± 61 × 10^3 *vs.* 104 ± 37 × 10^3 cells/mm³) and in neutrophils (7.6 ± 1.8 × 10^3 *vs.* 4.9 ± 2.1 × 10^3 cells/mm³) is observed.[28,29]

In humans, intratracheal administration of PAF-acether from 0.04 mg/kg to 1.2 mg/kg also causes an increase in the peak inspiratory pressure and of the airway pressure, indicating the development of a bronchoconstriction.[31] These functional changes are associated with a decrease in leukocyte and platelet counts probably related to their aggregation in the pulmonary vascular bed. Camussi et al.[21] have shown that instillation of PAF-acether (10μg/kg) to rabbits induces an acute pulmonary inflammatory reaction characterized by the accumulation of macrophages in the alveolar space, degenerative and necrotic changes of the alveolar epithelium, and accumulation of PMN and platelets in the alveolar capillary lumen. In addition, degenerative changes in endothelial cells are observed.

Therefore, it is conceivable that the PMN aggregation and activation induced by PAF-acether is responsible for the pulmonary lesions and functional changes occurring after administration of PAF-acether.

Aggregation and Adherence

PAF-acether from 1 nM to 10 μM evokes in vitro aggregation of rat peritoneal[30] and human[18,57,66] PMN. The nonacetylated molecule, 2-lyso PAF-acether, causes a small aggregation of rat PMN only at 2 mM.[30] The PMN aggregation to PAF-acether requires extracellular Ca^{2+} and Mg^{2+} and appears to proceed through ADP and arachidonic acid independent pathways.[18] These results are similar to those reported for the platelet aggregation induced by PAF-acether.[12]

The specificity of the interaction PAF-acether/neutrophils has been assessed (1) towards unrelated compounds known to activate neutrophils C_{5a}, N-formyl-methionyl-leucyl-phenylalanine (FMLP), phorbol myristate acetate (PMA), ionophore A 23187, and STZ, and (2) towards phospholipids close to the PAF-acether structure. When neutrophils are stimulated first with a stimulating agent in the absence of Ca^{2+} and Mg^{2+}, washed, and then rechallenged with the same agonist in the presence of the divalent cations, activation does not occur. However, if the first stimulation is carried out in the presence of a different agonist, activation will still take place. This phenomenon is referred to as a "desensitization" process. When desensitization does not occur, it indicates that PAF-acether and the other stimulating agents possess independent sites of action.

Preincubation of neutrophils with PAF-acether or its 2-ethyl analog desensitizes the cells to these phospholipids but not to C_{5a} or FMLP,[53] whereas cells densensitized to FMLP or C_{5a} exhibit a normal aggregation response to the two active phospholipids. These data support that C_{5a}, FMLP, and the two phospholipids represent three distinct classes of agonists that stimulate neutrophils probably through different receptors.

PAF-acether increases the adherence of PMN on columns of Sephadex G25 in a dose-related manner between 2 nM and 650 nM.[73] The maximal enhancement of PMN adherence (85%) evoked by 650 nM PAF-acether is identical in magnitude to that elicited with an optimal concentration of FMLP. PMN adherence increases within 1 minute after exposure of the leukocytes to PAF-acether and persists for over 30 minutes in spite of extensive washing of the cells.[73] Because of the persistent activation, functional desensitization never occurred. Thus, exposure of PMN to PAF-acether induces a permanent change in the capacity of the cells to adhere to foreign surfaces, perhaps by altering the expression of critical membrane proteins as it has been shown for the expression of C_3 receptors.[72]

Degranulation

PAF-acether from 1 nM to 10 μM induces the release of the granule-associated enzymes, lysosyme, β-glucuronidase and acid phosphatase, from rabbit[57] and human PMN[24,25,33,39,53,66] (Fig. 2) in a process that is dependent upon extracellular calcium.[54,69] This effect is observed with cells treated or untreated with cytochalasin B. PAF-acether[24,25,39] also enhances enzyme release from PMN stimulated with STZ. O'Flaherty et al.[57] and Wykle et al.[79] demonstrated that the 2-O-ethyl and the 2-O-methyl analogs of PAF-acether are also able to induce human PMN degranulation and are both selectively cross-desensitized with PAF-acether. In contrast, the enantiomer of PAF-acether and the deacetylated compound, 2-lyso PAF-acether, are inactive. The activity of analogs lacking oxygen at position 2 of the glycerol is reduced by 100–10,000 times.[80] These results demonstrate that the presence and the configuration of the short acyl chain at position 2 of the glycerol are critical for the degranulating activity of PAF-acether.

Chemotaxis and Chemokinesis

In vitro, semisynthetic PAF-acether prepared from beef heart plasmalogens induces human PMN chemotactic response in a range of concentrations from 0.1 to 10 μM but exhibits no chemokinetic activity.[33] The sensitivity of PMN to semisynthetic PAF-acether is enhanced when the cells are pretreated with cytochalasin B.[66] Under those conditions, PAF-acether induces chemotactic activity from 0.1 nM to 10 μM with a peak effect at 1 μM and a decreased effect at 10 μM. Czarnetzki and Benveniste[25,26] have also demonstrated an even more pronounced chemotactic effect of synthetic PAF-acether on human PMN. In contrast to the experiments carried out with semisynthetic PAF-acether, the synthetic one in the absence of cytochalasin B induces not only chemotaxis at a 10 nM concentration but also chemokinesis from 10 nM to 1 μM. 2-lyso PAF-acether is 1,000 times less potent than PAF-acether.[25,26] As for the aggregating and degranulating activities, the chemotactic activity of PAF-acether is also dependent on the nature of the 2-acyl substituent. The presence of the double bond of the 2-succinyl analog of PAF-acether results in an increased chemotactic potency as compared to the 2-maleyl PAF-acether analog.[33] Surprisingly, PAF-acether and 2-lyso PAF-acether deactivate each other, whereas their chemotactic activity is unaffected by preincubation of the cells with the other chemotactic factors, NFMP (an analog of FMLP) and the eosinophil chemotactic factor (ECF).[24] The cross-desensitization between PAF-acether

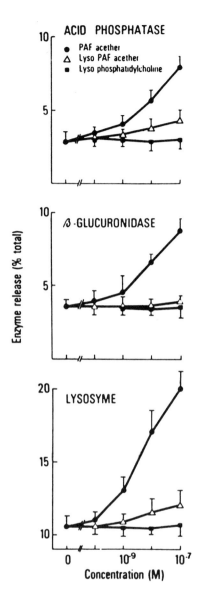

Figure 2: *Release of acid phosphatase, β-glucuronidase, and lysosyme from human neutrophils exposed to varying concentrations of PAF-acether, 2-lyso PAF-acether and lyso-phosphatidylcholine (from ref. 39, with permission from Birkhauser Verlag).*

and 2-lyso PAF-acether suggests that they share a common receptor structure that differs from the membrane receptor site for ECF or NFMP. The potent inhibition exerted by 2-lyso PAF-acether from 10 nM to 1 μM, which contrasts with its weak agonist effect, indicates that mechanisms other than binding to a receptor are involved in the deactivation process. The chemotactic effect of PAF-acether is enhanced by BW 755 C but not by indomethacin, suggesting that the products of the lipoxygenase pathway are inhibitory.[26] PAF-acether also modulates the effect of other chemotactic factors since it enhances up to tenfold the effect of ECF and causes an additive effect on NFMP (Fig. 3). The enhancing effect of PAF-acether occurred with concentrations from 10 nM to 1 μM and is

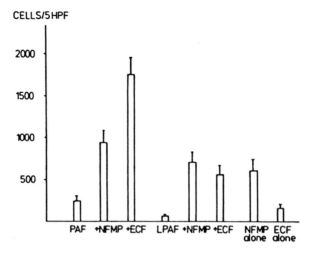

Figure 3: *Effect of PAF-acether (1 μM) and 2-lyso PAF-acether (1 μM) alone or in combination with different chemotactic factors on human neutrophil migration. All substances were placed on the chemoattractant side of the chemotaxis chamber. Results are expressed as number of cells that have migrated through the filter in five random microscopic fields (HPF). ECF (eosinophil-chemotactic factor) (100 μl) causes a synergistic enhancement and NFMP (N-formyl methionine peptide) (5 μM) an additive effect on PAF-acether and its lyso-derivative (from ref. 26, with permission from Elsevier Biomedical Press).*

totally inhibited upon addition of BW 775 C.[26] This result is puzzling in view of the enhancing effect of the drug on cell migration due to PAF-acether or ECF alone.

The chemotactic activity of PAF-acether on PMN is also observed in vivo. In rats, accumulation of PMN is observed 4 hours after intradermal injection of the mediator. Such an injection results in a plasma exudation in 2−5 minutes, which is therefore related neither to the presence of PMN nor to the presence of platelets.[37,59] Similar results are obtained in guinea pigs,[51] rabbits,[14,77] hamsters,[14,15] and humans.[5]

Superoxide Anions and Oxygen Radical Production

Semisynthetic PAF-acether from 10 nM to 10 μM is slightly active in generating superoxide anions from cytochalasin B-treated human PMN as assessed by the superoxide dismutase-inhibitable reduction of ferricytochrome C.[66] Goetzl et al.[33] did not observe any effect on untreated PMN, a result that is in contradiction with the data from Jouvin-Marche et al.,[39] who used synthetic PAF-acether (100 nM) and showed that it induces superoxide production from human PMN, even untreated with cytochalasin B. Synthetic PAF-acether from 100 nM to 10 μM also enhances the production by PMN of superoxide anions and other oxygenated free radicals, as detected by the very sensitive methods of luminol-dependent chemiluminescence (LDCL).[60,63] The cytochalasin B pre-treatment of PMN modifies the kinetics of the reaction but not the sensitivity of the cells to PAF-acether.[60]

PAF-acether appears to be less potent than other agents known to induce superoxide anion production by PMN, such as FMLP, STZ, and PMA (Fig. 4). However, PAF-acether exhibits a remarkable enhancing effect on the zymosan or STZ-induced oxygen radical production (Fig. 5), suggesting the independent sites of action of PAF-acether and the particles. The comparison of the effects of PAF-acether with those of several structurally related phospholipids on LDCL from PMN has allowed definition of the structural features of the molecule necessary for activation. Not only the presence and the configuration of the acetyl moiety but also the ether linkage at position 1 of the glycerol are necessary to insure activity. Again, these structural requirements are superimposable with those already published for platelet activation.[35,42,65]

The Effect of PAF-Acether on Synthesis of LTB₄

Besides its effects on several PMN functions, PAF-acether also induces the biosynthesis of newly formed lipid mediators derived from arachidonic acid.

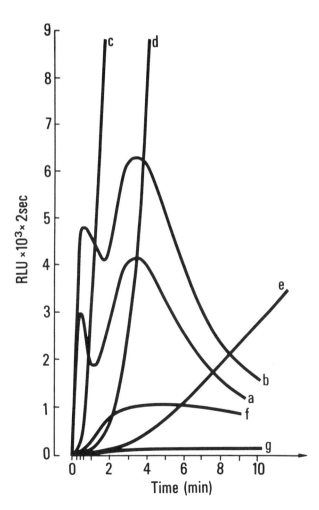

Figure 4: *Kinetics of the LDCL induced by* **(a)** *PAF-acether (10 μM);* **(b)** *FMLP (0.1 μM);* **(c)** *PMA (0.12 μM);* **(d)** *STZ (1 mg/ml);* **(e)** *zymosan (1 mg/ml);* **(f)** *latex particles (280 particles/cell);* **(g)** *control. Tracings were recorded from a single donor representative of 4 experiments (from ref. 60, with permission from Elsevier Biomedical Press).*

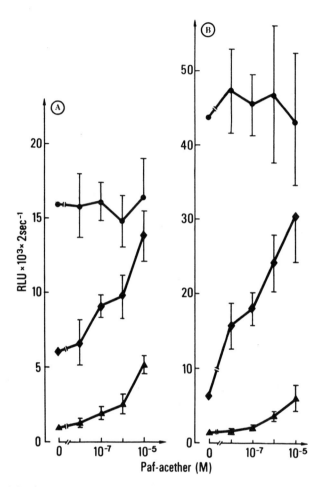

Figure 5: *Modulatory effects of PAF-acether used at various concentrations on the STZ (10 μg/ml) (A) or zymosan (100 μg/ml) (B) induced LDCL. LDCL was assessed at 5 min (▲———▲), 10 min (◆———◆), and at the plateau values (•———•———•), which are at 30 min for zymosan and 20 min for STZ. Results are expressed as means ± SEM of three experiments (from ref. 60, with permission from Elsevier Biomedical Press).*

PAF-acether induces 5-hydroxy-eicosatetraenoic acid (5-HETE) and LTB$_4$ formation from rabbit PMN obtained after intraperitoneal injection of glycogen.[23] This LTB$_4$ formation is observed on cytochalasin B-pretreated PMN, with a PAF-acether concentration as low as 20 nM.[23] A concentration of 1 μM PAF-acether is required to induce LTB$_4$ biosynthesis in human PMN.[43] PAF-acether appears to be a weak activator for LTB$_4$ biosynthesis from human PMN since it induced the release of 0.5% of the amounts of LTB$_4$ generated upon ionophore A 23187 activation.[50] However, the amounts of LTB$_4$ formed upon PAF-acether stimulation are sufficient to raise the question of whether or not part of the effects of PAF-acether are mediated through the generation of LTB$_4$, a potent PMN activator.

What Is the Mechanism of the PAF-Acether-Induced PMN Activation?

Role of LTB$_4$ Generation

Discrepant results have been obtained concerning the relationship between PAF-acether action and LTB$_4$ generation on the various PMN functions.

Regarding neutrophil aggregation, PAF-acether and LTB$_4$ cross-desensitized, suggesting that both mediators activate human PMN through a common mechanism.[56] The desensitization approach appears inadequate, since LTB$_4$-desensitized PMNs are also hyporesponsive to FMPL and C$_{5a}$ which have different receptors and thus probably different pathways of PMN activation.[63] Therefore a pharmacologic approach has been used, but with different results depending on the species. The PAF-acether-induced aggregation of human PMN is abrogated by previous treatment of the cells with an inhibitor of PLA$_2$[18] and by two inhibitors of the arachidonate lipoxygenase cascade, eicosatetraynoic acid (ETYA)[18,30,43] and nordihydroguaiaretic acid (NDGA),[30,43] but not by inhibitors of the cyclooxygenase pathway.[18] In rats, the aggregation of PMN by PAF-acether is unaffected by pretreatment of the cells with cyclooxygenase and lipoxygenase inhibitors.[30]

A role for LTB$_4$ generation in the PAF-acether-induced LDCL has also been suggested, since LTB$_4$-desensitized human PMNs are hyporesponsive to PAF-acether.[63]

With respect to PMN degranulation, NDGA and ETYA cause a concentration-dependent suppression of enzyme release from human PMN exposed to PAF-acether, whereas the cyclooxygenase inhibitor, indomethacin, is without effect.[56,68] These results favor a role for the major products of the lipoxygenase pathway, 5-HETE or LTB$_4$, in PAF-acether-induced PMN degranulation. Indeed, the effect of PAF-acether is potentiated by 5-HETE, which neither induces degranulation to a detectable level nor influences the degranulating action of C$_{5a}$, ionophore A 23187 or FMPL.[55] A role for LTB$_4$ in the PAF-acether-induced PMN degranulation is suggested by experiments showing that degranulation induced by both mediators is maximal in less than 5 minutes, requires intact pathways of arachidonic acid, and is dependent on the presence of cytochalasin B and on physiologic concentrations of extracellular calcium.[58] However, the following observations dispute a role for LTB$_4$ in the PAF-acether-induced degranulation of PMN. First, PMNs desensitized to LTB$_4$ degranulate normally when challenged to PAF-acether.[56] Second, the degranulating action of PAF-acether is susceptible only to antilipoxygenase drugs, whereas the degranulating action of LTB$_4$ is inhibited by antilipoxygenase and anticyclooxygenase drugs.[58] Third, PAF-acether produces a greater degranulation response than LTB$_4$.

Receptors for PAF-Acether

The existence of a specific receptor for PAF-acether was suggested by the specificity of PAF-acether action as compared to structurally related phospholipids and the cross-desensitization studies. Valone and Goetzl[72] have demonstrated the existence of a binding site specific for PAF-acether on human PMN. This site exhibits a high affinity (KD = 0.11 nM) and is saturable at 196 pmol PAF-acether. $5.2 \pm 1 \times 10^6$ sites are expressed per cell. As measured by the capacity of PAF-acether analogs to inhibit the binding of PAF-acether, these authors demonstrate that this binding site is specific for phospholipids with a 1-ether linkage and a 2-short-fatty-acid chain, but appears to lack stereo-specificity. PAF-acether binding sites have also been demonstrated on purified plasma membranes from bovine and guinea pig PMN with KD of 4.93 nM and 7.58 nM, respectively.[38] PAF-acether binding is not observed on membranes from erythrocytes and alveolar macrophages[38] which are probably not target cells for the mediator. Specific binding sites for PAF-acether have also been identified on rabbit platelet plasma membranes.[38,71]

Conclusions: A Role for PAF-Acether in Inflammatory Processes and Lung Diseases

Although a role for PAF-acether in pulmonary disease is not yet established, its numerous effects on various cell types including PMN may explain many of the features of the inflammatory reactions in lung. Alveolar macrophages release various mediators including PAF-acether when stimulated in vitro with phagocytosable particles such as zymosan or bacteria.[3,27] In addition, the generation of PAF-acether by alveolar macrophages from allergic patients is obtained in vitro upon stimulation with the specific allergen.[27] Consequently, the release of PAF-acether within lung tissues upon antigenic or nonantigenic stimulation may occur, strengthening the postulated role for the mediator in asthma and inflammatory lung diseases. Besides alveolar macrophages, other cell types present in lung tissue are also capable of releasing PAF-acether. Human endothelial cells in culture release PAF-acether when stimulated with angiotensin, vasopressin, or a rabbit antihuman factor VIII antiserum.[22] This release is likely to happen in vivo since PAF-acether is detected in plasma after administration of antibodies against the lung angiotensin-covering enzyme,[19] a marker of pulmonary endothelial cells.

Once released, PAF-acether will recruit PMN. Indeed, Pfister et al. (in preparation) have observed that the most remarkable feature after PAF-acether injection in the guinea pig is a margination of both PMN and platelets in lung tissue. A similar margination is observed when inducing PAF-acether release in vivo.[19] In addition to margination, PAF-acether will also induce PMN aggregation and degranulation, resulting in the obstruction of small vessels, the formation of a lesional pulmonary edema, and tissue injuries. Superoxide anion generation may participate in cell damage through lipid peroxydation and attack of the cell membrane. Finally, de novo formation of LTB_4 by PAF-acether-stimulated PMN will contribute to amplify and perpetuate the inflammatory reaction. PAF-acether also induces the formation and release of LTC_4 and LTD_4 from rat perfused lung,[76] and this may explain part of the bronchoconstrictive effect of PAF-acether if released in vivo from alveolar macrophages, endothelial cells, or PMN.

In conclusion, PAF-acether is not only a platelet-activating factor but also a potent PMN-activating factor. Since it is formed by and acting on PMN, PAF-acether may play a role as a "secondary messenger" of PMN activation. At the present time, only the development of new drugs capable of interacting specifically with its biosynthetic pathways or sites of action will allow definition of its role in various pathological situations including lung diseases.

REFERENCES

1. Albert, D.H. and Snyder, F.: Biosynthesis of 1-alkyl-2-acetyl-*sn*-glycero-3-phospho-choline (platelet-activating factor) from 1-alkyl-2-acyl-*sn*-glycero-3-phosphocholine by rat alveolar macrophages. *J. Biol. Chem.* 258:97–102, 1983.
2. Alonso, F., Gil, M.G., Sanchez-Crespo, M., et al.: Activation of 1-alkyl-2-lyso-glycero-3-phosphocholine acetyl-CoA transferase during phagocytosis in human polymor-phonuclear leukocytes. *J. Biol. Chem.* 257:3376–3378, 1982.
3. Arnoux, B., Cerrina, J., Jouvin, E., et al.: Release of platelet-activating factor (PAF-acether) from monocytes and alveolar macrophages in pulmonary diseases. *Eur. J. Clin. Invest.* 11:2, 1981 (Abstr.).
4. Barbaro, J.F. and Zvaifler, N.J.: Antigen-induced histamine release from platelets of rabbits producing homologous PCA-antibody. *Proc. Soc. Exp. Biol. Med.* 122: 1245–1247, 1966.
5. Basran, G.S., Morley, J., Page, C.P., et al.: Platelet-activating factor: A potential mediator of acute and chronic asthma. *Am. Rev. Respir. Dis.* 125:52, 1982 (Abstr.).
6. Benveniste, J., Henson, P.M., and Cochrane, C.G.: Leukocyte-dependent histamine release from rabbit platelets: The role of IgE, basophils and a platelet-activating factor. *J. Exp. Med.* 136:1356–1377, 1972.
7. Benveniste, J.: Platelet-activating factor, a new mediator of anaphylaxis and im-mune complex deposition from rabbit and human platelets. *Nature (London)* 249: 481–583, 1974.
8. Benveniste, J., Le Couedic, J.P., and Kamoun, P.: Aggregation of human platelets by platelet-activating factor. *Lancet* 1:344, 1975.
9. Benveniste, J., Le Couedic, J.P., Polonsky, J., et al.: Structural analysis of purified platelet-activating factor by lipases. *Nature (London)* 269:170 171, 1977.
10. Benveniste, J., Tencé, M., Varenne, P., et al.: Semi-synthèse et structure proposée du facteur activant les plaquettes (PAF): PAF-acéther, un alkyl-éther analogue de la lysophosphatidylcholine. *C.R. Acad. Sci. Paris* 289D:1037–1040, 1979.
11. Benveniste, J., Roubin, R., Chignard, M., et al.: Release of platelet-activating factor (PAF-acether) and 2-lyso PAF-acether from three cell types. *Agents Actions* 12: 711–713, 1982.
12. Benveniste, J. and Vargaftig, B.B.: An ether-lipid with biological activities: Platelet-activating factor (PAF-acether). In *Ether-Lipids: Biochemical and Bio-medical Aspects.* Mangold, H.K. and Paltauf, H., eds. New York, Academic Press, 1983, pp. 355–376.
13. Betz, S.J. and Henson, P.M.: Production and release of platelet-activating factor (PAF): Dissociation from degranulation and superoxide production in the human neutrophil. *J. Immunol.* 125:2756–2762, 1980.
14. Björk, J., Lindbom, L., Gerdin, B., et al.: PAF-acether (platelet-activating factor) increases microvascular permeability and affects endothelium-granulocyte interac-tion in microvascular beds. *Acta Physiol. Scand.* 119:305–308, 1983.
15. Björk, J. and Smedegard, G.: Acute microvascular effects of PAF-acether, as studied by intravital microscopy. *Eur. J. Pharmacol.* 96:87–94, 1983.
16. Blank, M.L., Snyder F., Byers, L.W., et al.: Antihypertensive activity of an alkyl ether analog of phosphatidylcholine. *Biochem. Biophys. Res. Commun.* 90:1194–1200, 1979.
17. Camussi, G., Aglietta, M., Coda, R., et al.: Release of platelet-activating factor (PAF) and histamine. II. The cellular origin of human PAF: Monocytes, polymorphonu-clear neutrophils and basophils. *Immunology* 42:191–199, 1981.
18. Camussi, G., Tetta, C., Bussolino, F., et al.: Mediators of immune complex-induced aggregation of polymorphonuclear neutrophils. II. Platelet-activating factor as the effector substance of immune induced aggregation. *Int. Archs. Allergy Appl. Immunol.* 64:25–41, 1981.

19. Camussi, G., Pawlowski, I., Bussolino, F., et al.: Release of platelet-activating factor in rabbits with antibody-mediated injury of the lung: The role of leukocytes and of pulmonary endothelial cells. *J. Immunol.* 131:1802–1807, 1983.

20. Camussi, G., Tetta, C., and Bussolino, F.: Inhibitory effect of prostacyclin (PGI$_2$) on neutropenia induced by intravenous injection of platelet-activating factor (PAF) in the rabbit. *Prostaglandins* 25:343–351, 1983.

21. Camussi, G., Pawlowski, I., Tetta, C., et al.: Acute lung inflammation induced in the rabbit by local instillation of 1-O-octadecyl-2-acetyl-*sn*-glyceryl-3-phosphorylcholine or a native platelet-activating factor. *Am. J. Pathol.* 112:78–88, 1983.

22. Camussi, G., Aglietta, M., Malavasi, F., et al.: The release of platelet-activating factor from human endothelial cells in culture. *J. Immunol.* 131:2397–2403, 1983.

23. Chilton, F.H., O'Flaherty, J.T., Walsch, E.C., et al.: Platelet-activating factor. Stimulation of the lipoxygenase pathway in polymorphonuclear leukocytes by 1-O-alkyl-2-O-acetyl-*sn*-glycero-3-phosphocholine. *J. Biol. Chem.* 257:5402–5408, 1982.

24. Czarnetzki, B.M.: Effect of platelet-activating factor on leukocytes. II. Enhancement of eosinophil chemotactic factor and β-glucuronidase release. *Chem. Phys. Lipids* 31:205–211, 1982.

25. Czarnetzki, B.M. and Benveniste, J.: Effect of synthetic PAF-acether on human neutrophil function. *Agents Actions* 11:549–550, 1981.

26. Czarnetzki, B.M. and Benveniste, J.: Effect of 1-O-octadecyl-2-O-acetyl-*sn*-glycero-3-phosphocholine (PAF-acether) on leukocytes: I. Analysis of the in vitro migration of human neutrophils. *Chem. Phys. Lipids* 29:317–326, 1981.

27. Demopoulos, C.A., Pinckard, R.N., and Hanahan, D.J.: Evidence for 1-O-alkyl-2-acetyl-*sn*-glyceryl-3-phosphorylcholine as the active component (a new class of lipid chemical mediators). *J. Biol. Chem.* 254:9355–9359, 1979.

28. Denjean, A., Arnoux, B., Masse, R., et al.: Acute effect of intratracheal administration of PAF-acether in baboons. *J. Appl. Physiol.* 55:799–804, 1983.

29. Denjean, A., Arnoux, B., Benveniste, J., et al.: Bronchoconstriction induced by intratracheal administration of platelet-activating factor (PAF-acether) in baboons. *Agents Actions* 11:567–568, 1981.

30. Ford-Hutchinson, A.W.: Neutrophil aggregating properties of PAF-acether and leukotrienes B$_4$. *Int. J. Immunopharmacol.* 1:17–21, 1983.

31. Gateau, O., Arnoux, B., Deriaz, H., et al.: Acute effects of intratracheal administration of PAF-acether (platelet-activating factor) in human. *Am. Rev. Respir. Dis.* (Abstr., in press), 1984.

32. Godfroid, J.J., Heymans, F., Michel, E., et al.: Platelet-activating factor (PAF-acether): Total synthesis of 1-O-octadecyl-2-O-acetyl–*sn*-glycerol-3-phosphorylcholine. *FEBS Lett.* 116:161–164, 1980.

33. Goetzl, E.J., Derian, C.K., Tauber, A.I., et al.: Novel effects of 1-O-hexadecyl-2-acyl-*sn*-glycero-3-phosphorylcholine mediators on human leukocyte function: Delineation of the specific roles of the acyl substituents. *Biochem. Biophys. Res. Commun.* 94:881–888, 1980.

34. Halonen, M., Palmer, J.D., Lohman, I.C., et al.: Differential effect of platelet depletion on the physiologic alterations of IgE anaphylaxis and acetyl-glyceryl-ether-phosphorylcholine infusion in the rabbit. *Am. Rev. Respir. Dis.* 124:416–421, 1981.

35. Hanahan, D.J., Munder, P.G., Satouchi, K., et al.: Potent platelet-stimulating activity of the enantiomer of acetyl-glyceryl-ether-phosphorylcholine and its metoxy analogues. *Biochem. Biophys. Res. Commun.* 99:183–188, 1981.

36. Henson, P.M.: Platelet-activating factor (PAF) as a mediator of neutrophil-platelet interaction in inflammation. In *Pharmacology of Inflammation and Allergy*. Russo-Marie, F., Vargaftig, B.B., and Benveniste, J., eds. Paris, Publications INSERM, vol. 100, 1981, pp. 63–81.

37. Humphrey, D.M., McManus, L., Hanahan, D.J., et al.: Morphologic basis of increased vascular permeability induced by acetyl glyceryl ether phosphorylcholine. *Lab. Invest.* 50:16–25, 1984.

38. Hwang, S.B., Lee, C.S.C., Cheah, M.J., et al.: Specific Receptor sites for 1-O-alkyl-2-O-acetyl-*sn*-glycero-3-phosphorylcholine (platelet-activating factor) on rabbit platelets and guinea pig smooth muscle membranes. *Biochemistry* 22:4763–4769, 1983.

39. Jouvin-Marche, E., Poitevin, B., and Benveniste, J.: Platelet-activating factor (PAF-acether), an activator of neutrophil functions. *Agents Actions* 12:716–720, 1982.

40. Jouvin-Marche, E., Cerrina, J., Coëffier, E., et al.: Effect of the Ca^{2+} antagonist nifedipine on the release of platelet-activating factor (PAF-acether), slow-reacting substance and β-glucuronidase from human neutrophils. *Eur. J. Pharmacol.* 89: 19–26, 1983.

41. Jouvin-Marche, E., Ninio, E., Beaurain, G., et al.: Biosynthesis of platelet-activating factor. VII. Precursors of PAF-acether and acetyltransferase activity in human leukocytes. *J. Immunol.* (In press) 1984.

42. Lalau Keraly, C. and Benveniste, J.: Specific desensitization of rabbit platelets by platelet-activating factor (PAF-acether) and derivatives. *Br. J. Haematol.* 51: 313–322, 1982.

43. Lin, A.H., Morton, D.R., and Gorman, R.R.: Acetyl glyceryl ether phosphorylcholine stimulates leukotriene B_4 synthesis in human polymorphonuclear leukocytes. *J. Clin. Invest.* 70:1058–1065, 1982.

44. Lotner, G.Z., Lynch, J.M., Betz, S.J., et al.: Human neutrophil-derived platelet-activating factor. *J. Immunol.* 124:676–684, 1980.

45. Lynch, J.M., Lotner, G.Z., Betz, S.J., et al.: The release of a platelet-activating factor by stimulated rabbit neutrophils. *J. Immunol.* 123:1219–1226, 1979.

46. McManus, L.M., Hanahan, D.J., Demopoulos, C.A., et al.: Pathobiology of the intravenous injection of acetyl glyceryl ether phosphorylcholine (AGEPC), a synthetic platelet-activating factor. *J. Immunol.* 124:2919–2924, 1980.

47. McManus, L.M., Pinckard, R.N., Fitzpatrick, F.A., et al.: Acetyl glyceryl ether phosphorylcholine. Intravascular alterations following intravenous infusion into the baboon. *Lab. Invest.* 45:303–307, 1981.

48. Mencia-Huerta, J.M., Akerman, C., and Benveniste, J.: Phospholipase A_2 (PLA_2), lipo (LO), cyclo (CO) oxygenases and release of platelet-activating factor (PAF) and slow-reacting substance (SRS) from rat macrophages. *Fed. Proc.* 39:905, 1980, (Abstr.).

49. Mencia-Huerta, J.M., Ninio, E., Roubin, R., et al.: Is platelet-activating factor (PAF-acether) synthesis by murine peritoneal cells (PC) a two-step process? *Agents Actions* 11:556–558, 1981.

50. Mencia-Huerta, J.M., Lee, C.W., Lee, T.H., et al.: Platelet-activating factor (PAF-acether): Generation from a mast cell subclass by an IgE-dependent mechanism. In *Platelet-Activating Factor and Structurally Related Ether-Lipids. INSERM Symposium 23.* Benveniste, J. and Arnoux, B., eds. Amsterdam, Elsevier Science Publishers, 1983, pp. 101–108.

51. Morley, J., Page, C.P., and Paul, W.: Inflammatory action of platelet-activating factor (PAF-acether) in guinea pig skin. *Br. J. Pharmacol.* 80:503–509, 1983.

52. Ninio, E., Mencia-Huerta, J.M., Heymans, F., et al.: Biosynthesis of platelet-activating factor (PAF-acether). I. Evidence for an acetyl-transferase activity in murine macrophages. *Biochim. Biophys. Acta* 710:23–31, 1982.

53. O'Flaherty, J.T., Lees, C.J., Miller, C.H., et al.: Selective desensitization of neutrophils: Further studies with 1-O-alkyl-*sn*-glycero-3-phosphocholine analogues. *J. Immunol.* 127:731–737, 1981.

54. O'Flaherty, J.T., Swendsem, C.L., Lees, C.J., et al.: Role of extracellular calcium in neutrophil degranulation response to 1-O-alkyl-2-O-acetyl-*sn*-glycero-3-phosphocholine. *Am. J. Pathol.* 105:107–113, 1981.

55. O'Flaherty, J.T., Thomas, M.J., Hamett, M.J., et al.: 5-L-hydroxy-6,8,11,14-eicosatetraenoate potentiates the human neutrophil degranulating action of platelet-activating factor. *Biochem. Biophys. Res. Commun.* 111:1–7, 1981.

56. O'Flaherty, J.T., Wykle, R.L, McCall, C.E., et al.: Desensitization of the human

neutrophil degranulation response: Studies with 5,12-dihydroxy-6,8,10,14-eicosate-traenoic acid. *Biochem. Biophys. Res. Commun.* 101:1290–1296, 1981.

57. O'Flaherty, J.T., Wykle, R.L., Miller, C.H., et al.: 1-O-alkyl-*sn*-glyceryl-3-phos-phorylcholines. A novel class of neutrophil stimulants. *Am. J. Pathol.* 103:70–79, 1981.

58. O'Flaherty, J.T., Wykle, R.L., Lees, C.J., et al.: Neutrophil degranulating action of 5-12-dihydro-6,8,10,14-eicosatetraenoic acid and 1-O-alkyl-2-O-acetyl-*sn*-glycero-3-phosphocholine. *Am. J. Pathol.* 105:264–269, 1981.

59. Pirotzky, E., Page, C.P., Roubin, R., et al.: PAF-acether-induced plasma exudation in rat skin is independent of platelets and neutrophils. *Microcirc. Endothel. Lymph.* 1:107–122, 1984.

60. Poitevin, B., Roubin, R., and Benveniste, J.: PAF-acether generates chemilumines-cence in human neutrophils in the absence of cytochalasin B. *Immunopharmacology* 7:135–144, 1984.

61. Polonsky, J., Tencé, M., Varenne, P., et al.: Release of 1-O-alkyl-glyceryl-3-phos-phorylcholine, O-deacetyl platelet-activating factor from leukocytes: Chemical ion-ization mass spectrometry of phospholipids. *Proc. Natl. Acad. Sci. USA* 77: 7019–7023, 1980.

62. Roubin, R., Tencé, M., Mencia-Huerta, J.M., et al.: A chemically defined monokine: Macrophage-derived platelet-activating factor (PAF-acether). In *Lymphokines*, Pick, E., ed. New York, Academic Press, 1983, vol. 8, pp. 249–276.

63. Salzer, W., McCall, C., and O'Flaherty, J.: Leukotriene B$_4$ (LTB$_4$) desensitizes human neutrophil PMN chemiluminescence. *Fed. Proc.* 42:522, 1983 (Abstr.).

64. Sanchez-Crespo, M., Alonso, F., and Egido, J.: Platelet-activating factor in anaphy-laxis and phagocytosis: Release from human peripheral polymorphonuclears and monocytes during the stimulation by ionophore A 23187 and phagocytosis but not from degranulating basophils. *Immunology* 40:645–655, 1980.

65. Satouchi, K., Pinckard, R.N., Ferrigni, K.S., et al.: Influence of alkyl ether chain length of acetyl glycerol ether phosphorylcholine and its ethanolamine analog on biological activity towards rabbit platelets. *J. Immunol.* 127:1250–1255, 1981.

66. Shaw, J.O., Pinckard, R.N., Ferrigni, K.S., et al.: Activation of human neutrophils with 1-O-hexadecyl/octadecyl-2-acetyl-*sn*-glyceryl-3-phosphorylcholine (platelet-activating factor). *J. Immunol.* 127:1250–1255, 1981.

67. Siraganian, R.P. and Osler, A.G.: Destruction of rabbit platelets in the allergic response of sensitized leukocytes. I. Demonstration of a fluid phase intermediate. *J. Immunol.* 106:1244–1251, 1971.

68. Smith, R.J. and Bowman, B.J.: Stimulation of human neutrophil degranulation with 1-O-octadecyl-2-O-acetyl-*sn*-glyceryl-3-phosphorylcholine: Modulation by in-hibitors of arachidonic acid metabolism. *Biochem. Biophys. Res. Commun.* 104: 1495–1501, 1982.

69. Smith, R.J., Bowman, B.J., and Iden, S.S.: Characteristics of 1-O-hexadecyl and 1-O-octadecyl-2-O-acetyl-*sn*-glyceryl-3-phosphorylcholine-stimulated granule en-zyme release from human neutrophils. *Clin. Immunol. Immunopathol.* 28:13–28, 1983.

70. Tencé, M., Polonsky, J., Le Couedic, J.P., et al.: Release, purification and characteri-zation of platelet-activating factor (PAF). *Biochimie* 62:251–259, 1980.

71. Valone, F.H., Coles, E., Reinhold, V.R., et al.: Specific binding of phospholipid platelet-activating factor by human platelets. *J. Immunol.* 129:1637–1641, 1982.

72. Valone, F.H. and Goetzl, E.J.: Specific binding by human polymorphonuclear leuko-cytes of the immunological mediator 1-O-hexadecyl/octadecyl-2-acetyl-*sn*-glycero-3-phosphorylcholine. *Immunology* 48:141–148, 1983.

73. Valone, F.H. and Goetzl, E.J.: Enhancement of human polymorphonuclear leuko-cyte adherence by the phospholipid mediator 1-O-hexadecyl-2-acetyl-*sn*-glycero-3-phosphorylcholine. *Am. J. Pathol.* 113:85–89, 1983.

74. Vargaftig, B.B., Lefort, J., Chignard, M., et al.: Platelet-activating factor induces a platelet-dependent bronchoconstriction unrelated to the formation of prostaglandin derivatives. *Eur. J. Pharmacol.* 65:185–192, 1980.

75. Virella, G., Lopes-Virella, M.F.L., Shuler, C., et al.: Release of PAF by human polymorphonuclear leukocytes stimulated by immune complexes bound to sepharose particles and human erythrocytes. *Immunology* 50:43–51, 1983.

76. Voelkel, N.F., Worthen, S., Reeves, J.T., et al.: Non-immunological production of leukotrienes induced by platelet-activating factor. *Science* 218:286–288, 1982.

77. Wedmore, C.V. and Williams, T.J.: Platelet-activating factor (PAF), a secretory product of polymorphonuclear leukocytes, increases vascular permeability in rabbit skin. *Br. J. Pharmacol.* 74:916–917P, 1981.

78. Wykle, R.L., Malone, B., and Snyder, F.: Enzymatic synthesis of 1-alkyl-2-acetyl-*sn*-glycero-3-phosphocholine, a hypotensive and platelet-aggregating lipid. *J. Biol. Chem.* 255:10256–10260, 1980.

79. Wykle, R.L., Miller, C.H., Lewis, J.C., et al.: Stereospecific activity of 1-O-alkyl-2-O-acetyl-*sn*-glycero-3-phosphocholine and comparison of analogs in the degranulation of platelets and neutrophils. *Biochem. Biophys. Res. Commun.* 100:1651–1658, 1981.

80. Wykle, R.L., Surles, J.R., Piantadosi, C., et al.: Platelet-activating factor (1-O-alkyl-2-O-acetyl-*sn*-glycero-3-phosphocholine. Activity of analogs lacking oxygen at the 2 position. *FEBS Lett.* 141:29–32, 1982.

CHAPTER 17

Platelet-Activating Factor (PAF) and Acute Lung Injury

Mohammad Mojarad,
Charles P. Cox, and
Sami I. Said

Introduction

Platelet-activating factor (PAF) is a potent phospholipid secreted by a variety of mammalian cells and tissues, including rabbit basophils,[5,34,52] hog leukocytes,[7] rat kidneys,[12] rat and mouse macrophages,[46] mouse platelets,[6] human neutrophils,[9] and alveolar macrophages[2]. It can also be detected in human blood,[20] saliva,[21] and urine.[10] The structure of PAF has been identified as 1-O-alkyl-2-acetyl-*sn*-glycero-3-phosphorylcholine.[7,12,25] This compound is also known as acetyl glyceryl ether phosphorylcholine (AGEPC) or as PAF-acether, both names referring to its unusual phospholipid structure. The historical background of PAF research and its broad spectrum of biological activities have been reviewed in detail by others[53,54,69] (see also Chapter 16 of this book). PAF aggregates and stimulates both leukocytes and platelets, and contracts pulmonary artery and airway smooth muscle in many species. These characteristics suggest a possible mediator role for PAF in acute lung injury.

Many factors are involved in the pathogenesis of acute lung injury, expressed clinically as the adult respiratory distress syndrome (ARDS). There is increasing evidence for the role of cellular elements of the blood such as leukocytes and platelets in this condition.[15,23,36,66] The pathogenetic contributions of humoral mediators such as histamine, serotonin, vasoactive peptides, free oxygen radicals, prostaglandins, leukotrienes, and thromboxanes are being actively investigated.[3,24,57,58]

Although PAF is biologically active in nanomolar quantities in vivo and in vitro, affecting a wide variety of cells and tissues, little is known about its possible role in relation to acute lung injury. Before PAF—or any other endogenous biologically active compound—can be said to have a mediator effect in the production of lung injury, certain criteria must be fulfilled. These criteria include:[58]

(1) the candidate mediator should be capable of mimicking, alone or with other compounds, the effects it is suspected of mediating;

From Said, S.I. (ed.): *The Pulmonary Circulation and Acute Lung Injury.* Mount Kisco, N.Y., Futura Publishing Co., Inc., 1985.

(2)   it should be released in sufficient concentrations, at or near the site of its postulated action;

(3)   its release should be detectable before, or at the onset of, the suspected effects;

(4)   measured levels should correlate with the intensity of the presumed response; and

(5)   inhibition of its release or of its actions should reduce or abolish these effects.

Can PAF Induce the Pathophysiologic Responses of Acute Lung Injury?

The main responses in acute lung injury against which the potential role of PAF will be examined include: high-permeability pulmonary edema, pulmonary vasoconstriction and pulmonary hypertension, bronchoconstriction and decreased lung compliance, as well as systemic hypotension, cardiac dysfunction, and other systemic complications.

High-Permeability Pulmonary Edema and Pulmonary Vasoconstriction

Pulmonary edema has been observed following administration of PAF in several animal models. Although it has been difficult to distinguish between high-permeability and high-pressure edema in some preparations, the use of large animal models, such as dogs and sheep, has helped clarify this issue by allowing the collection of pulmonary lymph and analysis of its protein content and flow characteristics.

Mojarad et al.[48] examined the effects of PAF on lung fluid balance, hemodynamics, and gas exchange in anesthetized dogs with right lymph duct cannulation. As shown in Figure 1, the flow of lymph (derived to a major degree from pulmonary lymph) and its total albumin and globulin content increased with the infusion of 50 ng/kg PAF into the pulmonary artery. The left atrial, pulmonary, and systemic arterial blood pressures, cardiac output and arterial blood pH, P_{CO_2} and P_{O_2} did not change after injection of this small dose of PAF. The wet/dry lung weight ratio was increased by 20% in these dogs, indicating formation of pulmonary edema. Since pulmonary edema induced by PAF was not associated with increased left atrial or pulmonary arterial pressure, nor with decreased lymph protein content, altered pulmonary microvascular permeability seemed the likely mechanism of pulmonary edema.

Cox et al.[19] studied the effects of PAF infusion into awake sheep with chronic lung lymph fistulas.[63] In order to eliminate the effects of increased surface area on lung lymph flow, left atrial pressure was raised to 20 to 25 mmHg prior to each experiment by inflation of a Foley balloon in the left atrium. The resultant increase in pulmonary lymph flow was associated with a decrease in pulmonary lymph protein content, indicating high-pressure pulmonary edema. After a new steady state was obtained (60−90 min), 0.5 µg/kg of PAF was infused into the pulmonary artery over a 2-minute period. The lymph flow further increased two to three times within 15 minutes and became grossly hemorrhagic, but neither the lymph/plasma protein ratio nor vascular pressures changed. Leukopenia and thrombocytopenia were observed within 1 minute after PAF infusion, with maximal falls of leukocyte and platelet counts of

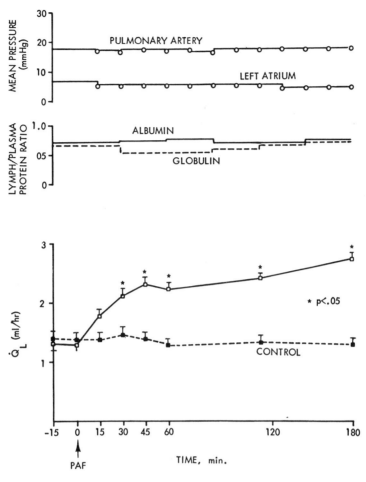

Figure 1: *The right lymph duct flow* ($\dot{Q}_L$) *increased following 50 ng/kg of PAF into the pulmonary artery at arrow. Lymph/plasma albumin and globulin ratios, pulmonary arterial and left atrial pressures remained unchanged. Asterisks indicate values significantly above basal level (P < 0.05). Data represent mean ± SEM in nine dogs.*

60% occurring at 5 minutes after the infusion. The cell counts returned to baseline levels within 15 minutes. These findings strongly suggested that PAF increased lung lymph flow by increasing pulmonary microvascular permeability, by a mechanism possibly related to leukocyte and platelet activation.

Hamasaki and colleagues[31] evaluated the effects of PAF on pulmonary vascular hemodynamics and pulmonary vascular permeability in isolated guinea pig lungs perfused in situ with cell-free Krebs solution. PAF (1–10 μg) infused into the pulmonary artery caused a dose-dependent increase in pulmonary arterial pressure up to 70% of baseline values. Extravascular lung water, as measured by wet/dry lung weight ratio, increased from a control value of 5.53 ± 0.02 to 7.13 ± 0.04 following infusion of 3 μg PAF. Concentrations of PAF less than 1 μg had no effect on pulmonary arterial pressure or lung weight. These results did not, however, identify the mechanism of formation of pulmonary edema, though it was apparently a direct effect and independent of the presence of leukocytes or platelets. Voelkel et al.[72] studied the effects of PAF on the pulmonary circulation of isolated rat lungs perfused with an albumin-free buffer solution. They reported that 1–2 μg PAF injected into the pulmonary artery increased pulmonary arterial pressure by 15 mmHg and increased the gravimetrically determined lung weight by 2.4 to 7.0 g.[72] Using isolated, perfused rabbit lungs, Heffner et al.[33] showed that 20 μg of PAF alone had no effect on lung edema formation, but in the presence of human platelets increased pulmonary arterial pressure by nine or ten times and lung weight by an average of 20 g.

Alterations in Lung Mechanics

Halonen et al.[30] demonstrated that the intravenous infusion of PAF (0.6 μg/kg) into rabbits increased total pulmonary resistance by 115 ± 14% and decreased dynamic compliance by 86 ± 10%. Vargaftig and co-workers[70] found that small intravenous doses of PAF (10 to 20 ng/kg) raised airway pressure by 6.7 ± 1.5 cm H_2O in anesthetized guinea pigs. In later studies,[67,68,71] these authors reported that the PAF-induced bronchoconstriction was histamine-independent, and could also be induced by slightly larger doses of aerosolized PAF (20 to 40 ng/kg). The responses of primates to PAF infusion and inhalation were similar to those of rabbits and guinea pigs. Patterson and Harris[51] administered aerosolized PAF (15 breaths of 2 to 10 μg/ml) to rhesus monkeys (*Macaca mulatta*), and observed an increase in pulmonary resistance of at least 25% and a decrease in dynamic compliance of at least 20%. These results did not determine whether the airway contraction resulted from a direct effect of PAF or from the release of other mediators. When PAF (60 μg/kg) was instilled intratracheally[26] in curarized and ventilated baboons (*Papio papio*), peak airway inspiratory pressure almost doubled within 60 seconds. Static pulmonary compliance did not change significantly, suggesting that in this study, PAF constricted predominantly large airways.

PAF also contracts airways in perfused lungs and constricts lung parenchymal strips. Infusion of PAF into the pulmonary artery of mechanically ventilated guinea pig lungs, perfused in situ with cell-free Krebs solution, increased peak airway pressure dose-dependently.[31] At the maximum dose used (10 μg), peak airway pressure was increased by 230%. PAF (0.54 to 54 ng/ml) induced a slowly developing contraction of isolated rabbit lung parenchymal strips[16,17] and a dose-dependent contraction of lung parenchymal strips with an ED_{50} value of 0.54 ng/ml in guinea pigs.[64] This contractile effect was not blocked by an H_1 histamine-receptor antagonist (pyrilamine), by cyclooxygenase inhibitors (indomethacin, aspirin, or sulfinpyrazone), by a lipoxygenase inhibitor (nordihydroguaiaretic acid), or by a leukotriene antagonist (FPL 55712).

Systemic Hypotension and Cardiac Dysfunction

PAF causes systemic arterial hypotension in dogs in a dose-dependent fashion.[37] At 0.1, 0.2, 0.4, and 0.8 μg/kg, PAF reduced mean arterial blood pressure by 9%, 32%, 39%, and 41%, repectively. The marked systemic hypotension occurred within 1 to 3 minutes after PAF infusion (from 98 to 52 mmHg). Blood pressure gradually returned toward the normal level, but remained about 10% below the baseline value for up to 1 hour. Systemic vascular resistance increased following a slight and transient decrease, which occurred within 5 to 30 seconds after PAF injection. The maximal increase in systemic vascular resistance (by 125%) occurred 3 to 10 minutes after PAF infusion, when the systemic blood pressure was near normal, and dP/dt and aortic blood flow were markedly reduced. Both aortic blood flow and left ventricular dP/dt, an index of ventricular contractility, decreased by 50% within 2 minutes after intravenous administration of 0.4 μg/kg PAF. Bessin et al.[8] described an acute cardiovascular failure in anesthetized, mechanically ventilated dogs following infusion of 5 to 20 μg/kg PAF. They used ^{51}Cr-labeled erythrocytes and showed a 43% decrease in plasma volume 30 minutes after the intravenous infusion of 5 μg/kg PAF. Immediately after the PAF infusion was started, pulmonary arterial pressure increased transiently from 15.0 ± 1.2 mmHg to 100 ± 13 mmHg and portal vein pressure increased transiently from 98 ± 8 mm H_2O to 185 ± 13 mm H_2O. Higher doses of PAF (20 μg/kg) infused into anesthetized open-chest dogs reduced coronary arterial blood flow by 56% within 10 minutes. These findings are similar to those observed in shock induced by endotoxin or histamine.[35] Sanchez-Crespo et al.[56] used ^{57}Co and ^{113}Sn-labeled microspheres to calculate cardiac output and systemic vascular resistance following PAF infusion in anesthetized rats. They showed a dose-dependent systemic hypotension and decreased peripheral vascular resistance at 0.5 and 5 μg PAF, although no changes in cardiac output were noted. In rabbits,[30,45] an initial bradycardia, systemic arterial hypotension, and decreased cardiac output was observed. Benveniste et al.[4] used an isolated guinea pig heart preparation to study the effects of PAF on cardiac muscle and reported that PAF (5.4 to 540 ng/ml) induced a dose-dependent decrease in both contractile force (maximum of 60%) and coronary flow (maximum of 75%), neither of which was blocked by atropine. Levi et al.[41] used a similar isolated heart preparation to compare the effects of exogenous PAF with those of endogenous PAF released during antigen-induced anaphylaxis and subsequent cardiac abnormalities. In both models, coronary flow decreased (by 5% to 85%), left ventricular contractile force decreased (by 5% to 85%), and the incidence of arrhythmias increased, suggesting that PAF may contribute to the heart failure resulting from systemic anaphylaxis.

Morphologic Evidence of Pulmonary Endothelial Injury

The major pathological change associated with ARDS is damage to pulmonary microvascular endothelial cells. This damage is often accompanied by platelet and leukocyte "plugs" in pulmonary capillaries. Similar findings have been reported in the lungs of laboratory animals after administration of PAF. Lewis et al.[42] examined alterations in pulmonary ultrastructure following intravenous infusion of 0.15 to 10 μg/kg PAF in rabbits, and found marked vacuolation and vesiculation of pulmonary capillary endothelial cells and lobular protrusion of these cells into the luminal spaces. Even at low doses of PAF, the alveolar septa appeared to be distorted, and capillaries were filled with platelet and leukocyte aggregates. Although they reported changes in both vesicle size and number as compared with control animals, there was no direct measurement of extravascular lung water. Intratracheal instillation of PAF in rabbits[18] also caused a dose-dependent acute inflammatory reaction, manifested by degenerative and necrotic changes in the epithelium and damage to alveolar walls. These inflammatory changes, seen as early as 2 hours post-instillation, were accompanied by marked cellular infiltration, predominantly of macrophages in the alveolar spaces and septa, and PMNs in the capillaries. Large aggregates of degranulated platelets within the capillaries, with some aggregates adherent to the endothelium, were also observed in these animals. Rabbits receiving relatively high doses of PAF (5 μg) had significant pulmonary fibrosis 30 days post-instillation. Due to the severe damage, the usual morphometric criteria for evaluating pulmonary edema were not helpful, but the data support the hypothesis that PAF can mediate pulmonary inflammation.

Is PAF Released During Acute Lung Injury?

Despite the convincing data summarized above that the administration of exogenous PAF can mimic the pathophysiologic changes associated with acute lung injury, the release of PAF during induction of acute lung injury in experimental animals has yet to be demonstrated. To date, there are no reports of either successful or unsuccessful attempts to recover PAF from animal models of acute lung injury. However, evidence suggesting the release of PAF into the bronchial lavage fluid during hypoxic vasoconstriction has been presented.[55] The major obstacle to the recovery of PAF from biological fluids is its short half-life, which is less than 30 seconds. PAF is rapidly degraded by a highly specific acetylhydrolase found in plasma[22,28] and in tissue microsomes.[11] The biologically inactive metabolite, 2-lyso-PAF, is a ubiquitous molecule that may also be the precursor for the de novo synthesis of PAF;[6,40] it is therefore not a particularly useful indicator of PAF release. The acetylhydrolase activity in plasma can, however, be eliminated by the immediate acidification of blood samples to pH 2.5 prior to phospholipid extraction,[13] allowing the recovery of PAF from whole blood.[20,22,25,28]

The inability to demonstrate PAF release may also be due to the limited sensitivity of currently available assay methods. The most widely used assay for PAF is the turbidimetric platelet aggregation method.[14] Although platelet-rich plasma (PRP) can be used directly, Ardlie[1] described a procedure for preparing washed, [³H]serotonin-labeled platelets that can be used to detect and quantify platelet secretion as well as platelet aggregation in response to various stimuli. The sensitivity of this bioassay is approximately 10^{-10}M, depending on the species of platelets used, whereas PAF may be present in vivo at concentrations as low as 10^{-12}M.[68] As with most bioassays, there may be considerable day-to-day variability in the platelet response to PAF, which in turn reflects inherent differences between washed platelet preparations. The development of a sensitive and specific radioimmunoassay will greatly increase the chance of detecting and measuring PAF release in acute lung injury.[50]

How Does PAF Induce Acute Lung Injury?

The precise mechanism of PAF-induced lung injury and pulmonary edema is unknown. Although some effects of PAF on pulmonary smooth muscle and microvasculature may be independent of circulating platelets and leukocytes, the biological effects of PAF are probably amplified by the presence of these cells. Current evidence suggests that substances released from activated neutrophils and platelets are major mediators of acute lung injury. These mediators include lysosomal enzymes, toxic O_2 radicals, thromboxane A_2 (TxA_2), and leukotrienes C_4 and D_4 (LTC_4 and LTD_4).

As noted above, PAF causes sequestration of leukocytes and platelets in the lung.[30,45,54] Strong evidence (presented elsewhere in this volume) suggests that accumulation of neutrophils in the lung plays an important role in the pathogenesis of experimental acute lung injury.[73] Neutrophil-mediated injury appears to be an extension of the two major mechanisms available to these cells for killing microorganisms, namely: release of proteinases that are capable of degrading lung tissue,[36,49] and production of toxic oxygen species.[27,38] PAF has been shown to initiate the oxidative burst in guinea pig macrophages[32] and in human neutrophils,[61,62] resulting in both degranulation and the release of superoxide anion and other toxic oxygen radicals.

The leukotrienes may also participate in mediating PAF-induced acute lung injury. Voelkel and co-workers[72] reported that isolated rat lungs perfused with cell-free media released LTC_4 and LTD_4 into the lung effluent following the infusion of PAF. Human PMNs stimulated by PAF in vitro also release leukotrienes.[29,43] Mojarad et al.[47] demonstrated that infusion of LTC_4 or LTD_4 into the pulmonary artery of unanesthetized sheep resulted in high-permeability pulmonary edema. It is thus possible that similar interactions between PAF and leukocytes occur in vivo, with secondary release of leukotrienes as an intermediate step in the production of acute lung injury.

Similarly, release of thromboxane A_2 (TxA_2) has been associated with PAF-induced acute lung injury both in vivo and in vitro. Hamasaki et al.[31] observed that the PAF-induced pulmonary edema and pulmonary hypertension in guinea pig lungs perfused with cell-free Krebs solution was accompanied by increased levels of thromboxane B_2 (TxB_2) and 6-keto-$PGF_{1\alpha}$, the respective metabolites of TxA_2 and prostaglandin I_2 (PGI_2). Pretreatment with 10 µg indomethacin attenuated these PAF-induced changes markedly (79% protection) at low doses of PAF (1 µg/kg), but provided only 35% protection when 3 µg/kg PAF was infused. The authors concluded that the PAF-induced platelet-independent pulmonary edema and pulmonary hypotension were partially mediated by TxA_2 or other cyclooxygenase products.

Specific antagonists of PAF are of considerable potential value in identifying the role of PAF in acute lung injury. Numerous structural analogs of PAF have been developed by altering the length of the alkyl chain[59] and the polar head group,[60] but these analogs have retained significant levels of PAF-like biological activity. Terashita and co-workers[65] recently developed a new structural analog of PAF, designated "CV-3988," which reportedly lacks intrinsic PAF-like activity and selectively blocks PAF-induced rabbit platelet aggregation in vitro and PAF-mediated hypotension in rats in vivo.[44] A recent report indicates that triazolobenzodiazapines (psychotropic drugs) are potent PAF inhibitors and are capable of inhibiting PAF-induced changes in human platelet shape, aggregation, and secretion.[39]

Is PAF A Mediator of Acute Lung Injury?

From the evidence presented above, based on the effects of exogenously administered PAF, it is clearly capable of causing most of the hallmarks of acute lung injury including: alveolar-capillary damage, high-permeability pulmonary edema, pulmonary vasoconstriction, and bronchoconstriction. Whether PAF causes acute lung injury by direct action on the pulmonary microvasculature or by the release of secondary mediators from activated platelets and neutrophils, or by both mechanisms, remains uncertain. Equally uncertain at present is whether PAF actually serves as a mediator of lung injury in the clinical condition of ARDS or its experimental counterparts. The development of a highly sensitive radioimmunoassay for PAF will make it possible to measure the release of picomolar concentrations of endogenous PAF in animal models of acute lung injury, as well as in patients with ARDS. The use of specific PAF antagonists should also provide new insights into the pathophysiologic role of this potent compound and should suggest effective means of counteracting its deleterious effects.

Acknowledgment

Supported in part by NIH research grant nos. HL30450 and HL31039, and by Veterans Administration medical research funds.

REFERENCES

1. Ardlie, N.G., Packham, M.A., and Mustard, J.F.: Adenosine diphosphate-induced platelet aggregation in suspensions of washed rabbit platelets. *Br. J. Hematol.* 19:7–17, 1970.
2. Arnoux, B., Duval, D., and Benveniste, J.: Release of platelet-activating factor (PAF-acether) from alveolar macrophages by the calcium ionophore A23187 and phagocytosis. *Eur. J. Clin. Invest.* 10:437–441, 1980.
3. Barie, P.S. and Malik, A.B.: Metabolic factors as mediators of pulmonary vascular injury. *Ann. N.Y. Acad. Sci.* 384:344–355, 1982.
4. Benveniste, J., Boullet, C., Brink, C., et al.: The actions of PAF-acether (platelet-activating factor) on guinea-pig isolated heart preparations. *Br. J. Pharmacol.* 80:81–83, 1983.
5. Benveniste, J., Henson, P.M., and Cochrane, C.G.: Leukocyte-dependent histamine release from rabbit platelets: the role of IgE, basophils and a platelet-activating factor. *J. Exp. Med.* 136:1356–1377, 1972.
6. Benveniste, J., Roubin, R., Chignard, M., et al.: Release of platelet-activating factor (PAF-acether) and 2-lyso PAF-acether from three cell types. *Agents Actions* 12:711–713, 1982.
7. Benveniste, J., Tence, M., Varenne, P., et al.: Semi-synthesè et structure proposeé du facteur activant les plaquettes (PAF): PAF-acether, un alkyl-ether analogue de la lysophosphatidylcholine. *C.R. Acad. Sci. (Paris)* 289D:1037–1040, 1979.
8. Bessin, P., Bonnet, J., Apffel, D., et al.: Acute circulatory collapse caused by platelet-activating factor (PAF-acether) in dogs. *Eur. J. Pharmacol.* 86:403–413, 1983.
9. Betz, S.J. and Henson, P.M.: Production and release of platelet-activating factor (PAF): Dissociation from degranulation and superoxide production in the human neutrophil. *J. Immunol.* 125:2756–2763, 1980.
10. Billah, M.M. and Johnston, J.M.: Identification of phospholipid platelet-activating factor (1-O-alkyl-2-acetyl-*sn*-glycero-3-phosphocholine) in human amniotic fluid and urine. *Biochem. Biophys. Res. Commun.* 113:51–58, 1983.
11. Blank, M.L., Lee, T.-C., Fitzgerald, V., et al.: A specific acetylhydrolase for 1-alkyl-

2-acetyl-*sn*-glycero-3-phosphocholine (a hypotensive and platelet-activating lipid). *J. Biol. Chem.* 256:175–178, 1981.

12. Blank, M.L., Snyder, F., Byers, L.W., et al.: Antihypertensive activity of an alkyl ether analog of phosphatidylcholine. *Biochem. Biophys. Res. Commun.* 90:1194–1200, 1979.

13. Bligh, E.G. and Dyer, W.J.: A rapid method of total lipid extraction and purification. *Can. J. Biochem. Physiol.* 37:911–917, 1959.

14. Born, G.V.R.: Aggregation of blood platelets by adenosine diphosphate and its reversal. *Nature* 194:927–929, 1962.

15. Brigham, K.L. and Meyrick, B.: Interactions of granulocytes with the lungs. *Circ. Res.* 54:623–635, 1984.

16. Camussi, G., Montrucchio, G., Antro, C., et al.: Platelet-activating factor-mediated contraction of rabbit lung strips: Pharmacologic modulation. *Immunopharmacology* 6:87–96, 1983.

17. Camussi, G., Montrucchio, G., Antro, C., et al.: In vitro spasmogenic effect on rabbit lung tissue of 1-0-octadecyl-2-acetyl-*sn*-glyceryl-3-phosphorylcholine (platelet-activating factor): Specific desensitization after in vivo infusion. *Agents Actions* 13:507–509, 1983.

18. Camussi, G., Pawlowski, I., Tetta, C., et al.: Acute lung inflammation induced in the rabbit by local instillation of 1-0-octadecyl-2-acetyl-*sn*-glyceryl-3-phosphorylcholine or of native platelet-activating factor. *Am. J. Pathol.* 112:78–88, 1983.

19. Cox, C.P., Mojarad, M., Attiah, A., et al.: Platelet-activating factor (PAF) increases pulmonary vascular permeability in awake sheep. *Am. Rev. Respir. Dis.* 129:334A, 1984.

20. Cox, C.P., Wardlow, M.L., Jorgenson, R., et al.: A substance similar to platelet-activating factor in human blood. *Fed. Proc.* 39:693A, 1980.

21. Cox, C.P., Wardlow, M.L., Jorgensen, R., et al.: The presence of platelet-activating factor (PAF) in normal human mixed saliva. *J. Immunol.* 127:46–50, 1981.

22. Cox, C.P., Wardlow, M.L., Meng, K.E., et al.: Substrate specificity of the phosphatide 2-acylhydrolase that inactivates AGEPC. *INSERM Symposia* 23:299–304, 1983.

23. Craddock, P.R., Fehr, J., Dalmasso, A.P., et al.: Hemodialysis leukopenia: Pulmonary vascular leukostasis resulting from complement activation by dialyzer cellophane membranes. *J. Clin. Invest.* 59:679–688, 1977.

24. Demling, R.H.: Role of prostaglandins in acute pulmonary microvascular injury. *Ann. N.Y. Acad. Sci.* 384:515–534, 1982.

25. Demopoulos, C.A., Pinckard, R.N., and Hanahan, D.J.: Platelet-activating factor: Evidence for 1-0-alkyl-2-acetyl-*sn*-glyceryl-3-phosphorylcholine as the active component (a new class of lipid chemical mediators). *J. Biol. Chem.* 254:9355–9358, 1979.

26. Denjean, A., Arnoux, B., Benveniste, J., et al.: Bronchoconstriction induced by intratracheal administration of platelet-activating factor (PAF-acether) in baboons. *Agents Actions* 11:567–568, 1981.

27. Drath, D.B. and Karnovsky, M.L.: Superoxide production by phagocytic leukocytes. *J. Exp. Med.* 141:257–261, 1980.

28. Farr, R.S., Cox, C.P., Wardlow, M.L., et al.: Preliminary studies of an acid-labile factor (ALF) in human serum that inactivates platelet-activating factor (PAF). *Clin. Immunol. Immunopathol.* 15:318–330, 1980.

29. Gorman, R.R., Morton, D.R., Hopkins, N.K., et al.: Acetyl glyceryl ether phosphorylcholine stimulates leukotriene B_4 synthesis and cyclic AMP accumulation in human polymorphonuclear leukocytes. In *Advances in Prostaglandin, Thromboxane and Leukotriene Research, Vol. 12.* Samuelsson, B., Paoletti, R., and Ramwell, P., eds. New York, Raven Press, 1983, pp. 57–63.

30. Halonen, M., Palmer, J.D., Lohman, C., et al.: Differential effects of platelet depletion on the physiologic alterations of IgE anaphylaxis and acetyl glyceryl ether phosphorylcholine infusion in the rabbit. *Am. Rev. Respir. Dis.* 124:416–421, 1981.

31. Hamasaki, Y., Mojarad, M., Saga, T., et al.: Platelet-activating factor raises airway

and vascular pressures and induces edema in lungs perfused with platelet-free solution. *Am. Rev. Respir. Dis.* 129:742–746, 1984.

32. Hartung, H.P., Parnham, M.J., Winkelmann, J., et al.: Platelet-activating factor (PAF) induces the oxidative burst in macrophages. *Int. J. Immunopharmacol.* 5: 115–121, 1983.

33. Heffner, J.E., Shoemaker, S.A., Canham, E.M., et al.: Acetyl glyceryl ether phosphorylcholine-stimulated human platelets cause pulmonary hypertension and edema in isolated rabbit lungs. Role of thromboxane A_2. *J. Clin. Invest.* 71:351–357, 1983.

34. Henson, P.M. and Pinckard, R.N.: Basophil-derived platelet-activating factor (PAF) as an in vivo mediator of acute allergic reactions: Demonstration of specific desensitization of platelets to PAF during IgE-induced anaphylaxis in the rabbit. *J. Immunol.* 119:2179–2184, 1977.

35. Hinshaw, L.B., Emerson, T.E., Jr., Iampetro, P.F., et al.: A comparative study of the hemodynamic actions of histamine and endotoxin. *Am. J. Physiol.* 203:600–606, 1962.

36. Jacob, H.S., Maldow, C.F., Flynn, J., et al.: Therapeutic ramifications of the interaction of complement, granulocytes and platelets in the production of acute lung injury. *Ann. N.Y. Acad. Sci.* 384:489–495, 1982.

37. Kenzora, J.L., Perez, J.E., Bergmann, S.R., et al.: Effects of acetyl glyceryl ether phosphorylcholine (platelet activating factor) on ventricular preload, afterload and contractility in dogs. *J. Clin. Invest.* 74:1193–1203, 1984.

38. Klebanoff, S.J.: Oxygen metabolism and the toxic properties of phagocytes. *Ann. Int. Med.* 93:480–489, 1980.

39. Kornecki, E., Ehrlich, Y.H., and Lenox, R.H.: Platelet activation-factor-induced aggregation of human platelets specifically inhibited by triazolobenzodiazepines. *Science* 226:1454–1456, 1984.

40. Lee, T.C., Malone, B., Wasserman, S.L., et al.: Activities of enzymes that metabolize platelet-activating factor (1-0-alkyl-2-acetyl-*sn*-glycero-3-phosphocholine) in neutrophils and eosinophils from humans and the effect of a calcium ionophore. *Biochem. Biophys. Res. Commun.* 105:1303–1308, 1982.

41. Levi, R., Burke, J.A., Gou, Z.G., et al.: Acetyl glyceryl ether phosphorylcholine (AGEPC) a putative mediator of cardiac anaphylaxis in the guinea pig. *Circ. Res.* 54:117–124, 1984.

42. Lewis, J.C., O'Flaherty, J.T., McCall, C.E., et al.: Platelet-activating factor effects on pulmonary ultrastructure in rabbits. *Exp. Molec. Pathol.* 38:100–108, 1983.

43. Lin, A.H., Morton, D.R., and Gorman, R.R.: Acetyl glyceryl ether phosphorylcholine stimulates leukotriene B_4 synthesis in human polymorphonuclear leukocytes. *J. Clin. Invest.* 70:1058–1065, 1982.

44. Masugi, F., Ogihara, T., Optsuka, A., et al.: Effect of 1-alkyl-2-acetyl-*sn*-glycero-3-phosphorylcholine inhibitor on the reduction of one-kidney, one-clip hypertension after unclipping in the rat. *Life Sci.* 34:197–201, 1984.

45. McManus, L.M., Hanahan, D.J., Demopoulos, C.A., et al.: Pathobiology of the intravenous infusion of acetyl glyceryl ether phosphorylcholine (AGEPC), a synthetic platelet-activating factor (PAF), in the rabbit. *J. Immunol.* 124:2919–2924, 1980.

46. Mencia-Huerta, J.M. and Benveniste, J.: Platelet-activating factor and macrophages. I. Evidence for the release from rat and mouse peritoneal macrophages and not from mastocytes. *Eur. J. Immunol.* 9:409–415, 1979.

47. Mojarad, M., Blalock, J., Cox, C.P., et al.: Leukotriene C_4 increases pulmonary lymph flow in awake sheep, probably by increasing vascular permeability. *Am. Rev. Respir. Dis.* 129:103A, 1984.

48. Mojarad, M., Hamasaki, Y., and Said, S.I.: Platelet-activating factor increases pulmonary microvascular permeability and induces pulmonary edema: A preliminary report. *Clin. Respir. Physiol.* 19:253–256, 1983.

49. Murphy, D.: *The Neutrophil.* New York, Plenum Medical Book Co., 1976.

50. Nishihira, J., Ishibashi, T., and Imai, Y.: Production and characterization of specific

antibodies against 1-0-alkyl-2-acetyl-sn-glycero-3-phosphocholine (a potent hypotensive and platelet-activating ether-linked phospholipid). *J. Biochem.* 95:1247–1251, 1984.

51. Patterson, R. and Harris, K.E.: The activity of aerosolized and intracutaneous synthetic platelet activating factor (AGEPC) in rhesus monkeys with IgE-mediated airway responses and normal monkeys. *J. Lab. Clin. Med.* 102:933–938, 1983.

52. Pinckard, R.N., Farr, R.S., and Hanahan, D.J.: Physiochemical and functional identity of platelet-activating factor (PAF) released in vivo during IgE anaphylaxis with PAF released in vitro from IgE-sensitized basophils. *J. Immunol.* 123:1847–1857, 1979.

53. Pinckard, R.N., McManus, L.M., and Hanahan, D.J.: Chemistry and biology of acetyl glyceryl ether phosphorylcholine (platelet-activating factor). In *Advances in Inflammation Research, Vol. 4.* Weissman, G., ed. New York, Raven Press, 1982, pp. 147–180.

54. Pinckard, R.N., McManus, L.M., Hanahan, D.J., et al.: Immunopharmacology of acetyl glyceryl ether phosphorylcholine (AGEPC). In *Immunopharmacology of the Lung.* Newball, H.H., ed. New York, Marcel Dekker, Inc., 1983, pp. 73–107.

55. Prevost, M.-C., Cariven, C., Simon, M.-F., et al.: Platelet activating factor (PAF-acether) is released into rat pulmonary alveolar fluid as a consequence of hypoxia. *Biochem. Biophys. Res. Commun.* 119:58–63, 1984.

56. Sanchez-Crespo, M., Alonso, F., Inarrea, P., et al.: Vascular actions of synthetic PAF-acether (a synthetic platelet-activating factor) in the rat: Evidence for a platelet-independent mechanism. *Immunopharmacology* 4:173–185, 1982.

57. Said, S.I.: Metabolic functions of the pulmonary circulation. *Circ. Res.* 50:325–333, 1982.

58. Said, S.I.: Peptides and lipids as mediators of acute lung injury. In *Acute Respiratory Failure.* Zapol, W.R., ed. In *Lung Biology in Health and Disease* series, Lenfant, C., ed. New York, Marcel Dekker, Inc., (In press).

59. Satouchi, K., Pinckard, R.N., Ferrigni, K.S., et al.: Influence of alkyl ether chain length of acetyl glyceryl ether phosphorylcholine and its ethanolamine analog on biological activity towards rabbit platelets. *J. Immunol.* 127:1250–1255, 1981.

60. Satouchi, K., Pinckard, R.N., McManus, L.M., et al.: Modification of the polar head group of acetyl glyceryl ether phosphorylcholine and subsequent effects upon platelet activation. *J. Biol. Chem.* 256:4425–4432, 1981.

61. Shaw, J.O., Pinckard, R.N., Ferrigni, K.S., et al.: Activation of human neutrophils with 1-0-hexadecyl/octadecyl-2-acetyl-*sn*-glyceryl-3-phosphorylcholines: A novel class of neutrophil stimulants. *Am. J. Pathol.* 103:70–79, 1981.

62. Smith, R.J., Bowman, B.J., and Iden, S.S.: Stimulation of the human neutrophil superoxide anion-generating system with 1-0-hexadecyl/octadecyl-2-acetyl-*sn*-glyceryl-3-phosphorylcholine. *Biochem. Pharmacol.* 33:973–978, 1984.

63. Staub, N.C., Bland, R.D., Brigham, K.L., et al.: Preparation of chronic lung lymph fistulas in sheep. *J. Surg. Res.* 19:315–320, 1975.

64. Stimler, N.P. and O'Flaherty, J.T.: Spasmogenic properties of platelet-activating factor: Evidence for a direct mechanism in the contractile response of pulmonary tissues. *Am. J. Pathol.* 113:75–84, 1983.

65. Terashita, Z., Tsushima, S., Yoshioka, Y., et al.: CV-3988: A specific antagonist of platelet-activating factor (PAF). *Life Sci.* 32:1975–1982, 1983.

66. Vaage, J.: Intravascular platelet aggregation and pulmonary injury. *Ann. N.Y. Acad. Sci.* 384:301–318, 1982.

67. Vargaftig, B.B.: Phospholipids, particularly platelet-activating factor (PAF-acether), in experimental bronchoconstriction. *Agents Actions* 13(suppl. 1):155–171, 1983.

68. Vargaftig, B.B. and Benveniste, J.: Platelet-activating factor today. *Trends Pharmacol. Sci.* 4:341–343, 1983.

69. Vargaftig, B.B., Chignard, M., Benveniste, J., et al.: Background and present status of research on platelet-activating factor (PAF-acether). *Ann. N.Y. Acad. Sci.* 370:119–137, 1981.

70. Vargaftig, B.B., Lefort, J., Chignard, M., et al.: Platelet-activating factor induces a platelet-dependent bronchoconstriction unrelated to the formation of prostaglandin derivatives. *Eur. J. Pharmacol.* 65:185–192, 1980.
71. Vargaftig, B.B., Lefort, J., Wal, F., et al.: Non-steroidal anti-flammatory drugs if combined with antihistamine and anti-serotonin agents interfere with the bronchial platelet "effects of platelet-activating factor" (PAF-acether). *Eur. J. Pharmacol.* 82:121–130, 1982.
72. Voelkel, N.F., Worthen, S., Reeves, J.T., et al.: Nonimmunological production of leukotrienes induced by platelet-activating factor. *Science* 218:286–288, 1982.
73. Wittels, E.H., Coalson, J.J., Welch, M.H., et al.: Pulmonary intravascular leukocyte sequestration: A potential mechanism of lung injury. *Am. Rev. Respir. Dis.* 109: 502–509, 1974.

CHAPTER 18

Complement-Induced Lung Injury

Gerd O. Till and
Peter A. Ward

Introduction

Trauma and/or infection may lead to activation of the complement system and the development of an inflammatory reaction. Activation products of the complement system can induce various biological functions that generally support host defenses against invasion by pathogenic microorganisms. In an acute inflammatory reaction to local bacterial infection, complement activation products may increase blood flow and vascular permeability, cause increased adherence of neutrophils to vascular endothelium, emigration, and directed migration (chemotaxis) into the inflamed tissue, and may facilitate phagocytosis and intracellular killing of the bacteria by neutrophils and tissue macrophages.

There is, however, an increasing body of clinical and experimental evidence suggesting that under certain circumstances complement activation can be harmful to the host. This may occur by two different means. First, complement activation may lead to irreversible damage of cell membranes via the "membrane attack" mechanism, either by interaction of complement proteins with antibody-coated cells or by complement reactions in close vicinity of cells leading to "innocent bystander" cell damage or lysis.[2] Secondly, complement activation products such as C5a may cause release from neutrophils and other phagocytic cells of enzymes and the generation of oxygen radicals, all of which may be harmful to the host's cells and tissues.[15]

Current interest in the pathophysiologic role of complement and neutrophils in acute inflammatory reactions has been stimulated by recent observations in experimental animals and patients. In 1974, McCall et al.[34] showed that systemic complement activation in the rabbit following intravenous injection of cobra venom factor (CVF) or inulin (both activators of the alternative complement pathway) could cause a profound but transient neutropenia that was followed by an extensive granulocytosis. The authors assumed that the neutropenia was related to a complement activation product that caused mar-

From Said, S.I. (ed.): *The Pulmonary Circulation and Acute Lung Injury.* Mount Kisco, N.Y., Futura Publishing Co., Inc., 1985.

gination and pulmonary sequestration of blood neutrophils. A complement-derived leukocyte-mobilizing factor, first described by Rother,[45] was postulated to be responsible for the observed granulocytosis. Similar alterations in neutrophil kinetics that could also be related to complement activation were observed in patients during hemodialysis with a cellophane-membrane apparatus.[12] A similar phenomenon was also described in normal donors during nylon fiber leukapheresis.[36] Furthermore, Craddock et al.[11] showed that reinfusion of complement-activated autologous plasma into experimental animals resulted not only in neutropenia and granulocytosis but also caused sequestration of neutrophils in the lungs and plugging of pulmonary vessels.

Although the mechanism of the neutrophil sequestration in pulmonary capillaries is not completely understood, data from in vitro experiments suggested that the complement activation products cause aggregation and trapping of neutrophils in the lung vasculature[13] and/or may increase adherence of neutrophils to vascular endothelium.[23] O'Flaherty et al.[37] demonstrated that the infusion of purified chemotactic peptides (C5a and N-formyl-met-leu-phe) could reproduce the neutropenia findings associated with the systemic infusion into rabbits of complement-activated serum. This complement-mediated sequestration of neutrophils in the lung vasculature was thought to be associated with pulmonary dysfunction[13] and possibly related to the development of adult respiratory distress syndrome (ARDS).[19] This is supported by in vitro findings suggesting that contact of granulocytes with complement-activated serum results in the release of ^{51}Cr from endothelial cells.[46]

These observations indicate a key role of the polymorphonuclear leukocyte in acute inflammatory reactions as a "response organ" to complement-derived biological products. Any discussion of the role of complement in acute inflammatory reactions inevitably has to include the polymorphonuclear leukocyte and its secretion products, such as neutral proteinases, oxygen-derived free radicals, and lipid mediators. We will focus on experimental models of complement-mediated pulmonary injury, discuss potential mediators and pathogenic mechanisms involved, and present some experimental approaches to prevention of complement-induced acute lung injury.

Induction of Complement-Mediated Lung Injury

Vascular Endothelial Cell Injury

Systemic Complement Activation

It is well accepted that a wide variety of factors and mechanisms contribute to the development of ARDS making an experimental analysis of its pathogenesis extremely difficult. However, activation of the complement system and generation of biologically active products such as C5a appear to play a central role. If this assumption is correct, it would imply that in vivo intravascular complement activation in experimental animals will lead to acute lung injury.

To answer this question, adult pathogen-free Long Evans rats received an intravenous bolus injection of CVF, resulting in an immediate and profound intravascular complement activation.[55] Serum hemolytic complement activity (CH50 values) was completely abolished within 2 to 3 minutes following CVF injection. This was paralleled by a sharp increase in serum levels of complement-derived chemotactic activity, reaching peak values at 5 minutes post-CVF injection. Incubation of the chemotactically active serum samples with antibody to human C5a abolished the chemotactic activity, indicating that the chemotactic activity was immunochemically related to C5. Coinciding with the appearance of C5-related chemotactic activity, a profound but transient neutropenia developed. At 20 minutes after CVF injection, extensive granulocytosis was evident. Morphological studies of the lung tissue under light microscopy showed an intracapillary sequestration of neutrophils along interstitial capillary channels (Fig. 1).

In order to determine whether systemic complement activation results in acute lung injury, morphological studies (transmission electron microscopy) and measurements of lung vascular permeability were performed. Radiolabeled bovine serum albumin (^{125}I-BSA) was injected together with CVF. Rats were sacrificed at different time intervals. The lung vasculature was then perfused free of remaining blood and the transudation of ^{125}I-BSA into lung tissue was measured and expressed as lung vascular permeability values.[55] Following the intravenous injection of CVF into rats, lung vascular permeability values increased with time, reaching peak values at 30 minutes after injection of CVF. Lung vascular permeability then gradually decreased to background values within 4 hours.[55] Morphological studies of lung tissue sections by transmission electron microscopy revealed focal destruction of endothelial cell lining of pulmonary capillaries, direct contact of neutrophils with vascular basement membrane, fibrin deposits, and erythrocytes within alveolar spaces (Fig. 2).

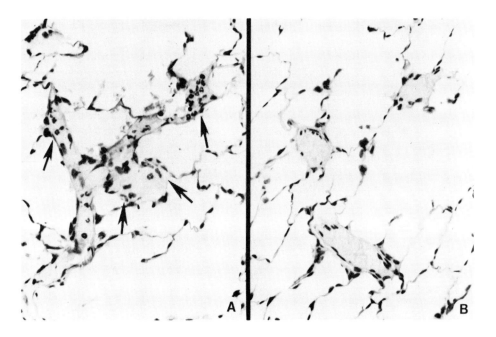

Figure 1: A: *Rat lung 30 minutes after intravenous injection of cobra venom factor dissolved in phosphate buffered saline. Interstitial capillaries contain large numbers of granulocytes.* **B:***Lung of rat that received intravenous injection of phosphate buffered saline only. Intravascular accumulates of granulocytes are not present. (Original magnification, ×100.)*

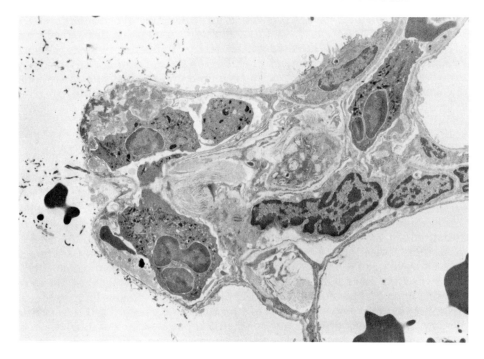

Figure 2: *Transmission electron micrograph of section from lung of rat injected with cobra venom factor 30 minutes previously. Several neutrophils with multilobed nuclei and electron-dense granules are present within pulmonary interstitial capillaries, often in intimate contact with vessel walls. In some areas, the endothelial cells are necrotic and appear as smudged, ill-defined, irregular densities. In addition, there is evidence of intraalveolar hemorrhage and fibrin deposition, as indicated by the electron-dense spicules of protein. The interstitial tissue also shows changes indicative of edema with a spreading apart of cross-linked collagen fibers. (Original magnification, ×6,500.)*

Similar observations of acute pulmonary injury following systemic complement activation were also made in CVF-treated mice[58] and in thermally injured rats.[54] When anesthetized rats were subjected to thermal injury, which was achieved by exposure of skin in the lumbosacral area to 70°C hot water for 30 seconds, systemic complement activation was observed. This could be documented by decreases in total hemolytic complement activity and the activity of individual complement components, with electrophoretic conversion of serum C3 and appearance in the circulation of C5-related chemotactic activity. As in CVF-treated rats, the presence in serum of C5-related chemotactic activity was short-lived; however, the appearance of the chemotactic activity was delayed (30 minutes after thermal injury). Consumption of total hemolytic and single component activities gradually increased over time, with a 30–40% drop in total hemolytic activity, which was most evident 3 to 4 hours after thermal injury. The rather slow and incomplete activation of complement may explain why the pulmonary injury secondary to skin burns was never as pronounced as in CVF-treated rats.

It should be noted that infusion of CVF into rabbits also caused sequestration of neutrophils in the lung vasculature but failed to produce evidence of lung injury.[20] Increases in lung vascular permeability were absent and lung endothelial cells appeared normal under transmission electron microscopy. Only when CVF infusion was combined with mild insults to the lung (hypoxia) or infusion of PGE_2 could increases in lung vascular permeability be observed. These effects could be explained by the fact that hypoxia causes release of prostaglandins into the lung[47] and the observation that permeability increases in rabbit skin are dependent on a synergistic action between C5a and PGE_2 and the presence of neutrophils.[64] The reason for the observed differences in lung vascular responses between rat and rabbit is not known. It should be mentioned, however, that injection of CVF into rats is followed by a striking increase in serum levels of PGE_2 (Till et al., unpublished data). Pretreatment of mice with indomethacin followed by intravenous injection of CVF caused a slight but significant decrease in lung vascular permeability.[58]

The important pathogenic role that neutrophils and complement play in the rat model of acute lung injury could be demonstrated by specific depletion experiments. Intraperitoneal injection into rats of rabbit antiserum against rat neutrophils 18–24 hours prior to CVF injection or thermal injury resulted in profound neutrophil depletion ($< 250/mm^3$) and almost completely prevented the development of acute pulmonary injury.[54,55] Similarly, when rats were depleted of their complement (C3) by intraperitoneal treatment with CVF at 24–36 hours prior to thermal injury or intravenous CVF injection, increases in lung vascular permeability were greatly attenuated. Furthermore, studies in C5-deficient mice indicated that C5 is required for the development of lung vascular injury although the complement product responsible for the lung injury in mice has not been identified.[58]

C5a may bind to specific receptors on neutrophils as has been shown for human granulocytes[6] and may cause increased adherence, margination, and sequestration of these cells in lung capillaries. Preferential binding of C5a to pulmonary endothelium[63] may further support the sequestration of neutrophils in the lungs. This uptake of C5a by circulating neutrophils and pulmonary endothelium may also explain the short lifespan of C5a in the circulation of CVF-treated or thermally injured rats.[54,55] Release of large numbers of neutrophils from bone marrow pools eventually triggered by the complement-derived leukocyte mobilizing factor[45] may further speed the C5a clearance. This interpretation is consistent with our observation that disappearance of C5a from serum of CVF-treated rats is immediately succeeded by a profound granulocytosis. Weisdorf et al.[65] demonstrated that the clearance of C5a des arg from the plasma of rabbits in vivo was affected by the number of circulating neutrophils. In neutropenic rabbits, the mean half-life of C5a des arg (3 minutes) was prolonged by almost 60%. Splenectomy and treatment of rabbits with epsilonaminocaproic acid also significantly lengthened the clearance rate.

The rapid disappearance of serum chemotactic activity may also be explained by the action of an inactivator that directly and irreversibly interacts with C5-derived chemotactic activity.[1,57] Recent evidence suggests that serum levels of chemotactic factor inactivator (CFI) can rapidly fluctuate in response to complement-mediated acute inflammatory reactions. In experimental rats with acute immune complex-induced vasculitis (Arthus reaction), the appearance of a short-lived serum peak of C5a was followed by a rapid increase in serum levels of CFI.[56] These observations were confirmed by others, showing a rapid increase in serum CFI when patients with pigeon breeder's disease received an aerosol challenge with pigeon serum.[30] An interpretation of these data is that sudden increases in serum levels of C5a may induce an increase in CFI activity which, in turn, may inactivate the C5-derived chemotactic activity.

Lung injury in CVF-treated rats was also of rather short duration. At 4 hours after intravenous injection of CVF, lung vascular permeability values had already dropped to background values. The reason for this brief duration and reversibility of the lung injury is not known. The bolus injection of CVF resulting in a one-time generation of large amounts of C5a could be a limiting factor. On the other hand, relatively small, focal lesions in pulmonary endothelium may cause rapid and extensive vascular leakage[24] but may easily be covered and sealed off by immigrating endothelial cells as shown in lesions of aortic endothelium.[42]

To summarize the experimental data described so far, it is obvious that many details regarding the in vivo interaction between C5a, neutrophils, and pulmonary endothelial cells are still not known. Our own observations in the experimental rat model, however, provide evidence to suggest that intravascular complement activation following thermal injury or vascular infusion of CVF results in acute lung injury. This has been determined by pathologic changes in lung morphology and increases in vascular permeability. The acute lung injury is associated with the early appearance of C5-derived chemotactic activity in the circulation coincident with the development of neutropenia that is followed by profound granulocytosis. The lung injury is dependent on complement-activated neutrophils sequestered in pulmonary capillaries.

Intravascular Infusion of Complement-Activation Products

Based on their clinical observations, Craddock and co-workers[11-13] were able to show that infusion of complement-activated plasma into rabbits caused pulmonary sequestration of neutrophils, which was accompanied by pulmonary dysfunctions. Morphologic examinations of lung tissue sections (under light microscopy) revealed interstitial pulmonary edema.[13] Experimental studies performed to answer the question as to whether intravenous infusion of complement-activation products can cause pulmonary injury in rabbits have produced conflicting results. Using the experimental approach that consisted of plasmapheresis and complement activation by zymosan with repeated reinfusion of the activated plasma into rabbits over a period of 4 hours, Hohn et al.[22] obtained morphological evidence of lung injury. Transmission electron micrographs showed **pulmonary** capillaries plugged with degranulated neutrophils and (in focal areas) intensive blebbing of endothelial cells associated with interstitial pulmonary edema and hemorrhage. Rabbits that had been treated with nonactivated autologous plasma or with nitrogen mustard (to produce leukopenia) did not show morphological changes on lung tissue sections. Bowers et al.[3] made similar observations showing that prolonged intravenous infusion of complement-activated plasma into rabbits caused modest pulmonary dysfunction and focal microvascular necrosis.

Other investigators claimed that an additional insult such as hypoxia might be necessary for induction of lung injury in rabbits following infusion of C5a or complement-activated plasma. Only when systemic complement activation was combined with experimental hypoxia which leads to release of prostaglandins[47] or PGE_2 treatment could pulmonary microvascular injury be demonstrated.[20] However, studies in sheep appear to indicate that prostanoids are not directly involved in the production of pulmonary microvascular injury following infusion of complement-activated plasma[10,18,40] since the development of hypoxemia and pulmonary hypertension, but not microvascular injury, appears to depend on cyclooxygenase products of arachidonic acid.[10,40]

The early observations by Hohn et al.[22] of pulmonary injury in the rabbit following infusion of complement-activated plasma have been confirmed and extended by other investigators utilizing the sheep as an experimental animal.[10,33,40,49] In an extensive study of structural and functional changes in the lung of sheep following a single intravenous infusion of complement-activated plasma, Meyrick and Brigham[33] could show a close correlation between the numbers of sequestered neutrophils in pulmonary capillaries and endothelial cell damage leading to increased vascular permeability. The kinetics of the lung injury observed in this animal model were almost identical to those seen in rats that had received a single intravenous injection of CVF.[55] Since it is well accepted that damage to pulmonary endothelium depends on the presence of sequestered neutrophils, the transience of microvascular injury might be explained by the fact that sequestered neutrophils leave the lung and recirculate within 2 to 4 hours after a single injection of CVF or activated plasma[33,55] as well as for the other reasons described above. Difficulties in the induction of complement-mediated lung injury in the rabbit as reported by some investigators[62] may also be explained by the transience of neutrophil sequestration when only a single injection of complement-activation products is given. Prolonged or multiple infusions of complement-activated plasma appear to be necessary to produce microvascular injury in the rabbit.[3,22]

In summary, experimental studies in rat, rabbit, and sheep have shown that both systemic complement activation and intravenous infusion of complement-activation products can cause acute lung injury. Sequestration of complement-activated neutrophils in pulmonary capillaries appears to be essential for the induction of microvascular injury. The transient vascular endothelial cell injury can lead to increased vascular permeability, interstitial pulmonary edema, and intraalveolar hemorrhage.

Alveolar Cell Injury

Immune Complex Deposition

There is an increasing body of clinical evidence that suggests a role for immune complexes in the pathogenesis of various types of human lung disease. However, most of our understanding of the pathogenic mechanisms involved in immune complex-induced pulmonary injury is based on data that had been obtained from experimental models.

One of the experimental approaches involved immunization of animals followed by challenge with the aerosolized antigen. Richerson[43] was the first to show that, within 4 to 6 hours, challenge of ovalbumin-immunized guinea pigs with the aerosolized immunogen could cause severe hemorrhagic pneumonitis. The reaction was dependent on the presence of complement-fixing antibodies in the circulation of the experimental animal. Roska et al.[44] established an animal model resembling hypersensitivity pneumonitis in humans (pigeon breeder's disease). The authors could show that guinea pigs, actively or passively immunized with pigeon serum protein, developed acute hemorrhagic alveolitis with extensive infiltrations of neutrophils following aerosol challenge with the immunogen. Experimental animals previously depleted of complement did not develop acute pulmonary inflammation following aerosol challenge. These observations were interpreted as being consistent with complement-dependent acute immune complex lung injury. In other studies, airway instillation of preformed immune complexes or individual applications of antigen and antibody were performed, which resulted in immune complex deposition along the alveolar walls.

Ten years ago, Johnson and Ward[28] developed a model of acute immune complex lung injury in the rat utilizing intratracheal administration of heterologous antibody via a catheter and the simultaneous intravenous injection of the antigen. By the use of this model, it was possible to show, in an antibody dose-dependent fashion, the development of acute inflammatory reactions in the lung characterized by acute hemorrhagic and neutrophil-rich exudate in alveolar and interstitial areas. The inflammatory reaction was most profound 4 to 6 hours after injection of the immune reactants. Immunofluorescence studies showed deposition of immune complexes along alveolar walls and in the lung interstitium. Prior depletion of experimental animals of complement or circulating blood neutrophils significantly attenuated the acute lung injury, indicating a dependency of this reaction on both neutrophils and complement. This is not surprising since this model of acute lung injury closely resembles the classic skin Arthus reaction that had previously been shown to depend on complement activation and infiltrating neutrophils.[9,60,61]

To determine the contribution of individual complement components to this type of lung injury, congenic C5-deficient and C5-sufficient mice were challenged by intrapulmonary administration of preformed immune complexes.[31] It was found that neutrophil infiltration, edema, and intraalveolar hemorrhage were more generalized and severe in lungs of C5-sufficient than in lungs of C5-deficient mice. These observations suggested that the C5 molecule and its phlogistic fragments (C5a, C5a des arg) may play a central role in the pathogenesis of acute immune complex lung injury. The prominent role of C5a in mediating pulmonary disease processes has also been documented by other investigators who introduced C5 fragments and other chemotactic peptides into lungs of experimental animals (see following section).

Sufficient activation and fixation of complement by immune complexes deposited in the alveolar space appears to be a prerequisite for induction of acute inflammation in immune complex lung injury. Scherzer and Ward[48] showed that instillation of preformed immune complexes into the airways of non-immune rats caused the most intense damage to lungs when the complexes were of large molecular weight and made up at the point of antigen-antibody equivalence. The phlogistic activity of these immune complexes correlated well with their complement-activating capacity in vitro. Changes in the ratio of antigen to antibody decreased the ability of the immune complexes to induce both complement activation in vitro and lung tissue injury in vivo.

It is generally assumed that once immune complexes have deposited or formed in the alveolar wall, complement activation occurs, with generation of chemotactic factor(s) and the chemotactic influx of neutrophils from the circulation. The neutrophil, in turn, may release activation products that may cause damage of lung tissue. It appears, however, that pathogenic events leading to immune complex lung injury may be more complex. For instance, instillation of

IgA-antibody into the airways of rats followed by intravenous injection of the corresponding antigen caused acute lung injury as characterized by increases in lung vascular permeability and morphological changes that were indistinguishable from lung damage caused by IgG-immune complexes.[25] Yet, the IgA-immune complex lung injury although complement-dependent, does not depend on the availability of neutrophils. The immunopathological mechanism of this new type of immune complex-mediated acute lung injury is as yet unexplained.

Airway Instillation of Chemotactic Factors

As already mentioned, complement-derived chemotactic activity (C5a, C5a des arg) appears to play a dominant role in the pathogenesis of acute pulmonary injury following intraalveolar deposition of immune complexes or intravenous infusion of CVF or zymosan-activated plasma. Requirement for C5 in complement-mediated acute lung injury has been documented in experimental studies utilizing C5-deficient mice[31,58] and by treatment of rats with CFI (chemotactic factor inactivator),[27] which irreversibly blocks the activity of chemotactic C5a.[57] Inactivation of C5a or congenital absence of C5 both resulted in significant protection from acute pulmonary injury. The ability of CFI to suppress immune complex-induced acute inflammatory reactions was associated with absence of infiltrates of neutrophils,[27] providing strong indirect evidence that C5-derived chemotactic factors are directly responsible for induction of immune complex-triggered and neutrophil-mediated acute tissue injury.

Direct evidence for the phlogistic potency of C5-derived chemotactic peptides in the lung was derived from studies utilizing intrapulmonary instillation of C5 or derivatives of C5.[14,32,50] Intratracheal instillation in hamsters of a chemotactic fragment isolated from human C5 produced acute inflammatory reactions that were characterized by early (at 5 min) intravascular margination of neutrophils followed (at 60 to 120 min) by extensive intraalveolar accumulation of granulocytes. Only modest increases in lung vascular permeability were observed although perivascular edema could be demonstrated. The chemotactic synthetic peptide N-formyl-met-leu-phe was shown to induce similar reactions. Interestingly, instillation of intact human C5 into hamster lungs also caused inflammatory reactions that were even more profound than those elicited with the C5-fragment. Lavage studies in hamsters provided evidence that the C5 was being enzymatically cleaved into chemotactically active fragments, which in turn may have caused the intraalveolar neutrophil accumulation. The hamster appears unique in this regard, since cleavage of C5 by bronchoalveolar lavage fluid does not occur with humans, rats, and rabbits.

Stimler et al.[52] showed that intrabronchial injection into guinea pigs of homologous anaphylatoxins (C3a, C5a, or a mixture of C5a and C5a des arg) causes immediate broncho- and vasoconstriction. Morphological studies showed aggregates of neutrophils and platelets in pulmonary vessels at 20 minutes after injection of C3a or C5a. Later time points were not included in this study. Evidence of acute pulmonary damage following intratracheal injection of C5-derived chemotactic fragments was reported by Shaw et al.[50] The morphological changes included injury of pulmonary vascular endothelium and endothelial basement membranes and damage to type I but not type II alveolar epithelial cells.

Under the assumption that, in vivo, most of the C5a molecules are rapidly converted to C5a des arg because of serum carboxypeptidase B,[5] the phlogistic potential of C5a and C5a des arg was tested in rabbit lungs.[32] Intratracheal instillation of human C5a des arg produced a marked inflammatory response that was most profound 6 hours later and characterized by intraalveolar accumulation of neutrophils, edema, hemorrhage, fibrin deposition, and damage to alveolar epithelium. Interestingly, similar treatment with human C5a did not cause significant lung injury. The reason for this differential effect of C5a and C5a des arg is as yet unexplained. Henson and co-workers[21] discussed the possibility that C5a des arg may induce alveolar macrophages to produce a neutrophil-directed chemotactic factor. The apparent increased neutrophil-attracting activity of C5a des arg over C5a in vivo may thus represent an indirect effect of the peptide. The chemotactic activity of C5a des arg may also be affected by an acidic plasma protein that has the capacity to interact with C5a des arg but not with C5a[38] to build a C5a des arg "helper factor" complex that may be more active in vivo compared to C5a.

As can be seen, there is good evidence to suggest that chemotactic C5 fragments play an important role in the pathogenesis of complement and neutrophil-mediated acute lung injury. In immune complex-triggered pulmonary injury, margination and sequestration of neutrophils in the lung vasculature as well as emigration and accumulation of these cells in the alveolar spaces appear to depend on availability of C5-derived chemotactic activity. Similarly, non-complement-activating immune complexes will not induce hemorrhagic pneumonitis.[43,48]

Whether neutrophil phagocytosis of C3b-opsonized immune complexes adds to the cell and tissue damage is not clear. In vitro observations by Wright and Silverstein[67] suggested that release of potentially tissue damaging oxygen metabolites from neutrophils following uptake of immune complexes may not depend on the presence of opsonizing C3b. These data are in accordance with observations by Weiss and Ward[66] who demonstrated in vitro that complement-fixing immune complexes were readily phagocytized and caused release of lysosomal enzymes, but induced only limited release of toxic oxygen species. Immune complexes pretreated with complement did not show increased effectiveness for activation of neutrophils. In the same studies, non-complement-fixing immune complexes, which were less effectively internalized, were shown to be more effective in causing release of toxic oxygen metabolites from neutrophils. It appears attractive to speculate that in an admixture of immune complexes of various sizes and composition, which probably occurs in vivo, complement-fixing (activating) immune complexes may trigger the generation of neutrophil chemotactic (C5a) activity, while the more soluble non-complement-fixing immune complexes may cause optimal activation of neutrophils to release toxic oxygen radicals. Our knowledge of the in vivo interactions between host–mediator systems such as immune complexes, complement, neutrophils, and endothelial cells (to name a few) and the molecular and subcellular responses that ultimately lead to acute inflammatory lung injury is still very limited.

Protection From Complement-Mediated Lung Injury

Effects of Catalase and Superoxide Dismutase

It has been known for many years that phagocytizing or chemotactically stimulated neutrophils respond by a large increase in oxygen consumption that is associated with production of highly reactive oxygen radicals including hydrogen peroxide (H_2O_2) and superoxide anion (O_2^-).[15] These products can be released into the extracellular environment and have been shown in vitro to display cytotoxic effects on a variety of cell types including erythrocytes,[29] eukaryotic cells such as fibroblasts,[51] tumor cells,[8] platelets,[7] and vascular endothelial cells.[46] In addition, the known ability of oxygen products from activated leukocytes to oxidatively inactivate α1-antiproteinase[4] as well as the recent observation that nanomolar amounts of H_2O_2 will interact with substrates such as fibrinogen, hemoglobin, and basement membrane to render them more susceptible to proteolysis (by trypsin and leukocytic extracts)[16] suggests additional ways in which oxygen products from activated leukocytes may cause tissue damage. These in vitro observations have opened up a new and promising avenue of experimental and clinical research, especially in the field of inflammation. During the last 3–5 years, considerable evidence has accumulated suggesting that oxygen-derived free radicals most likely derived from neutrophils may be responsible for acute complement-dependent lung injury.

As already described, systemic complement activation in the rat causes neutrophil-dependent acute pulmonary injury characterized by focal damage to capillary endothelium, and fibrin deposition and hemorrhage in alveolar spaces.[55] To test for possible involvement of toxic oxygen species in this type of lung injury, rats were treated with specific enzymes such as superoxide dismutase (SOD), which converts O_2^- to H_2O_2, and catalase, which converts H_2O_2 to molecular oxygen and water. It was found that both SOD and catalase protect the pulmonary vasculature from injury after systemic complement activation.[55] Similar protective effects were observed in thermally injured rats. Treatment with SOD or catalase significantly attenuated the development of the complement and neutrophil-dependent acute pulmonary injury.[54] An almost complete protection from lung injury was afforded by systemic treatment of thermally injured rats with a combination of SOD and catalase. SOD treatment was also shown to attenuate significantly pulmonary injury in sheep that had received repeated intravenous injections of complement-activated homologous plasma.[40] These data provide strong evidence that acute pulmonary injury following systemic complement activation or infusion of complement-activated plasma is closely linked to production by sequestered neutrophils of toxic oxygen metabolites.

Further evidence implicating a role for O_2^- and H_2O_2 in complement and neutrophil-dependent acute inflammatory reactions had been demonstrated by SOD and catalase-induced protection from immune complex-mediated lung injury.[26,35] It was found that protective effects of SOD were brief in duration. As assessed by measurement of lung vascular permeability, SOD almost completely suppressed pulmonary injury at 2 hours after application of the immunoreactants. However, by 4 hours, when the inflammatory reaction was at its height, suppressive effects of SOD were no longer evident.[35] Treatment of rats with SOD was associated with a decreased influx of neutrophils. This observation is consistent with experimental data showing that O_2^- can bring about generation of a chemotactic lipid,[39,41] which may serve as an important amplifier of inflammatory reactions. It is assumed that SOD blocks this amplification step in the early phase of acute lung injury. It would appear that once significant amounts of C5a have accumulated, the build-up of this chemotactic peptide obviates a role for the chemotactic lipid generated by O_2^-. Catalase did not block neutrophil accumulation in the lung following immune complex deposition, but prevented hemorrhage and intraalveolar edema.[26] Since lung damaging effects have been related to H_2O_2 (mainly associated with its derivatives),[27] this observation is consistent with the idea that catalase destroys H_2O_2 generated by complement and/or immune-complex-activated neutrophils, thus protecting the lung from injury by H_2O_2 or its conversion products.

Effects of Iron Chelators and Hydroxyl Radical Scavengers

Although experimental evidence suggests that H_2O_2 may play a role in complement and neutrophil-dependent acute lung injury (see above), there is little evidence to suggest that H_2O_2 is tissue toxic per se. It appears more likely that a conversion product of H_2O_2, perhaps hydroxyl radical ($^\cdot OH$), is the agent responsible for lung vascular injury. It is well accepted that iron plays an essential role in the classic Fenton reaction in which $^\cdot OH$ is formed from H_2O_2:

$$Fe^{3+} + O_2^- \longrightarrow Fe^{2+} + O_2$$
$$Fe^{2+} + H_2O_2 \longrightarrow Fe^{3+}\ OH^- + \ ^\cdot OH \text{ (Fenton reaction)}$$

With this in mind, we tested the effects of iron chelators and hydroxyl radical scavengers on acute pulmonary injury, using the model of systemic complement activation in rats as described above.

Pretreatment of experimental animals with iron chelators, such as human milk apolactoferrin (iron-free lactoferrin) or deferoxamine mesylate, provided significant dose-dependent protection against complement and neutrophil-mediated pulmonary injury.[59] Iron saturation of lactoferrin resulted in complete loss of its lung protective effects. The role of iron in this type of pulmonary injury could also be demonstrated by the fact that intravenous infusion of nanomolar amounts of ferric chloride into CVF-treated rats augmented lung injury in a dose-dependent fashion. Furthermore, treatment with the potent $^\cdot OH$ scavenger dimethyl sulfoxide (DMSO) also attenuated pulmonary injury. In CVF-treated rats protected with apolactoferrin, deferoxamine, or DMSO, morphological studies revealed leukoaggregates within interstitial capillaries but not endothelial cell damage, hemorrhage, or fibrin deposition. Similar protection from microvascular injury in the lung was observed in thermally injured rats. Pretreatment of rats with iron chelators (deferoxamine, 2,3 dihydroxybenzoic acid) or $^\cdot OH$ scavengers (DMSO, dimethyl thiourea, benzoate) significantly reduced pulmonary transudation of intravenously injected ^{125}I-labeled bovine serum albumin.[53] Morphological evaluations of protected thermally injured rats showed intrapulmonary sequestration of neutrophils but little evidence of microvascular injury. Furthermore, acute immune complex-induced vasculitis in rats was shown to follow a similar pattern with attenuation of the vascular injury by pretreatment of rats with iron chelators and with scavengers of $^\cdot OH$. Additionally, infusion of ferric chloride accentuated this injury, suggesting that the vascular injury is due to conversion of H_2O_2 to $^\cdot OH$.[17] These data support the concept that acute pulmonary injury that is complement- and neutrophil-dependent may be related to generation of $^\cdot OH$. This iron-catalyzed conversion product of H_2O_2 may be the key mediator related to lung microvascular injury following systemic complement activation.

The mechanism of $^\cdot OH$-related injury to lung vascular endothelial cells is not known. There is some evidence to suggest that generation of highly reactive hydroxyl radicals from neutrophil-derived hydrogen peroxide may lead to lipid peroxidation, which in turn may result in cell membrane damage. The observation that plasma from thermally injured rats contained increased levels of lipid peroxidation products that were dependent on the availability of neutrophils[53] seems to support this concept. Furthermore, treatment of thermally injured rats with iron chelators or ˙OH scavengers significantly decreased plasma levels of lipid peroxidation products.

Conclusion

There is increasing evidence that activation of the complement system either within or outside the vascular system results in a series of events ultimately leading to activation of neutrophils, vascular permeability changes, and cell damage/destruction. Within the lung, systemic activation of complement results in damage of vascular endothelial cells while complement activation products generated within the alveolar compartment (as during immune complex deposition) produce damage to both alveolar tissues and vascular endothelial cells. It now appears that toxic oxygen products of activated neutrophils are largely responsible for the acute tissue injury. The production of H_2O_2 followed by its reduction, which is facilitated by the presence of iron, results in the generation of ˙OH, which appears to be the oxygen product most immediately related to tissue injury. Accordingly, interventions with catalase, iron chelators, or scavengers of ˙OH are lung protective.

REFERENCES

1. Berenberg, J.L. and Ward, P.A.: The chemotactic factor inactivator in normal human serum. *J. Clin. Invest.* 52:1200–1206, 1973.
2. Biesecker, G.: Biology of disease. Membrane attack complex of complement as a pathologic mediator. *Lab. Invest.* 49:237–249, 1983.
3. Bowers, T.K., Ozolins, A.L., Ratliff, N.B., et al.: Hyperacute pulmonary vasculitis in rabbits receiving prolonged infusions of activated complement. *Inflammation* 7:1–13, 1983.
4. Carp, H. and Janoff, A.: In vitro suppression of serum elastase-inhibitory capacity by reactive oxygen species generated by phagocytosing polymorphonuclear leukocytes. *J. Clin. Invest.* 63:793–797, 1979.
5. Chenoweth, D.E. and Hugli, T.E.: Human C5a and C5a analogs as probes of the neutrophil C5a receptor. *Mol. Immunol.* 17:151–157, 1980.
6. Chenoweth, E.E. and Hugli, T.E.: Demonstration of specific C5a receptor on intact human polymorphonuclear leukocytes. *Proc. Natl. Acad. Sci. USA* 75:3943–3947, 1978.
7. Clark, R.A. and Klebanoff, S.J.: Myeloperoxidase-mediated platelet release reaction. *J. Clin. Invest.* 63:177–183, 1979.
8. Clark, R.A., Klebanoff, S.J., Einstein, A.B., et al.: Peroxidase-H_2O_2-halide system: Cytotoxic effect on mammalian tumor cells. *Blood* 45:161–170, 1975.
9. Cochrane, C.G., Muller-Eberhard, H.J., and Aikin, B.S.: Depletion of plasma complement in vivo by a protein of cobra venom: Its effect on various immunologic reactions. *J. Immunol.* 105:55–67, 1970.
10. Cooper, J.D., McDonald, W.D., Ali, M., et al.: Prostaglandin production associated with the pulmonary vascular response to complement activation. *Surgery* 88:215–221, 1980.

11. Craddock, P.R., Fehr, J., Dalmasso, A.P., et al.: Hemodialysis leukopenia: Pulmonary vascular leukostasis resulting from complement activation by dialyzer cellophane membranes. *J. Clin. Invest.* 59:879–888, 1977.

12. Craddock, P.R., Hammerschmidt, D., White, J.G., et al.: Complement (C5a)-induced granulocyte aggregation in vitro. A possible mechanism of complement-mediated leukostasis and leukopenia. *J. Clin. Invest.* 60:260–264, 1977.

13. Craddock, P.R., Fehr, J., Brigham, K.L., et al.: Complement and leukocyte-mediated pulmonary dysfunction in hemodialysis. *N. Engl. J. Med.* 296:769–774, 1977.

14. Desai, J., Kreutzer, D. L., Showell, H. J., et al.: Acute inflammatory pulmonary reactions induced by chemotactic factors. *Am. J. Pathol.* 96:71–83, 1979.

15. Fantone, J.C. and Ward, P.A.: Role of oxygen-derived free radicals and metabolites in leukocyte-dependent inflammatory reactions. *Am. J. Pathol.* 107:397–418, 1982.

16. Fligiel, S.E.G., Lee, E.C., McCoy, J.P., et al.: Protein degradation following treatment with hydrogen peroxide. *Am. J. Pathol.* 115:418–425, 1984.

17. Fligiel, S.E.G., Ward, P.A., Johnson, K.J., et al.: Evidence for a role of hydroxyl radical in immune complex-induced vasculitis. *Am. J. Pathol.* 115:375–382, 1984.

18. Gee, M.H., Perkowski, S.Z., Havill, A.M., et al.: Role of prostaglandins and leukotrienes in complement-initiated lung vascular injury. *Chest* 83:82S–85S, 1983.

19. Hammerschmidt, D.E., Weaver, L.J., Hudson, L.D., et al.: Association of complement activation and elevated plasma-C5a with adult respiratory distress syndrome: Pathophysiological relevance and possible prognostic value. *Lancet* I:947–949, 1980.

20. Henson, P.M., Larsen, G.L., Webster, R.O., et al.: Pulmonary microvascular alterations and injury induced by complement fragments: Synergistic effect of complement activation, neutrophil sequestration and prostaglandins. *Ann. N.Y. Acad. Sci.* 384:287–300, 1982.

21. Henson, P.M., McCarthy, K., Larsen, G.L., et al.: Complement fragments, alveolar macrophages, and alveolitis. *Am. J. Pathol.* 97:93–110, 1979.

22. Hohn, D.C., Meyers, A.J., Gherini, S.T., et al.: Production of acute pulmonary injury by leukocytes and activated complement. *Surgery* (St. Louis) 88:48–58, 1980.

23. Hoover, R.L., Briggs, R.T., and Karnovsky, M.J.: The adhesive interaction between polymorphonuclear leukocytes and endothelial cells in vitro. *Cell* 14:423–434, 1978.

24. Hurley, J.V.: Types of pulmonary microvascular injury. *Ann N.Y. Acad. Sci.* 384: 269–286, 1982.

25. Johnson, K.J., Wilson, B.S., Till, G.O., et al.: Acute lung injury in rat caused by IgA immune complexes. *J. Clin. Invest.* 74:358–369, 1984.

26. Johnson, K.J. and Ward, P.A.: Role of oxygen metabolites in immune complex injury of lung. *J. Immunol.* 126:2365–2369, 1981.

27. Johnson, K.J., Anderson, T.P., and Ward, P.A.: Suppression of immune complex-induced inflammation by the chemotactic factor inactivator. *J. Clin. Invest.* 59: 951–958, 1977.

28. Johnson, K.J. and Ward, P.A.: Acute immunologic pulmonary alveolitis. *J. Clin. Invest.* 54:349–357, 1974.

29. Klebanoff, S.J. and Clark, R.A.: Hemolysis and iodination of erythrocyte components by a myeloperoxidase-mediated system. *Blood* 45:699–707, 1975.

30. Kreutzer, D.L., McCormick, J.R., Thrall, R.S., et al.: Elevation of serum chemotactic factor inactivator activity during acute inflammatory reactions in patients with hypersensitivity pneumonitis. *Am. Rev. Respir. Dis.* 125:612–614, 1982.

31. Larsen, G.L., Mitchell, B.C., and Henson, P.M.: The pulmonary response of C5 sufficient and deficient mice to immune complexes. *Am. Rev. Respir. Dis.* 123: 434–439, 1981.

32. Larsen, G.L., McCarthy, K., Webster, R.O., et al.: A differential effect of C5a and C5a des arg in the induction of pulmonary inflammation. *Am. J. Pathol.* 100: 179–192, 1980.

33. Meyrick, B.O. and Brigham, K.L.: The effect of single infusion of zymosan-

activated plasma on the pulmonary microcirculation of sheep. Structure-function relationships. *Am. J. Pathol.* 114:32–45, 1984.

34. McCall, C.E., DeChatelet, L.R., Brown, D., et al.: New biological activity following intravascular activation of the complement cascade. *Nature* 249:841–843, 1974.

35. McCormick, J.R., Harkin, M.M., Johnson, K.J., et al.: Suppression by superoxide dismutase of immune-complex-induced pulmonary alveolitis and dermal inflammation. *Am. J. Pathol.* 102:55–61, 1981.

36. Nusbacher, J., Rosenfeld, S.I., MacPherson, J.L. et al.: Nylon fiber leukapheresis-associated complement component changes and granulocytopenia. *Blood* 51: 359–365, 1978.

37. O'Flaherty, J.T., Showell, H., and Ward, P.A.: Neutropenia induced by systemic infusion of chemotactic factors. *J. Immunol.* 118:1586–1589, 1977.

38. Perez, H.D., Goldstein, I.M., Chernoff, D., et al.: Chemotactic activity of C5a des arg: Evidence of a requirement for an anionic peptide "helper factor" and inhibition by a cationic protein in serum from patients with systemic lupus erythematosus. *Mol. Immunol.* 17:163–169, 1980.

39. Perez, H.D., Weksler, B.B., and Goldstein, I.A.: Generation of a chemotatic lipid from arachidonic acid by exposure to a superoxide-generating system. *Inflammation* 4:313–328, 1980.

40. Perkowski, S.Z., Havill, A.M., Flynn, J.T., et al.: Role of intrapulmonary release of eicosanoids and superoxide anion as mediators of pulmonary dysfunction and endothelial injury in sheep with intermittent complement activation. *Circ. Res.* 53: 574–583, 1983.

41. Petrone, W.F., English, D.K., Wong, K., et al.: Free radicals and inflammation: The superoxide dependent activation of a neutrophil chemotactic factor in plasma. *Proc. Natl. Acad. Sci. USA* 77:1159–1163, 1980.

42. Reidy, M.A. and Schwartz, S.M.: Endothelial regeneration. III. Time course of initial changes after small defined injury to rat aortic endothelium. *Lab. Invest.* 44:301–308, 1981.

43. Richerson, H.B.: Acute experimental hypersensitivity pneumonitis in the guinea pig. *J. Lab. Clin. Med.* 79:745–757, 1972.

44. Roska, A.K.B., Moore, V.L., and Abramoff, P.: Immune complex disease in guinea pig lungs: Elicitation with pigeon serum. *Am. Rev. Respir. Dis.* 120:129–136, 1979.

45. Rother, K.: Leukocyte mobilizing factor: A new biological activity derived from the third component of complement. *Eur. J. Immunol.* 2:550–558, 1972.

46. Sacks, T., Moldow, C.F., Craddock, P.R., et al.: Oxygen radical-mediated endothelial cell damage by complement-stimulated granulocytes. An in vitro model of immune vascular damage. *J. Clin. Invest.* 61:1161–1167, 1978.

47. Said, S.I., Yoshida, T., Kitamura, S., et al.: Pulmonary alveolar hypoxia. Release of prostaglandins and other humoral mediators. *Science* 185:1181–1183, 1974.

48. Scherzer, H. and Ward, P.A.: Lung injury produced by immune complexes of varying composition. *J. Immunol.* 121:947–952, 1978.

49. Sharkey, P., Judges, D., Driedger, A.A., et al.: The effect of infusion of zymosan-activated plasma on hemodynamic and pulmonary function in sheep. *Circ. Shock* 12:79–93, 1984.

50. Shaw, J.O., Henson, P.M., Henson, J., et al.: Lung inflammation induced by complement-derived chemotactic fragments in the alveolus. *Lab. Invest.* 42:547–558, 1980.

51. Simon, R.H., Scoggin, C.H., and Patterson, D.: Hydrogen peroxide causes fatal injury to fibroblasts exposed to oxygen radicals. *J. Biol. Chem.* 256:7181–7186, 1981.

52. Stimler, N.P., Hugli, T.E., and Bloor, C.M.: Pulmonary injury induced by C3a and C5a anaphylatoxins. *Am. J. Pathol.* 100:327–348, 1980.

53. Till, G.O., Tourtellotte, W., Jr., Lutz, M.J., et al.: Acute lung injury secondary to skin burns: Evidence for role of hydroxyl radical and lipid peroxidation products. *Circ. Shock* 13:76, 1984.

54. Till, G.O., Beauchamp, C., Menapace, D., et al.: Oxygen radical-dependent lung damage following thermal injury to rat skin. *J. Trauma* 28:269–277, 1983.
55. Till, G.O., Johnson, K.J., Kunkel, R., et al.: Intravascular activation of complement and acute lung injury. Dependency on neutrophils and toxic oxygen metabolites. *J. Clin. Invest.* 69:1126–1135, 1982.
56. Till, G., Debatin, M., and Gemsa, D.: Regulatory mediators in Arthus reactions: Demonstration of chemotactic factor inactivator and cell directed inhibitor activity. In *Inflammation: Mechanisms and Treatment.* Willoughby, D.A., and Giroud, J.P., eds. Lancaster, England, MTP Press, 1980, pp. 639–645.
57. Till, G.O. and Ward, P.A.: Two distinct chemotactic factor inactivators in human serum. *J. Immunol.* 114:843–847, 1975.
58. Tvedten, H.W., Till, G.O., and Ward, P.A.: Mediators of lung injury in mice following systemic activation of complement. (Submitted for publication) 1984.
59. Ward, P.A., Till, G.O., Kunkel, R., et al.: Evidence for role of hydroxyl radical in complement and neutrophil-dependent tissue injury. *J. Clin. Invest.* 72:789–801, 1983.
60. Ward, P.A. and Hill, J.H.: Biologic role of complement products. Complement-derived leukotactic activity extractable from lesions of immunologic vasculitis. *J. Immunol.* 108:1137–1145, 1972.
61. Ward, P.A. and Cochrane, C.G.: Bound complement and immunologic injury of blood vessels. *J. Exp. Med.* 121:215–233, 1965.
62. Webster, R. O., Larsen, G.L., Mitchell, B.C., et al.: Absence of inflammatory lung injury in rabbits challenged intravascularly with complement-derived chemotactic factors. *Am. Rev. Respir. Dis.* 125:335–340, 1982.
63. Webster, R.O., Larsen, G.L., and Henson, P.M.: Tissue distribution of human C5a and C5a des arg complement fragments in normal and neutropenic rabbits. *Am. Rev. Respir. Dis.* 123(2):41, 1981.
64. Wedmore, C.V. and Williams, T.J.: Control of vascular permeability by polymorphonuclear leukocytes in inflammation. *Nature* 289:646–650, 1981.
65. Weisdorf, D.J., Hammerschmidt, D.E., Jacob, H.S., et al.: Rapid in vivo clearance of C5a des arg: A possible protective mechanism against complement-mediated tissue injury. *J. Lab. Clin. Med.* 98:823–830, 1981.
66. Weiss, S.J. and Ward, P.A.: Immune complex induced generation of oxygen metabolites by human neutrophils. *J. Immunol.* 129:309–313, 1982.
67. Wright, S.D. and Silverstein, S.C.: Receptors for C3b and C3bi promote phagocytosis but not the release of toxic oxygen from human phagocytes. *J. Exp. Med.* 158:2016–2023, 1983.

CHAPTER 19

Mechanisms of Pulmonary Vascular Injury in Sepsis

Robert H. Demling

Introduction

Acute respiratory failure remains a leading cause of death in the critically ill patient. The syndrome has, however, changed since its widespread recognition during the Vietnam conflict where it was termed "shock lung." Now the term shock lung appears to be a misnomer since hemorrhagic shock by itself has little deleterious effect on the lung.[15]

Currently, the predominant form of adult respiratory distress syndrome (ARDS) in the trauma patient appears to be that caused by a septic insult in the postresuscitation period. Septicemia by itself leads to a 20% incidence of acute lung injury while the incidence is over twice as high with a combination of trauma and sepsis.[45,98] Lung injury is actually the first symptom of sepsis in one-third of trauma patients, which indicates that the lung is a target organ. In one group of trauma patients, namely the burn patient, sepsis-induced ARDS had an extremely high mortality rate approaching 100% in some series, indicating that injured tissue markedly accentuates the response of the lung to a septic insult.[57]

There are three major pulmonary abnormalities in sepsis-induced lung injury. The alterations in the pulmonary circulation include pulmonary artery hypertension and increased pulmonary microvascular permeability.[2] The degree of pulmonary hypertension and increased pulmonary vascular resistances have been found in man to correlate directly with subsequent mortality.[85] Although the majority of the increase in pulmonary vascular resistance appears to be arteriolar, there is also an increase in microvascular hydrostatic pressure, P_{mv}, as well. This is reflected by an increase in pulmonary capillary wedge pressure and an increase in protein poor lung lymph seen in a number of animal studies.[6,15] The pulmonary hypertension, when severe (mean pressure exceeding 30 mmHg) can lead to right ventricular dysfunction, resulting in ventricular septal deviation to the left. This, in turn, will lead to a decrease in left ventricular compliance and cardiac output.

Supported in part by NIH grants HL 30068 and GM 31662.

From Said, S.I. (ed.): *The Pulmonary Circulation and Acute Lung Injury.* Mount Kisco, N.Y., Futura Publishing Co., Inc., 1985.

An increase in protein permeability is also characteristic of sepsis or endo-toxin injury in most animal species.[6,15] There is less documentation that this occurs in man as well. Several studies directly sampling edema fluid have reported protein contents approaching the plasma value.[91] Preliminary clinical reports using the in vivo technique of computerized gamma scintigraphy have also indicated a lung capillary leak with sepsis.[94] A number of mechanisms in sepsis have been reported to be responsible for the hypertension and the increased permeability (Fig. 1). A number of these mechanisms will be discussed. It is also important to recognize that the combination of an increased P_{mv} and protein permeability markedly potentiates the increased fluid and protein flux seen with either injury separately (Fig. 2).

The third characteristic of septic injury is a ventilatory abnormality. Increased small airways resistance leading to decreased lung compliance, atelectasis, and ventilation perfusion mismatch is well described in animals after endotoxin.[41,89] The hypoxia in sepsis lung injury is, therefore, not totally the result of increased lung water. Altered airways play a major role. In fact, a number of studies have now verified that there is not a direct correlation between shunt fraction and measured water content in the sepsis-injured lung.[7,50]

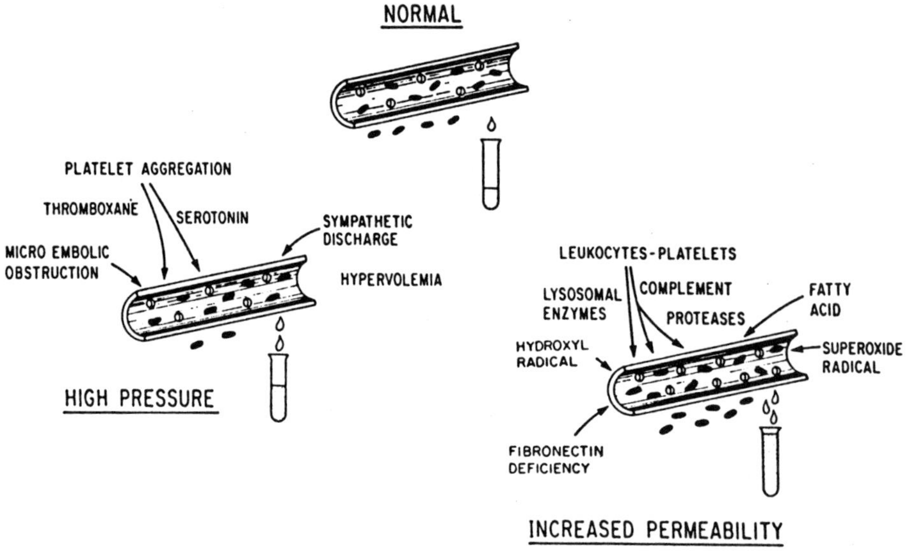

Figure 1: *The lung capillary under normal conditions leaks protein[1] and fluid through a number of holes or pores in the membrane. Increased transvascular fluid flux leading to increased lung water can occur if the capillary hydrostatic pressure is acutely elevated as a result of a number of insulting agents causing lung edema. Permeability does not appear to be altered significantly in pure "high pressure edema," thus the number of pores remains constant and the interstitial protein content decreases as it becomes diluted by the excess water. An increase in permeability is commonly seen with sepsis-induced ARDS. When protein permeability is altered, the number or size of the pores increases, resulting in greater quantities of both fluid and protein crossing the membrane. "Permeability edema" is generally of greater magnitude than "high pressure edema." Many of the ARDS states are a combination of these forms of injury, but one form usually predominates.*

RESPONSE TO INCREASED LEFT ATRIAL PRESSURE

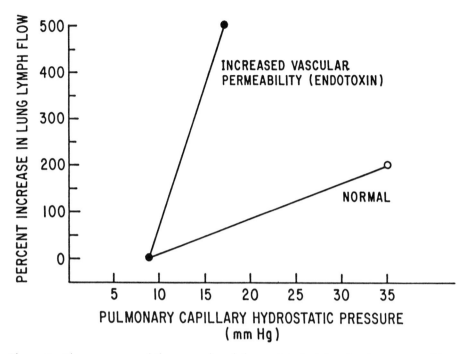

Figure 2: *The responses of the normal and the endotoxin-injured pulmonary capillary to changes in hydrostatic pressure are shown. Excess fluid crossing the capillary is reflected in the increased amount of lymph draining from the lung interstitium. Large increases in capillary pressure are required in the normal capillary to produce substantial increases in lung fluid leading to "high pressure edema." However, the capillary with increased permeability leaks large amounts of fluid in response to only minimal increases in pressure, resulting in the rapid onset of "permeability edema."*

There appears to be some common etiologic mechanisms in the ventilatory and circulatory abnormalities seen with sepsis lung injury. The concentration in this chapter will be on the pulmonary vascular injury; however, some attempts will be made to interrelate these components.

Pulmonary Vascular Injury

We and others have studied sepsis lung injury using endotoxin as the septic insult. Although controversy continues as to the validity of endotoxin as a model of sepsis, the pulmonary changes from bacteria and endotoxin in several animal models appear the same.[6,8] ARDS from burn wound sepsis is also probably endotoxin-induced in view of the frequent finding of negative blood cultures in burn patients with clear evidence of distant lung damage.[96]

The two characteristics of sepsis-induced ARDS that have been reported to be present in man, namely pulmonary artery hypertension and increased pulmonary capillary permeability, have been duplicated in a number of animal models given either endotoxin or bacteria. In the sheep, using lung lymph flow (Q_L) to monitor microvascular integrity, these characteristics of sepsis lung injury are separated in time course into two phases. Although somewhat artificial, this separation allows us to study the specific pathophysiology of each. The first phase is the hypertension phase, which is characterized by severe pulmonary artery hypertension, hypoxia, and increased Q_L with a decrease from baseline in lymph protein content relative to plasma, indicating an increase in capillary hydrostatic pressure. The second, or permeability phase, is characterized by moderate pulmonary hypertension, increased Q_L which is protein-rich, indicating increased protein permeability. This phase lasts for several hours. Again, it must be pointed out that the early hypoxia is not the result of lung edema as the measured increase in Q_L is usually not sufficient to significantly elevate lung water.

Most of our current information on sepsis and lung injury has been obtained from this type of animal model as only a modest amount of clinical data is available. A brief summary follows of what is currently known and not known about the pathophysiology. Current evidence indicates three interrelating elements to be causations of the pulmonary vascular injury: (1) products of arachidonic acid metabolism, (2) white cells and their byproducts, specifically oxygen radicals, and (3) platelets.

Arachidonic acid products, of course, can be divided into the well-studied cyclooxygenase products and the lipoxygenase pathway products, which are also of current interest.

Cyclooxygenase Products

Cyclooxygenase products of arachidonic acid, namely the prostaglandins (PGs) thromboxane (TxA$_2$) and prostacyclin (PGI$_2$) appear to be major factors in the pathophysiology of at least the hypertension and hypoxia phase. Thromboxane is released from platelets and stimulates further platelet aggregation.[6,63] This substance may well be the active mediator producing pulmonary damage from platelet emboli. Thromboxane is also released from leukocytes and from the lung itself in response to injury.[65] If the endothelium is significantly damaged, production of PGI$_2$ is impaired. This will allow platelets to adhere to the damaged wall and release TxA$_2$, promoting further platelet aggregation.

The mechanism of action of prostanoids on platelets and endothelial cells is felt to be through the alteration of intracellular cyclic adenosine monophosphate (AMP) and cyclic guanosine monophosphate (GMP), with the ratio of AMP to GMP determining cell stability.

A number of animal studies have now demonstrated that thromboxane release is, in large part, responsible for the early severe pulmonary hypertension and bronchoconstriction seen after endotoxin or bacterial infusion, as inhibition of thromboxane production by cyclooxygenase or thromboxane synthetase inhibitors markedly attenuates this aspect of the lung injury.[1,15,17,24,33] Several recent studies in man have now reported an increase in plasma TxA$_2$ during sepsis-induced ARDS.[74] It is interesting to note that a number of acute lung injuries such as an emboli, phorbol myristate acetate (PMA), infusion of complement-activated plasma,[35] and paraquat are characterized by a thromboxane-induced transient pulmonary hypertension indicating this to be a common pathway.[12,53,67] However, we and others have noted severe pulmonary hypertension in the later stages of sepsis or after repeated infusions of zymosan-activated plasma which are not TxA$_2$-induced. The role of TxA$_2$ in the more *sustained* pulmonary hypertension seen with sepsis in man also remains undetermined.

Prostacyclin, PGI$_2$, is also released after intravenous endotoxin. This compound is a potent vasodilator and is also reported to help maintain the stability of the microvascular membrane.[15] Prostacyclin infused into the normal lung increases fluid and protein flux, most likely as a result of its increase in cardiac output and vascular surface area.[30] PGI$_2$ does not appear to decrease vascular pressures in the normal lung. We have noted, however, a significant pulmonary vasodilator effect when PGI$_2$ infusion is begun prior to administration of endotoxin.[18] Endotoxin-induced changes in fluid and protein flux were markedly attenuated with PGI$_2$ (Fig. 3). We have not as yet determined whether the mechanism of action is via a decrease in capillary pressure or on permeability or both. PGI$_2$ release has also been reported to be responsible for increasing pulmonary dysfunction by causing the inhibition of hypoxic pulmonary vasoconstriction seen with endotoxin in dogs.[31]

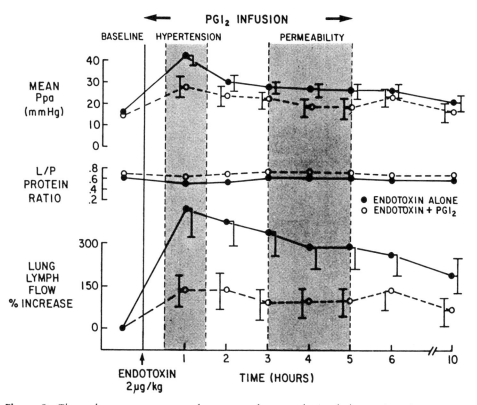

Figure 3: *The pulmonary response of a group of unanesthetized sheep given intravenous endotoxin is compared to a group given endotoxin along with an infusion of prostacyclin, PGI$_2$, at a rate of 0.2 μg/kg/min for a 5-hour period. Both phases of lung injury were attenuated with the PGI$_2$ infusion. (From Demling et al.,[18] with permission.)*

The difficulty of interpreting data on PGs is the fact that many cyclo-oxygenase inhibitors do more than inhibit PG synthesis and, therefore, the effects of the agent may not be due to PG inhibition. This is particularly true for the agent ibuprofen, which has an as yet poorly defined effect on neutrophils.[1,15]

In reference to potential therapy for man, infusions of PGI_2 or the less potent but more stable vasodilator prostaglandin, PEG_1, are very difficult to manage in view of (1) the variability of potency between batches of the compound making an infusion by *dose* virtually impossible, and (2) the significant systemic vasodilation that potentially occurs, which can lead to significant hypotension. Selective inhibitors of thromboxane synthesis would be more feasible, as this would alter the TxA_2/PGI_2 ratio in favor of the PGI_2 effect. We are currently hampered by the lack of suitable parenteral inhibitors in man that are available for human experimental use.

Prostaglandins do not appear to cause the increase in pulmonary capillary permeability that is also characteristic of ARDS. Cyclooxygenase inhibitors have shown no effect on this phase of injury in animal studies. In fact, this injury has actually increased with the use of some cyclooxygenase inhibitors. This latter effect has been felt to be due to shunting of arachidonic acid metabolism into the lipoxygenase pathway.[40] There is certainly an interrelationship between these two pathways.

Lipoxygenase Pathway

The end products of this pathway are the leukotrienes. These newly discovered agents, as well as their intermediates, hydroxy and hydroperoxy fatty acids, are potentially deleterious in that they are potent vaso- and broncho-constrictors.[5,13,52,103] This is particularly true of the leukotrienes LTC_4 and LTD_4. These two agents, when infused into animals, produce a transient pulmonary artery hypertension and a decrease in lung compliance. Interestingly, LTB_4, LTC_4 and LTD_4 have been shown to stimulate phospholipase activity and increase thromboxane production in animals, in particular, the guinea pig. Therefore, a significant portion of the smooth muscle constrictor action of the leukotrienes may be caused by TxA_2, again demonstrating the interaction between cyclooxygenase and lipoxygenase products.[71] The slow reactive substance of anaphylaxis SRS-A is now known to be the leukotrienes LTC_4 and LTD_4. Several of these products, in particular leukotriene LTB_4, are also potent neutrophil chemoattractants and are released in large quantities into inflammatory tissue. Neutrophils certainly play a major role in increasing lung vascular permeability. Neutrophils make large quantities of leukotrienes which, in turn, attract more granulocytes.

There remains some controversy as to the effects of the leukotrienes on microvascular permeability. A minimal to no increase in permeability in the lung has been noted with LTC_4 or LTD_4 in most in vivo animal studies.[92] However, both the agents appeared to increase systemic vascular permeability in the guinea pig systemic circulation.[75] Leukotriene B_4 has been less well studied as a permeability factor but, being a potent chemoattractant, may alter permeability indirectly through the action of the neutrophil.[58]

The role of the leukotriene in sepsis-induced lung injury remains undefined, in large part, due to the lack of assay techniques needed to determine their presence in disease.[87] There is evidence that 5-HETE, a product of the neutrophil lipoxygenase system, is present in high concentrations in sheep lung lymph during the increased permeability phase endotoxemia.[70] Preliminary data in the sheep model showed no effect on the pulmonary response to endotoxin with the use of LTC_4 and LTD_4 inhibitor FPL 55712.[9]

Lipoxygenase products are also released during inflammation[44] and, although they may not have a direct role in a pure endotoxin or sepsis lung injury, they may play a more important part in the accentuated sepsis lung injury that appears to be seen after soft tissue trauma or a burn, both of which result in an inflammatory focus.

White Cells

There is rapidly accumulating evidence that leukocytes are a major factor in a number of acute lung injuries, particularly sepsis.[93] Leukocytes can be seen sequestered in the pulmonary microcirculation after severe tissue trauma or resuscitation from shock.[77] Pulmonary leukostasis is particularly prominent during sepsis and is a characteristic of endotoxemia.[62,88] These cells, when activated, release factors such as proteases, lysosomal enzymes, and, of current interest, oxygen radicals which can injure the lung. We reported in a number of animal studies that the degree of permeability injury correlated well with the concentration of lung lysosomal enzymes.[19]

Neutrophils appear to play the predominant role in increasing lung vascular permeability in sepsis and other disease states such as oxygen toxicity[81] since removal of the neutrophils prior to the insulting agent has eliminated the increased permeability in a large number of animal studies.[37,59,82] Electron micrographic studies have also revealed pulmonary leukocytes in large numbers in patients with ARDS, particularly those with sepsis. Bronchoalveolar lavage in similar patients yielded fluid with increased numbers of polymorphonuclear neutrophils (PMNs), as well as high levels of neutrophil elastase.[51]

The presence of neutrophils in the lung by itself does not produce permeability damage. The cells must be activated to release products such as proteases and oxygen radicals. For example, animals rendered neutropenic had no lung injury with an infusion of C_{5a}.[39,101] A number of chemoattractants are released after trauma or sepsis, which may be responsible for the leukostasis. These include components of the complement cascade, specifically C_{5a} and the leukotriene LTB_4.

A potent chemotactic lipid produced by the action of superoxide anion on arachidonic acid has also been described.[76] This factor is considered to play a major role in inflammation.

Role of Chemotactic Factors

The formation and release of chemotactic factors has been reported to occur after endotoxin. Complement-derived agents such as C_{5a} have been reported to be released.[32] However, the cause and effect relationship between these factors and the leukostasis as well as any correlation with the degree of physiologic injury remains controversial. Are chemotactic factors a cause or simply an effect of sepsis lung injury? Also, the source of these factors has not been determined. The lung is a potentially rich source of these factors.[23] Chemoattractants can be liberated directly by the lung either from elements such as alveolar macrophages or from lung tissue through the action of proteases or oxygen radicals.[84] Increased concentrations of these agents relative to plasma have been measured in lymph draining the lung after a number of acute insults.[68] However, in other forms of leukocyte-induced injuries, these factors are not present. It is important to determine (1) whether chemotactic factors are liberated locally by the lung or systemically after endotoxemia, using the activity in lung lymph to reflect local productions, and (2) whether there is a cause and effect relationship between these factors and the physiologic injury during sepsis.

We and others have used the unanesthetized sheep with a chronic lung lymph fistula to monitor pulmonary microvascular injury considering Q_L and lymph protein content to reflect transvascular fluid flux and protein permeability, respectively. Horn et al.[42] measured chemotactic activity in lung lymph and plasma using the Boyden chamber technique. They reported increased chemotactic activity (CA) in plasma immediately after endotoxin infusion. Lung lymph CA also increased, but this did not occur until 1.5 hours postinfusion, which was well after the pulmonary leukostasis had occurred questioning the role of lung-derived chemotactic factors as a cause of early neutrophil sequestration. The CA was abolished with C_{5a} antibody, indicating the C5-derived peptides to be the measured chemoattractant. Still no cause and effect conclusion can be made from this data. We performed a similar study, but using the agarose-gelatin system for measurement of CA to human neutrophils.[65] We also noted an early increase in plasma CA but did not see an increase in the lung lymph activity[73] (Fig. 4, Table I). The role of the plasma CA factor in the permeability injury was further tested by the use of dimethylthiourea (DMTU).[26] This agent is a potent hydroxyl radical scavenger. The hydroxyl OH⁻ ion has been shown to be the cause of a number of granulocyte-induced lung injuries.[27,78] DMTU pretreatment was, in fact, able to prevent the liberation of plasma chemoattractants after endotoxin, but had no effect on either the leukocyte sequestration or on the lung injury. This indicates a lack of cause and effect between plasma CA and actual injury with endotoxin.

Neutrophil adherence or the stickiness of the cells is also an important property that contributes to the margination of these cells in the microcirculation.[55] Complement fragments have also been reported to increase neutrophil adherence to endothelial cells. Corticosteroids are considered to be beneficial in treating sepsis lung injury in that these agents increase the lipid fluidity of the neutrophil cell membrane and, thereby, decrease adherence.

Alveolar macrophages are also felt to play a significant role in ARDS. These cells are known to release potent chemotactic factors.[44] Macrophages are also the cells that are felt to initiate the interstitial inflammatory response.

Oxygen Radicals

Oxygen radicals are essential for killing of bacteria once phagocytized by the neutrophil. These extremely reactive agents can, however, be very destructive when released into tissues. The most reactive of these agents appears to be the hydroxyl (OH⁻) radical. Oxygen radicals can alter the lipid layer of the cell membrane by increasing peroxide formation[11,86] (Fig. 5). Increased lung lipid peroxidation has been reported in man after a number of insults, including oxygen toxicity[80] and paraquat poisoning. Paraquat is a herbicide that produces a severe acute lung injury as a result of oxygen radical release, leading

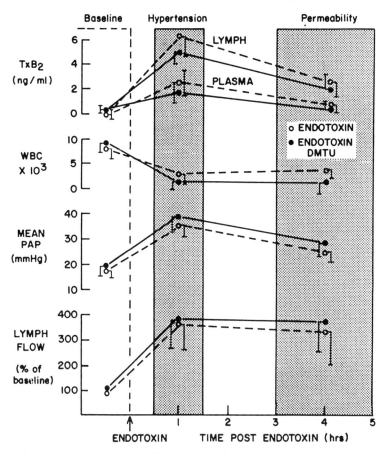

Figure 4: *The pulmonary response of a group of sheep given endotoxin alone (2 μg/kg) is compared to a group given endotoxin preceded by dimethylthiourea (DMTU) a hydroxyl radical scavenger (0.5 mg/kg). There was no effect on the preliminary response to endotoxin, despite therapeutic levels of DMTU present in plasma and lymph as determined by HPLC. The leukocyte sequestration was also comparable, despite suppression of increased plasma chemotactic activity.*

Table I
Chemotactic Generating Activity of Plasma and Lung Lymph
in E. Coli Sheep With Endotoxemia Pretreated DMTU

	Endotoxin only		Endotoxin + DMTU	
	% CA Lymph	% CA Plasma	%CA Lymph	%CA Plasma
Baseline Endotoxin	100	100	100	100
Hypertensive	80 ± 15	118 ± 14	104 ± 16	96 ± 12
Permeability	78 ± 16*	133 ± 13*	98 ± 12	102 ± 10

% CA = percent chemotactic activity of baseline
* Significantly different from baseline, $p < 0.05$
Lymph chemotactic activity remained baseline or decreased during endotoxemia while plasma activity was significantly increased. In the DMTU group, plasma CA remained at baseline, suggesting no cause and effect relationship of CA with leukocyte sequestration.

FREE RADICAL INJURY

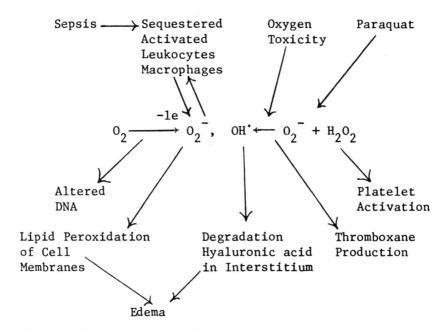

Figure 5: *Schema of potential mechanism of tissue damage from oxygen radicals.*

eventually to severe fibrosis.[107] Lipid peroxidation occurs in the liver after sepsis[80] and may likely occur in the lung as well. We have recently demonstrated increased lipid peroxidation in the sheep lung after endotoxin, with the increase occurring during the increased permeability.[104] This certainly does not demonstrate a cause and effect relationship. The permeability change could be the result of O_2 radical alteration in the basement membrane and interstitium rather than cell membrane changes. Oxygen radicals have been found to depolymerize enzymatically the hyaluronic acid in the lung interstitial space, thereby loosening the matrix and increasing edema formation.[28,60] (Fig. 5).

Although neutrophils are involved in sepsis lung injury and neutrophils release oxygen radicals, there is no definite proof that neutrophil-induced oxygen radical release causes sepsis lung injury. Evidence in support relates to data on a number of facets of sepsis. First, activation of the complement cascade, which is felt by some to be responsible for sepsis injury, produces a lung dysfunction that has been reported to be, in part, reduced by superoxide dismutase (SOD) indicating the superoxide anion, O_2^- is involved. As previously described, the relationship between complement and sepsis lung injury remains controversial.

Second, chemotactic factors are liberated from the lung and plasma by O_2 radicals. These chemoattractants are again felt to play a major role in sepsis injury by causing neutrophil sequestration and activation as well as further radical release. As pointed out in the previous section, chemotactic factors, although clearly playing a major role in producing inflammation at a septic focus, may not be responsible for initiating the pulmonary leukocyte sequestration of endotoxemia. We have not, as yet, been able to determine a cause and effect relationship between these factors and sepsis lung injury. Third, selective activation of neutrophils to release O_2 radicals with phorbol produces a lung injury characterized by increased protein permeability. The physiologic injury looks very similar to that seen after endotoxin. Fourth, there is evidence in patients and animals with sepsis lung injury that circulating neutrophils have been activated to release O_2 radicals. These last two points will be discussed further.

Phorbol myristate acetate is a compound that selectively activates white cells to release only O_2 radicals.[53] We and others have demonstrated that PMA infused into animals produces a lung injury identical to that seen after endotoxin[83] (Figs. 6 and 7). There is, again, a two-phase response. An initial thromboxane-induced pulmonary artery hypertension is seen. The TxA_2 release again points out the relationship between O_2 radicals and arachidonic acid metabolism.[29] An initial leukopenia occurs concomitant with the hyper-

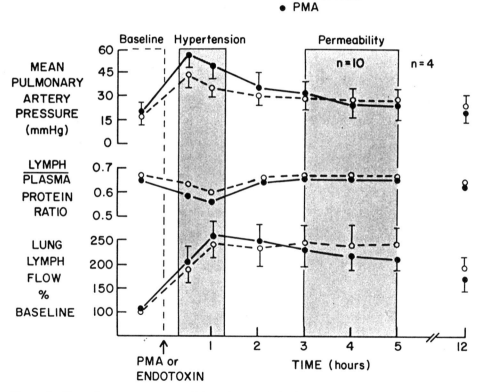

Figure 6: *The pulmonary response of the infusion of phorbol myristate acetate, PMA, 7 µg/kg, is compared with the response seen after endotoxin (1 µg/kg) infusion in unanesthetized sheep. A two-phase response was seen with both injuries, characterized by an initial hypoxia, severe pulmonary hypertension, and increased protein-poor lymph flow. This was followed by a steady state increase in protein-rich lung lymph with relatively normal pressures, which is characteristic of increased protein permeability.*

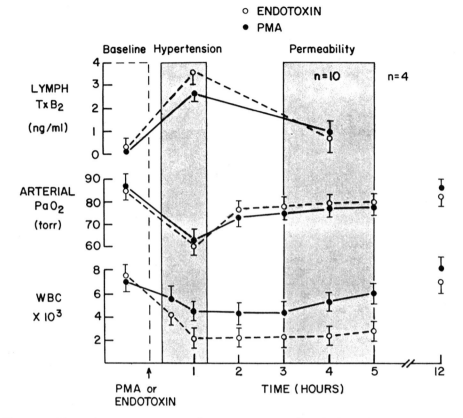

Figure 7: *The pulmonary response of PMA is compared with that of endotoxin in un-anesthetized sheep. In both injuries, there was an initial severe hypoxia and a significant increase in lymph thromboxane (TxB$_2$) production. Circulating white cell count fell in both groups but to a greater extent after endotoxin.*

tension and hypoxia. Several hours later, an increase in protein permeability is seen. We have recently reported that PMA injury is also characterized by a decrease in the large hyaluronic acid component of the interstitium and an increase in the smaller fragments, indicating damage to the lung interstitium.

Neutrophil Activation

It is extremely important to be able to measure neutrophil activation when studying sepsis lung injury since this process appears to be the key factor in the production of increased permeability.[25] Chemiluminescence is a technique currently used to monitor the release of O$_2$ radicals, which is seen with neutrophil activation.[46,102,109] A recent study in patients with sepsis indicated that when lung injury was present, there was evidence of increased chemiluminescent activity of circulating neutrophils.[109] This would indicate increased O$_2$ radical release.

We have analyzed lung lymph and plasma after endotoxin infusion in sheep to determine if an activator of neutrophil O_2 release was present. We studied this process using the chemiluminescence technique[108] and found that a factor in lymph was present early after endotoxin which increased neutrophil chemiluminescence activity. This factor is less than 30,000 molecular weight, but specific identity remains undetermined. We can, therefore, state that there is good evidence in animals and in man that activation of neutrophils to release O_2 radicals occurs. Whether this activation occurs in the lung and whether the released O_2 radicals are responsible for sepsis-induced ARDS remains to be determined.

We recently pretreated sheep with DMTU (0.5–0.75 µg/kg) prior to endotoxin. We selected an OH· radical scavenger because (1) OH· is the oxidant believed to be the source of tissue injury in most O_2 radical injuries, (2) PMA injury which is OH·-induced and blocked by DMTU has an identical physiological presentation to that seen with endotoxin, and (3) endotoxin liver damage has been reported to be OH·-induced. We were unable to attenuate the endotoxin lung injury with DMTU. This data would cast some doubt on the cause and effect relationship previously discussed. Another logical explanation would be that we selected the wrong oxidant to inhibit. To date, no other data on this topic is available.

Lipid Peroxidation

Lipid peroxidation is one characteristic of O_2 radical tissue damage. This is seen in the lung after several forms of acute lung injury from O_2 radicals and has been reported in the liver after endotoxemia. There are no studies on the lipid peroxide content of lungs injured from sepsis except for our recent study. We measured malondialdehyde (MDA) content of lung homogenate in control lungs and lungs injured by PMA infusion and by endotoxin infusion. We used MDA content as a reflection of the degree of lipid peroxidation.[3] We produced a comparable increase in protein permeability as reflected in protein-rich lung lymph flow with 7 µg/kg of PMA and 1 µg/kg of *E. coli* endotoxin. We found a significant increase in lung MDA content with phorbol but none with the endotoxin injury of comparable severity.[104] When we doubled the dose of endotoxin, MDA content increased. We can, therefore, state that lipid peroxidation occurs with severe endotoxin-induced lung injury but increased permeability can occur in the absence of increased lipid peroxidation. This data could be explained by the fact that O_2 radical-induced increased vascular permeability is not necessarily caused by cell membrane lipid peroxidation. Another process such as interstitial matrix O_2 radical damage may be causative.

Summary

There is, therefore, a considerable amount of indirect evidence that the release of O_2 radicals from activated neutrophils sequestered in the pulmonary circulation is responsible for a portion of the sepsis-induced ARDS. Our studies at the present time in the sheep would not support this hypothesis. Clearly this area needs further investigation before appropriate therapeutic modalities can be initiated.

Platelets

The role of the platelet in sepsis lung injury remains controversial.[97] This appears, in part, to be due to marked species variability in the platelet response to sepsis. Platelet count rapidly decreases in the dog and cat after endotoxin with evidence of fibrin platelet emboli in the lung. In the sheep, only a transient thrombocytopenia is seen, although we have noted that platelet count remains decreased with a more severe to fatal lung injury after endotoxin. This may, however, be more of an effect than a cause. The human platelet response appears to be somewhere between these two species.[36]

Platelets have also been found to release a number of factors that can alter lung function. Serotonin is a vasoactive agent found in high concentrations in platelets. When released, this substance results in bronchoconstriction, increased pulmonary venous pressure, and increased lung water.[10] Capillary pressure is increased because of increased venous resistance and the result is a "high pressure" form of edema. Platelet serotonin has also been recently found to accentuate neutrophil adherence and release of oxygen radicals, thereby augmenting the neutrophil-induced endothelial injury.[4] We have noted a significant increase in lung lymph serotonin levels after endotoxin with the increase beginning in the hypertensive phase (Fig. 8). Preliminary data, however, using the serotonin antagonist, Ketanserin, indicates that inhibition of serotonin smooth muscle constriction has no effect on either phase of the pulmonary vascular injury. Ketanserin, however, may not be effective in blocking the apparent accentuation of neutrophil-induced injury. Histamine is also found in platelets but not in particularly high levels in humans. Histamine infusion produces bronchoconstriction but no increase in pulmonary vascular permeability. Lung mast cells are probably the major source of the histamine, which is released rather than platelets. Thromboxane is also released by platelets. However, in preliminary findings, removal of platelets in the sheep prior to endotoxin (using rabbit antisheep platelet antibodies) has had no effect on the degree of initial hypertension, indicating that at least in the sheep, platelets are not the source of early TxA_2 release.

Platelet activating factor (PAF) is a compound that has generated considerable recent interest.[54,99,106] PAF is a glycerol phosphorylcholine that is liberated from neutrophils in response to activating agents such as C_{5a}. This substance is known to activate platelets to aggregate and release the agents just described. PAF also has a number of direct effects on the circulation, namely producing smooth muscle constriction and increased vascular permeability. Recent information indicates that PAF also is chemotactic to neutrophils and may be, in part, responsible for the initial neutrophil sequestration in the lung in response to sepsis. There also appears to be an interrelationship between PAF and the release of leukotrienes C_4 and C_5.

Sepsis and Trauma

Despite the fact that the trauma patient appears to be more susceptible to sepsis-induced lung injury, there is surprisingly little information available as to what these potentiating factors may be. We have demonstrated that hemorrhagic shock itself does not appear to be a major factor except for the increased fluid flux caused by the hypoproteinemia produced by fluid shifts and by resus-

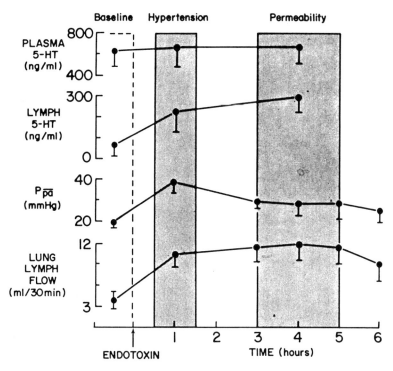

Figure 8: *Lymph and plasma serotonin levels are shown in a group of unanesthetized sheep given endotoxin 1 µg/kg. Plasma levels remained relatively constant while lymph levels increased significantly during both the hypertension and increased permeability phase.*

citation.[47,48] The addition of a hemorrhagic shock insult to an endotoxin insult does not potentiate the endotoxin lung injury.[105] This is the case as long as the hemorrhagic shock is totally volume resuscitated prior to intravenous endotoxin administration. Tissue trauma appears to be a major determinant in the accentuated lung response to sepsis. Both the incidence and severity of ARDS are increased in the septic trauma patient.

Teplitz et al.[96] and others have reported, in several large clinical series, minimal to no evidence of disseminated bacteremia in fatal cases of burn sepsis, indicating that absorbed bacterial byproducts are responsible for death. However, a number of studies have also indicated the lack of significant endotoxemia even after fatal burn sepsis.[64] It may be that burn patients are much more sensitive to the effects of endotoxin or that mediators released from the inflammatory focus are the cause of injury.

Thermally injured soft tissues have been reported to liberate large quantities of cyclooxygenase products, probably as a result of trauma-induced cell membranes.[34] Tissue injury and inflammation also result in increased leukocyte activation. We have previously demonstrated that lipoxygenase pathway products produce lung injury very similar to that seen with endotoxin administration.[87] Complement activation has also been reported to occur as a result of the soft tissue trauma.[38] This process can, of course, also activate leukocytes. It therefore appears quite possible that an exaggerated response to endotoxin could occur after a burn, since the elements that produce the actual injury are already activated or present in increased quantities.

We have devised and validated the use of an efferent lymphatic from the prefemoral lymph node to monitor microvascular fluid flux and protein permeability in the soft tissues, namely skin, subcutaneous tissue, and muscle drained by this node.[20] The addition of the systemic lymphatic to the lung lymphatic has three major advantages in allowing for a more accurate interpretation of our results for the study of acute lung injury. The first is that a comparison of the response of both the pulmonary and systemic microcirculations to a septic insult allows us to determine whether the vascular response is generalized or is specific to the lung.[21] The second advantage is the significance of the release of mediators in lung lymph, such as PGs, can be determined by the comparison with the content in systemic lymph and plasma. Is the process localized to the lung or generalized? And third, we can measure factors released in an area of tissue trauma such as burn or local infection, which may be responsible for the accentuated lung response to sepsis.

In a recent study, we produced a 25% total body surface third-degree burn. Animals were fluid resuscitated and were hemodynamically stable with no evidence of any lung abnormality at 3 days post-burn. A nonlethal dose of endotoxin (1 µg/kg) was given intravenously after 3 days and the response compared to that seen with endotoxin alone.[67]

We noted a marked accentuation of the pulmonary circulatory abnormalities with the combination of endotoxin and body burn. Four of nine burn animals died in this group as compared to no deaths in the endotoxin group. The predominant injury was clearly pulmonary, as evidenced by a marked increase in lung water and the histologic evidence of congestion, alveolar flooding, and leukocyte sequestration. Two factors were different between endotoxin alone and endotoxin plus burn. First, we noted that lung lymph thromboxane levels remained significantly increased during the permeability phase in post-burn endotoxin animals, particularly in those who later died. The increase may have been responsible for the greater degree of hypoxia and pulmonary hypertension. The thromboxane was probably not coming from the burn wound, in view of the normal TxB_2 levels in burn lymph.

Secondly, a progressive deterioration, beginning about 8 hours after endotoxin was noted in the four animals who died, characterized by a severe pulmonary hypertension, hypoxia, and clinical evidence of pulmonary edema, when TxB_2 levels were baseline. Evidence that this late phase reponse was, at least in part, leukocyte-induced, was the fact that a persistent leukopenia was seen in all burn animals who died as opposed to a rapid return to a normal count in surviving animals. The late deterioration may well be due to mediators released from the burn tissue which produce pulmonary venoconstriction or accentuate the endotoxin permeability change such as serotonin or the leukotrienes.

We have recently reported that microvascular integrity of nonburned tissue is not significantly altered with intravenous infusion of endotoxin (Fig. 9). A transient but modest increase in protein-poor systemic Q_L occurred during the early systemic hypertension seen immediately after endotoxin. This corresponded with an increase in venous TxA_2 levels. However, in contrast to the lung response, no increase was seen in protein permeability. We have also

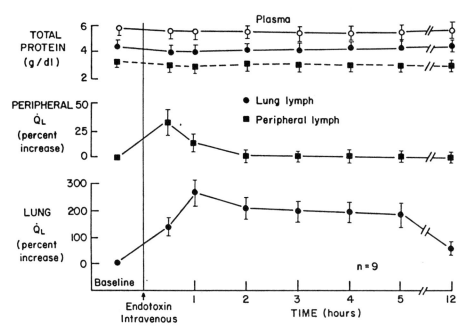

Figure 9: *A comparison is made between the lung and soft tissue microvascular response to intravenous endotoxin. Left atrial pressure, central venous pressure, and cardiac output were maintained constant during the study. Lung lymph flow increased significantly, lymph initially having a decreased protein content, followed at 2 – 3 hours by an increased content. Peripheral lymph flow increased transiently initially, with lymph being protein-poor. This was followed by a rapid return to baseline.*

infused *E. coli* endotoxin directly into the soft tissues of the flank in the drainage region of the cannulated prefemoral lymphatic, and again no increase in protein permeability is seen. We did, however, note a large increase in TxA_2 production in the flank injected with endotoxin tissue, as measured in lymph from this area. Plasma levels increased only modestly, as did lung lymph (Fig. 10). Lung values were equal to plasma while soft tissue levels were 10 – 20 times higher. We noted a pulmonary hypertension response with increased protein-poor lung Q_L but the lung was not the source of the TxA_2 as is seen with intravenous endotoxin.

These studies clearly point out the potential importance of local systemic tissue trauma or infection as the source of arachidonic acid metabolites and possibly factors that activate circulating neutrophils and subsequently affect lung function. Intravenous administration of bacteria or endotoxin is the most commonly used experimental septic insult, resulting in lung injury. The most common process of sepsis leading to ARDS in man, however, is trauma, infection, and inflammation in distant soft tissues.

Future Areas of Research

Most of the research on alterations in pulmonary microvascular fluid and protein flux have been concentrated on changes at the microvascular membrane

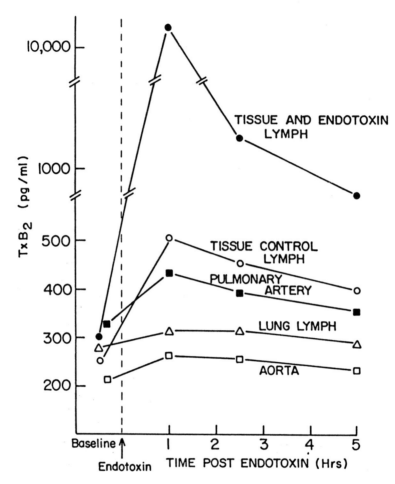

Figure 10: *Thromboxane release in lymph and plasma is shown for one animal in which endotoxin 2 µg/kg was injected beneath the hide of the flank. TxA$_2$ is measured as TxB$_2$. A marked increase in TxB$_2$ was seen in lymph draining the peripheral tissue injected with endotoxin. Tissue lymph TxB$_2$ was only modestly increased in lymph draining soft tissue on the side opposite that was injected with endotoxin. Pulmonary artery plasma TxB$_2$ increased as well to levels higher than that in aortic plasma and lung lymph, indicating that the peripheral tissues, rather than the lung, were the source of the TxB$_2$. Values were returning to baseline by 5 hours.*

itself. Current data, although limited, would indicate that the lung interstitium may play a major role in this process.[72,95,100]

The pulmonary interstitium is a complex network of collagen, elastic fibers, proteoglycans, and glycosaminoglycans.[14,43,79] The latter two components have the capability of swelling greatly when the tissue is hydrated. Included in the interstitium is the basement membrane, an important component of which is tissue fibronectin. Tissue fibronectin is the cement holding endothelial cells together.

Our understanding of the role of the interstitium in fluid and protein flux, both during normal and abnormal states, remains poorly defined. However, there is no doubt that the compliance or viscosity of this tissue is a very important determinant of fluid accumulation. Oppenheimer et al.[72] recently demonstrated that a significant portion of increased transvascular fluid flux is determined by the rate of water redistribution in the interstitium. Proteoglycans and glycosaminoglycans, in particular, hyaluronic acid, are now known to be major factors. For example, proteoglycans in the glomerular basement membrane form the major barrier to protein filtration. Enzymatic depolymerization of hyaluronic acid causes increased permeability in connective tissues. These compounds appear to maintain tissue impermeability because of their viscosity effects. Hyaluronic acid solutions have very high viscosities because of their highly polymerized state. The large hyaluronic acid molecules also occupy a large volume, thereby inhibiting water and solute accumulation.

Depolymerization of hyaluronic acid greatly decreases its viscosity. Also, the small hyaluronic fragments competitively interfere with intermolecular interaction between the larger hyaluronate molecule, leading to a further loss of viscosity and structure of the interstitium. Hyaluronic acid is known to be easily depolymerized to hydroxyl radicals. Hydroxyl radicals released from activated granulocytes are known to increase protein permeability. This process is inhibited by hydroxyl radical scavengers, superoxide dismutase, and catalase. Fox[28] produced a lung permeability injury with phorbol myristate acetate, which causes the release of oxygen radicals from granulocytes. An increase in protein-rich lymph flow resulted, an effect that has been attributed to an alteration at the endothelial cell membrane. These injured lungs also showed a severe depletion of the high molecular weight glycosaminoglycan hyaluronic acid compared to lungs of control subjects. This effect may also be responsible for the physiologic effect.

Hydration of these molecules, which, in turn, increases the space for protein distribution, certainly potentiates the compensatory decrease in interstitial protein content. This, then, helps to neutralize an increase in microvascular hydrostatic pressure, as previously described. We have also described the fact that interstitital space protein depletion increases fluid flux. I would hypothesize that the continued protein washout from the interstitial space decreases the matrix viscosity, thereby increasing compliance. It is possible that this expansion of the interstitial space has another protective effect in decreasing interstitial hydrostatic pressure, thereby protecting the alveolar membrane.

Interstitital components also appear to play an important role in permeability edema. Recent studies have indicated the importance of molecular charge on solute flux. The sulfated glycosaminoglycans are heavily anionically charged molecules. Alphanaphthyl thiourea causes a decrease in anionic charges in the lung and, in turn, an increase in permeability edema.

Another important component of basement membrane is tissue fibronectin.[22,61,69] Recent studies have indicated that a depletion of the circulating plasma fibronectin can accentuate the permeability injury from a number of insults. It has been hypothesized but not yet determined that there is an equilibrium between the plasma and the tissue form such that depletion of the former will lead to a depletion in the "cell cement," leading to an increase in protein permeability. Answers to this issue should be forthcoming.

It is clear that the interstitium and its components cannot be ignored in any discussion of lung fluid and solute flux after sepsis.

Future studies on the mechanism of lung injury in sepsis should continue to concentrate on the three interrelating elements that have been described, namely (1) products of arachidonic acid metabolism, (2) white cells and their byproducts, specifically oxygen radicals, and (3) platelets and their byproducts. Major gains in our knowledge of pathophysiology will be found in further defining the *interrelationship* that is clearly present among these elements, rather than studying each element separately. It may then become clear that one factor such as hydroxyl radical release may initiate the entire cascade involving all of the elements. At present, there are so many factors that appear to play a role in the disease that selection of appropriate therapeutic modalities remains nearly impossible.

The actual mechanism of cellular injury should be pursued by more emphasis on quantification of biochemical and subcellular alterations that may shed light on the specific causative agents, e.g., lipid peroxidation and oxygen radicals. The measurement of fluid and protein flux exclusively will yield limited data.

REFERENCES

1. Adams, T. and Traber, D.: The effect of a prostaglandin synthetase inhibitor ibuprofen on the cardiopulmonary response to endotoxin in sheep. *Circ. Shock* 9:481–489, 1982.
2. Anderson, R.R., Holliday, R.L., Driedger, A., et al.: Documentation of pulmonary capillary permeability in the adult respiratory distress syndrome accompanying human sepsis. *Am. Rev. Respir. Dis.* 119:869–877, 1979.
3. Asakawa, T. and Matsushita, S.: Thiobarbituric acid test for detecting lipid peroxides. *Lipids* 14:401–406, 1978.
4. Boegaert, M., Jacob, H., and Moldow, C.: Enhancement of granulocyte-endothelial adherence and granulocyte induced cytotoxicity by platelet release factors. *Proc. Natl. Acad. Sci.* 79:7019–7023, 1982.
5. Bray, M.A., Cunningham, F.M., Ford-Hutchinson, A.W., et al.: Leukotriene B$_4$: A mediator of vascular permeability. *Br. J. Pharmacol.* 72:483, 1981.
6. Brigham, K.L., Bowers, R, and Haynes, J.: Increased sheep lung vascular permeability caused by Escherichia coli endotoxin. *Circ. Res.* 45:292–297, 1979.
7. Brigham, K., Kariman, K., Harris, T., et al.: Correlation of oxygenation with vascular permeability-surface area but not with lung water in humans with acute respiratory failure and pulmonary edema. *J. Clin. Invest.* 1984 (In press).
8. Brigham, K.L., Owen, P.J., and Bowers, R.E.: Increased permeability of sheep lung vessels to proteins after pseudomonas bacteremia. *Microvasc. Res.* 11: 415–421, 1976.
9. Brigham, K.L.: Proceedings workshop on arachidonic acid metabolites and the pulmonary circulation. September 30-October, 1982. NIH publication.
10. Brigham, K.L. and Owen, P.J.: Mechanisms of the serotonin effect on lung transvascular fluid and protein management in awake sheep. *Circ. Res.* 36:761–770, 1975.
11. Brown, R.E., Craver, R., and Drake, R.M.: Lipid peroxidation and pulmonary hyaline membranes of the newborn. *Ann. Clin. Lab. Sci.* 11:25–30, 1981.
12. Cooper, J.D., McDonald, J., and Clement, P.: Prostaglandin production associated with the pulmonary vascular response to complement activation. *Surgery* 88: 215–22, 1980.
13. Dahlen, S.E., Bjork, J., Hedquist, P., et al.: Leukotrienes promote plasma leakage and leukocyte adherence in post-capillary venules: In vivo effects with relevance to the acute inflammatory response. *Proc. Natl. Acad. Sci.* 78:3887, 1981.

14. Day, T.D.: The permeability of interstitial connective tissue and the nature of interfibrillary substance. *J. Physiol.* 117:1–8, 1952.

15. Demling, R.H., Niehaus, G., and Will, J.A.: Pulmonary microvascular response to hemorrhagic shock, resuscitation and recovery. *J. Appl. Physiol.* 46:498–503, 1979.

16. Demling, R.H., Smith, M., Gunther, R., et al.: Pulmonary injury and prostaglandin production during endotoxemia in conscious sheep. *Am. J. Physiol.* 240:348–353, 1981.

17. Demling, R.H.: Role of prostaglandins in acute microvascular injury. *Ann. NY Acad. Sci.* 384:517–534, 1982.

18. Demling, R.H., Smith, M., Gunther, R., et al.: The effect of prostacyclin infusion on endotoxin induced lung injury. *Surgery* 89:257–263, 1981.

19. Demling, R.H., Proctor, R., Grossman, J., et al.: Lung injury and lung lysosomal enzyme release during endotoxemia. *J. Surg. Res.* 30:135–141, 1981.

20. Demling, R., Smith, M., and Gunther, R.: Use of a chronic prefemoral lymphatic fistula for monitoring systemic capillary integrity in unanesthetized sheep. *J. Surg. Res.* 31:136–141, 1981.

21. Demling, R.H., Wong, C., and Wenger, H.: Effect of endotoxin on the integrity of the peripheral (soft tissue) microcirculation. *Circ. Shock.* 1984 (In press).

22. Deno, D.C., Saba, T.M., and Lewis, E.P.: Kinetics of endogenously labelled plasma fibronectin incorporation into tissue. *Am. J. Physiol.* 245:564–579, 1983.

23. Fantone, J.C. and Ward, P.M.: Chemotactic mechanisms in the lung. In *Immunopharmacology of the lung*. Newball, H., ed. New York, Marcel Dekker, 1983, pp. 243–261.

24. Flynn, J. and Demling, R.: Inhibition of endogenous thromboxane synthesis by exogenous prostacyclin during endotoxemia in conscious sheep. *Adv. Shock Res.* 7:199–207, 1982.

25. Fountain, S.W., Martin, B.A., and Cooper, J.D.: Pulmonary leukostasis and its relationship to pulmonary dysfunction in sheep and rabbits. *Circ. Res.* 46:175–181, 1980.

26. Fox, R.B., Harada, R.N., Tate, R.M., et al.: Prevention of thiourea-induced pulmonary edema by hydroxyl radical scavengers. *J. Appl. Physiol.* 55:1456–1459, 1983.

27. Fox, R.B., Hoidal, J.M., Brown, D.M., et al.: Pulmonary inflammation due to oxygen toxicity: Involvements of chemotactic factors and polymorphonuclear leukocytes. *Am. Rev. Respir. Dis.* 123:521–523, 1981.

28. Fox, R.B., Demling, R.H., Wong, C., et al.: Role of glycosaminoglycan depolymerization in the pathogenesis of permeability pulmonary edema due to granulocyte oxidants. *Physiologist* 26:8, 1983.

29. Gurtner, G.H., Knoblauch, A., Smith, P.L., et al.: Oxidant and lipid induced pulmonary vasoconstriction mediated by arachidonic acid metabolites. *J. Appl. Physiol.* 55:949–954, 1983.

30. Gunther, R., Zaiss, C., and Demling, R.: Pulmonary microvascular response to prostacyclin (PGI_2) infusion in unanesthetized sheep. *J. Appl. Physiol.* 52:1338–1342, 1982.

31. Hamasaki, Y., Tai, H.-H., and Said, S.: Hypoxia stimulates prostacyclin generation by dog lung in vitro. *Prost. Leuk. Med.* 8:311–316, 1982.

32. Hammerschmidt, D.E., Weaver, L.J., Hudson, L.D., et al.: Association of complement activation and elevated plasma-C_{5a} with adult respiratory distress syndrome. *Lancet* 1:947–949, 1980.

33. Harlon, J., Winn, R., Weaver, J., et al.: Selective blockade of thromboxane A_2 synthesis during experimental E. coli bacteremia in the goat. *Chest* 83:75–77, 1983.

34. Harms, B., Bodai, B., Flynn, J., et al.: Prostaglandin release and altered microvascular integrity after burn injury. *J. Surg. Res.* 31:274–280, 1981.

35. Havill, A.M., Perkoinski, S.Z., Flynn, J.T., et al.: Complement initiated lung microvascular injury in anesthetized sheep. *Fed. Proc.* 41:1501, 1982.

36. Hechtman, H.B., Lonergan, E.A., Staunton, P.B., et al.: Pulmonary entrapment of platelets during acute respiratory failure. *Surgery* 83:277–283, 1978.

37. Heflin, A.J. and Brigham, K.L.: Prevention by granulocyte depletion of increased vascular permeability of sheep lung following endotoxemia. *J. Clin. Invest.* 58: 1253–1260, 1981.

38. Heideman, M.: A shared effect of abscesses and nonviable tissue influencing the development of sepsis and acute respiratory distress syndrome. *Acta Chir. Scand.* 508:295–302, 1982.

39. Henson, P.M., Larsen, G.L., and Webster, R.O.: Pulmonary microvascular alterations and injury induced by complement fragments: Synergistic effect of complement activation, neutrophil sequestration and prostaglandins. *Ann. NY Acad. Sci.* 384:287–299, 1982.

40. Higgs, G.A., Eakins, K.F., Mugridge, K.G., et al.: The effect of nonsteroid anti-inflammatory drugs on leukocyte migration in carrageenin-induced inflammation. *Eur. J. Pharmacol.* 66:81–89, 1980.

41. Hinson, J.M., Brigham, K.L., Hutchison, A.A., et al.: Granulocytes participate in the early changes in lung mechanics caused by endotoxemia. *Am. Rev. Respir. Dis.* 127:275–283, 1982.

42. Horn, J., Flick, M., and Goldstein, I.M.: Endotoxin induced lung injury in sheep: Complement (C_5)-derived chemotactic activity in plasma and lung lymph. *J. Surg. Res.* 1984 (In press).

43. Horwitz, A.L. and Crystal, R.G.: Content and synthesis of glycosaminoglycans in the developing lung. *J. Clin. Invest.* 56:1312–1318, 1975.

44. Hunninghake, G.W., Gallin, J.I., and Fauci, A.J.: Immunologic reactivity of the lung: The in vivo and in vitro generation of a neutrophil chemotactic factor by alveolar macrophages. *Am. Rev. Respir. Dis.* 117:15–21, 1978.

45. Kaplan, R.J., Sabin, S.A., and Petty, T.L.: Incidence and outcome of the respiratory distress syndrome in gram negative sepsis. *Arch. Intern. Med.* 139:867–869, 1979.

46. Kato, T., Wokalek, H., and Schopf, E.: Measurements of chemiluminescence in freshly drawn human blood. *Klin. Wochenschr.* 59:203–211, 1981.

47. Kramer, G.C., Harms, B.A., Gunther, R., et al.: The effect of hypoproteinemia on blood to lymph fluid transport in sheep lung. *Circ. Res.* 49:1173–1180, 1982.

48. Kramer, G.C., Harms, B.A., Bodai, B., et al.: Effect of hypoproteinemia and increased vascular pressure on lung fluid balance in sheep. *J. Appl. Physiol.* 55: 1514–1522, 1983.

49. Kuehl, F.A. and Egan, R.W.: Prostaglandins, arachidonic acid and inflammation. *Science* 210:978, 1980.

50. Lava, J., Rice, C., Moss, G., et al.: Pulmonary dysfunction in sepsis: Is pulmonary edema the culprit? *J. Trauma* 22:280–284, 1982.

51. Lee, C.T., Fein, A.M., Lippman, M., et al.: Elastolytic activity in pulmonary lavage fluid from patients with adult respiratory distress syndrome. *N. Engl. J. Med.* 304:192–196, 1981.

52. Leitch, A.G., Austen, K.F., Corey, E.J., et al.: Effects of indomethacin (indo) on the contractile response of guinea pig lung parenchymal stups (GPLS) to leukotrienes (LT) B_4, C_4, D_4, E_4. *Fed. Proc.* 41:4545, 1982.

53. Loyd, J., Newman, J., English, D., et al.: Lung vascular effects of phorbol myristate acetate in awake sheep. *J. Appl. Physiol.* 54:267–276, 1983.

54. Lynch, J.M., Lotner, G.Z., Betz, S.J., et al.: The release of platelet activating factor by stimulated rabbit neutrophils. *J. Immunol.* 123:1219–1223, 1979.

55. MacGregor, R.R.: Granulocyte adherence changes induced by hemodialysis, endotoxin, epinephrine and glucocorticosteroids. *Ann. Intern. Med.* 86:35–41, 1977.

56. Malik, A.B.: Pulmonary microembolism. *Physiol. Rev.* 63:1114–1207, 1983.

57. Marshall, W. and Dimick, A.: The natural history of major burns with multiple subsystem failure. *J. Trauma* 23:102–108, 1983.

58. Martin, T., Altman, L.C., Albert, R.K., et al.: Leukotriene B_4 production by the

human alveolar macrophage: A potential mechanism for amplifying inflammation in the lung. *Am. Rev. Respir. Dis.* 129:106–111, 1984.

59. McCord, J.M. and Fridovich, I.: The biology and pathology of oxygen radicals. *Ann. Intern. Med.* 89:122–127, 1978.

60. McCord, J.: Free radicals and inflammation: Protection of synovial fluid by superoxide dismutase. *Science* 185:529–531, 1974.

61. McDonald, J.A., Baum, B.J., and Rosenberg, D.M.: Destruction of a major extracellular adhesive glycoprotein (fibronectin) of human fibroblasts of neural proteases from polymorphonuclear leukocyte granules. *Lab. Invest.* 40:350–57, 1979.

62. Meyrick, B. and Brigham, K.L.: Acute effects of Escherichia coli endotoxin on the pulmonary microcirculation of anesthetized sheep. *Lab. Invest.* 48:458–470, 1983.

63. Moncado, S. and Vane, J.: Arachidonic acid metabolites and the interactions between platelets and blood vessel walls. *N. Engl. J. Med.* 300:1142–1147, 1979.

64. Moncrief, J.A.: Medical progress in burns. *N. Engl. J. Med.* 288:444–455, 1974.

65. Morley, J., Bray, M.A., and Jones, R.W.: Prostaglandin and thromboxane production by human and guinea pig macrophages and leukocytes. *Prostaglandins* 17:729–736, 1979.

66. Nelson, R.D., Quie, P.G., and Simmons, R.L.: Chemotaxis under agarose: A new and simplified method for measuring chemotaxis and spontaneous migration of human polymorphonuclear leukocytes and monocytes. *J. Immunol.* 115:1650–1656, 1975.

67. Nerlich, M., Flynn, J., and Demling, R.: Effect of thermal injury on endotoxin-induced lung injury. *Surgery* 93:298, 1983.

68. Newman, J., Loyd, J., English, D., et al.: Effect of 100% oxygen in lung vascular function in awake sheep. *J. Appl. Physiol.* 54:1379–1386, 1983.

69. Niehaus, G.D., Schumaker, P.T., and Saba, T.M.: Influence of opsonic fibronectin deficiency on lung fluid balance during bacterial sepsis. *J. Appl. Physiol.* 49:693–699, 1980.

70. Ogletree, M., Oates, J.A., Brigham, K.L., et al.: Evidence for pulmonary release of 5-hydroxyeicosatetranoic acid (5-HETE) during endotoxemia in unanesthetized sheep. *Prostaglandins* 23:459–468, 1982.

71. Omini, C., Falco, T., Vigano, T., et al.: Leukotriene C_4 induces generation of PGI_2 and TxA_2 in guinea pigs in vivo. *Pharmacol. Res. Commun.* 13:633–640, 1980.

72. Oppenheimer, L., Unruh, H.W., Skooj, C., et al.: Transvascular fluid flux measured from intravascular water concentration changes. *J. Appl. Physiol.* 54:64–72, 1983.

73. Palder, S., Wong, C., Hood, I., et al.: Effect of the hydroxyl radical (OH˙) scavenger dimethyl thiourea (DMTU) on chemotactic activity of lung plasma and lymph in endotoxic sheep. *J. Surg. Res.* 1984 (In press).

74. Parratt, J., Coker, S., Hughes, B., et al.: The possible role of prostaglandins and thromboxane in the pulmonary consequences of experimental endotoxic shock and clinical sepsis. In *Role of Chemical Mediators in the Pathophysiology of Acute Illness and Injury*. McConn, R., ed. New York, Raven Press, 1982, pp. 195–219.

75. Peck, M.J., Piper, P.J., and Williams, T.J.: The effect of leukotrienes C_4 and D_4 on the microvasculature of guinea pig skin. *Prostaglandins* 21:315–320, 1981.

76. Petrone, W.F., English, D., Wong, C., et al.: Free radicals and inflammation: The superoxide-dependent activation of a neutrophil chemotactic factor in plasma. *Proc. Natl. Acad. Sci.* 77:1159–1163, 1980.

77. Pratt, P.C.: Pathology of adult respiratory distress syndrome. In *The Lung Structure, Function and Disease*. Thurlbeck, W., Abell, M.R., eds. Baltimore, MD, Williams and Wilkins, 1978, pp. 43–57.

78. Repine, J.E., Eaton, J.W., Anders, M.W., et al.: Generation of hydroxyl radical by enzymes, chemicals and human phagocytes in vitro. *J. Clin. Invest.* 65:1642–1651, 1979.

79. Sahu, S.C. and Ulsamer, A.G.: Hyaluronic acid: An indicator of pulmonary injury? *Toxicol. Lett.* 5:283–286, 1980.

80. Sakaguchi, S., Kanda, N., Shui, C., et al.: Lipid peroxide formation and membrane damage in endotoxin poisoned mice. *Microbiol. Immunol.* 25:229–244, 1981.
81. Shasby, D.M., Van Bethuysen, K.M., and Tate, R.M.: Granulocytes mediate acute edematous lung injury in rabbits and in isolated perfused lungs perfused with phorbol myristate acetate: Role of oxygen radicals. *Am. Rev. Respir. Dis.* 125: 443–447, 1981.
82. Shasby, D.M., Fox, R.B., Harada, R.N., et al.: Mechanisms of pulmonary oxygen toxicity: Neutropenia protects against acute lung injury after hyperoxia. *J. Appl. Physiol.* 52:1237–1244, 1982.
83. Shasby, D.M., Shasby, S.S., and Peach, M.J.: Granulocytes and phorbol myristate acetate increase permeability to albumin of cultured endothelial monolayers and isolated perfused lungs. *Am. Rev. Respir. Dis.* 127:72–76, 1983.
84. Shaw, J.O., Hensen, P.M., Henson, J.E., et al.: Lung inflammation induced by complement-derived chemotactic fragments in the alveolus. *Lab. Invest.* 42: 547–548, 1980.
85. Sibbald, W., Paterson, N., and Holliday, R.: Pulmonary hypertension in sepsis. *Chest* 5:583–592, 1978.
86. Slater, T.F. and Benedetto, C.: Free radical reactions in relation to lipid peroxidation, inflammation and prostaglandin metabolism. In *The Prostaglandin System.* Berti, F., Veto, G.V., eds. New York, Plenum Press, 1979, pp. 109–126.
87. Smith, M., Gunther, R., Zaiss, C., et al.: Pulmonary microvascular injury from lipoxygenase infusion: Comparison with endotoxin. *Circ. Shock* 8:647–652, 1981.
88. Smith, M., Gunther, R., Flynn, J., et al.: Leukocytes, platelets and thromboxane A_2 in endotoxin-induced lung injury. *Surgery* 90:102–107, 1981.
89. Snapper, J., Hutchison, A., Ogletree, M., et al.: Effects of cyclooxygenase inhibitors on the alteration in lung mechanics caused by endotoxemia in the unanesthetized sheep. *J. Clin. Invest.* 72:63–76, 1983.
90. Snapper, J., Bernard, G., Hinson, J., et al.: Endotoxemia induced leukopenia in sheep: Correlation with lung vascular permeability and hypoxemia but not with pulmonary hypertension. *Am. Rev. Respir. Dis.* 127:306–309, 1983.
91. Staub, N.C.: Pulmonary edema due to increased microvascular permeability to fluid and protein. *Circ. Res.* 43:143–152, 1978.
92. Stenmark, K.R., James, S.L., Voekel, N.F., et al.: Leukotrienes C_4 and D_4 in neonates with hypoxemia and pulmonary hypertension. *N. Engl. J. Med.* 309: 77–80, 1983.
93. Tate, R.M. and Repine, J.E.: Neutrophils and the adult respiratory syndrome. *Am. Rev. Respir. Dis.* 128:552–561, 1983.
94. Tatum, J., Burke, S., Sugerman, H., et al.: Computerized scintigraphic techniques for the evaluation of adult respiratory distress syndrome: Initial clinical trials. *Nucl. Med.* 143:237–242, 1982.
95. Taylor, A.E., Parker, J.C., Kvietys, P.R., et al.: The pulmonary interstitium in capillary exchange. *Ann. NY Acad. Sci.* 384:146–166, 1982.
96. Teplitz, C.: The pathology of burns and the fundamentals of burn wound sepsis. In *Burns: A Team Approach.* Artz, C., Moncrief, C., Pruitt, B., eds. Philadelphia, PA, W.B. Saunders, 1979, pp. 45–94.
97. Vaage, J.: Intravascular platelet aggregation and acute respiratory insufficiency. *Circ. Shock* 4:279–290, 1977.
98. Vito, L., Dennis, R., Weisel, R., et al.: Sepsis presenting as acute respiratory insufficiency. *Surg. Gynecol. Obstet.* 138:896–901, 1974.
99. Voekel, N.F., Worthen, G.S., Reeves, J.M., et al.: Platelet activating factor causes leukotriene production in rat lungs. *Science* 218:286–287, 1982.
100. Wagensteen, D., Yankovich, R., Hoidal, J., et al.: Bleomycin-induced changes in pulmonary microvascular albumin permeability and extravascular albumin space. *Am. Rev. Respir. Dis.* 127:204–208, 1983.
101. Webster, R.P., Tarsen, G., Mitchell, B., et al.: Absence of inflammatory lung in-

jury in rabbits challenged intravascularly with complement-derived chemotactic factors. *Am. Rev. Respir. Dis.* 125:335–343, 1982.

102. Westrick, S. and Chatelet, D.: Generation of chemiluminescence by human neutrophils exposed to soluble stimuli of oxidative metabolism. *Infect. Immunol.* 30:385–392, 1980.

103. Williams, T.J. and Piper, P.J.: The action of chemically pure SRS-A on the micro-circulation in vivo. *Prostaglandins* 19:779, 1980.

104. Wong, C., Flynn, J., and Demling, R.H.: Role of oxygen radicals in endotoxin-induced lung injury. *Arch. Surg.* 119:77–83, 1984.

105. Wong, C., Huval, W., Hechtman, H., et al.: Effect of hemorrhagic shock on endotoxin-induced pulmonary hypertension and increased vascular permeability in unanesthetized sheep. *Circ. Shock* 12:61–72, 1984.

106. Worthen, G.S., Goins, A.J., Mitchell, B.C., et al.: Platelet activating factor causes neutrophil accumulation and edema in rabbit lungs. *Chest* 83:13–15, 1983.

107. Yasaka, T., Ohya, T., and Matsumoto, J.: Acceleration of lipid peroxidation in human paraquat poisoning. *Arch. Int. Med.* 141:1169–1172, 1981.

108. Zaiss, C.P., Misra, H.P., and Demling, R.H.: Chemiluminescence monitoring of endotoxin-induced lung injury. *Fed. Proc.* 41:3768, 1982.

109. Zimmerman, G.A., Renzetti, A.D., and Hill, H.R.: Functional and metabolic activity of granulocytes from patients with adult respiratory distress syndrome. *Am. Rev. Respir. Dis.* 127:290–300, 1983.

CHAPTER 20

Mediators of Pulmonary Vascular Injury and Edema After Thrombin

Asrar B. Malik

Introduction

This review summarizes our recent data concerning the mechanisms of the pulmonary vascular injury and pulmonary edema after thrombin-induced intravascular coagulation. I will discuss the roles of several blood components (i.e., fibrinogen, platelets, and granulocytes) in mediating the lung vascular injury after thrombin and also the interactions among these components and how these might influence the injury process.

We have chosen to examine specifically the pulmonary consequences of thrombin because it produces increased lung vascular permeability and pulmonary edema as well as arterial hypoxemia.[15] Moreover, these changes in lung fluid balance and gas exchange are associated with the well-described effects of thrombin on various blood components, the most prominent being the clotting of fibrinogen and its conversion to fibrin.

Effects of Thrombin on the Pulmonary Microvasculature

Morphological Alterations

There are fairly uniform pulmonary morphological changes following thrombin-induced intravascular coagulation in species (dogs and sheep) that have been studied.[15,23] Polymerized fibrin is present in pulmonary vessels up to 500 μm in diameter after infusion of α-thrombin (i.e., the native enzyme) (Fig. 1). Vessels are often partially occluded with fibrin, and thus allow some blood flow even to these regions. Fibrin is usually not present in larger vessels (>500 μm) but appears to be evenly distributed in small pulmonary arteries and veins. The amount of fibrin in the lungs decreases within 3 hours following

Supported in part by NIH HL-17355 and HL-26551.
From Said, S.I. (ed.): *The Pulmonary Circulation and Acute Lung Injury*. Mount Kisco, N.Y., Futura Publishing Co., Inc., 1985.

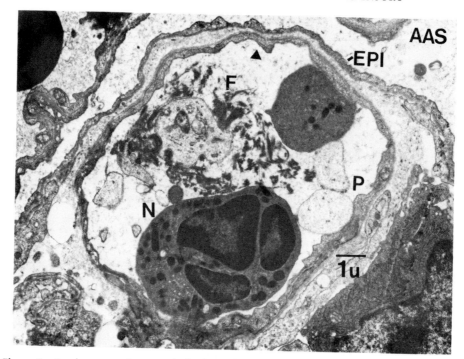

Figure 1: *A pulmonary microvessel of a sheep showing deposition of fibrillar protein (fibrin, F), degranulated platelets (P), and a marginated neutrophil (N) with granules at edge of the cell at 30 minutes after α-thrombin injection. The endothelium (arrowhead) appears normal and intact. Edema fluid is present in the perivascular interstitial space. Micrograph courtesy of Dr. F.L. Minnear.*

thrombin infusion (Fig. 2), probably reflecting the high plasminogen activity of endothelial cells.[19] Other agents that induce pulmonary microembolism, such as air, do not cause fibrin entrapment;[15] therefore, air-induced pulmonary microembolism is not a suitable model for studying the mechanisms of pulmonary edema after intravascular coagulation.

Platelets and neutrophils are also trapped in the pulmonary microcirculation after intravascular coagulation induced by α-thrombin (Fig. 1). The neutrophil sequestration in the lungs is transient occurring within 30 minutes to 3 hours after thrombin infusion (Fig. 2). Neutrophils are found close to the fibrin deposits and are often in end-stages of degranulation (Fig. 1). Fibrin may provide a "sticky" environment for neutrophil adherence or neutrophils may be drawn to the microthrombi by chemotaxins such as complement-derived peptides released during the processes of intravascular coagulation and fibrinolysis.[26] Platelet aggregation occurs early after thrombin infusion and there is clear evidence of degranulation (Fig. 1).

From these morphological observations, it is apparent that α-thrombin infusion induces a series of events that include intravascular coagulation and sequestration of neutrophils and platelets in pulmonary microvessels. A discussion follows of the importance of the interactions among these blood components in the development of lung vascular injury and pulmonary edema.

Species differences must be noted in the morphological alterations. Intersti-

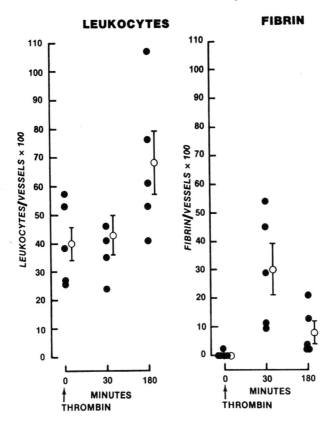

Figure 2: *Evaluation of fibrin and neutrophils in lungs of sheep after α-infusion. These are pulmonary vessels <500 μm in diameter. The uptake of fibrin is transient and there are increased numbers of neutrophils with time after thrombin.*

tial fibrin has been observed in dogs infused with thrombin and in patients with acute lung injury,[17,23] but this was not confirmed in the sheep lung. Interstitial fibrin, if present, may have consequences in the clearance of edema fluid by the lymphatic system in the lung.[25] In addition, even though interstitial and alveolar edema are present as early as 30 minutes after α-thrombin-induced intravascular coagulation, discrete endothelial lesions near the emboli as described after air embolism[15] are rarely seen. The increased fluid and protein fluxes in sheep after thrombin may result from increased endothelial junction "pore" dimensions rather than gross endothelial injury. In dog lungs, however, large interendothelial gaps developed after thrombin (Fig. 3); these may be the pathways of increased transvascular fluid and protein exudation that has been observed in this species.[16]

Effects of Thrombin on Hematological Parameters

Intravenous infusion of α-thrombin results in a rapid decrease in the arterial fibrinogen concentration presumably reflecting the conversion of fibrino-

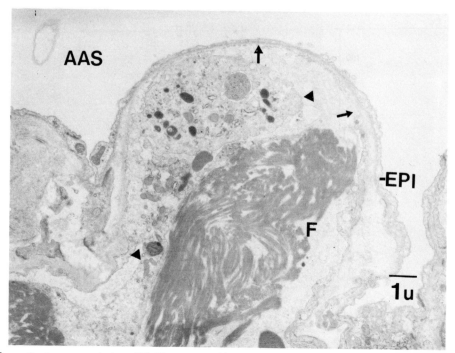

Figure 3: *An accumulation of fibrillar protein (fibrin, F) in a pulmonary microvessel of a dog that shows localized swelling (arrowheads) and degeneration (arrows) of the endothelium at 3 hours after α-thrombin injection. AAS = alveolar air space; EPI = type I alveolar epithelium. Magnification, × 7,300. Micrograph courtesy of Dr. F.L. Minnear.*

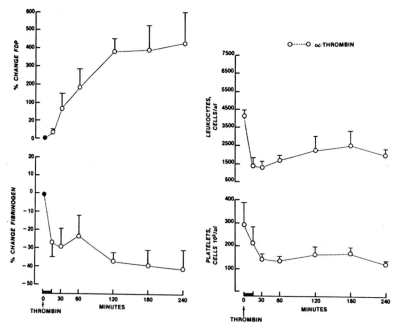

Figure 4: *Changes in the blood hematological parameters after α-thrombin infusion in sheep.*

gen to fibrin. In addition, there are characteristic rapid decreases in the arterial platelet and leukocyte counts (Fig. 4). Platelets are aggregated and activated in response to α-thrombin, which is a primary platelet-stimulating agent.[5] The rapid consumption of leukocytes is more difficult to explain. Thrombin may contribute directly to sequestration of leukocytes in the vascular bed because of the recently described chemotactic (Bizios et al., unpublished observation) and neutrophil-aggregating (Fenton et al., unpublished observation) properties of thrombin. Thrombin may also induce neutrophil sequestration by the release of aggregating substances (e.g., low molecular weight fibrin degradation products and complement-derived peptides[23] during the activation of clotting and fibrinolytic cascades.

The fibrinolytic pathway is clearly activated after thrombin infusion as evident by the generation of fibrin degradation products (Fig. 4). The fibrinolytic activation is delayed, indicating that it is secondary to fibrin deposition in the pulmonary microvessels. The activation of the fibrinolytic pathway has implications in the development of lung vascular injury as a result of the edemagenic effect of products released during the activation.[15]

Effects of Thrombin on Pulmonary Hemodynamics and Lung Fluid Balance

Intravenous infusion over 15 to 30 minutes of α-thrombin increases pulmonary vascular permeability to proteins in dogs and sheep.[14,16] Macromolecule permeability is used as a measure of vascular injury in animals, which morphologically may be the result of discrete endothelial cell membrane injury or alterations in interendothelial "pore" radius (e.g., "gap" formations).

The response in an anesthetized sheep to α-thrombin infusion is shown in Figure 5 (α-thrombin dosage of 100 clotting units per kg body weight). This dosage is physiological since thrombin concentration in blood is calculated to be 2 units/ml, which can occur locally during activation of the coagulation cascade.[5] Thrombin produced increases in pulmonary arterial pressure and pulmonary vascular resistance (PVR) (Fig. 5). Although not shown in this example, both parameters can remain elevated for up to several hours and then gradually decrease toward baseline. These hemodynamic changes reflect a decrease in the vascular cross-sectional area caused by vascular obstruction and the release of pulmonary vasoconstrictor substances secondary to intravascular coagulation, platelet aggregation, and leukostasis.[15]

The hemodynamic changes are associated with a large increase in pulmonary lymph flow (Q̇lym), reflecting an increase in the net transcapillary fluid filtration rate (i.e., the difference between fluid filtration and absorption). In addition, the lymph-to-plasma total protein concentration (L/P) ratio (a measure of the porosity of the capillary barrier) is elevated (Fig. 5), resulting in a marked increase in transvascular protein clearance (Q̇lym × L/P ratio). The elevated protein clearance in the face of mildly elevated pulmonary arterial pressure suggests that the increased protein transport is not due solely to a rise in pulmonary capillary pressure. An increase in permeability of pulmonary microvessels induced by thrombin is a likely explanation of the data. As proof of this, we have shown that increasing pulmonary capillary pressure (Pc) by inflating a balloon positioned in the left atrium after thrombin further increased Q̇lym, but the lymph protein concentration did not change from baseline (Fig. 6). This occurs if the pulmonary vascular permeability to proteins is increased.[25] A similar rise in Pc in the normal lung increases Q̇lym but

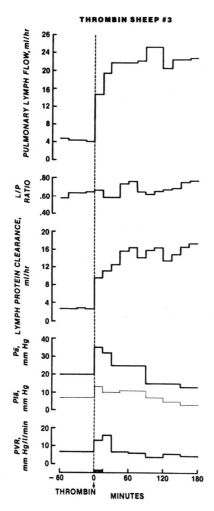

Figure 5: *The time course of changes in pulmonary arterial pressure ($P_{\overline{pa}}$), pulmonary vascular resistance (PVR), pulmonary lymph flow, lymph/plasma protein concentration ratio (L/P), and lymph protein clearance following α-thrombin in a sheep.*

decreases the lymph protein concentration (Fig. 6), a result that would be expected in hydrostatic edema because of ultrafiltration of protein-poor fluid.

In the dog, the approach to assessing lung vascular permeability has been to measure the protein reflection coefficient (σd) of pulmonary microvessels,[28] a measure of permeability. The normal σd in the dog lung is 0.72 (σd of 1 indicates that the microvascular barrier is impermeable to proteins and σd of 0 indicates that it is freely permeable to proteins).[28] After thrombin-induced intravascular coagulation, σd decreased to 0.48,[16] indicating an increased permeability. Pulmonary microembolism is associated with increased permeability in all species that have been examined, unlike other models of lung vascular injury, such as endotoxin,[3] in which the changes in lung vascular permeability are variable.[28]

It is important to note that the pulmonary edema that occurs with intravascular coagulation is the result of both increased vascular permeability and increased Pc.[23] Pc can increase if the pressure rise in the pulmonary arteries that occurs after microembolism is transmitted to the fluid-exchanging pulmo-

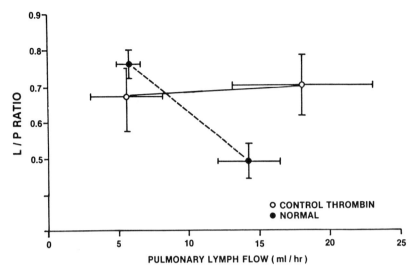

Figure 6: *The relationship between the increase in pulmonary lymph flow induced by left atrial hypertension after inflation of a left atrial balloon and the lymph-to-plasma protein concentration ratio. The studies were made in normal sheep and sheep challenged with α-thrombin.*

nary microvessels. If Pc increases in vessels with increased permeability, the net fluid filtration rate will be greatly enhanced.[15,28] This is explained by the Starling-Landis equation, because the rise in interstitial oncotic pressure (πi) (resulting from the increased protein permeation) produces a greater increase in filtration pressure (i.e., Pc + πi) than in the normal lung. Therefore, for a given increase in Pc, the extravascular water accumulation in the thrombin-embolized lung is expected to be greater than in the normal lung.

Dosage-Related Responses

The pulmonary lymph response is dependent on the dosage of α-thrombin (Fig. 7). This incremental response may result from dose-dependent increases in lung vascular permeability since it was associated with similar increases in pulmonary arterial pressure. The importance of this finding is that it may be possible to activate to different degrees the cellular and humoral mechanisms that are believed to mediate the response.[15] The dose-dependent response also has implications in design of experiments because it necessitates that fluid filtration and permeability changes be assessed at similar thrombin dosages. The studies described here dealing with mechanisms of lung vascular injury by thrombin were made at comparable thrombin dosages.

Response in Awake Sheep

Some interesting differences exist in the pulmonary vascular response to thrombin-induced intravascular coagulation between halothane-anesthetized acutely prepared sheep and the chronically instrumented awake animals. These

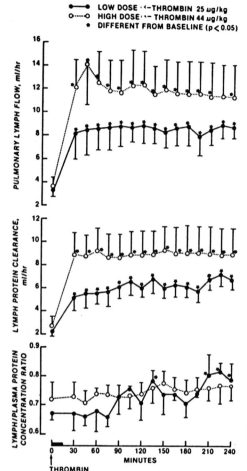

Figure 7: *Pulmonary lymph flow, lymph/ plasma protein concentration ratio, and lymph protein clearance and after low dose (22 µg/ kg) and high dose (44 µg/kg) α-thrombin infusion.*

differences may have a bearing in understanding the mechanism of the response. The same dosage of α-thrombin (110 U/kg body weight) that induces sustained increases in pulmonary arterial pressure and PVR in the anesthetized acutely prepared animal resulted in only transient responses in the awake animal (Fig. 8a). This may be explained by depression of fibrinolysis that occurs during surgical trauma and anesthesia.[23] Because the fibrinolytic capacity of these lungs is reduced, the vascular obstruction may be prolonged, resulting in a more sustained hemodynamic response. Pretreatment of awake sheep with tranexamic acid to partially inhibit fibrinolysis (i.e., to simulate the acutely prepared sheep) caused sustained increases in pulmonary arterial pressure and PVR; therefore, the differences in the fibrinolytic cascade between awake and anesthetized animals appear to be responsible for the different hemodynamic responses.

Qlym and transvascular protein clearance were also increased markedly for up to 10 hours after thrombin in the awake fibrinolysis-depressed as in the acutely prepared sheep, whereas the response was transient in the un-

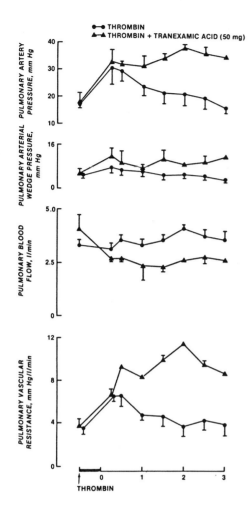

Figure 8a: *The pulmonary hemodynamic response to α-thrombin challenge in the awake sheep. One group received only thrombin and the other group received tranexamic acid to depress fibrinolysis prior to the thrombin infusion.*

treated awake sheep (Fig. 8b). These findings indicate that fibrinolytic activity is an important modulator of the increases in both pulmonary vascular resistance and pulmonary vascular permeability after intravascular coagulation. The prolongation of microthrombi in the pulmonary circulation as regulated by the fibrinolytic activity appears to be an important determinant of lung vascular injury.

Essential Role of Intravascular Coagulation in the Responses

Intravascular coagulation is necessary for the expression of the pulmonary hemodynamic and lymph responses associated with α-thrombin. The role of intravascular coagulation has been examined using the γ-thrombin molecule, which is a modified form of the enzyme. α-thrombin is the native enzyme with the fibrinogen recognition site and fibrinogen clotting activity as well as other known functions, platelet aggregation, and leukocyte chemotaxis.[5] In contrast,

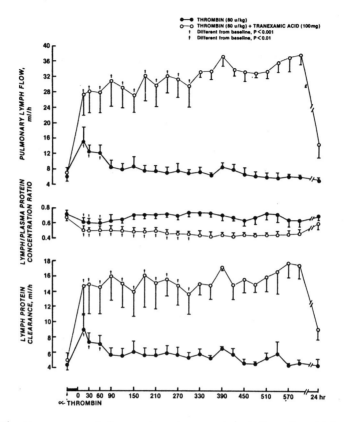

Figure 8b: *The time course of changes in pulmonary lymph flow, lymph/plasma protein concentration ratio, and transvascular protein clearance following α-thrombin challenge in awake sheep. A small amount of tranexamic acid was injected in the second group to depress the fibrinolysis.*

γ-thrombin, which is formed in vivo by autoproteolysis or in vitro by limited trypsin digestion of α-thrombin,[5] lacks the fibrinogen recognition site and clotting activity but retains the other thrombin-ascribed activities (Table I), although platelet aggregation and activation are an order of magnitude less for γ-thrombin.[15] The marked loss of fibrinogen clotting in γ-thrombin is attributable to destruction of the fibrinogen recognition site on the "fibrin side" of the catalytic site.[5] However, both forms of thrombin maintain their ability to cleave synthetic substrates and are inactivated by antithrombin III.[5] We exploited these biochemical differences to delineate the mechanisms of action of α-thrombin on the hematological parameters and the pulmonary circulation.

The biochemical properties of α- and γ-thrombin are reflected in their abilities to change the blood concentrations of platelets, leukocytes, and fibrinogen. Arterial fibrinogen concentration decreased markedly after infusion of α-thrombin, whereas the decrease was small after γ-thrombin (Fig. 9a). The lack of fibrinogen consumption is also reflected in the finding that concentration of fibrin degradation products increased after α-thrombin but not after γ-thrombin. The decrease in arterial platelet count after infusion of α-thrombin

Table I
Relative Activities of Human α- and
γ-Thrombins

Activity	α/γ-Ratio
Synthetic substrate cleavage	1
Antithrombin III inactivation	1
Factor XIII activation	<10
Platelet stimulatory	10
Fibrinogen clotting	3,000

was marked in contrast to the transient decrease after γ-thrombin (Fig. 9a), again reflecting the structural differences (Table I). The decrease in the arterial leukocyte count was greater after α-thrombin than after γ-thrombin (Fig. 9a). This does not conform to the in vitro data because both α- and γ-thrombin have similar chemotactic activities for sheep neutrophils with maximal chemotaxis on agarose plates at concentrations of 10^{-8}M (Bizios et al., unpublished observation) and similar neutrophil aggregatory activities (Fenton et al., unpublished observation). The different leukocyte consumption between α- and γ-thrombin may be related to differences in platelet aggregatory and fibrinogen clotting abilities between the two thrombin forms, i.e., greater intravascular

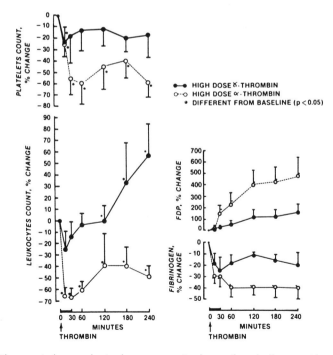

Figure 9a: *Changes in hematological parameters in sheep after challenge with α-thrombin and γ-thrombin infused at similar dosages.*

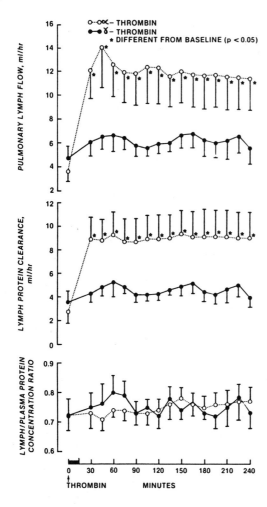

Figure 9b: *Pulmonary lymph flow, lymph/plasma protein concentration ratio, and lymph protein clearance after infusion of α-thrombin and γ-thrombin.*

coagulation and/or platelet aggregation occurring in vivo after α-thrombin may result in secondary generation of leukocyte-aggregating agent(s).

Infusion of γ-thrombin is not followed by increases in Qlym and transvascular protein clearance as is the case with α-thrombin (Fig. 9b), indicating that intravascular coagulation is required for increased lung vascular permeability response. Moreover, pulmonary arterial pressure and PVR did not increase appreciably after γ-thrombin, indicating that intravascular coagulation was also responsible for the hemodynamic changes associated with α-thrombin.

Role of Specific Blood Components in Thrombin-Induced Lung Vascular Injury

Fibrin

The contribution of fibrin was examined by fibrinogen depletion studies in sheep using Ancrod, a purified fraction of Malayan pit viper venom.[1,10] Chronic administration of this fraction resulted in plasma fibrinogen concentrations close to zero.[11] Administration of α-thrombin in these animals decreased the platelet count,[1] indicating that platelets aggregated in response to the thrombin. However, the leukocyte count did not decrease,[11] suggesting that leukocyte consumption is secondary to activation of the coagulation cascade and not to platelet aggregation as inferred from the above γ-thrombin study. The processes of intravascular coagulation and fibrinolysis may release leukocyte-aggregating agent(s), which may in turn be important to the development of lung vascular injury.

Pulmonary arterial pressure and PVR did not increase significantly after thrombin infusion in the defibrinogenated animals[11] (Fig. 10a); thus, pulmonary hypertension and increased PVR are probably also related to intravascular coagulation. Intravascular coagulation may induce these hemodynamic changes by partial obstruction of the pulmonary vascular bed with microthrombi and/or release of vasoactive humoral mediators such as thromboxane A_2 and serotonin from the lung mast cells, macrophages, and the sequestered neutrophils.[15,22,23]

Defibrinogenation (as with the γ-thrombin) prevented the thrombin-induced increases in Q̇lym and transvascular protein clearance[11] (Fig. 10b). Moreover, increasing Pc by inflation of left atrial balloon to test for an increase in lung vascular permeability resulted in a further increase in Q̇lym

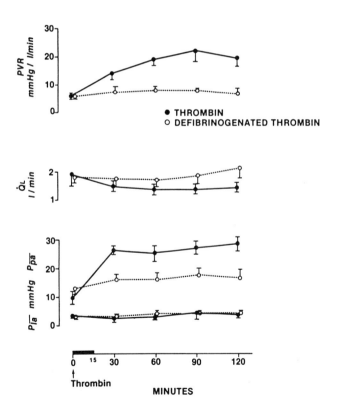

Figure 10a: *Pulmonary vascular resistance (PVR), pulmonary blood flow (Q̇$_L$), mean pulmonary arterial pressure (P$_{\overline{pa}}$), and mean left atrial pressure (P$_{\overline{la}}$) following α-thrombin infusion in control and defibrinogenated sheep.*

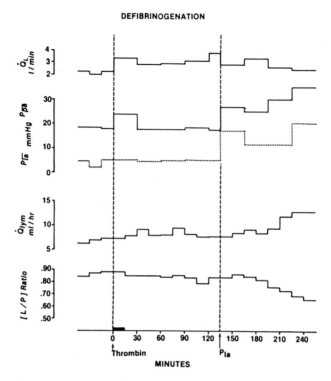

Figure 10b: *Pulmonary lymph flow (Q̇lym), lymph/plasma protein concentration ratio (L/P), pulmonary blood flow (Q̇_L), mean pulmonary arterial pressure (P_p̄a), and mean left atrial pressure (P_l̄a) following α-thrombin infusion in a defibrinogenated sheep. Note the effects of left atrial hypertension.*

and a decrease in L/P ratio (Fig. 10b), indicating that sieving properties of the pulmonary microvasculature remained normal despite α-thrombin infusion.[11] In the control thrombin group, however, the increase in Q̇lym after an elevation in Pc is associated with no change in L/P ratio.[11] This study indicates that thrombin causes the increase in lung vascular permeability by the initial step of converting fibrinogen to fibrin.

Leukocytes

The infusion of α-thrombin into sheep made neutropenic using hydroxy-urea (neutrophil count was 200 cells/ml) increased Q̇lym but, notably, the response was less than in controls (Fig. 11a). Moreover, the increased Q̇lym was associated with the decrease in L/P ratio (Fig. 11b), indicating that the increased fluid filtration was the result of elevated Pc and not due to increased permeability. Had there been an increase in vascular permeability in this group, this would have resulted in an unchanged or even higher L/P ratio during the increase in Q̇lym.

The increases in Q̇lym and protein clearance after α-thrombin were also

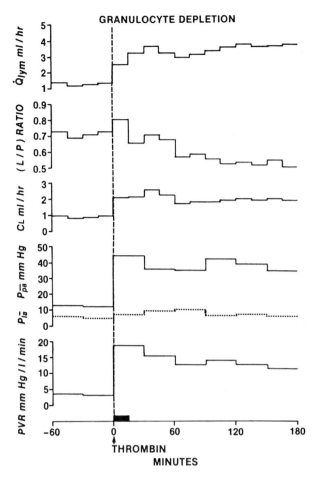

GRANULOCYTE DEPLETION

$\dot{Q}_{lym}$ ml / hr

(L / P) RATIO

C_L ml / hr

$P_{\overline{pa}}$ mm Hg

$P_{\overline{la}}$

PVR mm Hg / l / min

THROMBIN
MINUTES

Figure 11a: *Pulmonary lymph flow ($\dot{Q}$lym), lymph/plasma protein concentration ratio (L/P), lymph protein clearance (C_L), mean pulmonary arterial pressure ($P_{\overline{pa}}$), left atrial pressure ($P_{\overline{la}}$), and pulmonary vascular resistance (PVR) following α-thrombin infusion in a sheep made neutropenic with hyroxyurea.*

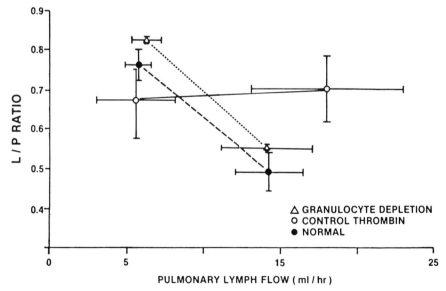

△ GRANULOCYTE DEPLETION
O CONTROL THROMBIN
● NORMAL

PULMONARY LYMPH FLOW (ml / hr)

Figure 11b: *The relationship between pulmonary lymph flow and lymph-to-plasma protein concentration ratio after left atrial hypertension in normal sheep, control sheep challenged with α-thrombin, and neutropenic sheep challenged with α-thrombin.*

attenuated by prior neutrophil depletion induced by sheep antineutrophil serum; therefore, the effects observed with hydroxyurea are not selective to this agent. Neutrophils appear to be the effector cells mediating the increased lung vascular permeability after thrombin-induced microembolism.

The neutrophil uptake kinetics after thrombin have been examined using [111]Indium oxine labeled neutrophils. α-thrombin infusion resulted in an increase in the lung gamma activity (Fig. 12); surprisingly, the increase in lung activity persisted for only 30 minutes. This would suggest that thrombin-induced lung vascular injury is an acute event resulting from transient sequestration of neutrophils. Further studies are needed in this area.

The oxygen radicals generated in the process of neutrophil activation[29] may be the ultimate agents responsible for mediating the lung vascular injury after thrombin. Leukocyte activation is associated with the production of toxic antibactericidal oxygen metabolites, superoxide anion (O_2^-), hydrogen peroxide (H_2O_2), and hydroxyl radical OH·),[4,21] all of which have been implicated in mediating endothelial injury.[15] These reactions are indicated in Figure 13. Enzymes such as superoxide dismutase and catalase are responsible for scavenging these oxygen radicals;[21,29] superoxide dismutase catalyzes the conversion of O_2^- to H_2O_2 and O_2, whereas catalase catalyzes the breakdown of H_2O_2 to H_2O and O_2. The production of these metabolites at the cellular level may overwhelm the scavenging abilities of these enzymes and leave the cell membranes susceptible to oxidant injury.[4]

Oxygen radicals may mediate or contribute to lung vascular injury by at least three mechanisms: direct oxidation damage of lipid membranes,[21] gener-

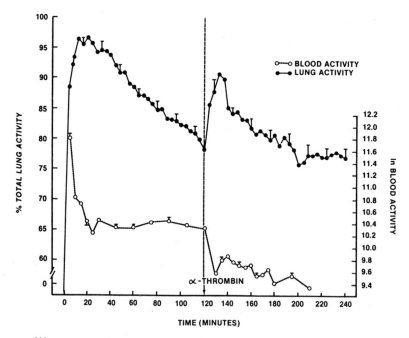

Figure 12: [111]Indium activities over the lung and in blood following injection of [111]Indium oxine labeled neutrophils. α-thrombin was infused at 120 minutes.

$$O_2^- + O_2^- + 2H^+ \xrightarrow{\text{SUPEROXIDE DISMUTASE}} H_2O_2 + O_2 \qquad (1)$$

$$H_2O_2 + H_2O_2 \xrightarrow{\text{CATALASE}} 2H_2O + O_2 \qquad (2)$$

$$H_2O_2 + 2GSH \xrightarrow{\text{PEROXIDASE}} 2H_2O + GSSG \qquad (3)$$

$$O_2^- + H_2O_2 \longrightarrow OH^{\cdot} + OH^- + O_2 \qquad (4)$$

Figure 13: *The major oxygen radical generating and scavenging reactions.*

ation of secondary chemotactic messengers from plasma, which recruit neutrophils into the affected areas,[21,29] and inactivation of antiproteases (i.e., α_1-antitrypsin).[4,21,29]

If O_2^- generation is indeed responsible for lung vascular injury, we reasoned that exogenous administration of superoxide dismutase would reduce the injury by scavenging the locally produced O_2^-. We studied the thrombin response in sheep infused with superoxide dismutase bound to Ficoll to prolong circulating life of the enzyme.[21] The increases in $\dot{Q}$lym and protein clearance were blunted in animals pretreated with superoxide dismutase-Ficoll (Fig. 14); this response was quite similar to that in neutropenic sheep challenged with α-thrombin. Because of the marked protection afforded by scavenging the O_2^- radicals, the results suggest that O_2^- generation (presumably from neutrophils) is an important metabolite producing the increased lung vascular permeability after thrombin. However, the most vasotoxic oxygen radical may be the $OH^{\cdot}$,[4,21,29] which is formed by the combination of H_2O_2 and O_2^- (Haber-Weiss reaction) (Fig. 13). The protective effect observed with superoxide dismutase-Ficoll may well be due to removal of O_2^- substrate from this reaction.

Platelets

Depletion of platelets (to a circulating count of less than 10,000 cells/μl) did not prevent the permeability increase after α-thrombin.[27] Infusion of thrombin into the platelet-depleted animals resulted in an increase in $\dot{Q}$lym (although it was less than the control group) and an increase in L/P ratio[27]

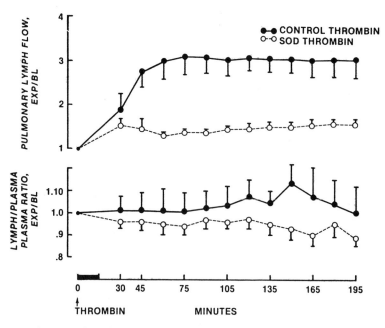

Figure 14: *Pulmonary lymph flow and lymph-plasma protein concentration ratio after α-thrombin challenge in control and superoxide dismutase-pretreated groups.*

(Fig. 15a). Moreover, raising Pc by inflating a left atrial balloon produced a further large increase in Q̇lym and unchanged L/P ratio, indicating increased protein sieving[27] (Fig. 15b).

Although platelet depletion did not prevent the permeability increase after thrombin, it did result in a smaller increase in Q̇lym.[27] A possible mechanism of this response is that the release of pulmonary vasoactive mediators such as thromboxane A_2 and serotonin would be less in the platelet-depleted animals, and thus Pc may not increase to the same extent as in normal lungs. By this means, it is possible that platelet aggregation contributes to pulmonary edema by increasing Pc.

Mechanisms of Neutrophil Sequestration and Activation After Thrombin

Since both thrombin and neutrophils are implicated in increasing lung vascular permeability after thrombin-induced intravascular coagulation, it is important to understand how fibrin and neutrophils interact in mediating this response. The following section discusses some of these interactions.

Plasminogen-Plasmin System

The role of plasminogen-plasmin system (i.e., fibrinolytic pathway) has been examined in animals by inhibiting plasminogen activation using tran-

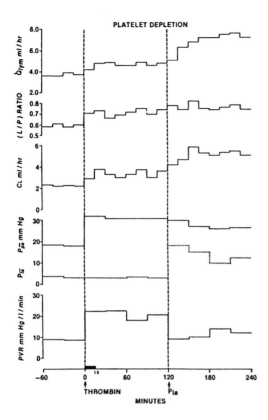

Figure 15a: *Pulmonary lymph flow (Q̇lym) lymph/plasma protein concentration ratio (L/P), transvascular protein clearance (C$_L$), mean pulmonary pressure (P$_{\overline{pa}}$), mean left atrial pressure (P$_{la}$), and pulmonary vascular resistance (PVR) after α-thrombin challenge in a thrombocytopenic sheep.*

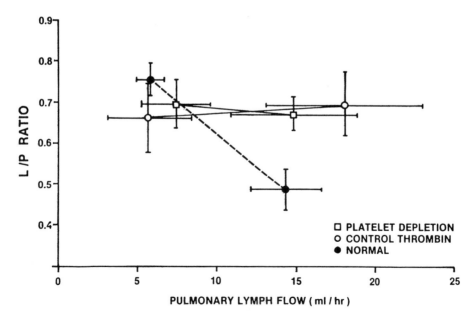

Figure 15b: *Pulmonary lymph flow versus the lymph/plasma protein concentration ratio (L/P) after left atrial hypertension in normal, control-thrombin, and platelet-depleted thrombin groups.*

examic acid, a substance that binds to tissue plasminogen activator and prevents the conversion of plasminogen to plasmin.[11,19] The hypothesis of this particular series of studies[11] was that plasmin generation (a potent serine protease) may contribute to the neutrophil-dependent increase in lung vascular permeability after thrombin by inducing the release of leukocyte-aggregating and -stimulating substances.

The concentration of fibrin degradation products did not increase in tranexamic acid-treated animals following α-thrombin infusion despite evidence of fibrinogen consumption[11] (Fig. 16a), indicating the effectiveness of fibrinolytic inhibition. The increase in $\dot{Q}$lym in these sheep after α-thrombin was delayed and, importantly, was associated with a decrease in L/P ratio[11] (Fig. 16b). Raising Pc resulted in a further increase in $\dot{Q}$lym and a further decrease in L/P ratio,[11] comparable to that seen in the normal lungs, suggesting that fibrinolysis inhibition was protective. This study suggests that fibrinolysis activation is required for the increase in lung vascular permeability after thrombin.

The fibrinolytic pathway may exert its deleterious effect via formation of fibrin degradation products[11,23] and/or by activation of other pathways such as the complement system.[12,23] Both fibrin degradation products and the complement-derived peptides have chemotactic and leukocyte aggregation properties.[19,26]

Interestingly, the leukocyte count in the tranexamic acid group did not decrease after thrombin as in the control group[11] (Fig. 16a), suggesting that somehow fibrinolytic inhibition prevented the neutrophil sequestration in the lung. This was confirmed by the observation that fibrinolytic inhibition abrogated the pulmonary uptake of [111]Indium oxine labeled neutrophils after α-thrombin infusion (Fig. 17). The effect of fibrinolytic inhibition in preventing the thrombin-induced lung vascular injury may be secondary to inhibition of pulmonary leukocyte sequestration. These studies point to an interaction between fibrinolytic activation and neutrophil sequestration in the lung.

Complement Activation

The activation of fibrinolysis may induce neutrophil sequestration through the activation of the complement system, which has been proposed as a key pathway in inducing lung vascular injury.[15] Generation of plasmin results in cleavage of complement proteins and formation of the complement-derived chemotactic and leukocyte-aggregating peptides, C3a and C5a.[18,22,26]

We examined the functional role of the complement system in sheep in thrombin-induced lung vascular injury by depleting the hemolytic complement activity to below 30% baseline by administration for several days of a phospholipase A_2-free cobra venom factor fraction.[9,18] α-thrombin infusion resulted in a transient increase in $\dot{Q}$lym and a decrease in the L/P ratio (Fig. 18), a response similar to that observed in neutropenic sheep. The protective effect of complement depletion may be the result of failure or reduction in neutrophil sequestration in the lungs. This is supported by the observation that the leukocyte count did not decrease markedly after α-thrombin infusion in the decomplemented sheep.[9]

In addition to plasmin-induced complement activation, the thrombin molecule has an independent complement-like activity.[8,31] Once activated,

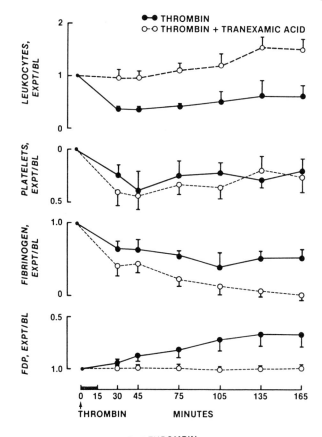

Figure 16a: *Leukocyte, platelet, fibrinogen, and fibrin degradation product (FDP) levels after α-thrombin infusion in the control sheep challenged with thrombin and fibrinolysis-inhibited sheep (tranexamic acid-treated) challenged with thrombin.*

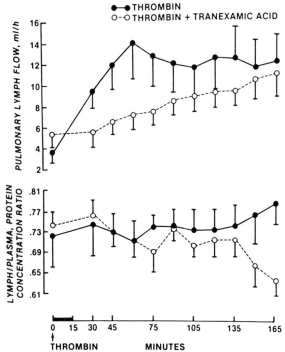

Figure 16b: *Pulmonary lymph flow and lymph/plasma protein concentration ratio after α-thrombin challenge in control sheep and fibrinolysis-inhibited sheep.*

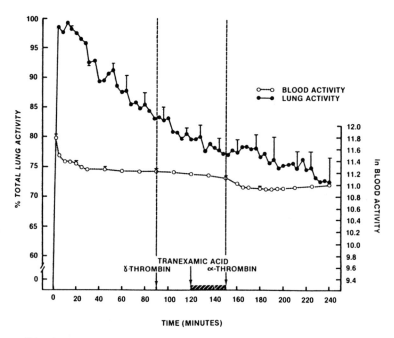

Figure 17: ^{111}Indium activities over the lung and in blood following injection of ^{111}Indium oxine labeled neutrohils. Note that γ-thrombin (unlike α-thrombin in Fig. 12) had no effect on neutrophil uptake. Also, fibrinolysis inhibition with tranexamic acid prevented the neutrophil uptake after injection of α-thrombin at 150 minutes.

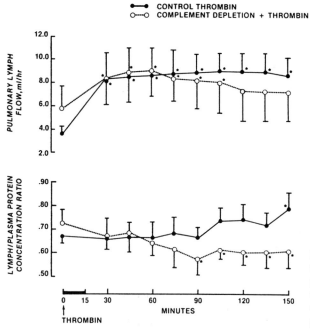

Figure 18: Alterations in pulmonary lymph flow and lymph/plasma protein concentration ratio after α-thrombin challenge in the control and decomplemented groups.

α-thrombin becomes entrapped in the fibrin clot where it is retained or degrades into nonclotting thrombin forms. The generation of plasmin releases the entrapped thrombin forms.[8,31] Both α- and γ-thrombins are known to have factor D activity in the alternate complement pathway,[5] which may augment complement-dependent processes.

The basis for leukocyte aggregation and activation after thrombin-induced intravascular coagulation is probably more complex than complement activation per se, because complement activation in vivo does not produce consistent or marked increases in lung vascular permeability. Leukocyte aggregation and activation after thrombin-induced intravascular coagulation also likely involves other important mediators, such as fibrin degradation products,[23] leukotriene B$_4$,[2,24] and platelet activating factor,[13,30] whose roles in inducing lung vascular injury is not well defined.

Direct Thrombin Effects

The thrombin molecule is a recently described chemotactic agent (Bizios et al., unpublished observation) and has been shown to induce neutrophil aggregation (Fenton et al., unpublished observation). Thus, the generation of α- thrombin may directly contribute to pulmonary leukostasis and play a part in the neutrophil-dependent lung vascular injury.

Conclusions

Figure 19 summarizes the pivotal role of leukocytes in increasing lung vascular permeability after thrombin. The leukocyte count decreases immedi-

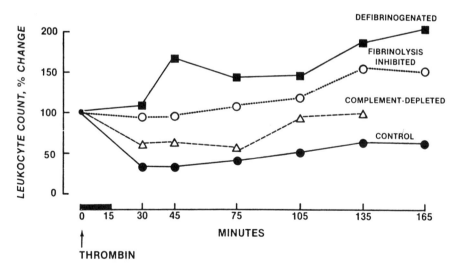

Figure 19: *Changes in leukocyte counts in the control and the treated groups showing prevention of the permeability-increase response.*

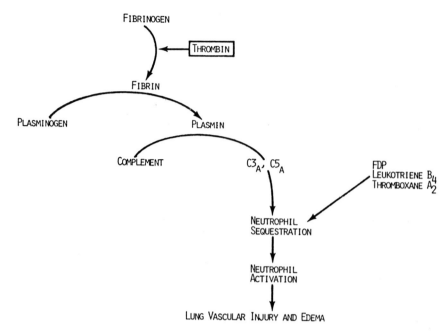

Figure 20: *Hypothesis of the mechanism of lung vascular injury and edema following intravascular coagulation with thrombin.*

ately after thrombin in control sheep, but the decrease is transient or does not occur in groups in which lung vascular permeability did not increase (i.e., neutropenia, complement depletion, and fibrinolytic inhibition groups). Although the initial drop in leukocyte count does not necessarily reflect leukocyte sequestration or activation, the finding does indicate an association between leukocytes and thrombin-induced lung vascular injury.

In the working hypothesis shown in Figure 20, α-thrombin proteolytically converts the clottable fibrinogen to fibrin and deposits fibrin thrombi in pulmonary microvessels. The clots may entrap the residual α-thrombin. Subsequent activation of plasminogen may directly activate the complement system, resulting in the formation of peptides (C3a and C5a), which induce neutrophil sequestration and activation in pulmonary microvessels. Activation of plasminogen also releases thrombin entrapped in clots, which may augment complement activation. In addition, α-thrombin contribute to neutrophil aggregation by direct effects of thrombin. Other factors generated during intravascular coagulation and fibrinolytic activation (e.g., fibrin degradation products, leukotriene B_4, thromboxane A_2, platelet activating factor) may also contribute to neutrophil sequestration and activation. It is clear that neutrophils are the final pathway of lung vascular injury after thrombin.

A greater understanding of the mechanisms of the lung vascular injury resulting from thrombin-induced intravascular coagulation requires the in vivo and in vitro descriptions of interrelationships among the clotting, fibrinolytic, and complement pathways and how these pathways affect neutrophil function.

Acknowledgments

I wish to thank my colleagues and collaborators Drs. Jeffrey Cooper, Arnold Johnson, Fred L. Minnear, Rene Garcia, Siu K. Lo, John Fenton, and Rena Bizios for allowing me to summarize their data. Also, I thank Kathleen Roche for her efforts in typing this manuscript.

REFERENCES

1. Bell, W.R., Shapiro, S.S., Martinez, J., et al.: The effects of Ancrod, the coagulating enzyme from the venom of the Malayan pit viper (A. rhodostoma) on prothrombin and fibrinogen metabolism and fibrin peptide A release in man. *J. Lab. Clin. Med.* 91:592–604, 1978.
2. Bizios, R., Minnear, F.L., van der Zee, H., et al.: Effect of cyclooxygenase and lipoxygenase inhibition on lung fluid balance after thrombin. *J. Appl. Physiol.* 55: 462–471, 1982.
3. Brigham, K.L., Woolverton, W.C., Blake, J.H., et al.: Increased sheep lung vascular permeability caused by Pseudomonas bacteremia. *J. Clin. Invest.* 54:792–804, 1974.
4. Del Maestro, R.F., Thaw, H.H., Bjork, J., et al.: Free radicals as mediators of tissue injury. *Acta Physiol. Scand.* 492:43–57, 1980.
5. Fenton, J.W.: Thrombin specificity. *Ann. N.Y. Acad. Sci.* 370:468–495, 1981.
6. Flick, M.R., Hoeffel, J.M., and Staub, N.C.: Superoxide dismutase combined with heparin prevents increased lung vascular permeability during air microembolism in sheep. *J. Appl. Physiol.* 55:1284–1291, 1983.
7. Flick, M.R., Perel, A., and Staub, N.C.: Leukocytes are required for increased lung vascular permeability after microembolization in sheep. *Circ. Res.* 48:344–351, 1981.
8. Francis, C.W., Markham, R.E., Jr., Barlow, G.H., et al.: Thrombin activity of fibrin thrombi and soluble plasmic derivatives. *J. Lab. Clin. Med.* 102:220–230, 1983.
9. Johnson, A., Blumenstock, F.A., Malik, A.B.: Effect of complement depletion on lung fluid balance after thrombin. *J. Appl. Physiol.* 55:1480–1485, 1983.
10. Johnson, A. and Malik, A.B.: Effect of defibrinogenation on lung fluid and protein exchange after glass bead embolization. *J. Appl. Physiol.* 53:895–900, 1982.
11. Johnson, A., Tahamont, M.V., and Malik, A.B.: Thrombin-induced lung vascular injury: Role of fibrinogen and fibrinolysis. *Am. Rev. Respir. Dis.* 128:38–44, 1983.
12. Johnson, A., Tahamont, M.V., Kaplan, J.E., et al.: Effects of pulmonary embolization induced by thrombin and fibrin microaggregates on lung fluid balance. *J. Appl. Physiol.* 52:1565–1570, 1982.
13. Jin, A.H., Merton, D.R., and Gorman, R.R.: Acetyl glyceryl ether phosphorylcholine stimulates leukotriene B$_4$ synthesis in human polymorphonuclear leukocytes. *J. Clin. Invest.* 70:1058–1065, 1982.
14. Malik, A.B. and van der Zee, H.: Lung vascular permeability following progressive embolization. *J. Appl. Physiol.* 45:590–597, 1978.
15. Malik, A.B.: Pulmonary microembolism. *Physiol. Rev.* 63:1114–1207, 1983.
16. Minnear, F.L., Martin, D., Taylor, A.E., et al.: Large increase in pulmonary lymph flow after thrombin-induced intravascular coagulation. *Fed. Proc.* 42:1274, 1983 (Abstr.).
17. MoCostabella, P.M., Lundquist, O., Kapanci, Y., et al.: Increased vascular permeability in the delayed microembolism syndrome. *Microvasc. Res.* 15:275–286, 1978.
18. Mueller-Eberhard, H.I. and Schreber, R.D.: Molecular biology and chemistry of the alternate pathway of complement. *Adv. Immunol.* 129:1–53, 1980.

19. Mulleretz, J.: The fibrinolytic system. *Scand. J. Haematol.* 34:15–34, 1979.
20. O'Brodovich, H., Andrews, M., and Coates, G.: Assessment of the coagulation cascade during air microembolization of the sheep and dog lung. *Am. Rev. Respir. Dis.* 127:309, 1983 (Abstr.).
21. Petrone, W.F., English, D.K., Wong, K., et al.: Free radicals and inflammation: Superoxide dependent activation of a neutrophil chemotactic factor in plasma. *Proc. Natl. Acad. Sci.* 77:1159–1163, 1980
22. Ryan, G.B.: Inflammation and localization of infection. *Surg. Clin. N. Am.* 56: 831–846, 1976.
23. Saldeen, T.: The microembolism syndrome. In *The Microembolism Syndrome* Saldeen, T., ed. Stockholm, Almquist and Wiksell International, 1979, pp. 7–44.
24. Samuelsson, B.: Leukotrienes: Mediators of immediate hypersensitivity reactions and inflammation. *Science* 220:568–575, 1983.
25. Staub, N.C.: Pulmonary edema. *Physiol. Rev.* 54:678–811, 1974.
26. Stormorhen, H.: Interrelations between the coagulation, fibrinolytic and the kallikrein-kinen system. *Scand. J. Haematol.* (Suppl.) 34:24–27, 1979.
27. Tahamont, M.V. and Malik, A.B.: Granulocytes mediate the increase in pulmonary vascular permeability after thrombin embolism. *J. Appl. Physiol.* 54:1489–1495, 1983.
28. Taylor, A.E., Parker, J.C., Granger, D.N., et al.: Assessment of capillary permeability using lymphatic protein flux: Estimation of the osmotic reflection coefficient. In *The Microcirculation.* Taylor, A.E., ed. New York, Academic Press, 1981, pp. 19–32.
29. Weissman, G., Smolen, J.E., and Korclak, H.M.: Release of inflammatory mediators from stimulated neutrophils. *N. Engl. J. Med.* 303:27–34, 1980.
30. Vaage, J.: Intravascular platelet aggregation and pulmonary injury. *Ann. N.Y. Acad. Sci.* 384:301–318, 1982.
31. Wilner, G.D., Danitz, M.P., Mudd, M.S., et al.: Selective immobilization of α-thrombin by surface-bound fibrin. *J. Lab. Clin. Med.* 97:403–411, 1981.

CHAPTER 21

Prostacyclin as a Modulator of Acute Lung Injury

Takahito Hirose

Introduction

Prostaglandin production has been found to be increased during a number of acute lung injuries. Prostaglandins of the E and F series,[25] as well as thromboxane A_2 and prostacyclin, are released after microembolic[15,23] and endotoxin-induced lung injuries.[8,26] Although it is likely that certain prostaglandins mediate or modify lung damage by their potent effects on hemodynamics and respiratory function, infusions of prostaglandins H_2, E_2, and $F_{2\alpha}$ do not alter lung vascular permeability.[3] Thromboxane A_2, however, may contribute to the increased permeability after thrombin,[15] although it does not mediate lung permeability changes after endotoxin.[42] The pulmonary vasodilator prostaglandin, PGE_1, reduced lung lymph flow by reducing perfused lung microvascular surface area, without changing permeability.[34]

Prostacyclin is a major product of arachidonic acid metabolism generated by vascular endothelium and a strong platelet antiaggregating substance,[1] as well as a strong relaxant of vascular smooth muscle and an inhibitor of thromboxane generation.[18] Prostacyclin also inhibits leukocyte aggregation and lysosomal enzyme release.[31] Thus, prostacyclin could modify or prevent acute lung injury following pulmonary microembolization and endotoxin shock by the interaction with these potential etiologic factors. The present work was undertaken to test this hypothesis in pulmonary microembolization and endotoxin shock in dogs.

Pulmonary Microembolization

Methods

Although the site of pulmonary edema after microembolization is a matter of debate, Lee and associates have reported that edema developed in the non-

From Said, S.I. (ed.): *The Pulmonary Circulation and Acute Lung Injury.* Mount Kisco, N.Y., Futura Publishing Co., Inc., 1985.

embolized as well as the embolized lung regions following unilateral micro-embolization.[30] Based on this report, we measured the filtration coefficient in the nonembolized lung using the gravimetric method after unilateral micro-embolization.

Mongrel dogs of either sex, weighing 12–15 kg, were anesthetized by intravenous administration of sodium pentobarbital (30 mg/kg body weight). Each dog was then intubated and ventilated with a Harvard respirator. We made a thoracotomy on the left side and the hilar tissues of the upper and middle lobes were then tied and the lobe removed. After a paper clip was attached to the ventral surface of the left lower lobe, we tied a string between the paper clip and a force displacement transducer mounted above the lobe to record continuously the changes in lobar weight. The filtration coefficient was estimated according to the method of Drake and associates.[10] The main pulmonary arterial, pulmonary vein, and aortic pressures were recorded using pressure transducers. We calculated microvascular pressure (Pmv) using the equation[14] $Pmv = Pv + 0.5$ $(Ppa - Ppv)$; where Ppa = mean pulmonary artery pressure, and Ppv = mean pulmonary venous pressure. Pulmonary blood flow to the left lower lobe was determined with an electromagnetic flow meter. The concentration of 6-keto $PGF_{1\alpha}$ in arterial blood was measured by radioimmunoassay according to the method of Jaffe and Behrman.[27] The siliconized glass beads, 0.1 g/kg (80–120 μm in diameter), were suspended in normal saline and injected into the right pulmonary artery.

Increase in Hydraulic Conductivity of Pulmonary Exchange Vessels in the Nonembolized Lung

The filtration coefficient (Kf) of nonembolized lobe increased significantly to 0.14 ± 0.02 ml/min/mmHg/100 g of the initial lobe weight from the baseline value of 0.07 ± 0.01 at 30 minutes after microembolization, followed by a decrease to near the baseline value at 60 minutes after infusion of glass beads (Fig. 1). As the filtration coefficient of a membrane is defined as the volume flow rate through the membrane divided by the pressure drop across the membrane, the most dramatic change should occur in the Kf, if permeability edema is a result of damage to the microvascular membrane and an increase in pore size, because Kf varies directly with the fourth power of the pore radius in cylindrical pores.[14] Although the filtration coefficient may vary with the change in effective surface area of microvascular bed, the increase in the filtration coefficient was not associated with any significant change in pulmonary vascular resistance (Table I). There were no significant changes in measured variables over 60-minute periods in dogs that had same operation and experimental procedures, but without infusion of glass beads.

Our results, therefore, could indicate that the vascular permeability of nonembolized lung increased following unilateral microembolization. We did not find any glass beads in suspended nonembolized lobes by digestion with concentrated sulfuric acid after experiment. Since we injected glass beads as a bolus, the increase in filtration coefficient was transient, as has been reported by Vaage and associates,[39] although Flick and associates have observed a sustained increase in vascular permeability following repeated administration of glass beads.[12] Even if the change in vascular permeability was transient or

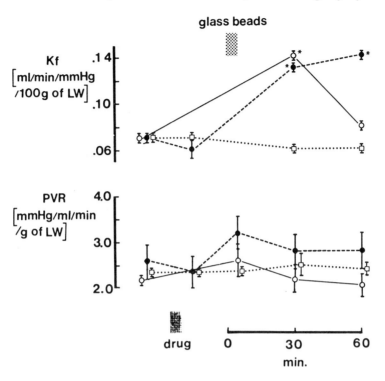

Figure 1: *Effects of unilateral microembolization on the filtration coefficient (Kf), pulmonary vascular resistance (PVR) in the nonembolized lung.* ○————○ = *microembolization alone;* ●————● = *Indomethacin + microembolization;* □·····□ = *PGI₂ methylester + microembolization. Values are mean ± SE;* * = *statistically significant (p < 0.05) compared to the baseline.*

Table I
Changes in Pulmonary Vascular Resistance(PVR), and Filtration Coefficient in Nonembolized Lobes Following Unilateral Pulmonary Microembolization

Group	N	Baseline	After drug infusion	Time after microembolization		
				5 min	30 min	60 min
PVR (mmHg/ml/min/g of the initial lobe weight) in LLL						
I	5	2.2 ± 0.5		2.6 ± 1.2	2.2 ± 0.6	2.1 ± 0.4
II	5	2.6 ± 0.8	2.3 ± 0.8	3.4 ± 0.9	2.8 ± 0.9	2.8 ± 0.9
III	5	2.3 ± 0.1	2.3 ± 0.2	2.3 ± 0.2	2.5 ± 0.4	2.4 ± 0.4
IV	5	2.3 ± 0.1	2.3 ± 0.2	2.4 ± 0.2	2.3 ± 0.1	2.4 ± 0.2
Filtration coefficient (ml/min/mmHg/100g of the initial lobe weight) in LLL						
I	5	0.07 ± 0.01			0.14 ± 0.02*	0.08 ± 0.02
II	5	0.07 ± 0.01	0.06 ± 0.02		0.13 ± 0.01*	0.14 ± 0.01*
III	5	0.07 ± 0.01	0.07 ± 0.01		0.06 ± 0.01	0.06 ± 0.01
IV	5	0.06 ± 0.01	0.06 ± 0.01		0.06 ± 0.01	0.05 ± 0.01

Group I: Microembolization alone; Group II: Indomethacin + Microembolization; Group III: PGI₂ Methylester + Microembolization; Group IV: Mepyramine maleate + Microembolization. LLL = Left lower lobe; N = number of animals. Values are mean ± SD. *Statistically significant by Student's *t*-test compared to the baseline (p < 0.05).

sustained, the mechanisms that initiate increased permeability could be similar.

Release of Prostacyclin into Arterial Blood

The concentration of 6-keto $PGF_{1\alpha}$ in arterial blood increased significantly to 4.15 ± 1.76 at 30 minutes and increased further to 5.76 ± 1.49 at 60 minutes from the baseline value of 1.90 ± 0.45 ng/ml following unilateral microembolization (Fig. 2). Although we could not conclude that prostacyclin was synthesized specifically in the lung in response to microembolization in this study, the pulmonary lymph 6-keto $PGF_{1\alpha}$ concentration increased after thrombin-induced pulmonary microembolization,[15] suggesting that lung tissue was the site of its origin. Since prostacyclin escapes pulmonary inactivation,[18] the increase in arterial concentration could occur by the locally increased synthesis of prostacyclin in response to microembolization.

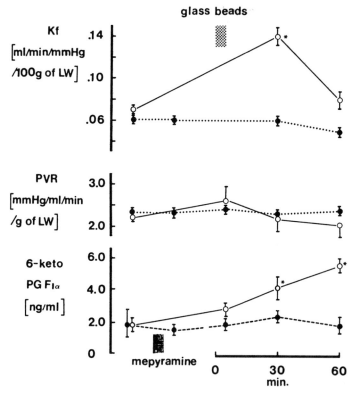

Figure 2: *Effects of mepyramine maleate on the increased filtration coefficient (Kf) in the nonembolized lung and 6-keto PGF₁ₐ in arterial blood following unilateral pulmonary microembolization. PVR = pulmonary vascular resistance in the nonembolized lung; ○———○ = microembolization alone; ●·····● = mepyramine + microembolization. Values are mean ± SE; *statistically significant (p < 0.05) compared to the baseline.*

Platelet Aggregation and Change in Leukocyte Count

The platelet count decreased from the baseline value of $13.3 \pm 3.2 \times 10^4$/cmm to 5.4 ± 1.1 within 5 minutes and increased toward baseline thereafter, although remaining below baseline at 30 minutes after microembolization. The white blood cell count did not change significantly from baseline.

Augmentation of the Increase in Fluid Conductivity by Indomethacin

Compared to a transient increase observed in nontreated animals, the filtration coefficient continued to increase even at 60 minutes following microembolization in dogs pretreated with indomethacin (10 mg/kg) (Fig. 1), although similar hemodynamic responses were observed (Table I). The increase in 6-keto $PGF_{1\alpha}$ in arterial blood was prevented completely and the platelet count did not decrease significantly by pretreatment with indomethacin. The white blood cell count did not change either in this group of animals. Because the inhibition of platelet aggregation by indomethacin was not associated with prevention of increase in the filtration coefficient following microembolization, platelet aggregation may not be essential for microembolic lung injury. Binder and associates were also unable to demonstrate a role for platelet aggregation in mediating lung vascular injury after glass-bead microemboli.[2] The release of thromboxane A_2 and serotonin[24] after platelet aggregation may account for the increase in filtration, but these substances did not increase lung vascular permeability.[5,42] Platelets may serve an augmenting function by trapping leukocytes in the pulmonary microvasculature.[12] Glass-bead microemboli induce intravascular coagulation by activating the Hageman factor, since the bead surface is negatively charged.[33] Intravascular coagulation is not only associated with fibrin entrapment and platelet aggregation, but also with pulmonary leukostasis through complement activation.[43] Further, indomethacin and aspirin increase leukocyte migration.[22] Although the number of circulating leukocytes did not change following microembolization, there was a trend toward an increase in this study. Johnson and Malik have suggested a release of the marginated leukocytes, as well as the reserves in bone marrow into the blood stream after embolization and reported that granulocytopenia prevents the accumulation of extravascular lung water after microembolization.[28]

Thus, an augmented lung vascular injury by indomethacin could indicate that thromboxane generation per se is not responsible for the increase in lung vascular permeability, but some prostaglandins with protective effect might be released following microembolization, although a role for the lipoxygenase pathway could not be ruled out.

Prevention of the Increased Pulmonary Vascular Permeability by the Infusion of PGI$_2$ Methylester

Exogenously administered prostacyclin, PGI_2 methylester (20 ng/kg/min), starting at 1 hour before microembolization to the end of the experiment, prevented the increase in the filtration coefficient following an infusion of glass beads (Fig. 1), although the changes in hemodynamics and blood cell counts were similar to those observed in nontreated animals (Table I). This result could indicate that prostacyclin released following microembolization plays an important role in the prevention of thromboembolic lung injury without its platelet antiaggregating activity. Although the mechanism whereby PGI_2 methylester prevents the increased hydraulic conductivity is not clear, it is unlikely that this effect depends on decreasing microvascular pressure, because hemodynamic responses in treated animals were quite similar to those in nontreated animals. An increase in prostacyclin could prevent the increase in lung vascular permeability by disaggregating leukocytes[4] lodged in the pulmonary microcirculation.

Interaction Between Histamine and Prostacyclin Release

To clarify the mechanisms of release of prostacyclin following microembolization, we investigated the effects of histamine H_1 blocker, mepyramine maleate, on the release of prostacyclin following microembolization, because histamine levels in the pulmonary venous blood were increased after embolization of the lung[36] and prostacyclin is released from the lung by histamine,[19] production of which is stimulated by complement activation after intravascular coagulation.[17] In animals pretreated with 3.0 mg/kg (bolus) + 1.5 mg/kg/h of mepyramine, an increase in 6-keto $PGF_{1\alpha}$ was prevented completely (Fig. 2). Mepyramine maleate also prevented the increase in the filtration coefficient following microembolization, although hemodynamic changes were similar to those in nontreated animals (Table I).

These results could indicate that a locally released endogenous histamine might be responsible for an endogenous release of prostacyclin. Histamine may play a role in the increased pulmonary vascular permeability in pulmonary embolism. Intravenous histamine infusion in sheep increased lung vascular permeability and an H_1-receptor antagonist, dephenhydramine, prevented the increase.[6] Antihistamines also prevented lung vascular injury after FDP infusion.[32] As histamine might be released from the embolized lung regions, histamine-induced released prostacyclin might be transmitted to the non-embolized lobe via bronchial circulation and blood recirculation and prevent the increase in vascular permeability following microembolization.

Endotoxin-Induced Lung Injury

Methods

To test a potential modifying effect of prostacyclin on fluid and solute exchange in the pulmonary vascular bed in endotoxin shock, dogs of either sex, weighing 9.5–24 kg, were anesthetized by intravenous administration of sodium pentobarbital (30 mg/kg body weight). Each animal was then intubated and ventilated with a Harvard respirator. The lung was hyperinflated periodically to prevent atelectasis. To cannulate the right lymph duct reliably, we used the method described by Vreim and associates.[40] Right duct lymph was collected into heparinized tubes containing 24 μg/ml of indomethacin for 15 minute intervals and flow was determined by weighing the tubes. Arterial blood samples were drawn every 30 minutes for determination of total protein using a refractometer. Lymph and plasma samples were assayed for prostanoids according to the method of Jaffe and Behrman.[27] To measure the pulmonary and systemic blood pressures with pressure transducers, a Swan-Ganz catheter and a hard rubber catheter were placed in the pulmonary artery and the abdominal aorta, respectively. Airway pressure was measured with a differential transducer. Polyethylene catheters were placed into both femoral veins for drugs and fluid administrations.

Evidence for Increased Pulmonary Vascular Permeability

In anesthetized artificially ventilated dogs, we observed the same biphasic response, pulmonary hypertension in the early phase and high flow of protein-rich lymph in the late phase, following endotoxin (1 mg/kg) administration as has been reported by others,[7,8] although the changes were smaller than in unanesthetized spontaneously breathing sheep. The reason for the difference could be due to the method of ventilation, as well as species differences. The lung lymph flow increased on an average of 1.5 times baseline in this study (Fig. 3). Brigham and associates have reported that the lymph/plasma (L/P) protein concentration ratio always decreased from baseline during increased lymph flow to $1.5-2.5$ times baseline using mechanically increased pressure study.[6] Thus, our finding of high lymph flow with a gradual increase in L/P ratio could be explained by an increase in vascular permeability (Table II).

Release of Prostacyclin into Lung Lymph and Arterial Blood

The concentration of 6-keto $PGF_{1\alpha}$ increased in the lung lymph and in arterial blood following endotoxin, associated with a transient increase in thromboxane B_2 in the early phase.[26] The concentration of 6-keto $PGF_{1\alpha}$ in the lung lymph increased significantly to 3.3 ± 1.0 ng/ml at 60 minutes and continued to increase to 8.2 ± 0.8 at 120 minutes after endotoxin, from a baseline value of 1.4 ± 0.4 ng/ml. Although there was a decreasing trend thereafter, the concentration remained elevated 5 hours after endotoxin. $PGF_{2\alpha}$ increased only in lymph. These changes in prostanoid concentration in the lung lymph are similar to those reported in sheep given endotoxin.[8] As the fraction of total lymph that is pulmonary in origin cannot be determined, we could not conclude from this study that these prostanoids were specifically synthesized in the lung. The right lymph duct lymph, however, contains, on the average, half of the total lung lymph.[40] Also, because the lung is the primary target organ of endotoxin[38] and pulmonary vascular endothelium is a rich source of prostacyclin,[18] the increase in 6-keto $PGF_{1\alpha}$ could be explained by the increased production of prostacyclin in the pulmonary vasculature. Although platelets in the lung could release thromboxane, the pulmonary artery also generates thromboxane A_2. Neutrophils are also a major source of thromboxane.[37] Removing the white cells prior to endotoxin, however, did not eliminate the pulmonary hypertension[21] that might be mediated by thromboxane A_2. Pretreatment with sulfinpyrazone also eliminated the hypertension but did not prevent the sequestration in the lung.[13] Thus, neutrophils may not be the source of thromboxane in endotoxin shock.

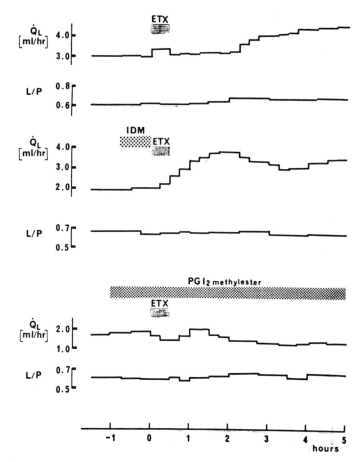

Figure 3: *Effects of indomethacin and PGI₂ methylester on the changes in lung lymph flow (Q̇ₗ) and lymph-to-plasma protein concentration ratio (L/P) following E. coli endotoxin administration. Values are mean of 18 dogs (endotoxin alone), of 9 dogs (pretreated with indomethacin), and of 6 dogs (treated with PGI₂ methylester).*

Aggregation of Platelets and Leukocytes

The platelet count decreased maximally to $7.0 \pm 0.8 \times 10^4$/cmm at 60 minutes and increased toward baseline thereafter from the baseline value of $23.3 \pm 1.8 \times 10^4$/cmm, although remaining decreased below baseline even 5 hours after endotoxin. The leukocyte count decreased also to $1.7 \pm 0.2 \times 10^3$/cmm after 60 minutes from the baseline value of $8.9 \pm 0.8 \times 10^3$/cmm and remained decreased below baseline for the study.

Accentuation of the Lymph Protein Clearance by Cyclooxygenase Inhibitors

Although the PG synthetase inhibitor, indomethacin (10 mg/kg), prevented the increase in pulmonary artery pressure and the increase in 6-keto PGF$_{1\alpha}$,[26]

Table II
Effect of Cyclooxygenase Inhibitor and PGI$_2$ Methylester on Endotoxin-Induced Pulmonary Hypertension and Increased Pulmonary Vascular Permeability

	Baseline	Drug	½ hr	1 hr	2 hr	3 hr	4 hr
			Group 1: Endotoxin alone				
PAP (mmHg)	16.2 ± 1.2		20.5 ± 1.3*		15.7 ± 1.2		16.2 ± 1.1
$\dot{Q}_L$ (ml/hr)	2.8 ± .5		3.2 ± .6	3.2 ± .6	3.4 ± .6*	3.6 ± .8*	4.0 ± .9*
L/P	.68 ± .03		.70 ± .03	.70 ± .03	.72 ± .03*	.72 ± .04*	.68 ± .04
$\dot{Q}_p$ (ml/hr)	2.0 ± .4		2.3 ± .5	2.4 ± .5	2.5 ± .5*	2.7 ± .6*	2.9 ± .7*
			Group 2: Cyclooxygenase inhibitor + Endotoxin				
PAP (mmHg)	13.4 ± 1.4	13.5 ± 1.4	14.9 ± 1.8		15.4 ± 2.2		15.8 ± 2.4
$\dot{Q}_L$ (ml/hr)	1.9 ± .6	1.9 ± .5	2.4 ± .5*¶	3.6 ± .6*¶	3.4 ± .6*¶	3.0 ± .5*	3.1 ± .5*
L/P	.68 ± .04	.68 ± .04	.67 ± .05	.66 ± .05	.66 ± .06	.63 ± .05	.66 ± .07
$\dot{Q}_P$ (ml/hr)	1.3 ± .4	1.4 ± .4	1.6 ± .4	2.5 ± .5*¶	2.3 ± .4*¶	2.0 ± .3*	2.1 ± .4*
			Group 3: PGI$_2$ Methylester + Endotoxin				
PAP (mmHg)	16.1 ± 1.0	15.2 ± 1.0	15.9 ± 1.4		16.4 ± 1.4		16.2 ± 1.4
$\dot{Q}_L$ (ml/hr)	2.7 ± .5	2.8 ± .5	2.5 ± .8	2.6 ± .8	2.8 ± .9	2.8 ± 1.0	2.9 ± 1.0
L/P	.66 ± .11	.66 ± .11	.65 ± .11	.67 ± .10	.68 ± .10	.69 ± .10	.68 ± .10
$\dot{Q}_P$ (ml/hr)	1.8 ± .3	1.8 ± .4	1.6 ± .6	1.7 ± .6	1.8 ± .8	1.9 ± .8	1.9 ± .9

Endotoxin was given to each group of animals at the dose of 1 mg/kg. Group 1: Administraton of endotoxin alone (18 dogs); Group 2: One of the cyclooxygenase inhibitors, indomethacin (5 dogs), phenylbutazone (2 dogs), or aspirin (2 dogs), was administered before endotoxin; Group 3: PGI$_2$ methylester was infused at a rate of 20 ng/kg/min 1 hour before endotoxin to the end of experiment into the central vein of 9 dogs. All values are mean ± SE. *Statistically significant by signed rank test (p<0.05) compared to baseline. ¶ Statistically significant by rank sum test (p<0.05) compared to the rate of increase in Group I. PAP = mean pulmonary artery pressure; $\dot{Q}_L$ = lymph flow; L/P = lymph-plasma protein concentration ratio; $\dot{Q}_p$ = lymph protein clearance (lymph flow × L/P).

the lymph protein clearance was accentuated after endotoxin (Fig. 3). The onset of the change in lymph protein clearance was rapid and the rate of the increase during 1–2 hour periods after endotoxin was higher than that observed in nontreated animals (Table II). Ogletree and Brigham also recently reported a greater increase in lung lymph flow with indomethacin and endotoxin compared to endotoxin alone.[34] As we observed the same degree of accentuation with phenylbutazone (30 mg/kg), and aspirin (30⁻ mg/kg), both of which are different in chemical structure but inhibit cyclooxygenase as a common feature, the accentuation of lymph protein clearance could be due to the blocking of the synthesis of some prostanoids with protective effects against lung injury, although a diversion of arachidonic acid substrate away from cyclooxygenase to lipoxygenase pathway could not be ruled out. Our finding of a protective effect of the inhibition of prostaglandin synthesis on endotoxin-induced pulmonary hypertension is similar to that reported by others.[20,35] Although the thromboxane synthetase inhibitor eliminates the early pulmonary hypertension in endotoxin-treated goats, thromboxane A$_2$ does not mediate endotoxin-induced permeability changes.[42] Because the aggregations of platelet and leukocyte were not inhibited by these cyclooxygenase inhibitors,[26] the mechanism of endotoxin-induced aggregation might be different from that in pulmonary embolism. Fletcher and Ramwell found that aspirin and indomethacin did not inhibit in vitro endotoxin-induced platelet aggregation.[11] Since prostacyclin inhibits leukocyte aggregation,[4] the inhibition of synthesis of prostacyclin might accentuate the leukocyte-dependent lung injury in endotoxin shock.

Prevention of Endotoxin-Induced Lung Injury by the Infusion of PGI_2 Methylester

The response to endotoxin was modulated by the administration of PGI_2 methylester (20 ng/min/kg). The lymph flow did not increase significantly, with stable lymph/plasma protein concentration ratio, so that lymph protein clearance did not change significantly after endotoxin (Fig. 3). The increase in pulmonary artery pressure in the early phase was also prevented by the infusion (Table II), although PGI_2 methylester had no apparent effect on platelet and leukocyte aggregation. Prostacyclin could counteract the vasoconstrictive thromboxane A_2 released mainly from the pulmonary vasculature.

The mechanisms whereby prostacyclin prevents the endotoxin-induced increase in protein clearance are not clear. This effect is unlikely to be related to the possible reduction of pulmonary microvascular pressure that might result from prostacyclin. If prostacyclin increased pulmonary microvascular surface area and enhanced blood flow to damaged microvasculature, an increase in lymph protein clearance should have been observed. Our results are consistent with those reported by Demling in sheep.[9] Although recent studies indicate that in the normal lung, fluid flux is significantly increased during a much larger dose of PGI_2 infusion in sheep,[34] a large dose of PGI_2 may increase the filtration by increasing the vascular surface area. We did not find any significant changes in hemodynamics with the dose of prostacyclin in this study before endotoxin.

Leukocytes have been implicated in mediating the endotoxin-induced lung injury. The increased permeability that occurs in sheep after endotoxin can be attenuated by rendering the sheep neutropenic, suggesting that neutrophils are necessary for the development of these permeability changes.[21] Endotoxin activates complement,[16] causing granulocytes to adhere to pulmonary vascular endothelium where activated granulocytes release lysosomal enzymes and toxic products of molecular oxygen, causing lung injury.[41] Demling found a lesser degree of lysosomal enzyme release by the infusion of prostacyclin after endotoxin.[9] Although PGI_2 methylester did not prevent leukocyte aggregation, the release of toxic agents from leukocytes might be inhibited by the stabilizing property of prostacyclin on leukocytes. Another reason for the protective effect of prostacyclin could be due to the inhibitory action on leukotriene production. The augmentation of acute lung injury with cyclooxygenase inhibitors in this study might also suggest the activation of the lipoxygenase pathway. Prostacyclin has been reported to diminish the adhesion of granulocytes to endothelial cells by the inhibition of the release of leukotriene B_4.[29] Prostacyclin released by leukotrienes can counteract the effects of leukotrienes C_4 and D_4,[29] which are putative mediators of increased pulmonary vascular permeability. The investigations on interactions between prostacyclin and leukotrienes will be needed to elucidate the mechanisms of the protective effect of prostacyclin and of the increased vascular permeability in acute lung injury.

Summary

Prostacyclin is released during a number of acute lung injuries with increased production of other prostaglandins. The concentration of 6-keto $PGF_{1\alpha}$ in arterial blood and in pulmonary lymph increased in pulmonary microembolism and in endotoxin shock. Since the use of cyclooxygenase inhibitors augmented and the infusion of PGI_2 methylester prevented the increased pulmonary vascular permeability, prostacylcin could be beneficial in maintaining pulmonary microvascular integrity during microembolic and endotoxin-induced lung injury. Although the mechanisms whereby prostacyclin prevents the increased vascular permeability are not clear, it is unlikely that this action is primarily due to vasodilation with a resultant decrease in microvascular hydrostatic pressure, or to antiaggregation of platelets and leukocytes. Prostacyclin also prevents pulmonary hypertension by counteracting the vasoconstrictive effect of thromboxane A_2. As leukocytes have been implicated in mediating the microembolic and endotoxin-induced lung injury, prostacylin might prevent the increased permeability by its stabilizing activity on leukocytes. Since pretreatment with cyclooxygenase inhibitors augmented the microembolic and endotoxin-induced lung injury, the activation of the lipoxygenase pathway could also be involved in the increased pulmonary vascular permeability. Another reason for the protective effect of prostacyclin, then, could be its inhibitory action on leukotriene production. Prostacyclin released by leukotrienes can counteract the putative mediators, leukotrienes C_4 and D_4, which can increase pulmonary vascular permeability.

REFERENCES

1. Best, L.C., Martin, T.J., Russell, R.G.G., et al.: Prostacyclin increases cyclic AMP levels and adenyl cyclase activity in platelets. *Nature (Lond.)*. 267:850–851, 1977.
2. Binder, A.S., Kagler, W., Perel, W., et al.: Effects of platelet depletion on lung vascular permeability after microemboli in sheep. *J. Appl. Physiol.* 48:414–420, 1980.
3. Bowers, R.E., Ellis, E.F., Brigham, K.L., et al.: Effects of prostaglandin cyclic endoperoxides on the lung circulation of anesthetized sheep. *J. Clin. Invest.* 63: 131–137, 1979.
4. Boxter, L.A., Allen, J.M., Schmidt, M., et al.: Inhibition of polymorphonuclear leukocytes adherence by prostacyclin. *J. Lab. Clin. Med.* 95:672–680, 1980.
5. Brigham, K.L., and Owen, P.J.: Mechanism of the serotonin effect on lung vascular fluid and protein movement in awake sheep. *Circ. Res.* 36:761–770, 1975.
6. Brigham, K.L., Bowers, R.E., and Owen, P.J.: Effects of antihistamines on the lung vascular response to histamine in unanesthetized sheep. Diphenhydramine prevention of pulmonary edema and increased permeability. *J. Clin. Invest.* 58:391–398, 1976.
7. Brigham, K.L., Bowers, R.E., and Haynes, J.: Increased sheep lung vascular permeability caused by Escherichia coli endotoxin. *Circ. Res.* 45:292–297, 1979.
8. Demling, R.H., Smith, M., Gunther, R., et al.: Pulmonary injury and prostaglandin

production during endotoxemia in conscious sheep. *Am. J. Physiol.* 240:H348–H353, 1981.

9. Demling, R.H.: Role of prostaglandins in acute pulmonary microvascular injury. *Ann. N.Y. Acad. Sci.* 384:517–534, 1982.

10. Drake, R.E., Smith, J.H., and Gabel, J.C.: Estimation of the filtration coefficient in intact dog lung. *Am. J. Physiol.* 238:H430–H438, 1980.

11. Fletcher, J.R. and Ramwell, P.W.: The effects of prostacyclin (PGI$_2$) on endotoxin shock and endotoxin-induced platelet aggregation in dogs. *Circ. Shock* 7:299–308, 1980.

12. Flick, M.R., Perel, A., and Staub, N.C.: Leukocytes are required for increased lung microvascular permeability after microembolization in sheep. *Circ. Res.* 48: 344–351, 1981.

13. Fountain, S.W., Martin, B.A., Masclow, E., et al.: Pulmonary leukostasis and its relationship to pulmonary dysfunction in sheep and rabbits. *Circ. Res.* 46:175–180, 1980.

14. Gabel, J.C., Drake, R.E., Arens, J.F., et al.: Unchanged pulmonary capillary filtration coefficients after Escherichia coli endotoxin infusion. *J. Surg. Res.* 25:97–104, 1978.

15. Garcia-Szabo, R.R., Peterson, M.B., Watkins, W.D., et al.: Thromboxane synthesis after thrombin: Protective effect of thromboxane synthetase inhibition of lung fluid balance. *Circ. Res.* 53:214–22, 1983.

16. Gewarz, H., Shin, H.S., and Mergenhagen, S.E.: Interactions of the complement system with endotoxin lipopolysaccharide: Consumption of each of the six terminal components. *J. Exp. Med.* 128:1049–1057, 1968.

17. Grant, J.A., Dupree, E., and Goldman, A.S.: Complement-mediated release of histamine from human leukocytes. *J. Immunol.* 114:1101–1106, 1975.

18. Gryglewski, J.H., Korbut, R., Ocetkiewicz, A., et al.: Lung as a generator of prostacyclin: Hypothesis on physiological significance. *Naunyn-Schmiederberg's Arch. Pharmacol.* 304:45–50, 1978.

19. Gryglewski, R.J., Splawinski, J., and Korbut, R.: Endogenous mechanisms that regulate prostacyclin release. In *Advance in Prostaglandin and Thromboxane Research.* Samuelsson, B., Ramwell, P.W., and Paoretti, R., eds. New York, NY, Raven Press, 1980, Vol. 7, p. 777–787.

20. Hales, C.A., Sonne, L., Peterson, M., et al.: Role of thromboxane and prostacyclin in pulmonary vasomotor changes after endotoxin in dogs. *J. Clin. Invest.* 68:497–505, 1981.

21. Heflin, A.C. and Brigham, K.L.: Prevention of granulocyte depletion of increased vascular permeability of sheep lung following endotoxemia. *J. Clin. Invest.* 68: 1253–1260, 1981.

22. Higgs, G.A., Eakins, K.E., Mugridge, K.G., et al.: The effects of non-steroid anti-inflammatory drugs on leukocyte migration in carrageenin-induced inflammation. *Eur. J. Pharmacol.* 68:81–86, 1980.

23. Hirose, T., Aoki, E., Ishibashi, M., et al.: The effect of prostacyclin on increased hydraulic conductivity of pulmonary exchange vessels following microembolization in dogs. *Microvas. Res.* 26:193–204, 1983.

24. Hirose, T., Yasutake, A., Tarabeih, A., et al.: Location of airway constriction following acute experimental pulmonary thromboembolism. *J. Appl. Physiol.* 34:431–437, 1973.

25. Hyman, A.L., Spannak, E.W., and Kadowitz, P.J.: Prostaglandins and the lung. *Am. Rev. Respir. Dis.* 117:111–136, 1978.

26. Ikeda, T., Hirose, T., Aoki, E., et al.: A pathophysiological role of endogenous prostacyclin in endotoxin-induced increase in lung vascular permeability in dogs. *Prostaglandins Leukotrienes and Medicine* 12:385–397, 1983.

27. Jaffe, B.M., Behrman, H., and Parker, C.W.: Radioimmunoassay measurement of prostaglandin E, A, and F in human plasma. *J. Clin. Invest.* 52:398–405, 1973.

28. Johnson, A. and Malik, A.B.: Effect of granulocytopenia on extravascular water after microembolization. *Am. Rev. Respir. Dis.* 122:561–566, 1980.
29. Kuehl, F.A., Dougherty, H.W., and Ham, E.A.: Interaction between prostaglandins and leukotrienes. *Biochem. Pharmacol.* 33:1–5, 1984.
30. Lee, B.C., Van Der Zee, H., and Malik, A.B.: Site of pulmonary edema after unilateral microembolization. *J. Appl. Physiol.* 47:556–560, 1979.
31. Lefer, A.M., Sollott, S.L., and Galvin, M.J.: Beneficial actions of prostacyclin in traumatic shock. *Prostaglandins* 17:761–767, 1979.
32. Manwaring, D., Thorning, D., and Curreri, P.W.: Mechanisms of acute pulmonary dysfunction induced by fibrinogen degradation product D. *Surgery* 84:45–54, 1978.
33. Nossel, H.J.: The contact system. In *Human Blood Coagulation. Haemostasis and Thrombosis*. Biggs, R., ed. London, Black Well Publications, 1976, pp. 81–142.
34. Ogletree, M.L.: Pharmacology of prostaglandins in the pulmonary circulation. *Ann. N.Y. Acad. Sci.* 384:191–206, 1982.
35. Parratt, J.R. and Sturgess, R.M.: Evidence that prostaglandin release mediates pulmonary vasoconstriction induced by E. coli endotoxin. *J. Physiol. (Lond.)* 246: 79–80, 1975.
36. Said, S.I.: Release induced by physical and chemical stimuli. In *Metabolic Functions of the Lung*, Bakhle, Y.S., Vane, J.R., and Lenfant, C., eds. NY, Marcel Dekker, 1977, pp. 297–320.
37. Spagnuolo, P.J., Ellner, J.J., Hassid, A., et al.: Thromboxane A_2 mediates augmented polymorphonuclear leukocyte adhesiveness. *J. Clin. Invest.* 66:406–414, 1980.
38. Tikoff, G., Kuida, H., and Chiga, M.: Hemodynamic effects of endotoxin in calves. *Am. J. Physiol.* 210:847–853, 1966.
39. Vaage, J., Nicolayson, G., and Waaler, B.A.: Aggregation of blood platelets and increased hydraulic conductivity of pulmonary exchange vessels. *Acta Physiol. Scand.* 98:175–184, 1976.
40. Vreim, C.E., Ohkuda, K., and Staub, N.C.: Proportions of dog lung lymph in the thoracic and right lymph ducts. *J. Appl. Physiol.* 43:874–889, 1977.
41. Ward, P.A., Till, G.O., Kunkel, R., et al.: Evidence for role of hydroxyl radical in complement and neutrophil-dependent tissue injury. *J. Clin. Invest.* 72:789–801, 1983.
42. Winn, R., Harlan, J., Nadir, B., et al.: Thromboxane A_2 mediates lung vasoconstriction but not permeability after endotoxin. *J. Clin. Invest.* 72:911–918, 1983.
43. Zimmerman, T.S., Fierrei, J., and Roghberger, H.: Blood coagulation and the inflammatory response. *Semin. Hematol.* 14:391–408, 1977.

Abbreviations Used in This Book

ACE = angiotensin converting enzyme
ACTH = adrenocorticotropic hormone
ADP = adenosine diphosphate
AMP = adenosine monophosphate
ANTU = alpha-naphthylthiourea
ARDS = adult respiratory distress syndrome
BPD = bronchopulmonary dysplasia
CCK = cholecystokinin
CFI = chemotactic factor inactivator
CGD = chronic granulomatous disease
CSF = cerebrospinal fluid
DMSO = dimethyl sulfoxide
DMTU = dimethylthiourea
DPC = dipalmitylphosphatidyl choline
DSA = digital subtraction angiography
EAV = extra-alveolar vessel
ECF = eosinophil chemotactic factor
ETYA = eicosatetraynoic acid
EVLW = extravascular lung water
FMLP = N-formyl-methionyl-leucyl-phenylalanine
GMP = guanosine monophosphate
GRP = gastrin-releasing peptide
HDL = high-density lipoproteins
IgE = immunoglobulin E
LDCL = luminol-dependent chemoluminescence
LDH = lactate dehydrogenase
LDL = low-density lipoproteins
LT = leukotriene
MDA = malondialdehyde
MLB = multilamellar bodies
NBT = nitroblue tetrazolium
NDGA = nordihydroguaiaretic acid
NMR = nuclear magnetic resonance
P_A = alveolar pressure
PAF = platelet-activating factor
PAP or P_{PA} = pulmonary arterial pressure
PDGF = platelet-derived growth factor
PEG = polyethylene glycol
PG = prostaglandins
PHI/PHM = peptide histidine isoleucine/peptide histidine methionine
PLA_2 = phospholipase A_2
PMA = phorbol myristate acetate
PMN = polymorphonuclear leukocyte
Pmv = microvascular hydrostatic pressure
Ppl = pleural pressure
Ppmv = permicrovascular hydrostatic pressure
Ppv = pulmonary venous pressure
Pvas = vascular pressure
PVR = pulmonary vascular resistance
$\dot{Q}_L$ = lung lymph flow
RBC = red blood cells
RVH = right ventricular hypertrophy
SOD = superoxide dismutase
SRS-A = slow reacting substance of anaphylaxis
VIP = vasoactive intestinal peptide

Index

Author Index

473